# Emergencies of the Orbit and Adnexa

Bipasha Mukherjee • Hunter Yuen
Editors

# Emergencies of the Orbit and Adnexa

Springer

*Editors*
Bipasha Mukherjee
Medical Research Foundation
Sankara Nethralaya
Chennai
India

Hunter Yuen
Hong Kong Eye Hospital
Hong Kong
China

ISBN 978-81-322-1806-7 ISBN 978-81-322-1807-4 (eBook)
DOI 10.1007/978-81-322-1807-4

Library of Congress Control Number: 2016956850



Printed on acid-free paper

This Springer imprint is published by Springer Nature
The registered company is Springer (India) Pvt. Ltd
The registered company address is: 7th Floor, Vijaya Building, 17 Barakhamba Road, New Delhi 110 001, India

*Dedicated to my father, Dr. Satyamay Mukherjee, from whom I inherited the love for books, reading and teaching.*

Dr. Bipasha Mukherjee

# Foreword

In a world of ever-faster communications and information exchange, it is a particular privilege to have been involved – both as an advisor and an author – in the publication of a book that focuses on the importance of clinical care in the diagnosis and treatment of disease. Whilst there are many texts and other media that cover the broad spectrum of orbital, lacrimal, eyelid and socket disease, Dr. Bipasha Mukherjee and Dr. Hunter Yuen are to be congratulated on providing a wide-ranging book that addresses the more specific issues associated with clinical emergencies and acute conditions within this field. Finding guidelines for the care of such patients – who often present without notice and at awkward times – can be difficult and only few physicians have any significant practical experience in this specialist area; the editors have successfully overcome this difficulty by assembling contributions from a worldwide group of experienced authors, who together have extensive experience of working in very diverse clinical settings.

For ophthalmic surgeons with an interest in periocular disease, this compact book serves as an interesting read and a valuable handbook for the office shelf – ready to be consulted when facing an unexpected patient with the acute onset of severe ocular adnexal disease. Likewise, it provides a suitable synopsis of the complex care of patients with ocular adnexal disease for ophthalmic nurses and paramedical care workers.

The editors are to be congratulated on their foresight in the concept of a book focussing on this area of adnexal disease, their determination to get the project underway in the face of practical difficulties and their industry in getting it assembled from such a diverse worldwide team of authors – and all within a very acceptable time frame.

London, UK Geoffrey E. Rose, MS, DSc, MRCP, FRCS, FRCOphth
September 2015

# About the Editors

Dr. Bipasha Mukherjee is currently the director of the Department of Orbit, Oculoplasty, Reconstructive and Aesthetic Surgery at the Medical Research Foundation, Sankara Nethralaya, in Chennai, India. Her areas of interest include diseases of the orbit and adnexa including tumours, lacrimal and cosmetic eyelid surgery, cosmetic rehabilitation and reconstruction of anophthalmic socket and traumatic eyelid and adnexal injuries. She takes active interest in training of postgraduate residents and fellows at her institute. She has published more than 35 papers in peer-reviewed journals and has made presentations at more than 100 national and international conferences.

Dr. Hunter Yuen Kwok-Lai (FRCOphth, FRCSEd) graduated from the Chinese University of Hong Kong. He is the consultant ophthalmologist and coordinator of the Orbital and Oculoplastic Surgery at Hong Kong Eye Hospital. He has more than 60 peer-reviewed international publications and has delivered numerous oral and posters presentations in numerous international meetings. Dr. Yuen is the current president of the Asia-Pacific Society of Ophthalmic Plastic and Reconstructive Surgery (APSORPS) and president of the Hong Kong Society of Ophthalmic Plastic and Reconstructive Surgery (HKSOPRS) in the year 2016. He is the recipient of many awards, including one of Ten Outstanding Young Persons of Hong Kong in 2007, Hong Kong Volunteer Award in 2011, Asia-Pacific Academy of Ophthalmology Achievement Award and Distinguished Service Award in 2012.

# Preface

An emergency situation where inappropriate management can rapidly worsen the condition leading to blindness or even death is every ophthalmologist's nightmare. Unfortunately, barring some well-structured programmes, ophthalmology residents are barely exposed to orbital and adnexal disorders, let alone emergencies. As a result, most clinicians are inexperienced, and perhaps rightly so, uncertain and anxious about managing these situations.

There is a scarcity of teachers with the necessary experience of handling these patients, as well as books imparting theoretical knowledge on this subject. We have attempted to draw on the collective knowledge and expertise of renowned specialists to provide a thorough and comprehensive overview of the current practice standards in orbital and adnexal emergencies. This handbook has chapters that have been contributed by over 50 specialists hailing from more than 15 countries across the world.

We have tried to cover most of the common as well as lesser-known but important and interesting emergencies of the adnexa. The chapters are grouped to include all the aspects of traumatic and non-traumatic emergencies. The chapters cover both accepted techniques and the newer and innovative modifications by the skilled surgeons. We have described in detail the current diagnostic and surgical techniques. Surgical principles have been illustrated by high-quality clinical photos and professional illustrations.

We believe this knowledge would be beneficial to not only ophthalmologists but also to intensivists, general physicians, radiologists, craniofacial surgeons, neurologists and neurosurgeons, oculofacial plastic surgeons, orofaciomaxillary surgeons, otolaryngologists and general plastic surgeons. We trust that this collaborative handbook will address all levels of medical personnel, from medical and nursing students to experienced physicians and surgeons. We hope that this compilation of ideas from a diverse and respected group of superspecialists will benefit the reader and ultimately the patients.

Chennai, India — Bipasha Mukherjee, MS, DNB(Ophth.), FICO
Hong Kong, China — Hunter Kwok-Lai Yuen, FRCOphth, FRCSEd

# Acknowledgement

It has been a wonderful journey, made possible by many beautiful souls from all over the world coming together for this collaborative project.

We would like to convey our deep appreciation and gratitude to all the contributors for their diligence in preparing the individual chapters, for their patience through the grinding process of converting the manuscript to text and above all for their generosity in sharing their knowledge with the readers.

We would especially like to thank Dr. Geoffrey E. Rose, Moorfields Eye Hospital, UK, for his encouragement, help and guidance in this project from its inception. The credit for conceptualising the thoughtful and comprehensive list of chapters belongs to him.

We would also like to thank our family members for their understanding and support. It is their sacrifice of personal time, which enabled us to indulge in these academic pursuits.

We are grateful to Springer Publications and their associates for undertaking the publication of this handbook. We would, in particular, like to thank Mr. Naren Aggarwal, executive editor, Springer India, and Ms. Jessica Gonzalez, associate developmental editor, for their unstinting assistance in every step.

We are grateful to our institutes and our patients who have willingly allowed us to share the information with the readers.

# Contents

# Contributors

**Md. Shahid Alam, MS** Orbit Oculoplasty Reconstructive and Aesthetic Services, Sankara Nethralaya, Chennai, Tamil Nadu, India

**Mohammad Javed Ali, FRCS, FRCGP** Ophthalmic Plastic Surgery, L.V. Prasad Eye Institute, Hyderabad, Telangana, India

**Mamta Agarwal, MBBS, DNB(Ophthalmology)** Uvea & Cornea, Sankara Nethralaya, Chennai, Tamil Nadu, India

**Shweta Agarwal, MS(Ophthalmology)** Cornea, Refractive Surgery, Ocular Surface, Sankara Nethralaya, Chennai, Tamil Nadu, India

**Shaloo Bageja, DNB, MNAMS** Ophthalmology, Sir Ganga Ram Hospital, New Delhi, Delhi, India

**Manabjyoti Barman, DO, DNB** Vitreo-Retina, Sri Sankaradeva Nethralaya, Guwahati, Assam, India

**Harsha Bhattacharjee, MS, FRCP** Comprehensive Ophthalmology, Sri Sankaradeva Nethralaya, Guwahati, Assam, India

**Kasturi Bhattacharjee, MS, DNB, FRCS** Orbit, Ophthalmic, Plastic and Reconstructive Surgery, Sri Sankaradeva Nethralaya, Guwahati, Assam, India

**Priti Bhoutekar, MD** Orbit, Oculoplasty & Ocular Oncology, Aravind Eye Hospital, Madurai, Madurai, Tamil Nadu, India

**Harish Bora, MD** Anaesthesia, Vision Eye Centre, New Delhi, Delhi, India

**Cat N. Burkat, MD, FACS** Department of Ophthalmology and Visual Sciences, University of Wisconsin Hospitals and Clinics, Madison, WI, USA

**Andy C.O. Cheng, MMedSc, FRCSEd** Ophthalmology, Hong Kong Sanatorium & Hospital, Hong Kong, Hong Kong SAR, China

**Kelvin Kam-lung Chong, MB, ChB (Hon), FHKAM, FCOphth** Ophthalmology and Visual Science, The Chinese University of Hong Kong, Prince of Wales Hospital, Alice Ho Miu Ling Nethersole Hospital, Hong Kong, Hong Kong SAR, China

**Debleena Dey, MBBS, DO** Orbit, Ophthalmic Plastic and Reconstructive Surgery, Sankara Nethralaya Kolkata, Kolkata, West Bengal, India

**Mangesh Dhobekar, MBBS, MS, FMRF** Orbit, Oculoplasty and Ocular Prosthetic Services, Shri Ganapati Netralaya, Jalna, Maharashtra, India

**Yousef Ahmed Fouad** Ain Shams University Hospitals, Cairo, Egypt

**Suzanne K. Freitag, MD** Ophthalmic Plastic Surgery Service, Department of Ophthalmology, Massachusetts Eye and Ear Infirmary, Harvard Medical School, Boston, MA, USA

**Lora Rabin Dagi Glass, MD** Ophthalmic Plastic Surgery Service, Department of Ophthalmology, Massachusetts Eye and Ear Infirmary, Harvard Medical School, Boston, MA, USA

**Tjahjono D. Gondhowiardjo, PhD.** Corneal & Refractive Surgery, Jakarta-Eye-Center, Jakarta, Indonesia

Eye Department, Cipto Mangunkusumo – Kirana Hospital, Jakarta, Indonesia

**Seanna R. Grob, MD, MAS** Ophthalmology, Massachusetts Eye and Ear Infirmary, Harvard Medical School, Boston, MA, USA

**Ashok K. Grover, MD, MNAMS, FRCS, FICO, FIMSA** Ophthalmology, Sir Ganga Ram Hospital, New Delhi, Delhi, India

**Yasmin Ashraf Hamza** Ain Shams University Hospitals, Cairo, Egypt

**Jason N. Harris, MD** Neuro-Ophthalmology, Johns Hopkins, Baltimore, MD, USA

**Dov Hersh, BCom, MBBS, MMed, FRANZCO** Orbital Unit, Moorfields Eye Hospital, London, UK

**Lorenzo Iuliano, MD** Ophthalmology, San Raffaele Scientific Institute, Vita-Salute University, Milan, Italy

**Geetha Iyer, FRCS** Cornea, Refractive Surgery & Ocular Surface, Sankara Nethralaya, Chennai, Tamil Nadu, India

**Shannon S. Joseph, MD, MSc** Ophthalmology, Johns Hopkins, Baltimore, MD, USA

**Bokkwan Jun, MD** Neuro-Ophthalmology, University of Missouri, Columbia, MO, USA

**Tomoyuki Kashima, MD, PhD** Oculoplastic Service, Department of Ophthalmology, Gunma University, Maebashi, Gunma, Japan

**Saurbhi Khurana, MD, FICO** Ophthalmology, Medanta, Gurgaon, Haryana, India

**Usha R. Kim, DO, DNB** Orbit, Oculoplasty & Ocular Oncology, Aravind Eye Hospital, Madurai, Madurai, Tamil Nadu, India

**Seah Lay Leng, MBBS, FRCS, FRCOphth, FAMS** Oculoplastics, Singapore National Eye Centre, Singapore, Singapore

**Emmy Yuen Li, MBBS,MPH, FRCS, FCOphthHK, FHKAM** Ophthalmology, Hong Kong Eye Hospital, Hong Kong, Hong Kong SAR, China

**Neil R. Miller, MD** Ophthalmology, Neurology and Neurosurgery, Johns Hopkins, Baltimore, MD, USA

**Elisabetta Miserocchi, MD** Ophthalmology, San Raffaele Scientific Institute, Vita-Salute University, Milan, Italy

**Giulio Modorati, MD** Ophthalmology, San Raffaele Scientific Institute, Vita-Salute University, Milan, Italy

**Bipasha Mukherjee, MS, DNB(Ophthalmology), FICO** Orbit, Oculoplasty, Reconstructive & Aesthetic Services, Sankara Nethralaya, Chennai, Tamil Nadu, India

**Milind N. Naik, MD** Ophthalmic Plastic Surgery, L.V. Prasad Eye Institute, Hyderabad, Telangana, India

**Akshay Gopinathan Nair, MBBS, DNB** Ophthalmic Plastic Surgery, L.V. Prasad Eye Institute, Hyderabad, Telangana, India

**Ravija Patel, MBBS, MS** M & J Institute of Ophthalmology, Ahmedabad, Gujarat, India

**Marian Pauly, MBBS, MS, DNB** Orbit, Oculoplasty and Aesthetics, Giridhar Eye Institute, Kochi, Kerala, India

**Raymond Nelson C. Regalado, MD, DPBO** Department of Visual Sciences, Philippine General Hospital, Quezon City, Metro Manila, Philippines

**Geoffrey E. Rose, MS, DSc, MRCP, FRCS, FRCOphth** Orbital, Lacrimal and Oculoplastic Service, Moorfields Eye Hospital NHS Trust, London, UK

**Yvette Marie B. Santiago, MB, DPBO** Eye Institute, St. Luke's Medical Center, Quezon City, Philippines

**Manpreet Singh, MS, DNB** Orbit, Ophthalmic Plastic and Reconstructive Surgery, Sri Sankaradeva Nethralaya, Guwahati, Assam, India

**Darmayanti Siswoyo** Oculoplastic & Eye Reconstructive Surgery, Jakarta-Eye-Center, Jakarta, Indonesia

**Bhaskar Srinivasan, MS(Ophthalmology)** Cornea, Refractive Surgery & Ocular Surface, Sankara Nathralaya, Chennai, Tamil Nadu, India

**Hernawita Soeharko** Oculoplastic and Eye Reconstructive Surgery, Jakarta-Eye-Center, Jakarta, Indonesia

Eye Department, Cipto Mangunkusumo – Kirana Hospital, Jakarta, Indonesia

**Gangadhara Sundar, DO, FRCSEd, FAMS, AB Ophth(USA)**
Department of Ophthalmology, National University Hospital, Singapore, Singapore

**Hatem A. Tawfik, MD** Ophthalmology, Ain Shams University Hospitals, Cairo, Egypt

**Ann Q. Tran, BSc** Department of Ophthalmology and Visual Sciences, University of Wisconsin – Madison School of Medicine and Public Health, Madison, WI, USA

**Meghana Anika Varde, MS, FEBO, FMRF(Oculoplasty)** Ophthalmology, Klinikum Region Hannover, Hannover, Germany

**David H. Verity, MD, MA, FRCOphth** Adnexal Service, Moorfields Eye Hospital, London, UK

**Leslie A. Wei, MD** Department of Ophthalmology and Visual Sciences, University of Wisconsin Hospitals and Clinics, Madison, WI, USA

**Stephanie Ming Young, MBBS, MMed(Ophthalmology), FAMS, FRCOphth** Department of Ophthalmology, National University Hospital, Singapore, Singapore

**Hunter Kwok-Lai Yuen, FRCOphth, FRCSEd** Department of Ophthalmology and Visual Sciences, The Chinese University of Hong Kong, Hong Kong Eye Hospital, Hong Kong, Hong Kong SAR, China

# 1 Introduction: General Approach to Patient with Trauma

Geoffrey E. Rose

When a person suffers ophthalmic trauma, they are very vulnerable – both physically and psychologically – and there is a major risk that the injury is worsened by the incautious actions of the patient or well-intentioned bystanders. It is, therefore, extremely important that a clear leadership is established in caring for such patients – this leader not only showing the compassion and care required at such stressful times but also having the quiet wisdom and firm authority needed to assume the leading role in difficult circumstances.

Periocular trauma will occur either as a solely ophthalmic event – in which case the patient might be able to explain the nature of injury and, once calmed somewhat, be able to cooperate with treatments – or as part of a widespread, multiple-system injury. Ophthalmic injuries may be due to mechanical trauma, chemical injuries, thermal damage, electrical injuries or the more insidious effect of radiation injury. Mechanical trauma – by far the commonest type of injury – tends to be due to impact by missiles or fists, falls onto sharp objects or hard surfaces or avulsion of the eyelids or globe. Dog-bite injuries are particularly problematic in the younger patient.

G.E. Rose, MS, DSc, MRCP, FRCS, FRCOphth
Orbital, Lacrimal and Oculoplastic Service,
Moorfields Eye Hospital NHS Trust, London, UK
e-mail: geoff.rose@moorfields.nhs.uk

When first assessing the patient with periocular trauma, there are three key questions: First, "Is this solely ocular trauma or are there other injuries that demand urgent intervention?"; secondly, "Is there an open eye injury?"; and thirdly, "Does the patient have any other disease – such as insulin-dependent diabetes or epilepsy – that might suddenly manifest a problem during their acute care?". A history from the patient or observers will often give a good indication of the likely answers to these three questions, but the physician should continually remain aware of the risk of systemic disease becoming evident during the hours after major injury – either consequent to a premorbid condition (such as hypoglycaemia in an unconscious diabetic) or due to systemic deterioration from occult injuries (such as circulatory collapse due to a ruptured spleen or loss of consciousness due to subacute intracranial haemorrhage).

Closed eye injuries are most likely if there has been blunt trauma, such as a blow to the orbit, and in some cases will be associated with a blow-out fracture of the orbital floor or medial wall. Such closed eye injuries will typically present as a red eye with an enlarged or irregularly shaped pupil and reduced vision. Gross ocular hypotony, a large subconjunctival haemorrhage, major hyphaema or significant vitreous haemorrhage (with loss of the pupillary reflex) should alert the clinician to the presence of an occult rupture of the globe, this tending to occur near the equator



B. Mukherjee, H. Yuen (eds.), *Emergencies of the Orbit and Adnexa*,
DOI 10.1007/978-81-322-1807-4_1

or at the optic nerve head. Ocular and optic nerve function should be checked early where there is suspicion of injury to the globe: some form of visual acuity assessment is imperative in the cooperative patient, even where no formal test chart is available, and can be usefully be performed using newsprint, the distance at which finger counting can be performed or the directional perception of light. The presence and severity – mild, moderate or marked – of a relative afferent papillary defect (RAPD) should be recorded in all patients (whether conscious or not) and also whether this was a direct or consensual assessment of the injured eye; where extreme miosis precludes assessment of an RAPD – due, for example, to opiate analgesia – this should be noted contemporaneously. Ocular assessment is difficult in the presence of a large periocular haematoma or oedema but is generally possible after sustained compression of the swollen lids against the neighbouring brow ridge or cheek (totally avoiding any orbital pressure) and with the use of a suitable retractor, such as Desmarres; a suitably bent paper clip can be used to elevate the eyelid margin if a suitable retractor is unavailable.

Where vision is poor, it is safest to assume occult globe rupture until full examination is complete, and a suitable cover is placed to prevent inadvertent pressure on the eyeball – this being a Cartella shield if available or otherwise a cut-down disposable cup that will suffice. Any manifest globe rupture should obviously be protected in a like manner. Open eye injuries generally result from flying missiles and high-speed foreign bodies, stabbings with weapons or shards of glass and avulsion injuries and should be suspected wherever there are lacerations of the eyelids or conjunctiva or where there is a suggestive history; appropriate imaging should be considered in such cases, with magnetic resonance imaging being avoided where metallic foreign bodies might be present. It is always worthwhile asking relatives of the injured person about the possibility of foreign bodies as, in some cases, they will have the remains of the offending object with them at the time of attendance.

Acute chemical and thermal periocular injuries result in severe ischaemia. Materials causing thermal injury – such as splashes of molten metal – will have dissipated their energy by the time of ophthalmic assessment, and the acute treatment should be directed to removing any foreign bodies and reducing the inflammatory response that will exacerbate ocular ischaemia. In contrast, even where ocular irrigation has been given in the workplace, chemical injuries will often be associated with persistent contamination: because of this problem, all such patients should have immediate sustained irrigation – with special attention to the conjunctival fornices – until the tear film is shown to have near-neutral pH. Where ocular injury has involved solids (such as granular sodium hydroxide, cement powders or wet mortar), particular attention should be given to examination (and manual cleaning) of the conjunctival recesses where such materials tend to sequester; such cleansing is best performed after application of topical anaesthesia.

Reduced ocular motility should raise the suspicion of a blowout fracture – particularly the white-eyed blowout fracture of children – and a quick check for infraorbital hypoaesthesia will often confirm this clinical suspicion. Epistaxis is also a useful symptom of blowout fracture, and the patient should be warned not to blow their nose. Disruption of the orbital rim causes gross periocular ecchymosis and is often evident as an irregular orbital rim, as an unstable zygoma having pain when upward pressure is applied to the zygomatic arch or as altered dental occlusion.

The unconscious patient with periocular injury generally requires systemic intervention before any eye-specific therapy, and the ophthalmologist's role is to get the best possible baseline assessment of visual function and to protect the injured globe by placement of suitable shields. Clearly, should the ophthalmologist be the only person available to support the victim at the time of injury, it is appropriate to check the vital functions ("A, B, C") and consider hypoglycaemia, hypovolaemic shock, intracranial events or major intrathoracic injury (e.g. tension pneumothorax or haemothorax) as the cause for deteriorating conscious levels; in such circumstances, first-aid measures should be given as efficiently as possible until further assistance arrives.

All patients with periocular injury or sinus fractures should be considered for systemic antibiosis, particularly where trauma is due to contaminated missiles or animal (including human) bites. The status for tetanus prophylaxis is also important with open injury, and a booster dose of tetanus toxoid is prudent in many such cases.

Overall, the care of the patient with an acute periocular injury can be summarised in a few key phrases: first, prevent further damage to the patient, the patient's eye and the helpers; secondly, maintain the composure of friendly authority to help the patient face a difficult psychological time; thirdly, determine whether there is systemic injury or disease for which treatment takes priority over the eye condition; and, lastly, restore the structures of the eye and periocular region as soon as possible.

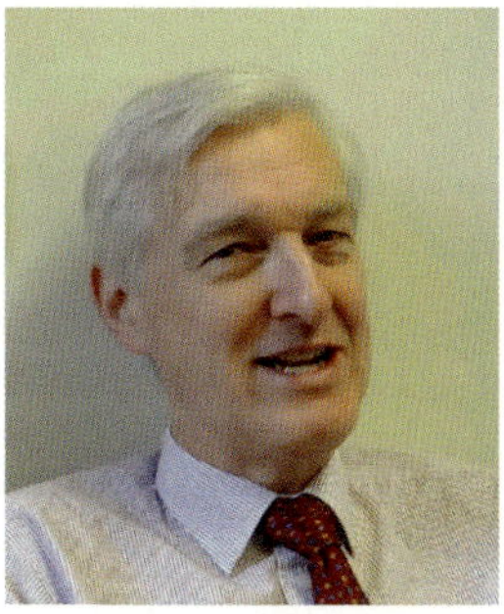

**Geoffrey E. Rose** Geoffrey Rose graduated BSc Pharmacology, MBBS, and MRCP. His postgraduate ophthalmic training culminated in award of FRCS in 1985 and FRCOphth at its foundation in 1988. In 1990, the University of London granted an MS doctorate for corneal research and, in 2004, a Doctor of Science in Ophthalmology and Ophthalmic Surgery.

Professor Rose was appointed consultant to Moorfields Eye Hospital, London, in 1990 and is also a Senior Research Fellow of the NIHR Biomedical Research Centre of the Institute of Ophthalmology. He served as the British Council member of the European Society of Ophthalmic Plastic and Reconstructive, is a Past-President of the British Oculoplastic Surgical Society, and is President of the European Society of Oculoplastic and Reconstructive Surgeons.

# Systemic Management in Orbital and Adnexal Emergencies

2

Ashok K. Grover, Saurbhi Khurana, and Harish Bora

Periorbital and ocular trauma can often be associated with intracranial trauma or other systemic problems. In a case of trauma, assessment is different from that of a usual patient. It is important to ensure patient's survival and tackle any other life-threatening complications first. It is therefore imperative to first assess the "ABCs" (airway, breathing, and circulation) of the patient before addressing the periorbital trauma (Fig. 2.1).

## Primary Assessment [1, 2]

The primary survey should take 2–5 min and consists of:

- *A = Airway*
- Establishing and maintaining an airway is always the first priority.
- Important signs of obstruction include snoring or gurgling, stridor, and paradoxical chest movements.
- The presence of a foreign body should be considered in unconscious patients.
- Advanced airway management (such as endotracheal intubation, cricothyrotomy, or tracheostomy) is indicated if there is apnea, persistent obstruction, severe head injury, maxillofacial trauma, a penetrating neck injury with an expanding hematoma, or major chest injuries.
- *B = Breathing and ventilation*
- Assessment of ventilation is best accomplished by the look, listen, and feel approach.
- Look for cyanosis, use of accessory muscles, flail chest, and penetrating chest injuries.
- Listen for the presence, absence, or diminution of breath sounds.

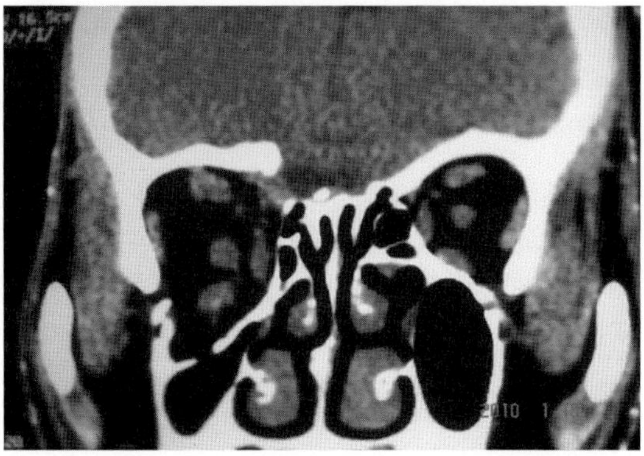

**Fig. 2.1** Coexisting orbital roof fracture with intracranial hematoma in a patient with eyelid injury

A.K. Grover, MD, MNAMS, FRCS, FICO, FIMSA
Ophthalomology, Sir Ganga Ram Hospital,
New Delhi, Delhi, India
e-mail: akgrover55@yahoo.com

S. Khurana, MD, FICO (✉)
Ophthalmology, Medanta,
Gurgaon 122001, Haryana, India
e-mail: saurbhi.khurana@gmail.com

H. Bora, MD
Anaesthesia, Vision Eye Centre,
New Delhi 110049, Delhi, India
e-mail: visioneyecentre21@gmail.com


B. Mukherjee, H. Yuen (eds.), *Emergencies of the Orbit and Adnexa*,
DOI 10.1007/978-81-322-1807-4_2

- Feel for subcutaneous emphysema, tracheal shift, and broken ribs.
- *C = Circulation*
- Adequacy of circulation is based on pulse rate, pulse fullness, blood pressure, and signs of peripheral perfusion.
- Signs of inadequate circulation include tachycardia, hypotension, weak or impalpable peripheral pulses, or cool, cyanotic extremities.
- The first priority in restoring adequate circulation is to stop any bleeding.
- The second priority is to replace the intravascular volume.
- *D = Disability*
- Evaluation for disability consists of a rapid neurological assessment. Because there is usually no time for a Glasgow Coma Scale (*GCS*), the *AVPU system* is used: *a*wake, *v*erbal *r*esponse, *p*ainful response, and *u*nresponsive.
- Multiple injuries may coexist, and the injuries that appear most dramatic may not be those that pose the most risk. Any intervention required for systemic injuries will have precedence over the ocular injury. Moreover, it is important to address these before we plan to take up a patient for eyelid repair under general anesthesia [3].

The secondary survey begins only when the ABCs are stabilized. In the secondary survey, the patient is evaluated from head to toe, and the indicated studies (e.g., radiographs, laboratory tests, invasive diagnostic procedures) are obtained [2].

## Investigations

Basic laboratory analysis includes a complete blood count (or hematocrit or hemoglobin), electrolytes, glucose, blood urea nitrogen (BUN), and creatinine.

Arterial blood gases may also be extremely helpful.

A chest X-ray should be obtained in all patients with major trauma.

The possibility of cervical spine injury is evaluated by examining all seven vertebrae in a cross-table lateral radiograph and a swimmer's view.

Depending on the injuries, hemodynamic status of the patient and history, other imaging techniques (e.g., chest computed tomography [CT] or angiography, CT head), or diagnostic tests such as diagnostic peritoneal lavage (DPL) may also be indicated [2].

Children involved in trauma are often uncooperative for systemic as well as ocular assessment. A detailed systemic evaluation is important so as to not miss out on any subtle visceral trauma/fractures. The extent of ocular and periocular injuries will often have to be assessed either in sedation or when the child is taken up for repair under general anesthesia. Moreover, certain injuries like white eye orbital floor fracture or foreign bodies in orbit or adnexa that can go undetected in children and cause chronic symptoms later need to be ruled out. An imaging is accordingly advised.

Hence, in trauma, assessment of systemic injuries and their management take precedence over ocular injuries.

## References

1. Wilson WC, Grande CM, Hoyt DB. Trauma: emergency resuscitation, perioperative anesthesia, vol. 1. Boca Raton: CRC Press; 2007. p. 267.
2. Newman MF, Fleisher L, Fink MP. Perioperative medicine: managing for outcome. Philadelphia: Saunders; 2008. p. 37.
3. Kuhn F, Pieramici DJ. Ocular trauma: principles and practice. New York: Thieme; 2011. p. 73.

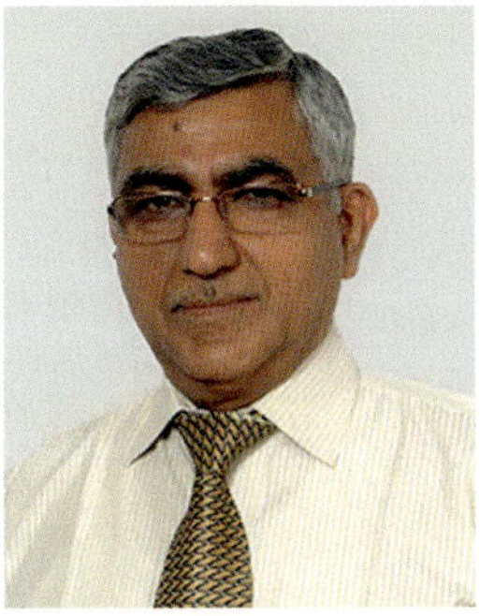

**Ashok K. Grover** Dr. A.K. Grover is recipient of Padmashri Award, one of the highest civilian awards by the President of India for his services to Ophthalmology. He is Chairman, Department of Ophthalmology at Sir Ganga Ram Hospital and Vision Eye Centre in New Delhi.

Dr. Grover is Chairman of Subspecialty Education Committee, International Council of Ophthalmologist (ICO), Councilor at large of the Asia Pacific Academy of Ophthalmology (APAO), Board Member of the Afro Asian Council of Ophthalmology (AACO), and Vice President of the Ocular Trauma Society of India (OTSI). He is Past President of the Asia Pacific Society of Ophthalmic Plastic and Reconstructive Surgery (APSOPRS), Oculoplastics Association of India (OPAI), and All India Ophthalmological Society (AIOS).

Dr. Grover serves on the Editorial Board of the *Asia Pacific Journal of Ophthalmology, Indian Journal of Ophthalmology, Nepalese Journal of Ophthalmology, Journal of International Medical Science Academy, Ocular Surgery News* (Asia Pacific Edition), and is a reviewer for several international/national journals. He is an examiner for FRCS (Glasgow).

Dr. Grover has received numerous prestigious Awards and Orations including the Distinguished Service Award from Asia Pacific Academy of Ophthalmology, Honorary FRCS, Honorary Fellowship of International Council of Ophthalmology (FICO), Col. Rangachari Award for the best paper from the All India Ophthalmological Society, and other numerous International and National Orations.

Dr. Grover has authored/edited 4 books, written over 60 chapters in textbooks, has over 75 publications, and over 1000 presentations at international and national levels. He has chaired sessions, been Guest Speaker, and done live surgery all over the globe including the World Congress, APAO, Afro Asian Academy, American Academy, APSOPRS, and National meetings.

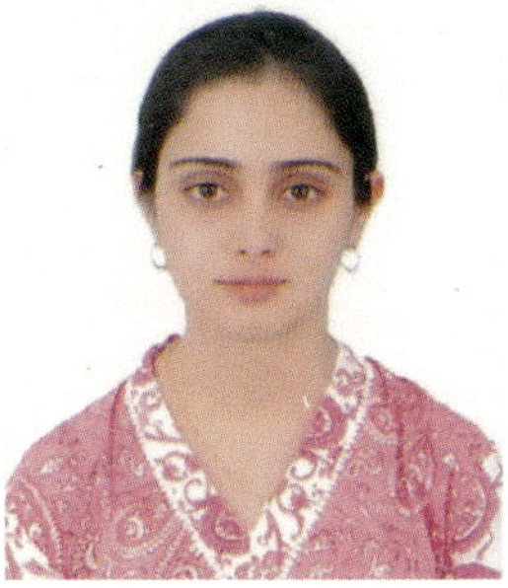

**Saurbhi Khurana** Dr. Saurbhi Khurana got her MBBS degree from the Maulana Azad Medical College in the year 2006. She did her MD in ophthalmology from Dr. Rajendra Prasad Centre for Ophthalmic Sciences, AIIMS, New Delhi in the year 2009. She was a senior resident at the same institute in the Department of Oculoplasty and Pediatric Ophthalmology till 2012. Following her senior residency, she did an oculoplasty fellowship at the Leicester University, UK. She has authored many peer-reviewed articles and is an invited faculty at various conferences. She is a skilled oculoplastic and aesthetic surgeon.

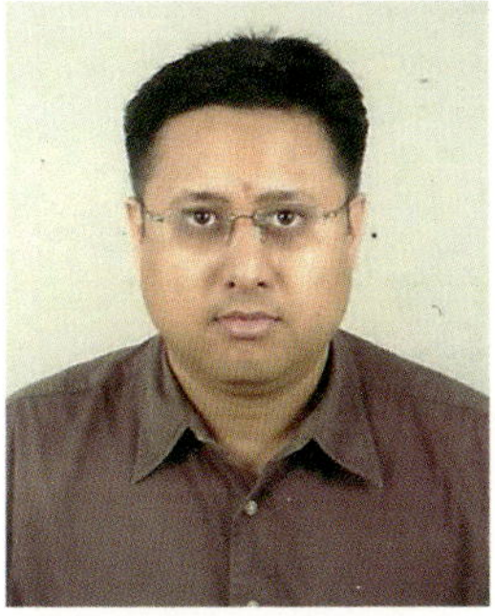

**Harish Bora** Harish Bora is a practicing Anesthetist with an experience of 25 years. He did his MBBS from Maulana Azad Medical College, New Delhi, and postgraduation from Safdarjung Hospital, New Delhi. Currently, he is a visiting consultant to various hospitals, namely, Vision Eye Centre, New Delhi; Shanti Mukand Hospital, Delhi; Mohan Eye Institute, New Delhi; and Agarwal Eye Clinic, New Delhi. He is certified by American Heart Association for BLS and ACLS. He is a Member of Indian Society of Anaesthesiologists and Member of Delhi Medical Council. Dr. Bora has special interest for Ophthalmology Anaesthesia and Paediatric Anaesthesia and Critical Care. He has edited textbook for paramedical and ORA technicians

# Globe Rupture

# 3

Harsha Bhattacharjee, Manabjyoti Barman, and Kasturi Bhattacharjee

## Introduction

Ocular trauma accounts for a major cause of worldwide visual morbidity that especially affects the young population. Ocular trauma comprises a wide field with varied mode and settings of injury. The Birmingham Eye Trauma Terminology (BETT) system has described specific terminology and assessment describing different eye injuries [1] (Table 3.1). This system has been endorsed by the International Society of Ocular Trauma, United States Eye Injury Registry, the Hungarian Eye Injury Registry, the Vitreous Society, the Retina Society, and the American Society of Ophthalmology.

While laceration and rupture are both open-globe injuries; a laceration generally implies full-thickness wound of the eye wall caused by a sharp object, and rupture is described as full-thickness wound of the eye wall caused by blunt trauma. The eye wall gives way at its weakest point which may or may not be at the site of impact. Some exceptions are like pellet and blast injuries, which have significant blunt force, still considered lacerations. The sole purpose of this section is to discuss details of presentation and management of globe rupture.

## Pathophysiology

Globe rupture may occur when a blunt object hits the globe, which compresses it anteroposteriorly along the horizontal axis, causing sudden rise of intraocular pressure to a point that the sclera tears. Ruptures from blunt trauma are most common at the anatomically thinner parts of the

**Table 3.1** Eye injury (Birmingham Eye Trauma Terminology system) [1]

| |
|---|
| Closed globe |
| Contusion |
| Lamellar laceration |
| Open globe |
| Rupture |
| Laceration |
| Penetrating |
| IOFB |
| Perforating |



H. Bhattacharjee, MS, FRCP
Comprehensive Ophthalmology, Sri Sankaradeva Nethralaya, Guwahati 781028, Assam, India
e-mail: drharshabhattacharjee@gmail.com

M. Barman, DO, DNB (✉)
Vitreo-Retina, Sri Sankaradeva Nethralaya, Guwahati 781028, Assam, India
e-mail: BARMANMJ@GMAIL.COM

K. Bhattacharjee, MS, DNB, FRCS
Orbit, Ophthalmic, Plastic and Reconstructive Surgery, Sri Sankaradeva Nethralaya, Guwahati 781028, Assam, India
e-mail: kasturibhattacharjee44@hotmail.com


B. Mukherjee, H. Yuen (eds.), *Emergencies of the Orbit and Adnexa*,
DOI 10.1007/978-81-322-1807-4_3

sclera, such as at the site of insertions of the extraocular muscles, at the limbus, or at the site of previous ocular surgery [2, 3].

## Epidemiology

The global pattern of eye injuries and their consequences emerging from a review of data compiled from the ophthalmic literature and WHO's Blindness Data Bank by Négrel AD et al. suggest that globally approximately 55 million people are exposed to ocular trauma each year, restricting activities more than one day; 750,000 cases require hospitalization each year, including some 200,000 open-globe injuries; and approximately 1.6 million people become blind from injuries, wherein bilateral low vision is found in 2.3 million people and unilateral low vision in almost 19 million [4].

Most of the epidemiological data of ocular trauma are based on information from more developed countries. The incidence rates of ocular trauma requiring hospitalization for those with definite ocular trauma (principal diagnosis) were 13.2 per 100,000 population and for total ocular trauma (principal or secondary diagnoses) 27.3 per 100,000 population per year in the United States [5, 6], 8.1 per 100,000 persons per year in Scotland [7], 12.6 per 100,000 persons per year in Singapore [8], and 15.2 per 100,000 persons per year in Australia [9]. In the United States alone, eye injuries cost >$300 million per year due to loss of productivity, medical expenses, and workers' compensation [10]. Developing countries, where the actual incidence may be much more, suffer the worst brunt of the problem.

The major risk factors for ocular trauma include age, gender, socioeconomic status, and lifestyle.

Open-globe injuries occur at a relatively younger age in men (median age 36 year) than in women (median age 73 year). Approximately one third of patients with eye trauma are children. Because of occupational and recreational predilection, open-globe injuries are common in men (78.6 %). However, men are more likely to have lacerations (69.9 %), whereas women present more frequently with globe rupture (68.1 %). Projectile-related injuries are more common in men (54.9 %). Compared to men, falls accounted for majority of globe injuries in women (8.1 % versus 55.3 %) [11].

## Causes

- Globe rupture in adults is common after blunt injury during motor vehicle accident, recreational activity, assault, or industrial or workplace-related accidents.
- One third of eye injuries occurring in children and adolescents are sports related [12].
- Eye injuries from paintball weapons are becoming frequent, with globe rupture occurring in 5 % of cases [13].
- Women commonly suffer from such injuries due to domestic accidents.

## Approach to a Patient with Globe Rupture

As ocular injuries causing globe rupture are more frequent in the workplace or during recreational activities; co-workers, co-players, or bystanders can play an important role in the management of such cases by giving initial support and bringing the victim to emergency care service at the earliest. Appropriate and timely management plays a significant role in the final outcome of these cases.

Usually an emergency department physician is the first skilled person to receive such cases. Approach to such a patient depends to a large extent on the age as well as mental and physical condition of the patient. While children are more prone for trauma, they usually are less cooperative for clinical examination. Often subtle injuries are missed in such cases. So these cases need more careful monitoring and evaluation whenever there is doubt of eye trauma. If necessary, examination under sedation or general anesthesia may be appropriate. A gentle and organized approach is essential.

Essential steps to be followed in the emergency department are:

- Rule out potentially life-threatening systemic injury. If ocular trauma is associated with any serious physical injury, like cardiovascular, respiratory, or neurological trauma; the patient should be immediately referred for appropriate care after initial eye protection with an eye shield or other rigid devices.
- Once major systemic injury is ruled out, a thorough history should be taken.
- Medicolegal aspect of such cases should be kept in mind, and necessary formalities should be accomplished.
- Brief eye examination should be performed and should be referred for ophthalmic care if necessary for further management.

## Emergency Department Care

- The injured eye should be kept covered with an eye shield or other rigid devices when not being examined (e.g., bottom of a polystyrene foam cup). Pad and bandage should better be avoided. Eye manipulation should be minimized as this may increase intraocular pressure with potential extrusion of intraocular contents.
- Antiemetics may be administered to prevent Valsalva maneuver.
- Analgesics should be given if necessary. However, sedatives should be avoided.
- Instillation of topical eye medication is contraindicated.
- Prophylactic systemic antibiotics may be administered to prevent endophthalmitis.
- Anti-rabies prophylaxis should be done if indicated.
- Tetanus immune status should be documented and updated if necessary.
- An intravenous line should be positioned depending upon physical condition of the patient or if the patient needs to be transferred.
- Patient should be advised to remain nil orally.
- The decision regarding referral to an ophthalmologist depends upon the condition of the eye and the expertise of the primary physician handling the case. All information along with any diagnostic test performed should accompany the patient.

Once the patient reaches the ophthalmologist's care, a quick review of the primary physician's note and the test reports should be done. A brief systemic evaluation to detect any change in vital systemic status should be done. Thereafter a systematic examination to the patient's injuries should be done to develop a logical treatment plan. Examination should be carried out promptly and comprehensively, as the details of internal structures of the eye may be obscured soon by edema or media opacity. The uninjured eye should also be thoroughly examined. Photographic documentation is invaluable not only for comparison of treatment outcome but also for medicolegal purpose. If photographic documentation is not possible, detailed drawing of all the injuries should be done. It should be assumed that any periocular or ocular trauma could include a ruptured globe.

## Relevant History and Ophthalmic Examination

- Details regarding the time, circumstance, and mechanism of injury should be obtained.
- Preexisting medical condition, prior history of ocular surgery, medications, allergy to any medication, tetanus immune status, and time of last meal should be recorded.
- Pain is not a useful guide to assess severity of injury, as it may not be severe in sharp injuries. Also it may be a misleading symptom in apprehensive patients.
- Visual acuity estimation is the most initial step of examination, as it can help in formulating treatment plan and prognosis. This may be hampered by lid and periorbital swelling. A lid speculum should be used gently in such situation. If immediate vision examination is not possible, the reason for not assessing the visual acuity should be noted with a recommendation for reassessment whenever possible.

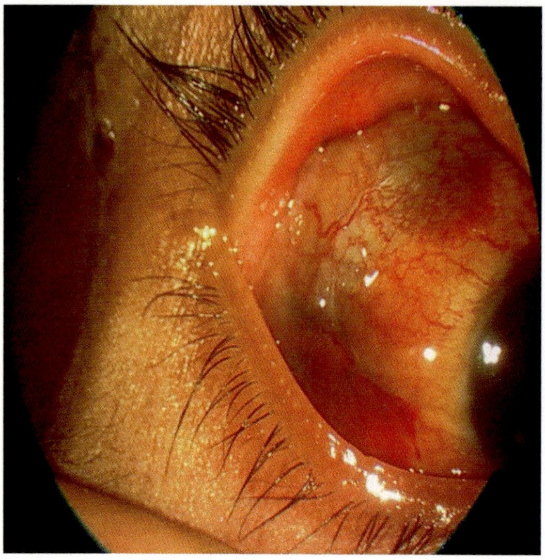

**Fig. 3.1** Globe rupture at equatorial area

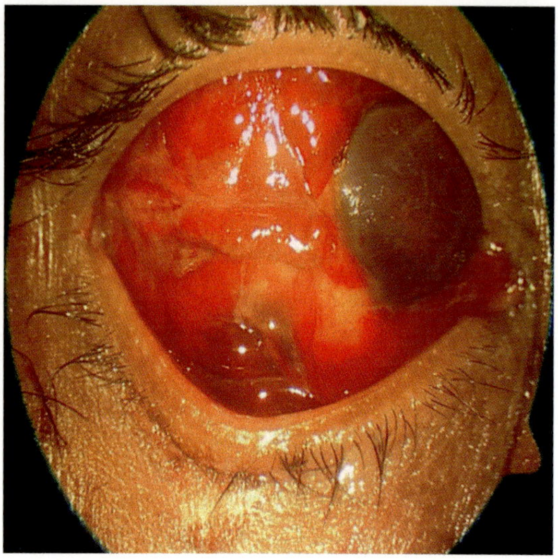

**Fig. 3.2** Conjunctival laceration with subconjunctival hemorrhage overlying a ruptured globe

- Extraocular movement should be evaluated to rule out entrapment or extraocular muscle injury with associated orbital floor fracture. Motility disorder may also be due to traumatic cranial nerve palsy.
- Orbital examination should be done to rule out fracture or bony deformity. Presence of orbital soft tissue crepitus signifies subcutaneous emphysema. A ruptured globe may present as enophthalmos. However, an associated retrobulbar hemorrhage may present as proptosis, even in the presence of an occult globe rupture.
- A general inspection of the eyeball is to be done to find out obvious signs of globe injury. The eye can be misshapen with prolapsed ocular contents. However, globe rupture may often be occult on presentation.
- With significant lid or periorbital edema, lid speculums or lid retractors should be used to expose the eyeball taking care not to press over it.
- Eyelid and lacrimal injuries should be evaluated with the goal of identifying possible deep injuries to the globe (Fig. 3.1). Lid repairs should be deferred until globe injury is ruled out.
- Conjunctival lacerations may sometimes overlie serious scleral injuries (Fig. 3.2). Large conjunctival hemorrhage may be an indication of underlying globe rupture.
- Localized scleral bulge or dark discoloration is often indicative of rupture. Subconjunctival dislocation of the lens (phacocele) is an evidence of scleral dehiscence at the limbus.
- Prolapse of the iris through a corneal or limbal wound may be visible at the site of injury (Fig. 3.3). More subtle or partially self-sealing wounds may be confirmed by fluorescein dye test (Fig. 3.4).
- Anterior chamber examination may show associated injuries such as iris transillumination defect, hyphema, and lens damage, including dislocation or subluxation. Shallow anterior chamber may be a sign of globe rupture. A posterior rupture, on the other hand, may present with a deep anterior chamber due to vitreous loss.
- Pupils should be checked for size, configuration, symmetry, and relative afferent defect. An injured pupil is usually oval and middilated. However, a dilated or a pinpoint pupil along with history of head injury warrants immediate neurological consultation. Any irregularity in the papillary shape may be a sign of globe rupture. An afferent pupillary defect indicates optic nerve injury, severe vas-

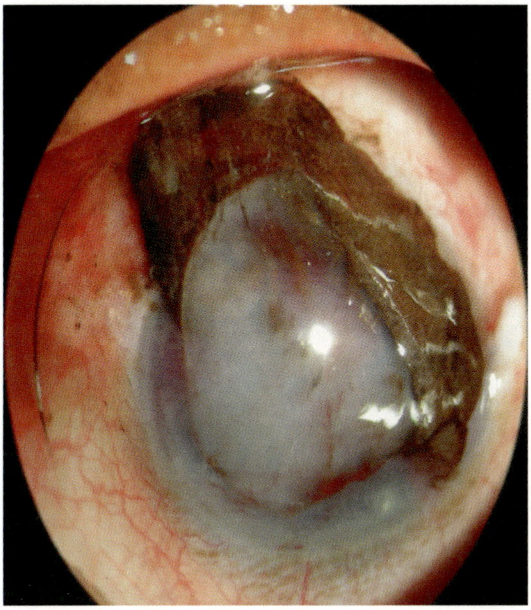

**Fig. 3.3** Corneal rupture with uveal tissue prolapsed (Courtesy Dr J Medhi, SSN. Guwahati)

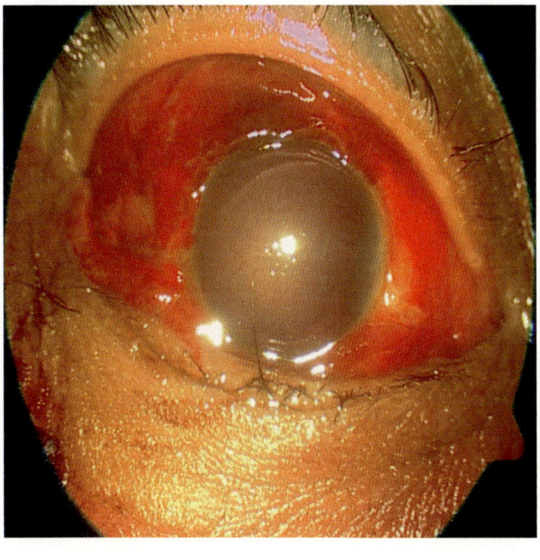

**Fig. 3.4** Corneal haze with globe rupture at the superior limbus extending temporally

cular damage, or extensive retinal damage. If the pupil cannot be visualized in the traumatized eye due to media opacity, check for an afferent pupillary defect in the fellow eye.

- Posterior segment examination may reveal vitreous hemorrhage, optic nerve avulsion, foreign body, retinal tear, edema, or detachment. Vitreous tract with localized hemorrhage may indicate globe rupture.
- Intraocular pressure measurement is contraindicated to avoid mechanical pressure if globe rupture is suspected. If felt necessary, a non-contact tonometer should be used. Intraocular pressure is usually low in a ruptured globe.

## Investigation

### Laboratory Studies

Laboratory studies are primarily needed for anesthesia purposes. Tests may be done as appropriate for coexisting trauma and to rule out other medical problems.

### Electrophysiology

In selected cases, where visual acuity assessment is not reliable, VEP may be helpful to confirm visual potential in the injured eye.

### Ultrasonography

Ultrasonography can detect irregularity in the ocular coats, lens dislocation, retrobulbar hemorrhage, retinal detachment, and intraocular foreign body. Visualization of periorbital gas in ultrasonography is an indication of orbital fracture. However, ultrasonography is better to be avoided in cases of open-globe injury.

### Computerized Tomography

CT scanning of the eye is the preferred imaging modality for assessment of occult open-globe injuries [14]. It is highly sensitive to detect an occult globe rupture, associated optic nerve injury, small foreign bodies, as well as to visualize the anatomy of the orbit. Sensitivity and specificity of ocular CT in determining occult open-globe injury range from 56 to 70 % and 70–100 %, respectively [15, 16]. Axial and coronal views of

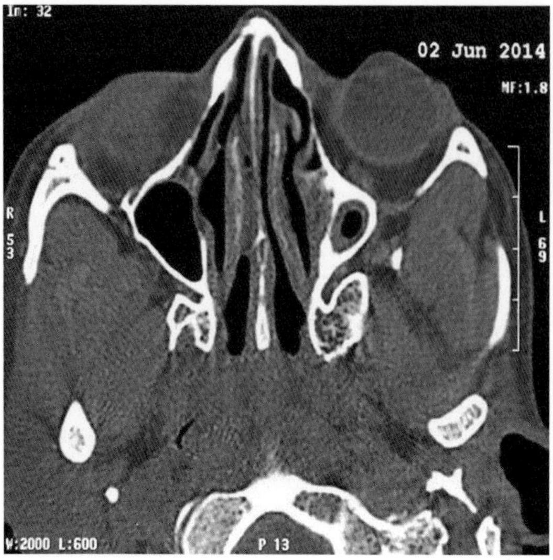


**Fig. 3.5** CT scan showing a ruptured right eyeball. Note small eyeball with irregular ocular coats

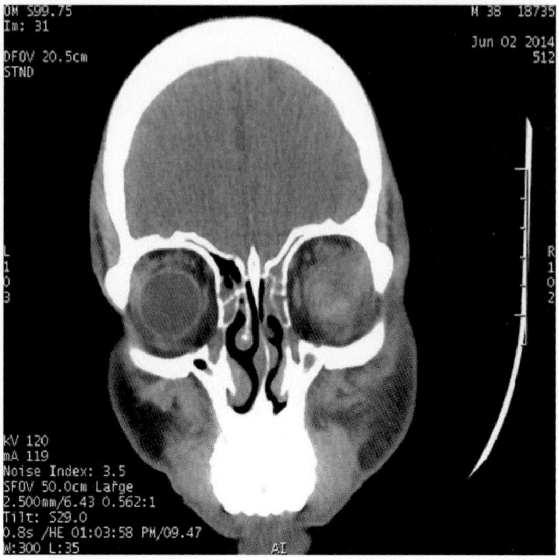


**Fig. 3.6** CT scan showing a ruptured right eyeball. Note small eyeball with irregular ocular coats

the brain and orbits without contrast utilizing 1–2 mm cuts should be obtained. Some nonmetallic foreign bodies, such as wood, glass, or plastic, may be missed in CT scan.

CT findings that can be present in a globe rupture include:

- Collapse of the globe (flat-tire appearance) (Fig. 3.5)
- Detect intraocular air or foreign body
- Deep AC with posterior movement of the lens
- Thickening of the posterior sclera
- Hazy and ill-defined outline of the globe (Fig. 3.6)

### MRI

MRI is of limited usefulness in the acute stages of ocular trauma and is contraindicated if possibility of metallic intraocular foreign body exists. However, MRI is excellent in identifying details of the soft tissues of the globe, optic nerve, and orbit and in localizing organic foreign bodies.

### X-ray

X-ray of the orbits and sinuses is rarely used for diagnosis in orbital trauma. A three-view plain film series is useful in evaluating the bony orbits and the sinuses and in identifying radiopaque foreign bodies. Water view provides details of the orbital floor and detects air-fluid level in the maxillary sinuses. Caldwell or anteroposterior view visualizes the medial orbital wall, the lateral and superior orbital rims, and the ethmoid and frontal sinuses. A lateral view is useful in visualizing the orbital roof, maxillary and frontal sinuses, zygoma, and sella turcica.

## Treatment

### Medication

The goal of medical therapy is to prevent infections and other pathophysiologic complications. The frequency of endophthalmitis after open-globe injury has been estimated to be about 6.8 % [17]. Prophylactic systemic antibiotics should be given to cover organisms commonly associated with post-traumatic endophthalmitis, including *bacillus* species, *s. aureus*, *pseudomonas*, gram-negative bacilli, anaerobes, corynebacteria, and streptococci. Special attention should be given to species-specific pathogens if injury is due to animal bites or if organic material is likely to have been introduced.

## Surgical Repair

As the diagnosis of globe rupture is not always clear-cut, a low threshold for surgical exploration should be maintained in case of any doubt of such injury. General anesthesia is indicated. Depolarizing paralytic agents should better be avoided due to possible risk of increased IOP. The main principle in the treatment of open-globe injury is to restore the physical integrity of the globe wall. Attempt should be made to reposit prolapsed intraocular structures.

Basic wound closure principles must be strictly observed. In cases where watertight closure cannot be achieved with sutures alone, tissue adhesive glue may be used. Foreign bodies in the anterior chamber or within easy reach can be removed. Disrupted lens material or prolapsed vitreous may be removed at the discretion of the surgeon. However, procedures that need more time and manipulation, such as posterior segment foreign body removal, retinal detachment repair, or intraocular lens implantation, are not advisable during primary repair. Intraocular air may be found in some open-globe injuries. Also air or gas may be injected during surgery to form the globe. This may be a concern if the patient needs to undergo air travel, due to possible risk of expansion of gas at high altitude. However, rise in IOP is not significant in the eyes with less than 10 % gas fill (0.6 ml). Also the half-life of air in the human eye is only 1.3 days, and most open globes, including those that have undergone recent repair, are hypotonus and can accommodate moderate rise in IOP [18].

## Sympathetic Ophthalmia

An uncommon but potentially devastating complication of open-globe injury leading to blindness in the fellow eye is sympathetic ophthalmia.

It is a diffuse bilateral granulomatous uveitis, believed to represent an autoimmune response to the exposed uveal or retinal antigens previously sequestered within the blood-aqueous or blood-retinal barrier. Incidence of sympathetic ophthalmia after open-globe injury varies widely from 0.02 to 56 % as reported in different studies [19]. In severely damaged eyes where repair is technically not possible, enucleation should be performed preferably within 2 weeks of injury to prevent sympathetic ophthalmia [20]. Though there is no definite evidence, yet evisceration is discouraged in such cases, due to the risk of potential presence of uveal antigens within the emissary channels of the scleral shell.

## Globe Repair Versus Enucleation: Decision-Making

Repair of open-globe injuries should be attempted whenever technically possible even with slightest possibility of survival of the globe. However, when a globe is so severely damaged that repair is not technically possible, enucleation must be performed at the earliest to prevent sympathetic ophthalmia. There is another group of patients, in whom repair is possible, but the ultimate prognosis for vision or globe survival is nonexistent. In such cases, also, repair should be attempted as this assures the patient that a reasonable effort was made to try to save the eye. Also the lack of visual function is demonstrated to the patient, thus allowing the patient to get involved in further decision-making process.

## Prognosis and Prognostic Models

Visual outcome following globe rupture is affected by multiple factors. Wound location and size, visual acuity at presentation, intraocular pressure, anterior chamber status, pupillary changes, posterior segment status, and time of management are prognostic determinants.

In a retrospective review, Esmaeli et al. studied 176 cases of ruptured globe to identify factors that may predict ocular survival and final visual acuity. According to the study, predictors of excellent final visual acuity (20/60 or better) were initial visual acuity of 20/200 or better, wound location anterior to the plane of insertion of the four recti muscles, wound length 10 mm or less, and sharp mechanism of injury [21].

Kuhn et al. developed a prognostic model, the Ocular Trauma Score (OTS), to predict the visual outcome of patients after ocular trauma. The OTS is estimated based on six variable factors each being assigned with certain numerical points: initial visual acuity, globe rupture, endophthalmitis, perforating injury, retinal detachment, and RAPD. The scores are stratified into five categories that give the probabilities of attaining a range of post-injury visual acuities [22].

More recently, Schmidt et al. proposed another prognostic model, the classification and regression tree (CART), to predict visual outcome in patients with open-globe injuries [23]. According to the classification tree, the presence of RAPD and poor initial visual acuity were the most predictive of visual loss; lid laceration and posteriorly located wound can also predict poor visual outcome. The study created another regression tree looking at the difference in vision survival based on age. Patients under the age of 38 had significantly higher chances of vision survival. This prognostic model has been found to have 85.7 % sensitivity and 91.9 % specificity to predict vision survival correctly. While validity of the regression tree model has been established, the Ocular Trauma Score (OTS) system has been found to have higher prognostic accuracy [24].

## Prevention

Awareness among people about risk of ocular trauma and proper use of protective eyewear is the mainstay of prevention of all ocular injuries. At industrial sites, at-risk workers should be provided with compulsory protective shields.

## References


1. Kuhn F, Morris R, Witherspoon CD, Mester V. The Birmingham Eye Trauma Terminology system (BETT). J Fr Ophtalmol. 2004;27(2):206–10.
2. Sharma R, Brunette DD. Ophthalmology. In: Marx, editor. Rosen's emergency medicine. Vol 2, 7th ed. 2009; Chap 69. Saunders (Elsevier), Philadelphia, USA.
3. Olitsky S, Hug D, Smith L. Injuries to the eye. In: Kliegman R, editor. Nelson textbook of pediatrics. 18th ed. 2007; Chap 634. Mosby (Elsevier), Philadelphia, USA.
4. Négrel AD, Thylefors B. The global impact of eye injuries. Ophthalmic Epidemiol. 1998;5(3):143–69.
5. Klopfer J, Tielsch JM, Vitale S, et al. Ocular trauma in the United States: eye injuries resulting in hospitalization, 1984 through 1987. Arch Ophthalmol. 1992; 110(6):838–42.
6. Tielsch JM, Parver L, Shankar B. Time trends in the incidence of hospitalized ocular trauma. Arch Ophthalmol. 1989;107(4):519–23.
7. Desai P, MacEwen CJ, Baines P, Minassian DC. Incidence of cases of ocular trauma admitted to hospital and incidence of blinding outcome. Br J Ophthalmol. 1996;80(7):592–6.
8. Wong TY, Tielsch JM. A population-based study on the incidence of severe ocular trauma in Singapore. Am J Ophthalmol Clin N Am. 1999;128(3):345–51.
9. Fong LP. Eye injuries in Victoria, Australia. Med J Aust. 1995;162(2):64–8.
10. Kanoff JM, Turalba AV, Andreoli MT, Andreoli CM. Characteristics and outcomes of work-related open globe injuries. Am J Ophthalmol. 2010;150(2):265–9.
11. Koo L, Kapadia MK, Singh RP, et al. Gender differences in etiology and outcome of open globe injuries. J Trauma. 2005;59(1):175–8.
12. Rodriguez JO, Lavina AM, Agarwal A. Prevention and treatment of common eye injuries in sports. Am Fam Physician. 2003;67(7):1481–8.
13. Listman DA. Paintball injuries in children: more than meets the eye. Pediatrics. 2004;113(1):15–8.
14. Harlan Jr JB, Pieramici DJ. Evaluation of patients with ocular trauma. Ophthalmol Clin North Am. 2002;15(2):153–61.
15. Arey ML, Mootha VV, Whittemore AR, et al. Computed tomography in the diagnosis of occult open-globe injuries. Ophthalmology. 2007;114(8):1448–52.
16. Hoffstetter P, Schreyer AG, Schreyer CI, et al. Multidetector CT (MD-CT) in the diagnosis of uncertain open globe injuries. Rofo. 2010;182(2):151–4.
17. Essex RW, Yi Q, Charles PG, Allen PJ. Post-traumatic endophthalmitis. Ophthalmology. 2004;111(11): 2015–22.
18. Mills MD, Devenyi RG, Lam WC, et al. An assessment of intraocular pressure rise in patients with gas filled eyes during simulated air flight. Ophthalmology. 2001;108(1):40–4.
19. Albert DM, Diaz-Rohena R. A historical review of sympathetic ophthalmia and its epidemiology. Surv Ophthalmol. 1989;34(1):1–14.
20. DeBacker CM, Holck DEE. Enucleation in orbital trauma. In: Holck DEE, Ng JD, editors. Evaluation and treatment of orbital fractures: a multidisciplinary approach. 2nd ed. Philadelphia: Elsevier Saunders; 2006. p. 365–8.
21. Esmaeli B, Elner SG, Schork MA, Elner VM. Visual outcome and ocular survival after penetrating trauma. A clinicopathologic study. Ophthalmology. 1995; 102(3):393–400.
22. Kuhn F, Maisiak R, Mann L, et al. The ocular trauma score (OTS). Ophthalmol Clin North Am. 2002;15(2): 163–5.
23. Schmidt GW, Broman AT, Hindman HB, Grant MP. Vision survival after open globe injury predicted by

classification and regression tree analysis. Ophthalmology. 2008;115(1):202–9.
24. Yu Wai Man C, Steel D. Visual outcome after open globe injury: a comparison of two prognostic models – the ocular trauma score and the classification and regression tree. Eye (Lond). 2010;24(1):84–9.

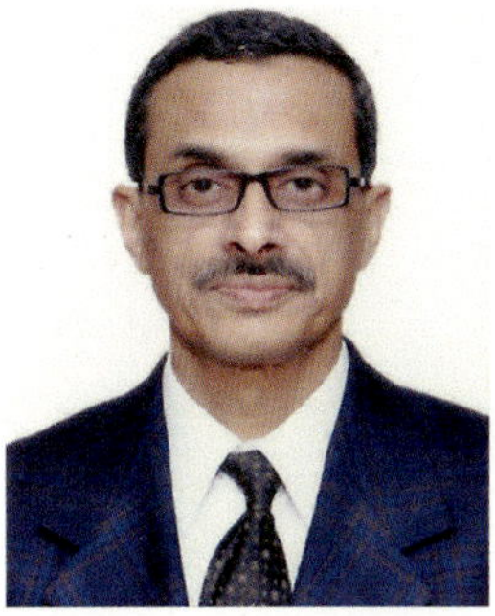

**Harsha Bhattacharjee** Dr. Harsha Bhattacharjee MS, FRCP is the founder Medical Director and trustee of Sri Sankaradeva Nethralaya, Guwahati, India. He has numerous publications in indexed journals and has trained more than 80 fellows. He is a post graduate examiner in Ophthalmology for national and international colleges.

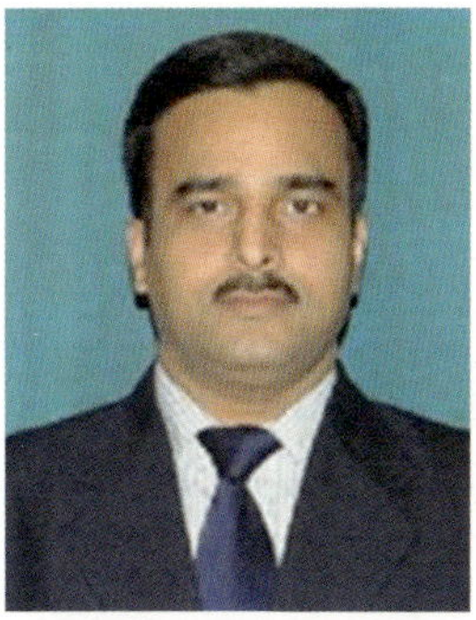

**Manabjyoti Barman** Dr. Manabjyoti Barman is currently working as senior consultant in Vitreo-Retina and Oncology Service of Sri Sankaradeva Nethralaya, Guwahati (India). He has done his ophthalmic postgraduation from Sri Sankaradeva Nethralaya (Guwahati) in 2006 followed by specialized fellowship in Vitreo-Retina from Sankara Nethralaya, Chennai (India) and in Ocular Oncology from New York Eye and Ear Infirmary (USA). Along with his primary field of interest in vitreoretinal disease and tumor management, he is also actively involved in ocular trauma management. He has made multiple national and international presentations and publications in the respective fields.

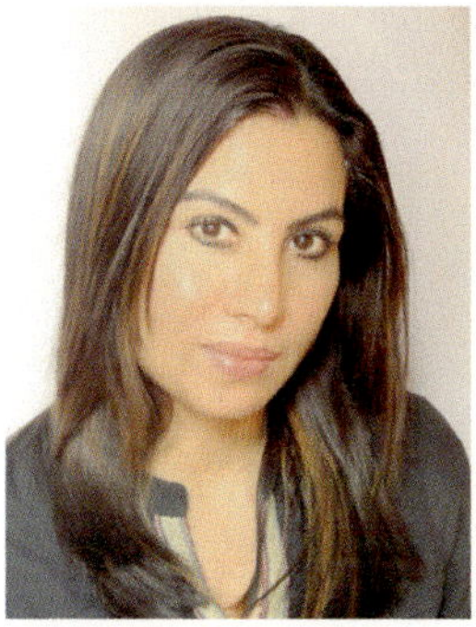

**Kasturi Bhattacharjee** Dr. (Mrs) Kasturi Bhattacharjee, MS, DNB, FRCS is the Head, Deptt. of Orbit, Ophthalmic Plastic & Reconstructive Surgery and Cataract & Refractive Surgery at Sri Sankaradeva Nethralaya, India. She is the recipient of more than 23 awards for her work in Ophthalmology and has more than 47 publications in National and International journals.

# Subluxated Globes

# 4

Kasturi Bhattacharjee, Harsha Bhattacharjee, Manpreet Singh, and Debleena Dey

## Introduction

Globe subluxation is a rare clinical entity. Although first reported in 1907 by Tucker, yet so far, the understanding of its pathomechanism is still limited [1]. It is described as partial (subluxation) or complete (dislocation) displacement of the eyeball from its normal anatomical position. Though rare, its occurrence can lead to a grievous impact in the form of irreversible vision loss which usually affects the younger and productive individuals of society.

The globe subluxation can be accompanied by avulsion or evulsion injury to the globe. The prefix 'e' suggests the pulling 'out' of the eyeball most commonly associated with optic nerve and muscle lacerations. The avulsion injury is described as pulling 'away' of any structure which is generally not associated with complete severing of optic nerve and muscles [2, 3]. However, out of the two, avulsion injuries have more often been described in literature. It is frequently used in conjunction with trauma to the optic nerve with partial or complete injury to it. The term globe 'luxation' is used for forward displacement of eyeball along with the spasmodic contraction of eyelids secondary to orbicularis oculi spasm [4]. In such situation, the equator of the globe crosses the orbital rim, often leading to severe pain, restriction of ocular movements and sometimes vision loss (Figs. 4.1 and 4.2).

**Etiologies:**

- Traumatic (most common)
- Spontaneous
- Voluntary or self inflicted (rare)

**Fig. 4.1** Etiologies of globe subluxation

**Predisposing factors for globe subluxation:**

- Severe cranio-facial trauma
- Shallow bony orbital cavity
- Lax eyelid, canthal tendons and periocular tissues
- Increased retrobulbar soft tissue volume
- Raised retrobulbar pressure
- Psychiatric disorder

**Fig. 4.2** Predisposing factors for globe subluxation

K. Bhattacharjee, MS, DNB, FRCS (✉)
M. Singh, MS, DNB
Orbit, Ophthalmic, Plastic and Reconstructive Surgery, Sri Sankaradeva Nethralaya, Guwahati 781028, Assam, India
e-mail: kasturibhattacharjee44@hotmail.com; drmanu83@gmail.com

H. Bhattacharjee
Comprehensive Ophthalmology, Sri Sankaradeva Nethralaya, Guwahati 781028, Assam, India
e-mail: drharshabhattacharjee@gmail.com

D. Dey, MBBS, DO
Orbit, Ophthalmic Plastic and Reconstructive Surgery, Sankara Nethralaya Kolkata, Kolkata 700099, West Bengal, India
e-mail: debleena82@gmail.com


B. Mukherjee, H. Yuen (eds.), *Emergencies of the Orbit and Adnexa*,
DOI 10.1007/978-81-322-1807-4_4

## Pathomechanism

The globe lies within a pyramid-shaped bony orbital cavity which is held in its position by the extraocular muscles, fascial sheaths, orbital fat volume and eyelid ligaments. These are externally well supported by bony orbital walls and act as a padded support which absorbs and dissipates the blunt trauma force. Hence, a force causing bony orbital wall fracture generally does not cause eyeball injury. If the fracture is large enough and the force to the globe is also significant, the subluxation of the globe into the maxillary sinus, ethmoidal sinus (see Fig. 4.3a, b) and cranial cavity can be seen [5–8].

*Traumatic* – Various types of mechanical injuries (major or minor) have been reported leading to globe subluxation, majority being motor vehicle accidents, finger poking, sports related (basketball, golf, snooker, swimming, cricket, etc.), kicked by animals and fall from height. The severity of impact and the direction of force contribute significantly in the pathomechanism of globe subluxation. The proximity of spacious bony cavities like maxillary and ethmoidal sinuses provides enough room for the orbital soft tissue to migrate into these through the fractured portions of the inferior and medial wall, respectively [5–13]. The different mechanisms proposed are mentioned in Fig. 4.4. Acute- and

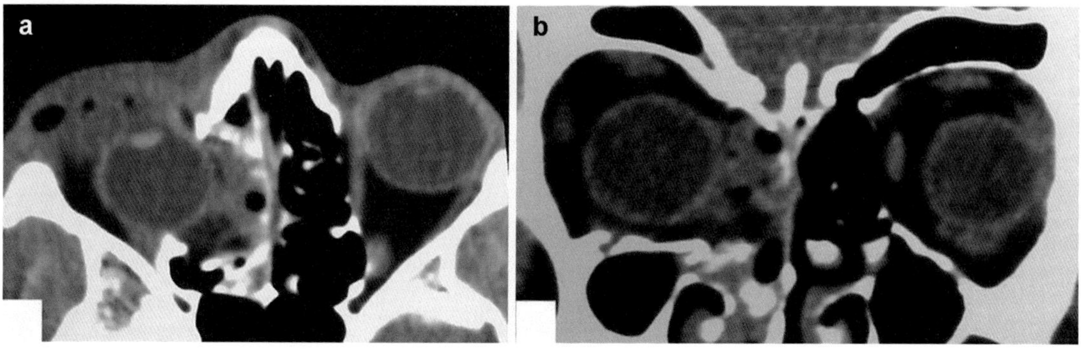


**Fig. 4.3** (**a**, **b**) (Axial and coronal views) Right globe subluxation into ethmoidal sinus cavities after road traffic accident, associated soft tissue hyperdensity and hypodensity reveals oedema and emphysema

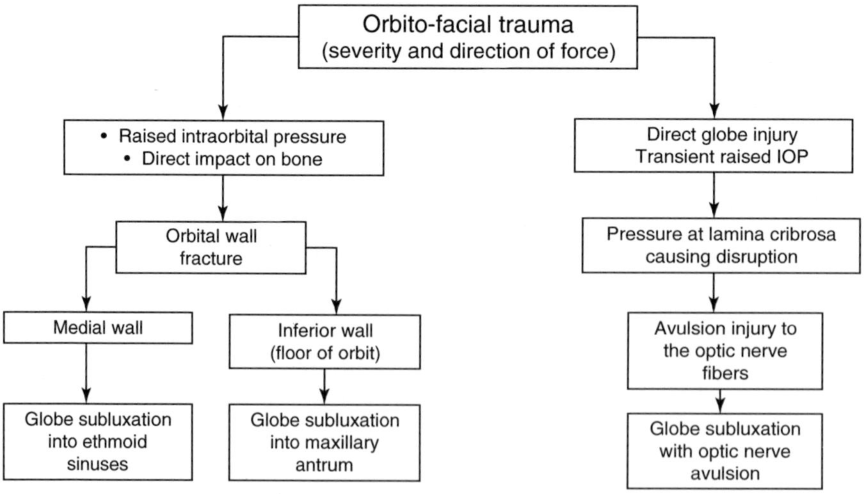


**Fig. 4.4** Orbito-facial trauma flowchart

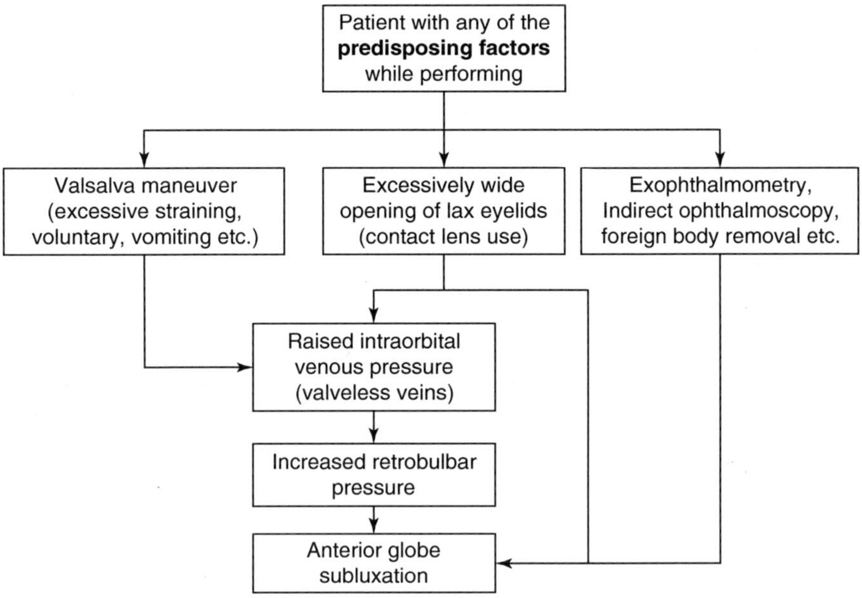


**Fig. 4.5** Pathomechanisms of globe subluxation

severe-forced medial rotation of the globe may also tear the optic nerve from the posterior sclera, causing the globe to luxate [14].

Morris et al. described three mechanisms of optic nerve injury leading to globe evulsion out of the orbital cavity. Firstly, total severance of optic nerve and its sheath due to *direct* sharp-edged object induced laceration. Secondly, *wedge effect* causing anterior push of the globe against lateral wall with stretch laceration of the optic nerve and its sheath. Thirdly, a *lever and fulcrum effect* can be caused by the object entering medially and as anterior nasal bone acting the fulcrum, anterior push by vector force, thus totally disrupting the optic nerve [15].

Besides trauma, globe subluxation can occur by voluntary effort, spontaneously or by self-mutilation. The pathomechanisms are described in Fig. 4.5. Spontaneous globe luxation has been reported in association with contact lens use, general anaesthesia, congenital craniofacial malformations, chronic obstructive pulmonary disease and thyroid-associated orbitopathy [16–18]. Rare cases have been reported in patients with histiocytosis X and Engelmann's disease [19, 20] (Fig. 4.6).

**Special risk factors in TAO:**

1. Increased retrobulbar fat volume
2. Raised retrobulbar venous pressure
3. Compliance of extraocular muscles
4. Upper and lower eyelid retraction
5. Stretched eyelids and tarsal plates
6. Africo-americans with shallow orbit and lax ligaments, cigarette smoking and high myopia

**Fig. 4.6** Special risk factors in TAO

Partial or total globe luxation can occur following auto-enucleation of the globe in functional psychosis like chronic psychotic depression and schizophrenia exhibiting clear paranoid traits. Historically, it has been linked to a method to achieve salvation after committing adultery. Though in general such self-mutilation is unilateral, bilateral self-enucleation has been reported up to 39 % without any gender preponderance. Patients abusing hallucinogenic drugs are also prone for inflicting such injuries to them [21].

## Clinical Features

Globe subluxation has variable presentations from being completely asymptomatic to total loss of vision which could be sudden and permanent, sudden with gradual partial recovery or chronic and progressive vision loss. In patients of traumatic globe subluxation, apart from a thorough ocular examination, orbital and surrounding area should be carefully examined for periocular emphysema and orbital rim defect. Both of these signs suggest medial or inferior orbital wall fracture. Important external signs include eyelid oedema, ecchymosis, conjunctival chemosis/haemorrhage, gross proptosis or severe enophthalmos (see Fig. 4.7). Restricted ocular motility and diplopia can also be associated with the latter. On fundus examination, an absent optic disc, scleral excavation at the optic disc site and circumferential retinal haemorrhages suggest an optic nerve avulsion injury, which is a very rare phenomenon [22, 23].

Severely reduced visual acuity, absent direct pupillary reaction, defective colour vision and abnormal confrontation suggest optic nerve injury attributing to poor prognosis. Floppy eyelids, corneal superficial punctate keratitis, corneal opacity, Descemet's folds and corneal oedema favour voluntary or routine spontaneous globe luxation [24–26]. In psychiatric patients, we should examine for multiple irregular cut injuries in periorbital region, wrists, arms and legs. The abnormal status of nails and hairs can provide a hint about patient's mental condition.

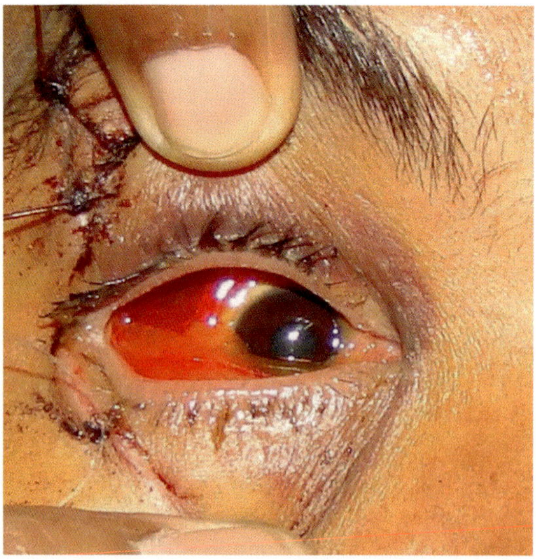

**Fig. 4.7** Clinical picture of the patient with globe subluxation into ethmoidal sinus with severe enophthalmos and soft tissue features

## Investigations

Radiological investigations have a limited role in the atraumatic group [27]. Thyroid function tests or sleep study should be advised in suspected patients. Computerised tomography (CT) highlights the status of bony orbital cavity and surrounding paranasal sinuses in relation to globe, while magnetic resonance imaging (MRI) better defines extraocular muscles, optic nerve (avulsion or laceration) and surrounding soft tissue. Other coexisting intraorbital pathologies, exact dimensions of bony fractures and foreign bodies can be quantitatively analysed on CT scan by adequate axial, coronal and saggital cuts which helps the surgeon to confirm the diagnosis, plan the treatment (conservative or surgery) and prognosticate the case. Imaging of the brain is vital in all trauma patients [18]. Photographic documentation is vital for records and medicolegal purpose and postoperative comparison.

## Treatment

Any globe subluxation should be managed as an emergency. The initial systemic assessment should be conducted for all patients to evaluate the adequacy of cardiovascular, nervous and respiratory system. In triage, the neurosurgical management remains supreme while handling the patients with severe craniofacial trauma. Combined surgery in a multi-speciality set-up should be planned for safer pre- and postoperative patient care [27–29] (Fig. 4.8).

In patients with globe subluxation, immediate repositioning of the globe back into the orbit is of paramount importance to alleviate patient's anxiety and pain and to prevent permanent vision loss due to corneal and optic nerve compromise (see Fig. 4.9a, b). Eyeball can be repositioned digitally as an office procedure, taking the points mentioned in the box into consideration. David Tse described his technique without anaesthesia in which the upper eyelid is pinched and pulled away from the globe while the patient is looking down. This simultaneously is accompanied by depression of the globe from scleral surface with the index finger of the other hand, and as soon as the equator passes beyond the eyelid, the patient is asked to look up, and the eyelid is positioned over the cornea [30].

The Desmarres retractor, bent paper clip or a tissue forceps can be used for the holding and retracting manoeuvre. Lateral tarsorrhaphy is thought to increase the intraorbital pressure leading to increased risk of luxation and hence should be avoided. The narrowed palpebral aperture further complicates the subsequent repositioning of the eyeball in recurrence [31].

The surgical management of globe subluxation into sinus cavities presents a significant challenge to most orbital surgeons. The surgery demands knowledge of orbital and paranasal sinus anatomy, orbital fat decompression and eyelid retraction management. The choice of surgical procedure is dictated by the severity and extent of globe displacement along with the condition of adnexal tissue. Patient needs to be hospitalised, and intravenous corticosteroids should be administered to minimise the sequelae of optic nerve injury. Prophylactic antibiotics can be given in a setting of old and infected laceration.

**POINTS FOR MANAGING GLOBE SUBLUXATION:**

1. Counsel the patient before globe reposition
2. Anesthetise the cornea with topical drops (relaxes the efferentarm of reflex causing orbicularis spasm)
3. Facial nerve regional block can provide orbicularis and facial relaxation
4. General anesthesia (for children, highly anxious and psychiatric patients)
5. Tse's maneuver

**Fig. 4.8** Points for managing globe subluxation

Open reduction and internal fixation of the periorbital bones and support for wall fractures are vital to achieve desirable results. This is done after reposting the globe and soft tissue via transorbital or transantral route. Most authors have suggested resurgery for the lost extraocular muscle within 7–10 days to avoid the muscle contracture [31].

Rarely, when the globe gets dislocated into maxillary or ethmoidal sinuses, utmost care should be taken while performing diligent manipulations to recover the globe as the scleral coats might be firmly stuck into the bony fractured edges of the orbital wall. This might lead to scleral perforation demanding a gentle pushing and pulling manoeuvre of the sinus and orbit, respectively. Our ENT colleagues can become vital as they can reach the sinus cavities without causing further iatrogenic trauma.

Reposting a traumatically evulsed globe into the orbit can provide a good psychological and cosmetic satisfaction to the patient even if the

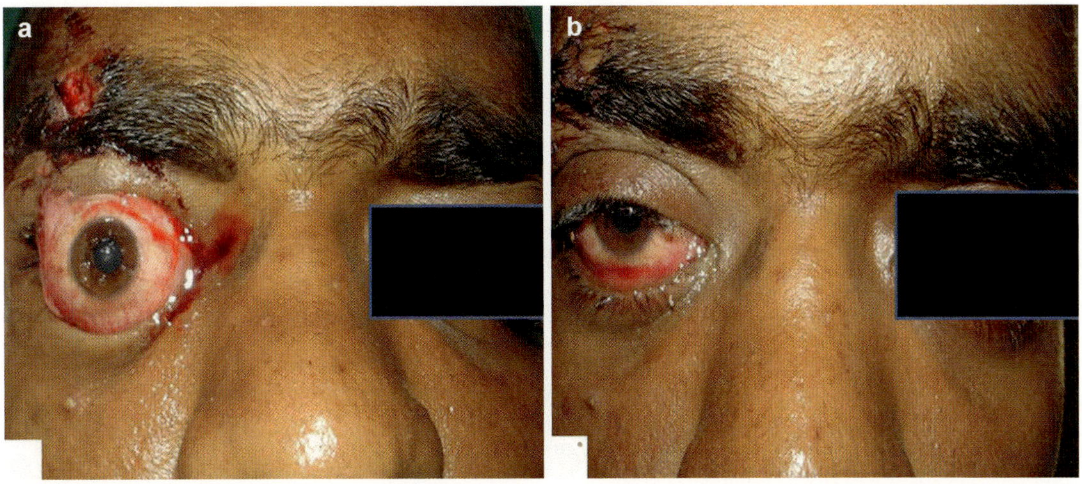


**Fig. 4.9** (**a**, **b**) Manual repositioning of the globe in a patient with anterior subluxation after road traffic accident (Courtesy of Dr. B L Sujatha Rathod, Dr. Preeti Sharma and Dr. Kumar Ravi of Minto Ophthalmic Institute, Regional Institute of Ophthalmology, Bangalore)

function is lost [32, 33]. Gupta et al. had reported definite advantage of timely globe repositioning without delay over primary enucleation in terms of organ preservation and better fitting of ocular prosthesis [34].

## Prevention

Proper counselling has an immense role to relax an anxious patient who presented with globe subluxation for the first time. The best method to prevent voluntary globe subluxation is to provide good psychiatric counselling and adequate treatment. In the patients presenting with spontaneous globe luxation, the predisposing factors should be addressed, and the patients can be educated and trained for self-globe reposition in case it occurs at home or work.

## Summary

Although the diagnosis of globe subluxation is not difficult, its exact position in a traumatic case needs proper imaging evaluation. Spontaneous globe luxation can be managed conservatively with good results; however there is paucity of literature regarding the surgical management of globe subluxation. Expertise in the management of polytrauma cases as well as evolving techniques in the field of facio-maxillary and neurosurgery allows better outcome in traumatic cases. Any form of globe subluxation is an emergency and should be treated accordingly to preserve vision and salvage the globe.

## References


1. Tucker B. Two cases of dislocation of the eyeball through the palpebral fissure. J Nerv Ment Dis. 1907;34(1):391–7.
2. Dorland's Illustrated Medical Dictionary. 28th ed. Philadelphia: WB Saunders; 1994. p. 589.
3. Dorland's Illustrated Medical Dictionary. 28th ed. Philadelphia: WB Saunders; 1994. p. 166.
4. Chhabra HN, Kawuma AMS. Luxation of the eyeball. Br J Ophthalmol. 1986;70(2):150–1.
5. Pelton RW, Rainey AM, Lee AG. Traumatic subluxation of the globe into the maxillary sinus. Am J Neuroradiol. 1998;19(8):1450–1.
6. Abrishami M, Aletaha M, Bagheri A, et al. Traumatic subluxation of the globe into the maxillary sinus. Ophthal Plast Reconstr Surg. 2007;23(2):156–8.
7. Ramstead C, McCabe J, Alkahtani M, et al. Traumatic dislocation of the globe into the maxillary sinus. Can J Ophthalmol. 2008;43(3):364–6.
8. Janfaza P. Surgical anatomy of the head and neck. New York: Lippincott Williams & Wilkins; 2001.
9. Haggerty CJ, Roman P. Repositioning of a traumatically displaced globe with maxillary antrostomy: review of the literature and treatment recommendations. J Oral Maxillofac Surg. 2013;71(11):1915–22.
10. Risco JM, Stratas BA, Knott RH. Prolapse of the globe into the ethmoid sinus. Am J Ophthalmol. 1984;97(5):659–60.
11. Tranfa F, Di Matteo G, Di Salle F, et al. Traumatic displacement of the globe into the ethmoid sinus. Am J Ophthalmol. 2000;130(2):253–4.
12. Nezami N, Sadighi A, Rahimi-Ardabili B. Magnetic resonance imaging of intact globe superior subluxation into the intracranium. Indian J Ophthalmol. 2012;60(1):69–70.
13. Shimia M, Sayyahmelli S. Traumatic displacement of the globe into brain. RMJ. 2009;34(2):234–5.
14. Kiratli H, Tümer B, Bilgic S. Management of traumatic luxation of the globe. A case report. Acta Ophthalmol Scand. 1999;77(3):340–2.
15. Morris WR, Osborn FD, Fleming JC. Traumatic evulsion of the globe. Ophthal Plast Reconstr Surg. 2002;18(4):261–7.
16. Kunesh JC, Katz SE. Spontaneous globe luxation associated with contact lens placement. CLAO J. 2002;28(1):2–4.
17. Kumar MA, Srikanth K, Pandurangan R. Spontaneous globe luxation associated with chronic obstructive pulmonary disease. Indian J Ophthalmol. 2012;60(4): 324–5.
18. Rubin PAD, Watkins LM, Rumelt S, et al. Orbital computed tomographic characteristics of globe subluxation in thyroid orbitopathy. Ophthalmology. 1998;105(11):2061–4.
19. Wood CM, Pearson AD, Craft AW, Howe JW. Globe luxation in histiocytosis X. Br J Ophthalmol. 1988;72(8): 631–3.
20. Brodrick JD. Luxation of the globe in Engelmann's disease. Am J Ophthalmol. 1977;83(6):870–3.
21. Krauss HR, Yee RD, Foos RY. Autoenucleation. Surv Ophthalmol. 1984;29(3):179–87.
22. Albert DM, Jakobiec FA. Principles and practice of ophthalmology, clinical practice. Vol. 5. Philadelphia: W. B. Saunders; 1994. p. 3359.
23. Duke–Elder S. System of ophthalmology, vol. 13. London: Henry Kimpton; 1974. p. 1233–4.
24. Alexandrakis G, Tse DT, Chang WJ, Fla M. Spontaneous globe luxation associated with floppy eyelid syndrome and shallow orbits. Arch Ophthalmol. 1999;117(1):138–9.
25. Clendenen SR, Kostick DA. Ocular globe luxation under general anaesthesia. Anesth Analg. 2008; 107(5):1630–1.

26. Apostolopoulos M, Papaspirou A, Damanakis A, et al. Bilateral optic neuropathy associated with voluntary globe subluxation and floppy eyelid syndrome. Arch Ophthalmol. 2004;122(10):1555–6.
27. Lyle DJ, McGavic JS. The cause of voluntary forward luxation of the eyeball. A case report with anatomical findings at necropsy. Am J Ophthalmol. 1936;19(1):316–20.
28. Offenbach B. Dislocation (luxation) of the eyeball. N Engl J Med. 1954;251(9):338–9.
29. Carlson RE, Scheribel KW, Hering PJ, Wolin L. Exophthalmos, global luxation, rapid weight gain: differential diagnosis. Ann Ophthalmol. 1982;14(8):724–9.
30. Tse DT. A simple maneuver to reposit a subluxed globe. Arch Ophthalmol. 2000;118(3):410–1.
31. Kelly EW, Fitch MT. Recurrent spontaneous globe subluxation: a case report and review of manual reduction techniques. J Emerg Med. 2013;44(1):17–20.
32. Song A, Carter KD. Bilateral traumatic globe subluxation. Ophthal Plast Reconstr Surg. 2006;22(2):136–7.
33. Srinivasan S, Gaskell A, McWhinnie H, et al. Conservative management of globe luxation with congenital orbital venous anomaly. J Pediatr Opthalmol Strabismus. 2003;40(3):170–1.
34. Gupta RC, Gupta P. Complete globe protrusion post trauma: a case report. J Dent Med Sci. 2013;6(5):28–9.

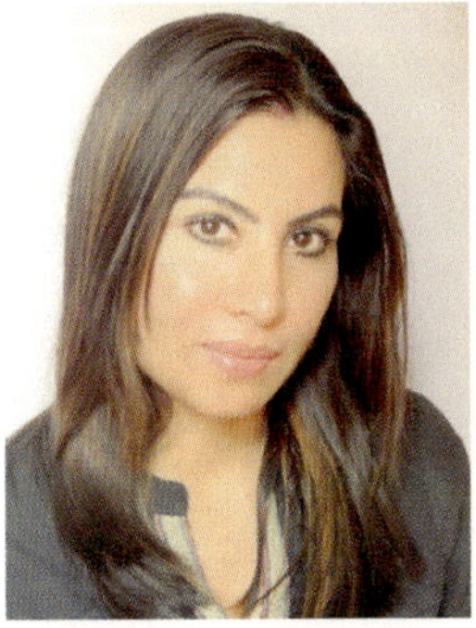

**Kasturi Bhattacharjee** Dr. (Mrs) Kasturi Bhattacharjee, MS, DNB, FRCS is the Head, Deptt. of Orbit, Ophthalmic Plastic & Reconstructive Surgery and Cataract & Refractive Surgery at Sri Sankaradeva Nethralaya, India. She is the recipient of more than 23 awards for her work in Ophthalmology and has more than 47 publications in National and International journals.

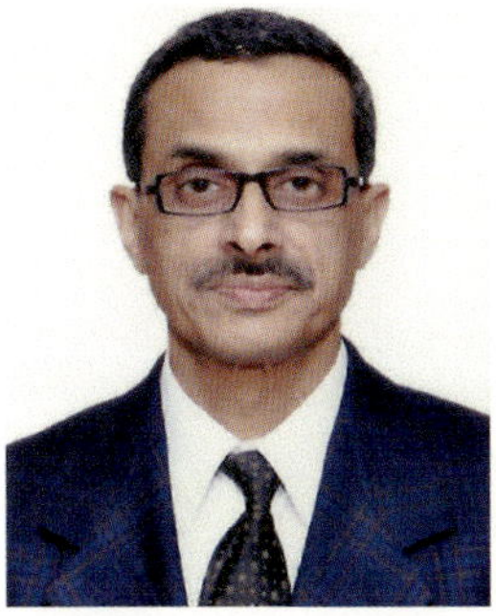

**Harsha Bhattacharjee** Dr. Harsha Bhattacharjee MS, FRCP is the founder Medical Director and trustee of Sri Sankaradeva Nethralaya, Guwahati, India. He has numerous publications in indexed journals and has trained more than 80 fellows. He is a post graduate examiner in Ophthalmology for national and international colleges.

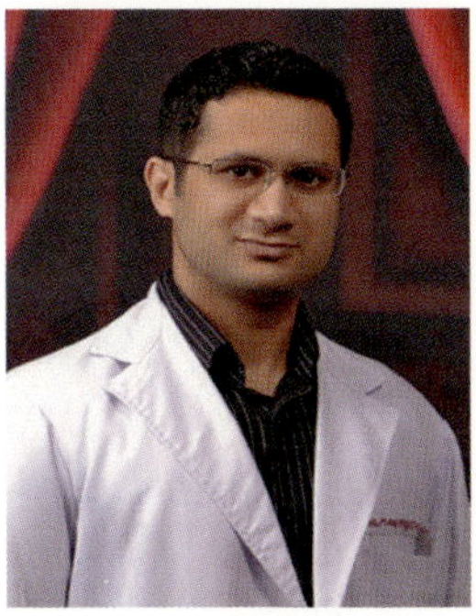

**Manpreet Singh** Dr. Manpreet Singh, MS, DNB, FAICO (Oculoplastic Surgery), is working as an Ophthalmic Plastic Surgeon in Chandigarh, India. He has published 20 National and International papers and has been active in academics and research. His special interests are Dacryology and Oculofacial aesthetics.

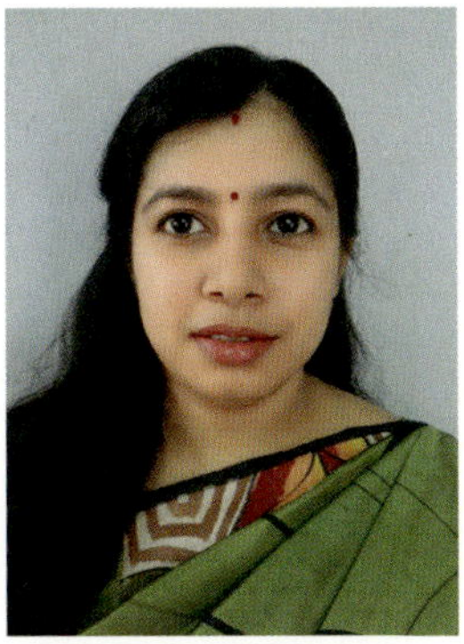

**Debleena Dey** Dr. Debleena Dey, MBBS, DO is working as an Ophthalmic Plastic Surgeon in Kolkata, India.

# 5 Exposure Keratopathy Due to Absent or Avulsed Eyelids

Hernawita Soeharko and Darmayanti Siswoyo

## Introduction

Eyelid avulsion is an injury in which the eyelid is forcibly detached from its natural position caused by trauma such as motor vehicle collisions, animal bites, and human bites. It can occur with or without eyelid tissue loss (Fig. 5.1a–c). Both of those conditions can lead to lacrimal pump disorders and corneal exposure with all of the consequences ranging from dryness of the cornea, exposure keratopathy, and ending with corneal perforation if not treated properly. Because the primary function of the eyelid is to protect the eyeball from the outside and because it is also an important part of the tear pump mechanism, surgical repair is required to manage eyelid avulsion and prevent exposure keratopathy. Exposure keratopathy due to avulsed/absent lids should be managed medically (see Chap. 29 "Management of Severe Exposure Keratopathy"); then as soon as possible, the avulsed/ absent lid should be repaired surgically to restore eyelid function. It is important to know about the basic rules of eyelid repair so that both cosmetic appearance and physiological function can be preserved [1, 2].

H. Soeharko
Oculoplastic & Eye Reconstructive Surgery, Jakarta-Eye-Center, Jakarta 10310, Indonesia

Eye Department, Cipto Mangunkusumo – Kirana Hospital, Jakarta 10310, Indonesia
e-mail: hernawita@jec.co.id; hernawita_suharko@yahoo.com

D. Siswoyo (✉)
Oculoplastic & Eye Reconstructive Surgery, Jakarta-Eye-Center, Jakarta 10310, Indonesia
e-mail: darmayanti_spm@yahoo.com; yanti@jec.co.id

## Treatment

### Timing of Repair

Although optimum repair for eyelid injuries is within 24 h after their occurrence, these injuries can easily be repaired up to several days later.

But the best time to repair eyelid avulsion is as soon as possible, especially if eyelid avulsion is accompanied by tissue loss and resulting corneal exposure. In order to get the best result, the surgery should be done by an oculoplastic surgeon [3, 4].

### Anesthesia

Eyelid avulsion can be repaired under local anesthesia. However, eyelid avulsion with tissue loss, which needs considerable time for reconstruction, should preferably be repaired under general anesthesia [4].


B. Mukherjee, H. Yuen (eds.), *Emergencies of the Orbit and Adnexa*,
DOI 10.1007/978-81-322-1807-4_5

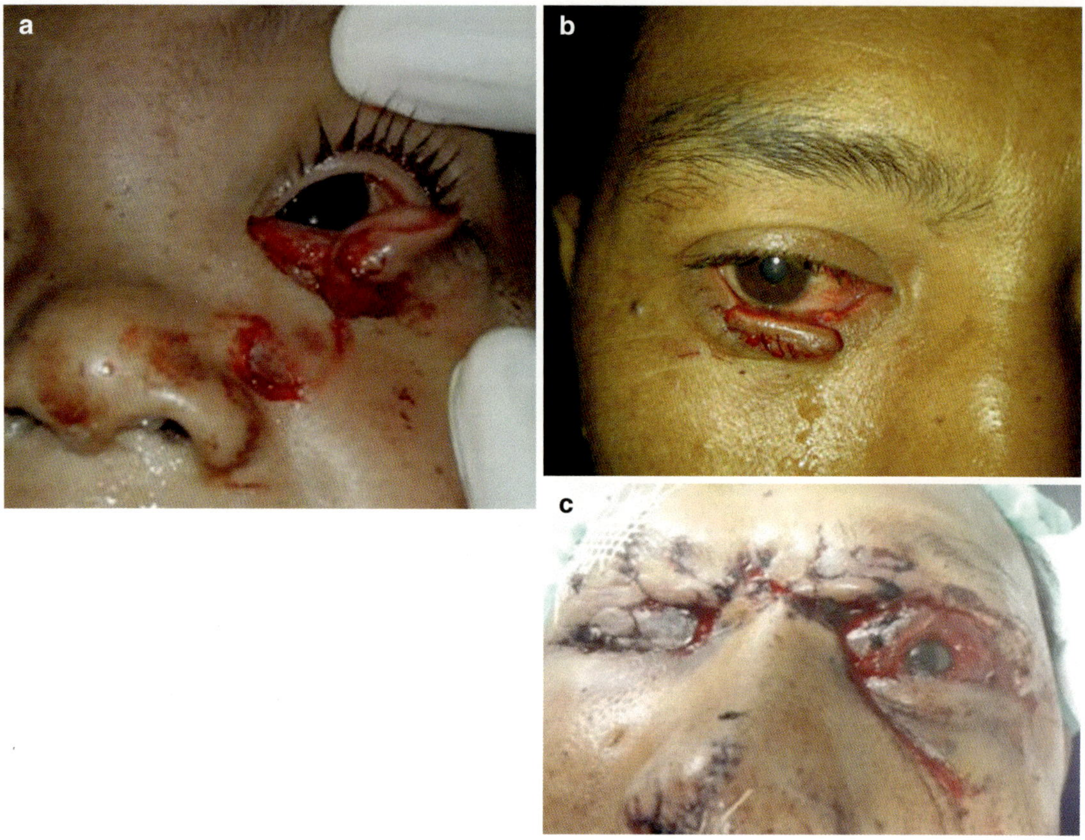

**Fig. 5.1** (**a**) Eyelid avulsion without tissue loss. (**b**) Eyelid avulsion without tissue loss. (**c**) Eyelid avulsion with tissue loss (part of superior eyelid)

## Treatment in Emergency Room

- Wound debridement.
- Toxoid/tetanus injection.
- Systemic antibiotic (oral or intravenous).
- Saline-moistened dressing should be placed over eyelid laceration/avulsion if there will be a delay between evaluation and surgical intervention [4].

## Surgical Technique

1. Eyelid avulsion without tissue loss (Fig. 5.2a, b):

   We can suture the wound directly layer by layer with the first step, repair of the lid margin with suture at the grayline, tarsus, orbicularis muscle, and skin. We use Vicryl 6-0 for the tarsus and orbicularis muscle and Prolene 6-0 for the grayline and skin [1, 2, 5].
2. Eyelid avulsion with tissue loss:

   It depends upon the degree and location of the defect.

   Degree of the defect are classified by size (small if the defect is <25 %, moderate if defect is 25–50 %, and large if the defect is >50 %). Small defects are amenable to direct closure, while moderate and large ones require flap advancement (Tenzel procedure), reconstruction with graft, and sometimes lid sharing procedure [2, 5].

1. Small eyelid defect (defect <25 %) → direct closure technique (Fig. 5.3):

   In the first step, we repair the lid margin with a suture through the grayline of the eyelid margin using Prolene 6-0 followed by suture of the tarsus, conjunctiva, orbicularis muscle using Vicryl 6-0, and suture of the skin using Prolene 6-0 [4–7].
2. Moderate eyelid defect (defect 25–50 %) → Tenzel procedure (Fig. 5.4):

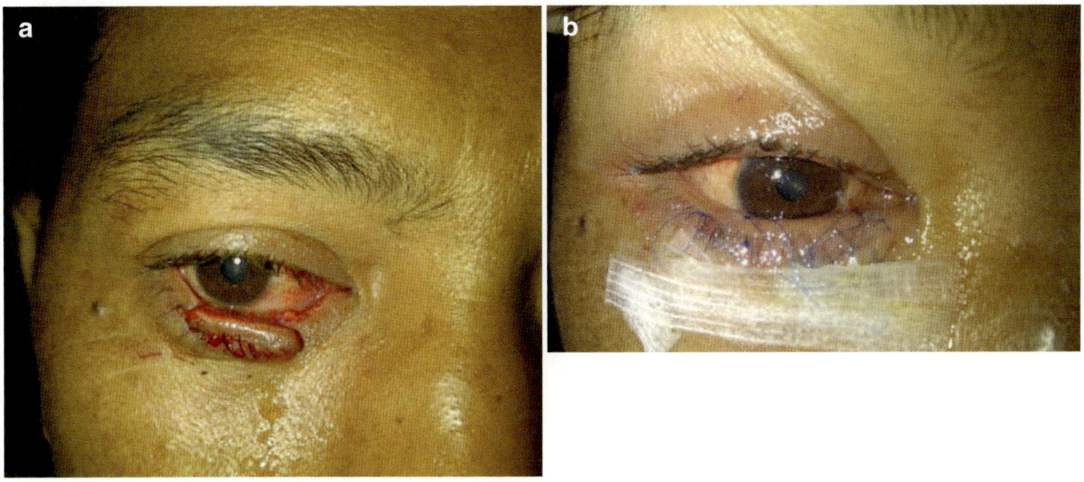


**Fig. 5.2** (**a**) Eyelid avulsion without tissue loss: preop. (**b**) Eyelid avulsion without tissue loss: postop

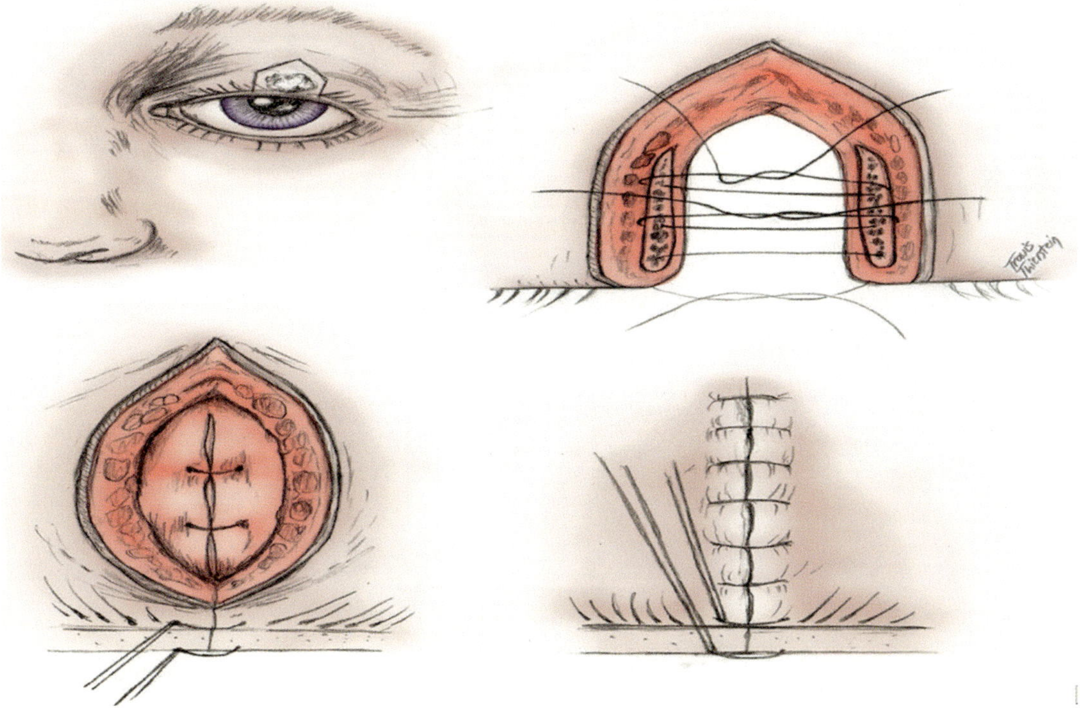

**Fig. 5.3** Schematic of direct closure technique

The first step is to make semicircular incision, lateral canthotomy and cantholysis. Closure of the eyelid margin followed by lateral canthoplasty and closure of the skin [4–7].

3. Large eyelid defect (defect >50 %) (Fig. 5.5a):

   Large eyelid defect >50 % of the eyelid width can be closed using skin flap (temporal or glabellar flap) combined with posterior lamellar graft (oral mucous graft), rotation cheek flap (Mustarde) combined with posterior lamellar graft, or lid sharing (Hughes procedure or Cutler-Beard procedure).

   Temporal/glabellar flap combined with oral mucous graft (Figs. 5.5b, c and 5.6):

   The first step is to take oral mucous graft and place into the eyelid defect, suture to the rest of the conjunctiva, and cover the graft with temporal flap/glabellar flap [4–7].

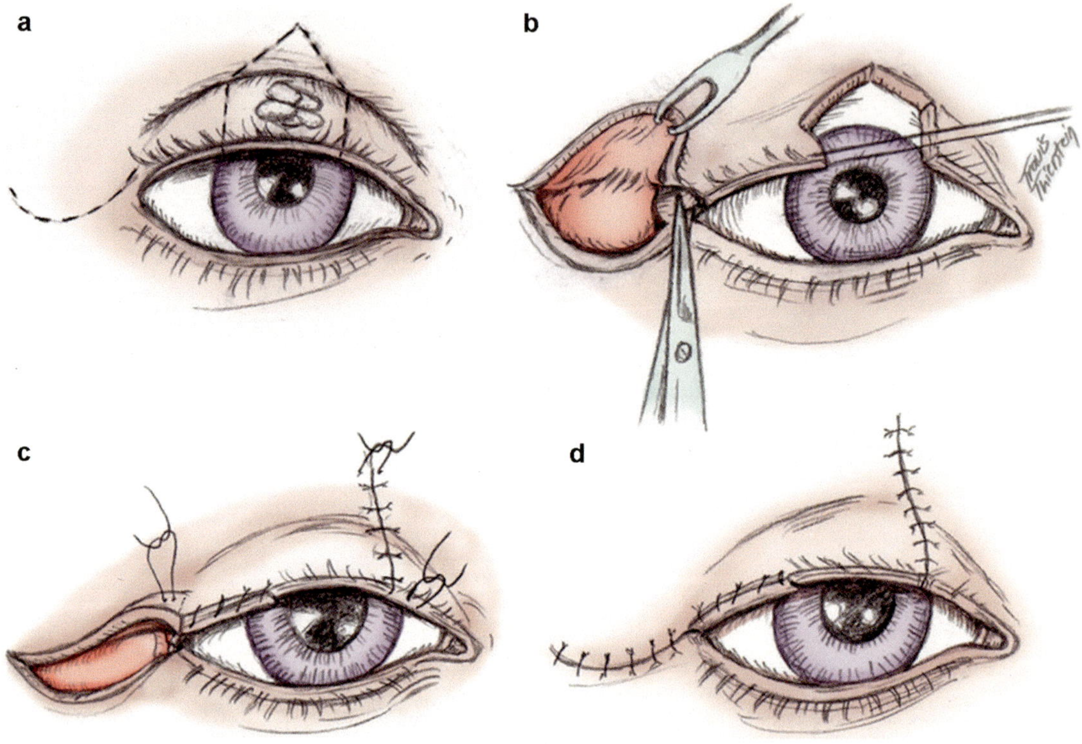


**Fig. 5.4** Schematic of semicircular flap technique (Tenzel procedure)

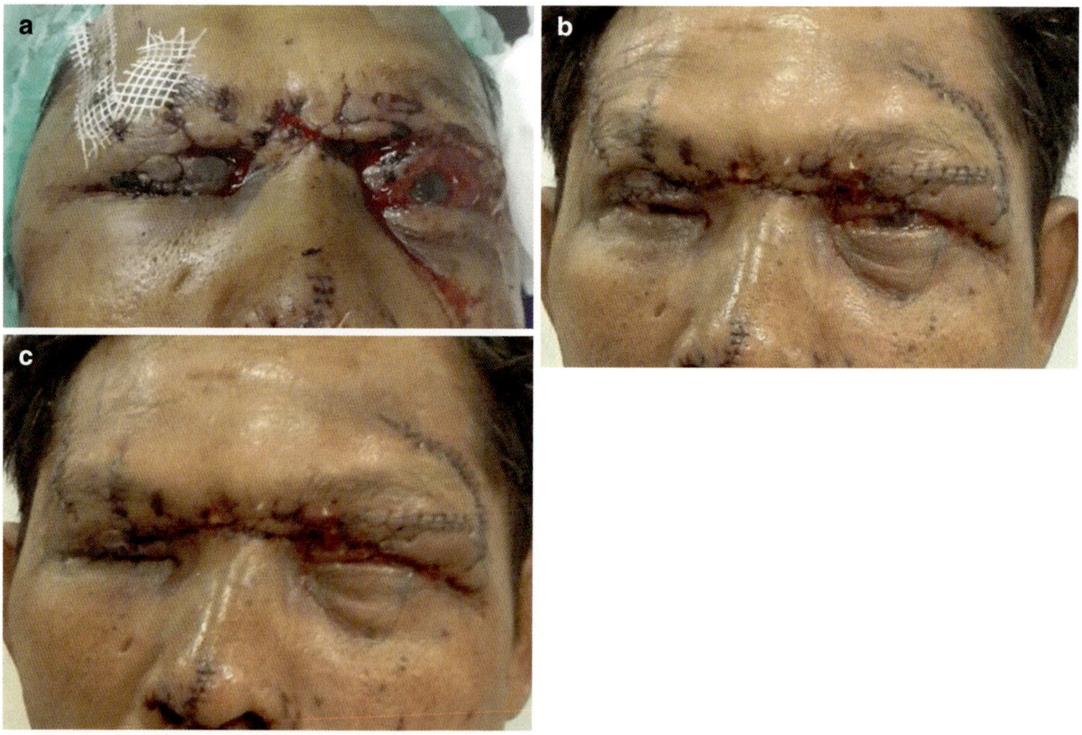


**Fig. 5.5** (**a**) Preoperative picture of eyelid avulsion with superior eyelid defect >50%. (**b**) Postoperative picture with temporal skin flap combined with oral mucosal graft technique. (**c**) Postoperative picture with temporal skin flap combined with oral mucosal graft technique

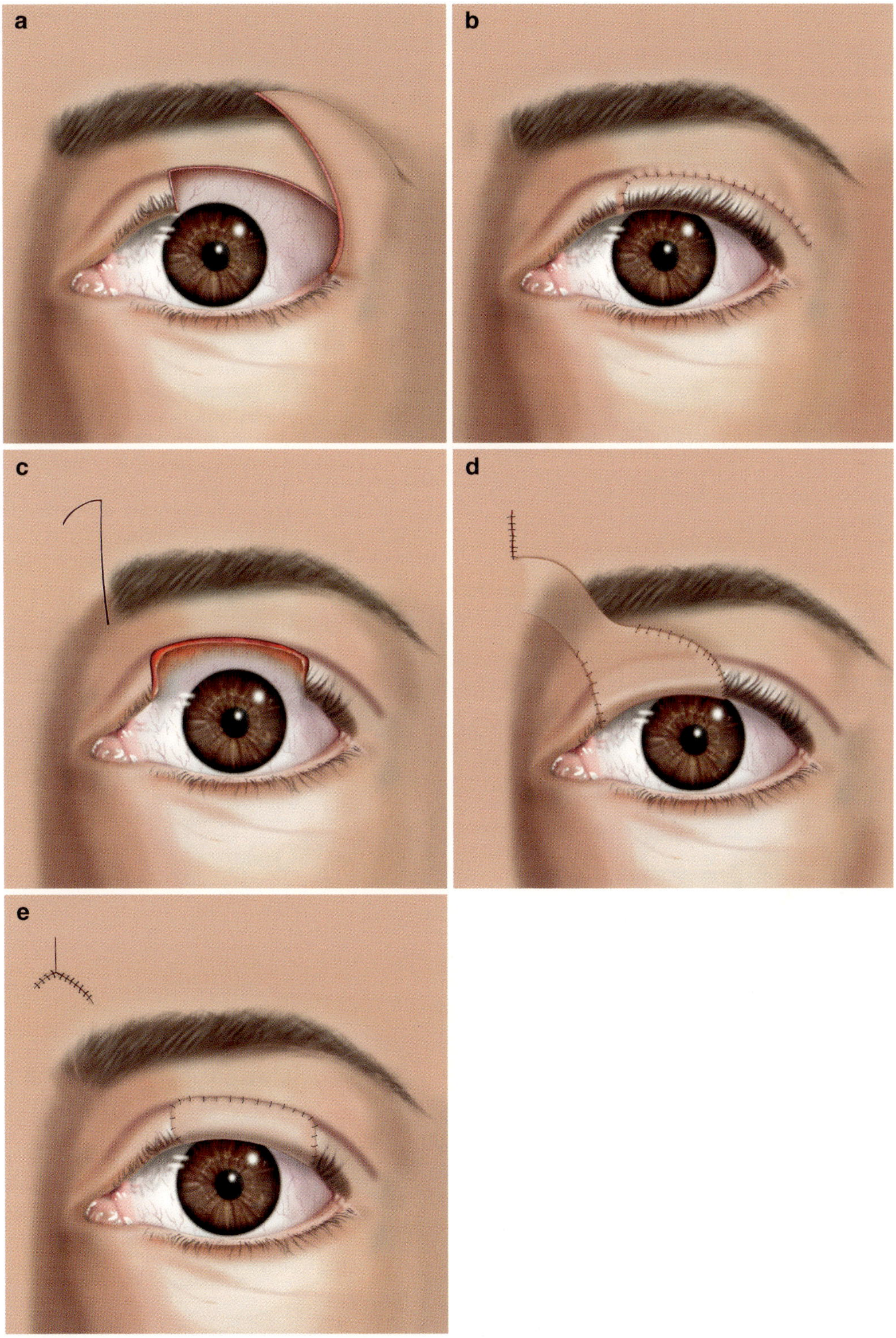


**Fig. 5.6** (**a**) Schematic of temporal flap combined with oral mucosal graft technique, step 1. (**b**) Schematic of temporal flap combined with oral mucosal graft technique, step 2. (**c**) Schematic of glabellar flap combined with oral mucosal graft technique, step 1. (**d**) Schematic of glabellar flap combined with oral mucosal graft technique, step 2. (**e**) Schematic of glabellar flap combined with oral mucosal graft technique, step 3

## References


1. Suryadevara AC, Moe KS. Reconstruction of eyelid defects. Facial Plast Surg Clin N Am. 2009;17:419–28.
2. Herford AS, Cicciu M, Clark A. Traumatic eyelid defects: a review of reconstructive options. J Oral Maxillofac Surg. 2009;67:3–9.
3. Nelson CC. Review: management of eyelid trauma. Aust N Z J Ophthalmol. 1991;19(4):357–63.
4. Miyamoto J, Nakajima T, Nagasao T, Konno E, Okabe K, et al. Full-thickness reconstruction of the eyelid with rotation flap based on orbicularis oculi muscle and palatal mucosal graft: long term results in 12 cases. J Plast Reconstr Aesthet Surg. 2009;62:1389–94.
5. Karesh JW. The evaluation and management of eyelid trauma. In: Tasman W, Jaeger EA, editors. Duane's ophthalmology. Philadelphia: Lippincott William Wilkins; 2012. p. 23–32.
6. Thornton JF, Kenkel JM. Eyelid reconstruction. In: Thornton JF, Kenkel JM, editors. Selected readings in plastic surgery. Dallas: Southwestern Medical Center; 2005. p. 1–23. 10(8).
7. Rubin PAD, Shore JW. Penetrating eyelid and orbital trauma. In: Albert DM, Jakobiec FA, editors. Principles and practice of ophthalmology. Philadelphia: WB Saunders; 1994. p. 3426–40.


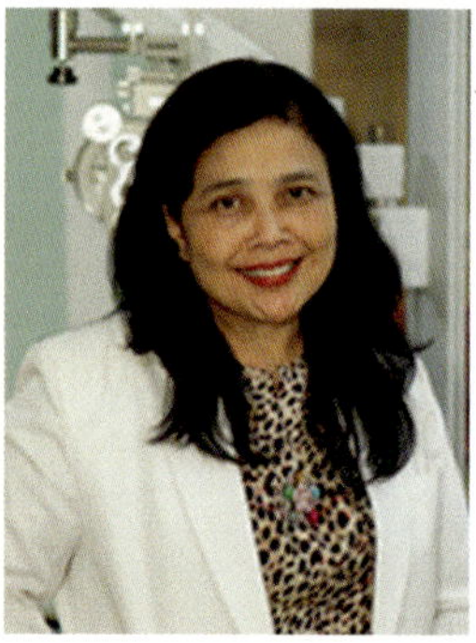

**Hernawita Soeharko** Dr. Hernawita Soeharko is currently Consultant of Ophthalmic Plastic & Reconstructive Surgery, Jakarta Eye Center Hospital, Indonesia.

She is currently Head of Ophthalmic Plastic & Reconstructive Surgery Division, Department of Ophthalmology, Faculty of Medicine, University of Indonesia (2006–now).

She is the past Head of Indonesian Ophthalmic Plastic & Reconstructive Surgery & Eye Tumor Surgery Association.

She graduated from the Department of Ophthalmology University of Indonesia in 1994.

She studied oculoplastic and reconstructive surgery at Moorefield Eye Hospital, London in 1995.

She is also contributed in various International and National Ophthalmology meetings as participant, speaker as well as instructor in oculoplastic courses.

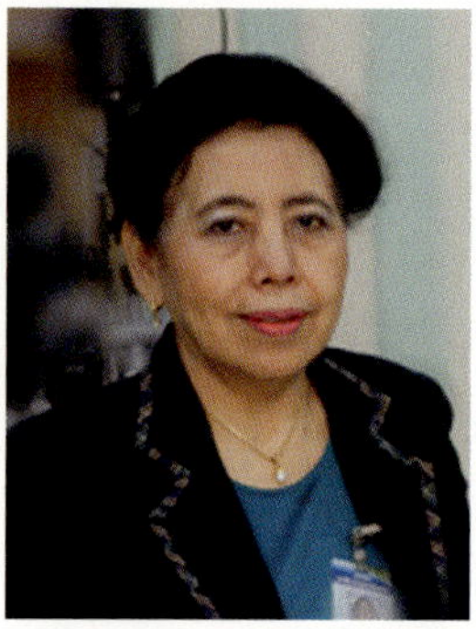

**Darmayanti Siswoyo** Dr. Darmayanti Siswoyo is currently consultant of Ophthalmic Plastic & Reconstructive Surgery, Jakarta Eye Center Hospital, Indonesia.

She is the past Head of Ophthalmic Plastic & Reconstructive Surgery Division, Department of Ophthalmology, Faculty of Medicine, University of Indonesia.

She is also the past Head of Indonesian Ophthalmic Plastic & Reconstructive & Eye Tumor Surgery Association. She graduated from Department of Ophthalmology University of Indonesia in 1987.

She underwent orbital reconstruction training at Cranio Facial Center, Department of Plastic surgery, Royal Adelaide Hospital, South Australia in 1987.

She also underwent Oculoplastic & Reconstructive Surgery training at Department of Plastic Surgery, Kansai Medical Faculty and Department of Ophthalmology, Hamamatsu Hospital, Japan in 1992.

She is a Observer at Moorfield Eye Hospital London, England, 1993.

She is also National Speaker, Didactic Course Instructor, Wet Lab Instructor in Oculoplastic and Reconstructive Surgery in Indonesia since 1988 and International Speaker in Oculoplastic & Reconstructive Surgery since 1996.

# Periocular and Adnexal Injuries Due to Animal Bites

6

Akshay Gopinathan Nair and Bipasha Mukherjee

Animal bite injuries to the face are seen in emergency rooms across the world. Mammalian bites account for nearly 10 % of patients who present with orofacial trauma. Animals commonly responsible for bites include dogs, cats, horses, rabbits, rats, and humans [1, 2]. Of these, dog bites constitute 60–80 % of all animal bite injuries and cat bites – 20–40 % [3]. Children are often the target of animal attacks, primarily due to their behavior, which may be perceived as provocative by animals and also their small stature, which makes them vulnerable and accessible. Facial injuries constitute nearly 10–15 % of all animal bite trauma, and children are involved in nearly half of them [2, 4]. It has been reported that children under the age of 4 years receive injuries to the head, face, and neck in 63 % of cases, whereas children who are over 4 years of age suffer extremity injuries 78 % of the time [5]. Since majority of animal bites are dog related and given the complexities of canine-related trauma, this chapter would focus largely on periocular dog bites. The principles of successfully managing periocular dog bites are thorough wound toilet, debridement, and subsequent reconstructive surgery. Concurrent immunization against rabies and adequate infection control too are equally important. Early management of complex periocular injuries usually guarantees satisfactory outcomes.

## Types of Injuries

Anecdotal evidence suggests that dogs preferentially attack the central face. This often results in trauma to the nose and eyelids. In addition to trauma to the globe, dog bites can present with a spectrum of periocular injuries such as lid abrasions, canthal avulsions, eyelid lacerations, canalicular tears, and trauma to extraocular muscles (Fig. 6.1). Fractures are relatively uncommon with one study reporting six cases of facial fractures associated with dog bites and reviewing ten other previously reported cases in literature [6].

## Treatment

It is important to obtain all relevant history to ascertain if the dog responsible for the bite was rabid or not, to check if the bite was provoked or

A.G. Nair, MBBS, DNB (✉)
Ophthalmic Plastic Surgery, L V Prasad Eye Institute, Hyderabad, Telangana 500034, India
e-mail: akshaygn@gmail.com

B. Mukherjee, MS, DNB(Ophthalmology), FICO
Orbit, Oculoplasty, Reconstructive & Aesthetic Services, Sankara Nethralaya, Chennai, Tamil Nadu 600006, India
e-mail: drbpm@snmail.org


B. Mukherjee, H. Yuen (eds.), *Emergencies of the Orbit and Adnexa*,
DOI 10.1007/978-81-322-1807-4_6

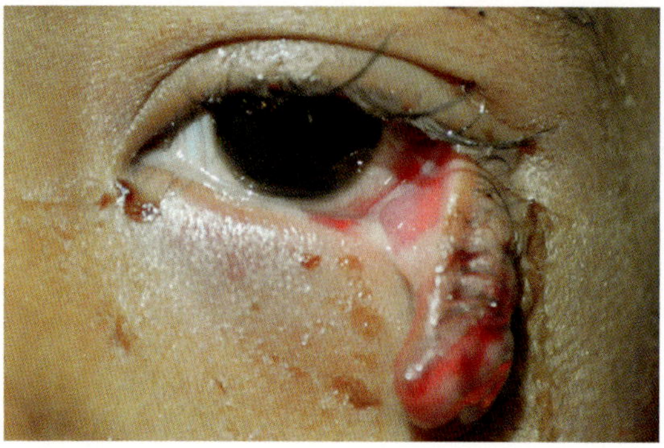

**Fig. 6.1** A 2-year-old male child who gave a history of a dog bite while playing with his pet dog, showing the most common form of eyelid trauma following dog bite. There is a lower lid avulsion with obvious canalicular trauma

unprovoked, to check if there were similar dog bites in the neighborhood on the same day or recent times involving the same dog.

The aims of treatment of such injuries can be broadly enlisted as:

- Adequate wound toilet to prevent wound infection
- Rabies prophylaxis
- Exploration and surgical reconstruction of normal anatomy with maximum restoration of function

## Primary Care

Facial bites are classified as category III dog bites which indicate single or multiple transdermal bites or scratches. This warrants both local treatment of the wound and complete postexposure prophylaxis measures including immunoglobulin and vaccination.

The initial management of any periocular animal bite-related trauma is thorough cleaning and debridement. The wound can be washed with soap and water, although ideally, a virucidal agent like povidone-iodine, if available, should be used. If required, this may be done under general anesthesia especially in smaller children. It is extremely important to debride the wound site of all devitalized tissue, remove all foreign bodies, and expose the surrounding healthy tissue [7]. The Center for Disease Control (CDC) guidelines recommend that 20 IU/kg of human rabies immunoglobulin (RIG) should be injected around the wound site after cleaning. Furthermore, any remaining RIG can be administered intramuscularly at an anatomical site distant from vaccine administration. Of particular importance is to ensure that while injecting RIG, it should not be administered in the same syringe as the vaccine. This is because there is a possibility that RIG might partially suppress the active production of antibody. Following this, human diploid cell rabies vaccine (HDCV) or purified chick embryo cell vaccine (PCECV) 1.0 mL intramuscularly, one each on days 0, 3, 7, and 14 should be administered [8]. Tetanus vaccine may also be given simultaneously after checking the patient's vaccination status.

Posttraumatic stress disorder following dog bites is a known phenomenon, especially in children [9]. Appropriate counseling should be provided in such cases.

## Surgical Management

Prior to any surgical treatment, it is a worthwhile clinical practice to routinely photograph the wound before and after cleaning [10]. Look for any associated trauma such as occult globe rupture, trauma to the canaliculi, levator muscle, and extraocular muscles and also for bony fractures [11]. There has been a controversy regarding primary closure of dog bite wounds. However, Ruifeng and colleagues reported that facial laceration of dog bite wounds should be primary closed immediately after formal and thorough debridement. Primary closure shortens the healing time of the wounds without increasing the rate of infection [7]. The eyelids are so well vascularized that the majority of these injuries may be primarily closed with superficial sutures (see Chap. 11).

Periocular dog bites have a propensity for involvement of the lacrimal canaliculus. In the largest series of periocular dog bites, 45 patients out of 68 (66 %) had canalicular involvement. Of these, 16 % involved only the superior canaliculus, whereas 73 % involved only the inferior

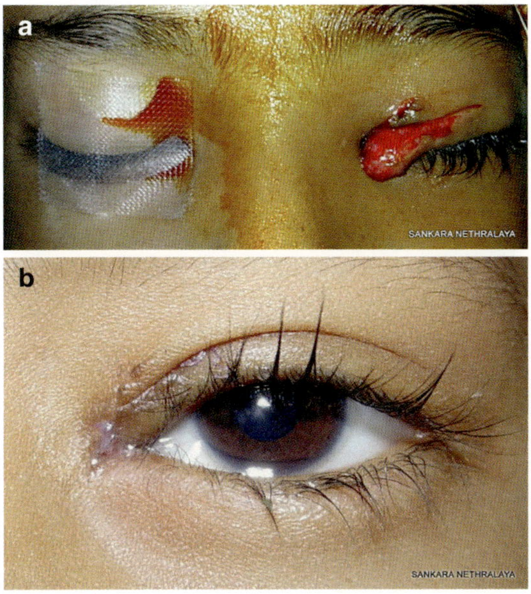


**Fig. 6.2** (**a**, **b**) A 5-year-old boy with left upper lid trauma with canalicular damage repaired with absorbable sutures and Mini-Monoka intubation

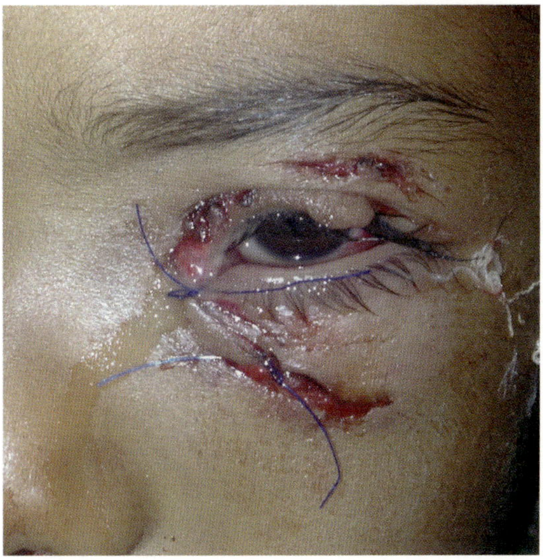

**Fig. 6.3** A 3-year-old boy with upper and lower lid trauma and canthal disinsertion and tissue loss. The wound had been crudely sutured together necessitating a revision surgery

canaliculus, and 11 % of the cases involved both [12] (Fig. 6.2a, b).

Canalicular tears should be addressed as early as possible to prevent scarring, which might preclude identification and intubation. For mono-canalicular trauma, a Mini-Monoka is preferred and usually results in good results after tube removal at 3 months. For bicanalicular trauma, bicanalicular intubation may be performed (see Chap. 12).

Canthal disinsertion may require reattachment to the periosteum in addition to canalicular repair. If the upper lid shows extensive damage, it is best to repair in such a way that the anatomy is maintained: the levator must be identified, and if found severed, the cut ends must be sutured to prevent ptosis. In large defects, primary closure may not be possible, in which case healing by secondary intention and subsequent reconstruction may be the preferred option, as long as exposure keratopathy is prevented.

Burroughs et al. have very succinctly presented the "Rule of 50s" which state that ≤50 % of all dog bites leave significant scarring, ≤50 % infection rate reduction with prophylactic antibiotics, and ≤50 % wounds are culture positive for pathogens [11].

Injuries caused by cats may present different patterns as their sharp teeth promote a small but deep puncture wound that might allow bacterial growth. On the other hand, dog bites usually present as crush injuries associated with lacerations, especially for bigger dogs [3] (Fig. 6.3).

## Infection Control

Wound infections can easily occur given the variety of resident flora in the oral cavity of animals. An average of five species of organisms was found in a prospective study of dog and cat bites by Talan et al. [13]. The most common isolates that they reported were *Pasteurella*, *Streptococci*, *Staphylococci*, *Moraxella*, *Corynebacterium*, and *Neisseria*. This underscores the importance of antibiotic prophylaxis.

Other animals such as horses, donkeys, and even humans have been documented to inflict bite injuries to the face and cause periocular injury. The management remains the same except the need for postexposure rabies prophylaxis which is recommended for bites from raccoons, bats, domestic cats, foxes, wolves, bobcats, skunks, and

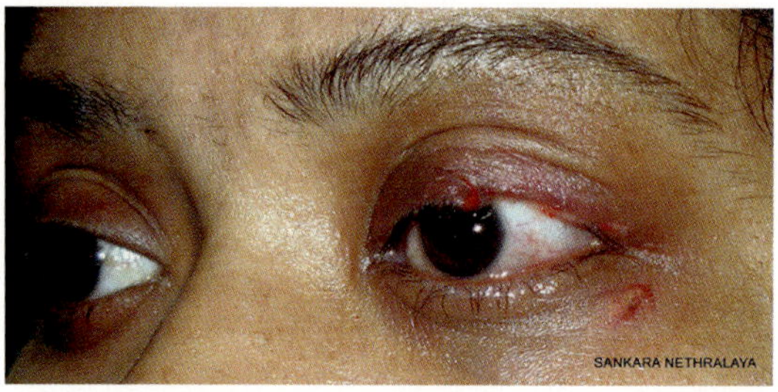


**Fig. 6.4** A 35-year-old female with loss of temporal upper lid margin due to human bite during an alleged fight with her spouse

otters (not an exhaustive list). Of particular interest are snakebites; where antivenom must be a part of the treatment plan. Human bite injuries may lead to loss of function, infection, and gross disfigurement. Human bites can be associated with interpersonal and sexual violence and may have subsequent medicolegal connotations (Fig. 6.4). Photographic documentation and detailed history recording is mandatory in these cases. Non-accidental injuries and child abuse should be kept in mind in pediatric patients. The unique nature of teeth and the bite marks are invaluable in forensic pathology. These bite wounds can get infected very rapidly from oral contaminants. Management includes wound debridement, surgery to repair or replace damaged tissue, and long-term antibiotic therapy [14]. Rarely, hepatitis B virus can be transmitted by mucosal exposure to saliva; hence all patients and perpetrators of human bites require hepatitis B follow-up. The risk of HCV-HIV transmission is biologically possible, and the patients and their biters need HCV-HIV testing after bloody bites. If the biter is found to be HIV positive, the patients need to be administered postexposure prophylaxis [15].

In conclusion, prompt medical management and appropriate surgical intervention can give good results in periocular trauma due to an animal bite.

## References


1. MacBean CE, Taylor DM, Ashby K. Animal and human bite injuries in Victoria. 1998–2004. Med J Aust. 2007;186(1):38–40.
2. Patil PD, Panchabhai TS, Galwankar SC. Managing human bites. J Emerg Trauma Shock. 2009;2(3): 186–90.
3. Simao NR, Borba AM, da Silva AL, Vieira EM, Carvalhosa AA, Bandeca MC, Borges AH. Animal bite injuries to the face: a case report. J Int Oral Health. 2013;5(4):68–72.
4. Morgan M. Hospital management of animal and human bites. J Hosp Infect. 2005;61(1):1–10.
5. Mathews JR, Lattal KA. A behavioral analysis of dog bites to children. J Dev Behav Pediatr. 1994;15: 44–52.
6. Tu AH, Girotto JA, Singh N, Dufresne CR, Robertson BC, Seyfer AE, Manson PN, Iliff N. Facial fractures from dog bite injuries. Plast Reconstr Surg. 2002; 109(4):1259–65.
7. Rui-feng C, Li-song H, Ji-bo Z, Li-qiu W. Emergency treatment on facial laceration of dog bite wounds with immediate primary closure: a prospective randomized trial study. BMC Emerg Med. 2013;13 Suppl 1:S2.
8. http://www.cdc.gov/rabies/medical_care/vaccine.html. Accessed 10th Feb 2014.
9. Peters V, Sottiaux M, Appelboom J, Kahn A. Posttraumatic stress disorder after dog bites in children. J Pediatr. 2004;144(1):121–2.
10. Mukherjee B, Nair AG. Principles and practice of external digital photography in ophthalmology. Indian J Ophthalmol. 2012;60:119–2.
11. Burroughs JR, Soparkar CN, Patrinely JR, Williams PD, Holck DE. Periocular dog bite injuries and responsible care. Ophthal Plast Reconstr Surg. 2002; 18(6):416–9.
12. Savar A, Kirszrot J, Rubin PA. Canalicular involvement in dog bite related eyelid lacerations. Ophthal Plast Reconstr Surg. 2008;24(4):296–8.
13. Talan DA, Citron DM, Abrahamian FM, et al. Bacteriologic analysis of infected dog and cat bites. Emergency medicine animal bite infection study group. N Engl J Med. 1999;340:85–92.
14. Liston PN, Tong DC, Firth NA, Kieser JA. Bite injuries: pathophysiology, forensic analysis, and management. N Z Dent J. 2001;97(428):58–63.
15. Lohiya GS, Tan-Figueroa L, Lohiya S, Lohiya S. Human bites: bloodborne pathogen risk and postexposure follow-up algorithm. J Natl Med Assoc. 2013; 105(1):92–5.

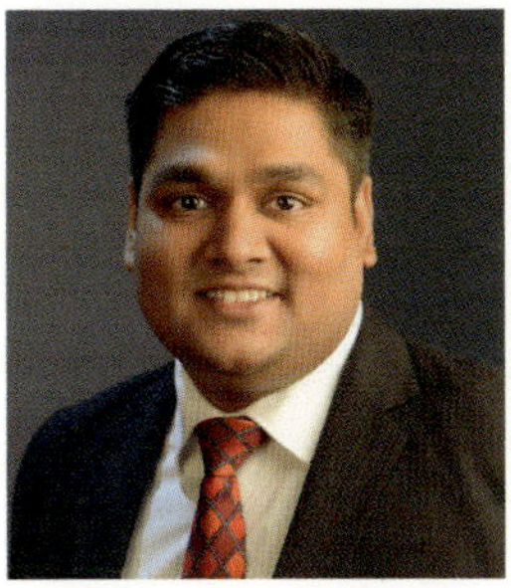

**Akshay Gopinathan Nair** Akshay Gopinathan Nair received his medical degree from Maharashtra University of Health Sciences, India and completed his residency training in ophthalmology from Sankara Nethralaya in Chennai, India. Following this, he underwent fellowship training in ophthalmic plastic surgery, ocular oncology and facial aesthetics at L V Prasad Eye Institute, Hyderabad, India and New York Eye & Ear Infirmary of Mount Sinai, USA. Dr. Nair has over 50 peer-reviewed publications, 8 book chapters in ophthalmology. His areas of special interest are ocular surface and eyelid tumours, ophthalmic imaging and neuroimaging. Dr. Nair is a faculty member at Lokmanya Tilak Municipal Medical College, Mumbai, India and is also affiliated with Advanced Eye Hospital & Institute and Aditya Jyot Eye Hospital in Mumbai.

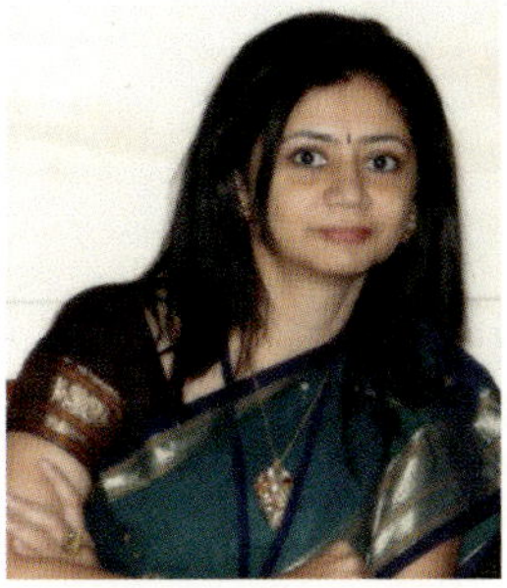

**Bipasha Mukherjee** Dr. Bipasha Mukherjee is a fellow in Orbit & Oculoplasty from Aravind Eye Hospitals, India, and ICO fellow from University Hospital of Limoges, France, under Prof. Jean-Paul Adenis. She has undergone clinical observerships with stalwarts like Jack Rootman, Richard Collins, Geoff Rose, Mark Duffy, and Robert Goldberg.

She currently heads the department of Orbit, Oculoplasty, Aesthetic & Reconstructive services in Medical Research Foundation, Chennai. She has numerous presentations in national and international conferences and publications in peer-reviewed journals and text books. Her areas of interest include diseases of the orbit and adnexa including tumors, lacrimal surgery, socket reconstruction, traumatic lid and adnexal injuries, training residents and fellows, and photography.

# Chemical and Thermal Injuries

# 7

Ravija Patel and Bipasha Mukherjee

## Introduction

The function of the eyelids is protection of the eyes. Burns to the eyelids may be caused by thermal, electrical or chemical sources, or ionizing radiation. Eyelid burns occur in less than 10 % of all thermal injuries, but are very common in patients with burns involving the face [1]. The loss of an eye primarily from a thermal injury is rare. This is due to protective mechanisms such as the reflex closure of the eyes and Bell's phenomenon. The initial corneal or ocular surface injury can be quite trivial compared to the injury sustained to the eyelids [2]. Chemical injuries on the other hand usually involve both the ocular surface and the eyelids. The most common sequelae of eyelid burns are ectropion or lid retraction and lagophthalmos. These, if not treated adequately and in timely fashion, may result in exposure keratopathy, corneal ulceration, and ultimately permanent visual impairment. Hence the role of an ophthalmologist and oculoplastic surgeon is vital in the management of these patients.

In thermal injuries, the degree of the injury is a function of two factors: temperature and exposure time. There is an inverse relationship between the intensity of a thermal exposure and the amount of time required to produce a burn. The common causes of thermal burns include fires (flame), liquid thermal burns either with hot water or combustible liquids like gasoline, and exposure to hot gas. While in chemical burns, the extent of injury varies according to the agent: acid burns are usually self-limiting, and alkali burns, on the other hand, cause much more extensive tissue destruction. In electrical burn, the damage is caused as a result of heat and electrical current itself. The amount of damage is related to the intensity of the current, to its voltage, and to the resistance of the areas through which it travels. The characteristic feature of electrical burns is that the damage is progressive [3]. In radiation injury, it is not possible to establish an exact dose-response relationship as it depends on multiple factors like age the of patient, the condition of tissue, any concurrent illness, dose, dose rate, medications, etc. [4].

R. Patel, MBBS, MS (✉)
M & J Institute of Ophthalmology,
Ahmedabad 380016, Gujarat, India
e-mail: ravijapatel@yahoo.com

B. Mukherjee, MS, DNB(Ophthalmology), FICO
Orbit, Oculoplasty, Reconstructive & Aesthetic
Services, Sankara Nethralaya,
Chennai 600006, Tamil Nadu, India
e-mail: drbpm@snmail.org


B. Mukherjee, H. Yuen (eds.), *Emergencies of the Orbit and Adnexa*,
DOI 10.1007/978-81-322-1807-4_7

## Classification of the Severity of Thermal Burns (Fig. 7.1)

### First-Degree Burns

Only the epidermis of the skin is involved resulting in mild erythema of the lids. Edema of the lid may impair eye opening but this is only transient. There is no blister formation. These injuries, though painful, heal usually within 7 days without any residual scar formation. Severe sunburns are the most common first-degree burns (Fig. 7.2a).

### Second-Degree Burns (Partial-Thickness Burns)

The entire depth of the epidermis and a part of the dermis are involved (Fig. 7.2b). These are usually more painful than first-degree burns. Depending on the depth of the penetration it can be further divided as:

1. Superficial partial thickness: involves the epidermis and superficial papillary dermis. There is erythematous appearance of the skin with blister formation and it is usually associated with edema. It heals within 2 weeks with minimal or no scarring unless it becomes infected; in which case the depth of tissue destruction and inflammation will result in a clinical course more similar to deep partial-thickness or third-degree burns.
2. Deep partial thickness: characterized by a pale white or mottled base under the blister. The clinical course varies from minimal tissue shrinkage and good skin healing within 1–3 weeks to significant contracture requiring a release and grafting procedure. Epithelialization occurs in about

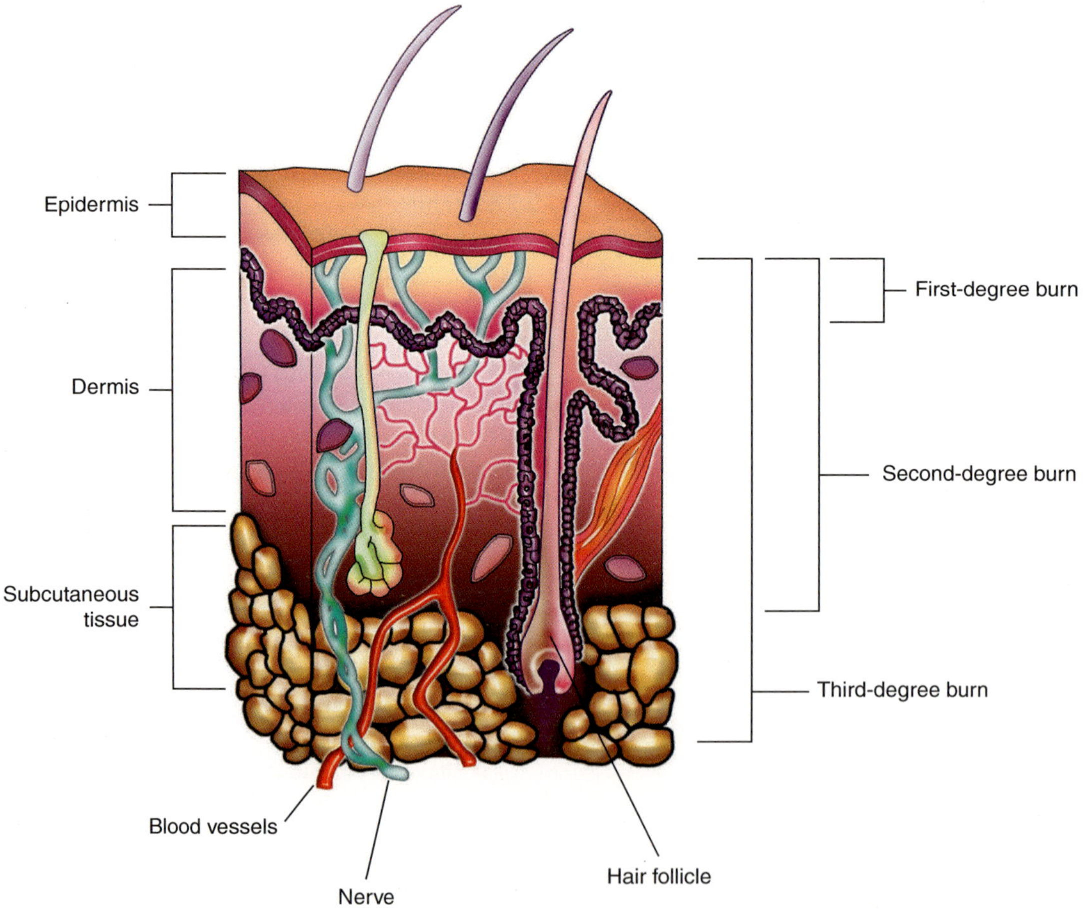


**Fig. 7.1** Classification of severity of thermal burns

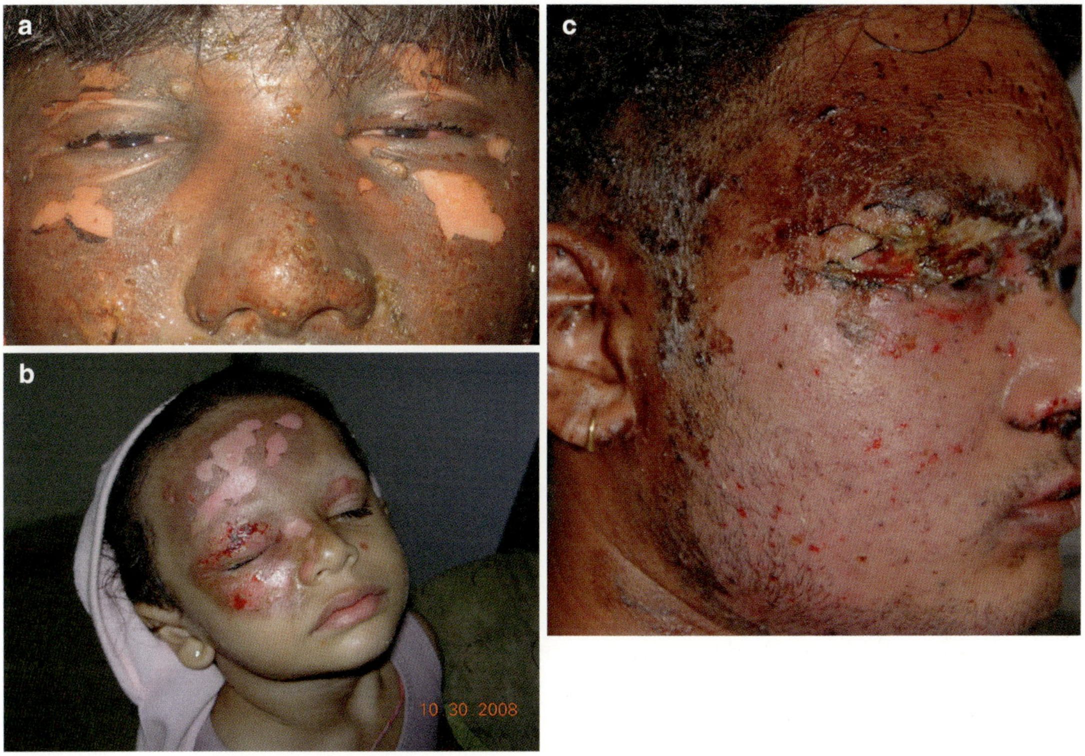


**Fig. 7.2** (**a**) First-degree burns – involvement of the epidermis without blister formation. (**b**) Second-degree burns – involvement of the epidermis and a part of the dermis. (**c**) Third-degree burns involving the epidermis and deep dermis with superimposed infection

14–28 days. Contracture can occur even after epithelialization occurs but slows down considerably. Deep second-degree burns may progress to third-degree burns if there is extension of avascularity in the transition zone between the viable and the nonviable tissue.

## Third-Degree Burns (Full-Thickness Burns) (Fig. 7.2c)

These involve both the epidermis and the dermis as well as all the regenerative elements. There is little or no pain. The skin is dry and leathery and because of heat coagulation of dermal vessel, the affected tissue is avascular and white. Healing only occurs from the edges and is associated with significant contracture. Early excision of the affected tissue and skin grafting is almost always required to prevent secondary corneal complications.

## Fourth-Degree Burns

These are full-thickness burns with destruction of the underlying muscle, bone, and vital structures. Such burns require extensive and complex management and invariably result in severe contracture and prolonged disability.

## Early Ophthalmic Evaluation

Life-threatening problems like asphyxia, shock, and associated trauma such as head injury and spinal cord injury if present should be taken care of.

In case of facial burns, ophthalmic evaluation should be done early before the ensuing conjunctival and eyelid edema prevents a detailed examination.

A thorough history should be taken, as early treatment depends on the etiological factor. For

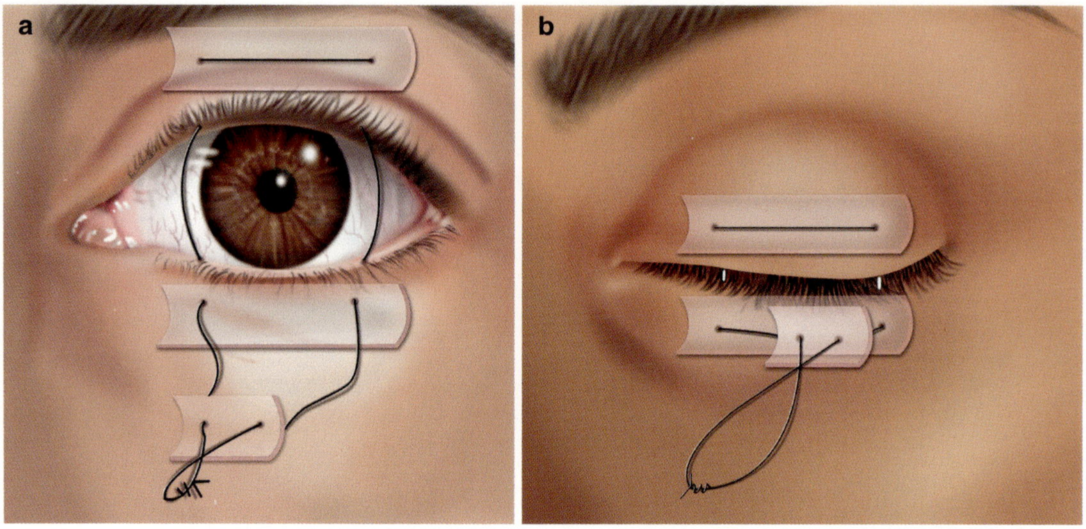


**Fig. 7.3** (**a**) Draw string tarsorrhaphy. (**b**) Draw string tarsorrhaphy

example, a chemical burn should be treated by continuous copious irrigation, and thermal injury should be treated by application of cold compresses.

Complete and detailed ophthalmic assessment should be done. The visual acuity should be recorded if possible. The extent and severity of eyelid burns is to be documented. Clinical photographs can be taken for documentation. Presence of eyelashes should be noted as it indicates intact lid margin. Injury to the globe should be ruled out. Fluorescent staining should be done to rule out corneal epithelial defects. If epithelial defect is present along with significant lagophthalmos special mention must be made about the Bell's phenomenon as it plays an important role in deciding the management. Fundus examination should be performed if possible especially in electrical burns where electrical damage can cause optic nerve and retinal injury and late cataract formation. Computerized tomography (CT) scan may be requested if there is suspicion of orbital or intraocular foreign body.

## Initial Management

1. Head elevation helps to reduce the eyelid edema.
2. Cool compresses should be given in case of thermal burns.
3. Copious continuous irrigation with saline has to be done in cases of chemical burns.
4. Foreign bodies and debris should be removed if present.
5. Prophylactic lubricating eye drops should be started three to four times a day. In case of patients with epithelial defects, more frequent lubrication should be initiated with prophylactic topical antibiotics providing gram-negative bacterial coverage to prevent corneal infection.
6. Singed eyelashes should be removed and trimming should be done with scissors coated with antibiotic so that the eyelashes do not fall in the eye and cause discomfort.
7. Orbital compartment syndrome has been reported in patients who undergo large volumes of fluid resuscitation particularly in patients with burn size greater than 25% of the total body surface area. Urgent canthotomy and cantholysis may be required in such patients [2].
8. Dressing: The eyelids should be cleaned with saline-soaked gauze. First-degree burns can be kept open. Second- and third-degree burns require moist dressing or dressing with antibiotic ointment. Dressing the wound decreases desiccation and wound necrosis. Superficial burns heal within 5–7 days, while the partial-thickness burns form a black eschar within this period. At this stage, loose

wet soaks should be applied to facilitate separation of the eschar and cleansing of the sloughing wound. In third-degree burns, the eschar is usually thick and its separation is slower – between 14 and 21 days. A layer of the granulation tissue will develop beneath the separating eschar and this needs to be resurfaced by skin grafting [3].

9. Tarsorrhaphy:

   In case of eyelid burns, the first and probably the most controversial decision to make is whether to perform a tarsorrhaphy, and if yes, whether temporary or suture tarsorrhaphy. Most authors do not prefer to use tarsorrhaphy [2, 3, 5].

   In the early phase of most partial-thickness eyelid burns, tarsorrhaphy is not required as these burns are associated with lid edema; hence the eyelid is closed naturally protecting the cornea. Also tarsorrhaphy is difficult to perform in an edematous eyelid with friable lid margins and it may cut through. If it does hold, tarsorrhaphy can result in deformities of the lid margin.

   After around 2 weeks, lid contracture and lagophthalmos develop. A tarsorrhaphy done at this stage however does not play any role in the prevention of this contracture of the eyelid and subsequent development of ectropion. Also, it interferes with the examination of the eyes. In patients with healthy skin on the brow or cheek, a simple frost suture may be helpful in patients with severe lagophthalmos awaiting definitive management. Some authors propose the use of drawstring tarsorrhaphy which allows lid closure, examination of the eye, as well as instillation of topical medications (Fig.7.3a, b).

   In case of severe burns involving both the lids, masquerade procedure (Fig.7.4) could be done to protect the cornea till definitive management is undertaken. In this procedure, all the necrotic tissue is debrided; the conjunctiva is mobilized from both upper and lower lids and sutured together so that the epithelial surface faces the cornea. It is then covered by split-thickness skin graft (STSG) leaving small gaps at the medial and lateral ends. This flap is divided after 1–3 months [2].

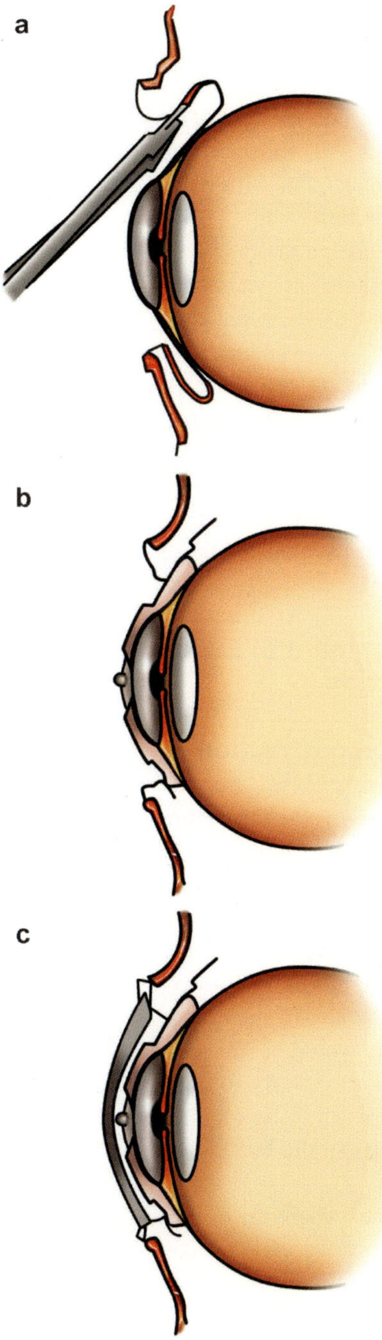


**Fig. 7.4** Masquerade procedure. The conjunctiva is mobilized (**a**), sutured together (**b**), and covered by a split-thickness skin graft (**c**)

If only the lower lid sloughing is present, then a tarsoconjunctival flap like modified Hughes can be fashioned which acts as a vascularized bed for a skin graft. Loss of upper lid is a greater problem as there is less tissue in lower lid to mobilize and the opening and closing functions of the eye are impaired. In case of sloughing of entire upper lid and part of lower lid, levator advancement with a full-thickness graft has been described. The levator advancement provides a good vascular bed for graft and also helps in eye opening [5].

10. Tenoplasty: In patients where conjunctival flaps cannot be made, tenoplasty can be done to provide vascularization and promote corneal epithelialization. In this procedure, Tenon's layer is advanced in a flap-like fashion and sutured at the limbus of the cornea. Split-thickness dermal grafts can also be used in such patients [2].

## Management of Ectropion/Lid Retraction

### Early Reconstruction

In general, eyelid burn debridement is performed at a later time compared to burns elsewhere. If the patient has extensive skin loss of one or both the eyelids, it is usually advisable to perform a graft as soon as the necrotic tissue sloughs and the granulation tissue begins to form [5].

Contracture in such cases is relentless and lid distortion would be greater if grafting is delayed. Also it is necessary to understand that multiple procedures may be required as the contracture progresses in the eyelids and surrounding facial tissue.

In cases where the eyelid contracture and lagophthalmos results in corneal exposure, the release of contracture followed by a graft should be planned.

The graft can be of two types, full-thickness skin graft (FTSG) or split-thickness skin graft (STSG). Thin full-thickness graft is preferred as it is associated with less contracture and does not compromise mobility or appearance [2]. Thin full-thickness skin can be taken from retroauricular, supraclavicular, infraaxillary, even groin, or scrotal skin or the foreskin [5]. However, in cases of more advanced burns, full-thickness skin may be insufficient and must be saved for later reconstruction. In these cases STSG can be used. Ideal donor areas should have good color match and should be a non-hair-bearing area like the inner thigh.

#### Technique (Fig. 7.5)

Traction sutures are taken at the lid margin. The incision is placed at the lid crease for the upper eyelid (Fig. 7.5b) and subciliary incision is placed for the lower eyelid [2]. The incision in the lower lid extends from canthus to canthus and is fashioned in upward direction for about 1.5 cm beyond the lateral canthus [3]. All the scar tissue is removed until complete eyelid release is achieved. Complete hemostasis of the graft bed is achieved (Fig. 7.5c). The graft should always be overcorrected to account for secondary contracture. Graft is sutured with silk suture and the ends are held long so that a tie-over dressing can be placed (Fig. 7.5d). FTSG is sutured edge to edge with the recipient bed, while STSG is anchored over the edge to the bed [5]. The lid margin sutures are used to give traction and are taped to the cheek or forehead. Tie-over dressing gives better graft to bed apposition and is left undisturbed for 5–7 days (Fig. 7.5e). After the dressing is removed, the graft can be left open with daily application of antibiotic ointment.

When both the upper and lower lids of one eye are involved, it is preferable to correct one lid at a time. However if two upper eyelids or two lower eyelids necessitate surgery, they can be corrected at the same time [3].

### Late Reconstruction

Late reconstruction may be required because of continued wound contracture in the eyelid itself as well as contracture of the adjacent tissue of the face.

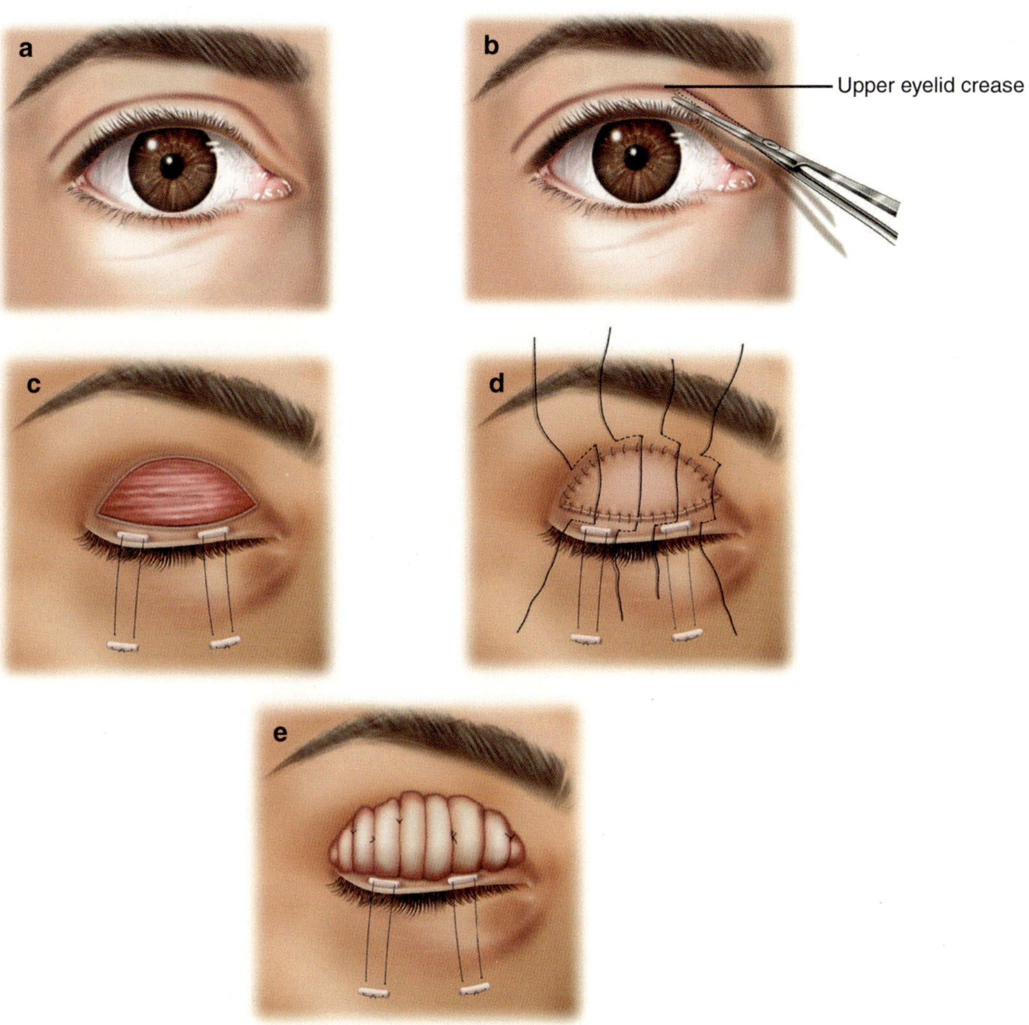


**Fig. 7.5** Full-thickness skin graft for the upper eyelid. (**a**) Upper eyelid contracture. (**b**) Superior lid crease incision. (**c**) Release of contracture. Lid is held down by traction sutures. (**d**) Graft sutured onto recipient area (**e**) Tie-over dressing in situ

Once lid closure is restored, it is preferable if possible, to wait till all the inflammation subsides and the contracture is complete and the tissue is as supple as possible before any final surgery is performed [5]. Definitive reconstruction surgery should be done 1 year after the burn injury. By this time the hypertrophic scars become pale and soft, and there is some degree of mobility of scars or grafted areas on the underlying tissues [3].

The principles of late reconstruction are the same as those of early reconstruction but the results are much more predictable.

The role of flaps for the reconstruction of postburn eyelids is limited because of lack of adjacent normal skin. The use of temporal-based orbicularis oculi myocutaneous flap for correction of the lower lid postburn ectropion has been described in cases where the upper eyelid is available for harvest [7]. Another potential source may be an island pedicle flap, and a free flap for total eyelid reconstruction following deep facial burn has also been reported [2].

In the recurrent ectropion of the burned lower eyelid, lower eyelid fascial sling (LEFS) with a temporalis fascial strip to create a suspension sling for the lower eyelid has been described. The lower eyelid sling opposes the vertical forces of contraction, which cause recurrent ectropion in the burned eyelid [8].

In case of chemical burns, as the ocular surface is involved as well, amniotic membrane graft can be used for bulbar conjunctiva, and mucous membrane graft can be used for palpebral conjunctiva after the release of symblepharon. The use of preputial skin to replace conjunctiva and to correct ectropion has been decribed in cases of chemical injury [6].

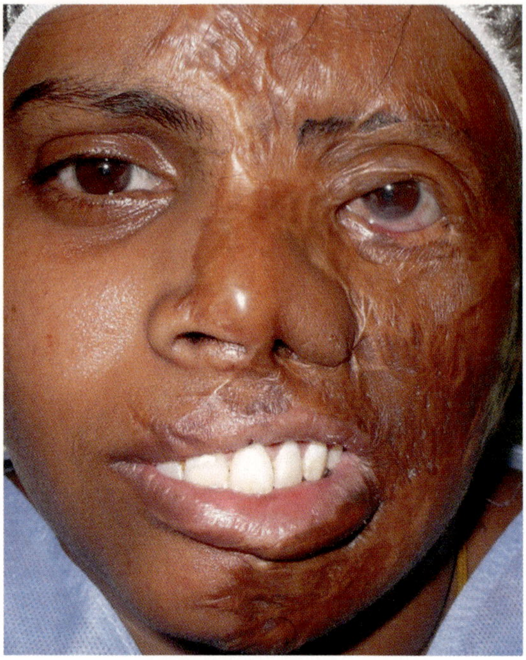

**Fig. 7.6** Webbing of the left medial canthal tissue in a patient with deep thermal burns

## Management of Other Sequelae

### Canthal Deformities (Fig.7.6)

Canthal webbing with psuedoepicanthal folds is seen frequently in patients with deep nasal burns. If the folds are supple and caused by contracture on the nose, then multiple Z-plasties work well. If the webs are densely scarred, excising the entire scarred web and replacing it with full-thickness graft gives good results.

### Lacrimal Obstruction

Lacrimal involvement in case of burns involving the medial canthal area usually includes punctal stenosis or canalicular obstruction. These may actually be beneficial in burns patients as they tend to have dry eyes. In symptomatic patients, these can be treated by the standard procedures like punctal dilatation followed by snip procedure for punctal stenosis and intubation or conjunctivodacryocystorhinostomy (CDCR) for canalicular obstruction.

### Eyebrow Deformities

The cicatricial damage to the brow varies from partial to complete alopecia depending on the severity and depth of the burn. Reconstruction can be done either by a composite graft of hair-bearing scalp or by a scalp island flap. Micrograft technique of hair transplantation also has some success but it is time consuming and may require a repeat procedure.

### Scar Management

Control of scarring directly around the eyelids can be difficult and requires intralesional steroid injection. Adjacent tissues may be better controlled by the use of compression techniques. The correction of the surgical scar from chemical cicatricial ectropion repair with injection of autologous fat has been reported [9]. Silicone gel sheets have been shown to be use-

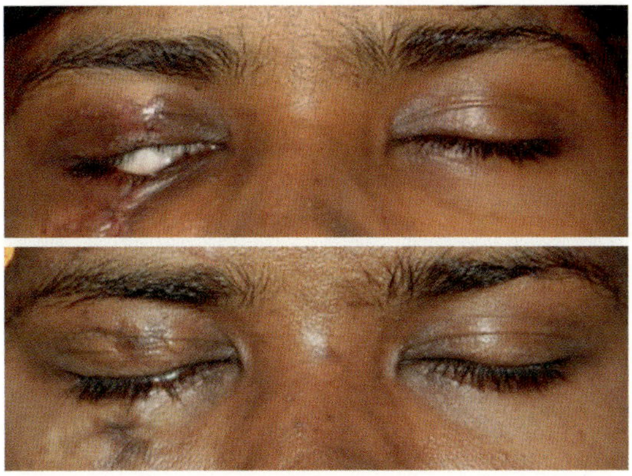

**Fig. 7.7** Patient with contracted lid scars (*above*) and 6 months following silicone gel sheet application for 12 h/ day along with scar massage (*below*)

ful for treatment of hypertrophic scars. They have to be worn for 24 hr a day with particular care to be taken of local hygiene to avoid the development of contact dermatitis. The exact mechanism of action of silicone gel is not known [10] (Fig.7.7).

## Radiation Injury

Radiotherapy represents a major problem in facial surgery, because it suppresses skeletal growth and induces contraction of the remaining soft tissues in the orbit. Complications related to radiation therapy can be acute or chronic. Acute reactions are rapid in onset and typically reversible. Chronic changes are delayed in onset and may not improve. Skin changes associated with radiation therapy include acute erythema, depigmentation, atrophy, telangiectasias, hair loss, and ectropion or entropion of the eyelid. The management of these patients has never been standardized. A combined approach of surgery and lipofilling to restore the orbital deformity and dystrophy respectively, has been described which significantly improve the functional and cosmetic outcome of shortened and dystrophic eyelids [11]. Also, adipose tissue is considered as a reservoir of mesenchymal cells which brings about improvement of skin appearance in such cases.

**Conclusion**

Management of eyelid burns requires prompt and timely intervention by ophthalmic and oculoplastic surgeon; otherwise it may result in high morbidity and loss of vision. The initial aim is to protect the cornea thereby preventing vision loss. The lid contracture in early phase can be treated by skin graft following debridement or release of scar tissue. Secondary contracture is common in the graft as well as the surrounding tissue which may require further management, but it is necessary to overcorrect keeping these in mind. Later reconstruction is aimed at better functional and cosmetic results which can be planned after the inflammation subsides and scar maturation is complete.

## References


1. Mandrekas AD, Zambacos GJ, Anastasopoulos A. Treatment of bilateral severe eyelid burns with skin grafts: an odyssey. Burns. 2002;28(1):80–6.
2. Malhotra R, Sheikh I, Dheansa B. The management of eyelid burns. Surv Ophthalmol. 2009;54(3):356–71.
3. Tsur H. Eyelid burns: a general plastic surgeon's approach. In: Hornblass A, Haing CJ, editors. Oculoplastics, orbital and reconstructive surgery. Baltimore: Williams & Wilkins; 1988. p. 448–54.
4. Finger PT. Radiation therapy for orbital tumors: concepts, current use and ophthalmic radiation side effects. Surv Ophthalmol. 2009;54(5):545–68.
5. Marrone AC. Thermal eyelid burns. In: Hornblass A, Haing CJ, editors. Oculoplastic, orbital and reconstructive surgery. Baltimore: Williams & Wilkins; 1988. p. 433–47.
6. Parkash S. The use of preputial skin to replace conjunctiva and to correct ectropion. Br J Plast Surg. 1982;35:206–8.
7. Kostakoglu N, Ozcan G. Orbicularis oculi myocutaneous flap in reconstruction of postburn lower eyelid ectropion. Burns. 1999;25:553–7.
8. De la Torre J, Simpson RL, Tenenhaus M, Bourhill I. Using lower eyelid fascial slings for recalcitrant burn ectropion. Ann Plast Surg. 2001;46(6):621–4.

9. Caviggioli F, Klinger F, Villani F, Fossati C, Vinci, Klinger M. Correction of cicatricial ectropion by autologous fat graft. Aesthetic Plast Surg. 2008;32:555–7.
10. Goel A, Shrivastava P. Post-burn scar and scar contractures. Indian J Plast Surg. 2010;43(Suppl):S63–71.
11. Tarallo M, Rizzo MI, Monarca C, Fanelli B, Parisi P, Scuderi N. Optimal care for the eyelid contraction after radiotherapy: case report and literature review. J Oral Maxillofac Surg. 2012;70:2459–65.

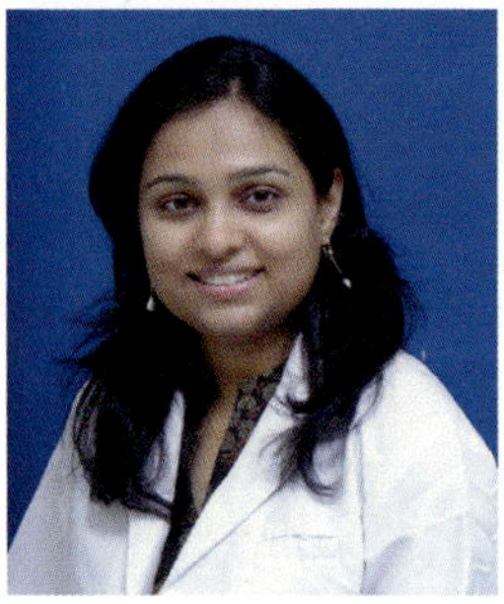

**Ravija Patel** Ravija Patel did fellowship in Orbit, oculoplasty and reconstructive services from Sankara Nethralaya, Chennai, India, after having finished graduation from Baroda Medical College, Gujarat, India. She was awarded gold medal for the best outgoing fellow. Being interested in academics as well as clinical practice, currently she is working as assistant professor at M & J Institute of Ophthalmology in Ahmedabad, India.

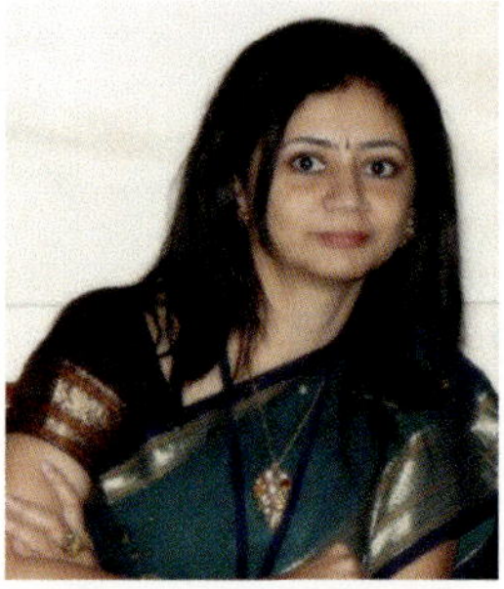

**Bipasha Mukherjee** Dr. Bipasha Mukherjee is a fellow in Orbit & Oculoplasty from Aravind Eye Hospitals, India, and ICO fellow from University Hospital of Limoges, France, under Prof. Jean-Paul Adenis. She has undergone clinical observerships with stalwarts like Jack Rootman, Richard Collins, Geoff Rose, Mark Duffy, and Robert Goldberg.

She currently heads the department of Orbit, Oculoplasty, Aesthetic & Reconstructive services in Medical Research Foundation, Chennai. She has numerous presentations in national and international conferences and publications in peer-reviewed journals and text books. Her areas of interest include diseases of the orbit and adnexa including tumors, lacrimal surgery, socket reconstruction, traumatic lid and adnexal injuries, training residents and fellows, and photography.

# 8 Endophthalmitis

Yvette Marie B. Santiago
and Raymond Nelson C. Regalado

Endophthalmitis, one of the most dreaded ocular complications, is defined as an inflammatory condition of the inner contents of the globe affecting the aqueous and the vitreous (Fig. 8.1). This condition is typically caused by infection with bacteria or fungi.

## Classification

Infectious endophthalmitis may be classified according to inciting event, chronicity, etiologic agent, and source of infection as summarized in Table 8.1.

Postsurgical endophthalmitis occurs after ocular surgery (e.g., post-cataract surgery, post-vitrectomy, post-intravitreal injection, filter-bleb associated), while post-traumatic endophthalmitis occurs after open-globe injury or trauma with or without intraocular foreign body (IOFB).

Sources of infection for exogenous endophthalmitis are the skin flora or other external contaminants. Endogenous endophthalmitis, on the other hand, is seen in immunocompromised individuals and those with underlying systemic infection.

### Incidence

Open-globe injury has about a tenfold higher rate of infection compared to intraocular surgery. Among infectious endophthalmitis, post-traumatic endophthalmitis comprises up to 31 % of cases. Several reviews have reported higher rates of infection with vegetable or organic IOFB than metallic ones [1]. However, a report from the National Eye Trauma System (NETS) Registry did not see significant difference

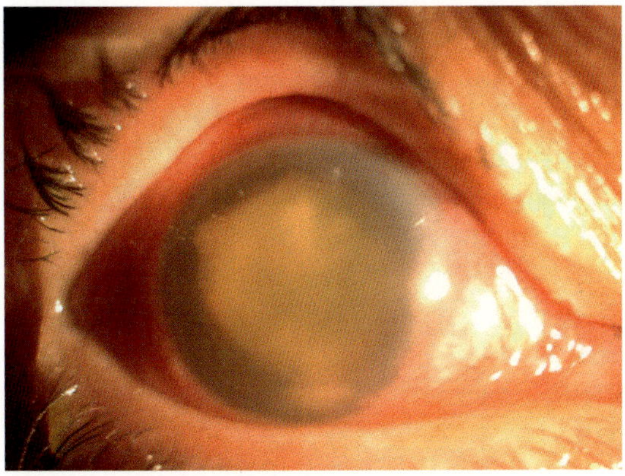

**Fig. 8.1** Endophthalmitis

Y.M.B. Santiago, MB, DPBO (✉)
R.N.C. Regalado, MD, DPBO
Eye Institute, St. Luke's Medical Center,
Quezon City 1122, Metro Manila, Philippines
e-mail: yvettesantiago@me.com;
monherbert@hotmail.com


B. Mukherjee, H. Yuen (eds.), *Emergencies of the Orbit and Adnexa*,
DOI 10.1007/978-81-322-1807-4_8

**Table 8.1** Classification of infectious endophthalmitis

| Basis | Classification |
|---|---|
| Inciting event | (a) Postsurgical endophthalmitis: occurs after ocular surgery (e.g., post-cataract surgery, post-vitrectomy, post-intravitreal injection, filter-bleb associated) |
| | (b) Post-traumatic endophthalmitis |
| Chronicity | (a) Acute |
| | (b) Subacute |
| | (c) Chronic |
| Etiologic agent | (a) Bacterial |
| | (b) Fungal |
| Source of infection | (a) Exogenous |
| | (b) Endogenous |

among various types of IOFB [2]. The number of reported endophthalmitis has decreased through the years with the development of more effective antibiotics and improved prophylactic management.

**Table 8.2** Risk factors of infectious endophthalmitis

| |
|---|
| *Postsurgical endophthalmitis* |
| *Patient factors*: |
| (a) Conjunctival and periocular flora |
| (b) Pre-existing periocular infections |
| (c) Systemic infection |
| (d) Diabetes and other immunocompromised states |
| *Surgical factors*: |
| (a) Bacterial contamination of the aqueous during surgery |
| (b) IOL material |
| (c) Incision type |
| (d) Prolonged and complicated surgery |
| *Postoperative factors*: |
| (a) Vitreous wick |
| (b) Wound leaks |
| (c) Infected wound edges |
| *Post-traumatic endophthalmitis* |
| (a) Retained intraocular foreign body |
| (b) Delayed primary wound closure of more than 24 h |
| (c) Lens rupture |
| (d) Rural setting |

## Postsurgical Endophthalmitis

### Risk Factors

Risk of postsurgical endophthalmitis can be due to factors inherent in the patient, surgical technique, and postoperative course as enumerated in Table 8.2 [3].

Among factors inherent to the patient, pre-existing periocular infections such as bacterial blepharitis and dacryocystitis can increase the risk of aqueous contamination during surgery.

Bacterial contamination of the aqueous may also occur from improperly sterilized instruments, contaminated surgical field and fluids, and use of intraocular lenses (IOLs) with polypropylene haptics and silicone implants. IOLs made from the aforementioned materials have a higher risk of bacterial adherence compared to polymethyl methacrylate and acrylic hydrophobic IOLs [4–6].

Clear corneal incision, likewise, increases the risk two- to threefold more than corneoscleral incision (0.13 %) [7]. Prolonged and complicated surgery with posterior capsular rent and/or vitreous loss may increase risk of aqueous bacterial contamination. Postoperative factors that increase likelihood of endophthalmitis are due to wound abnormalities such as vitreous wick, wound leaks, and infected wound edges (Fig. 8.2).

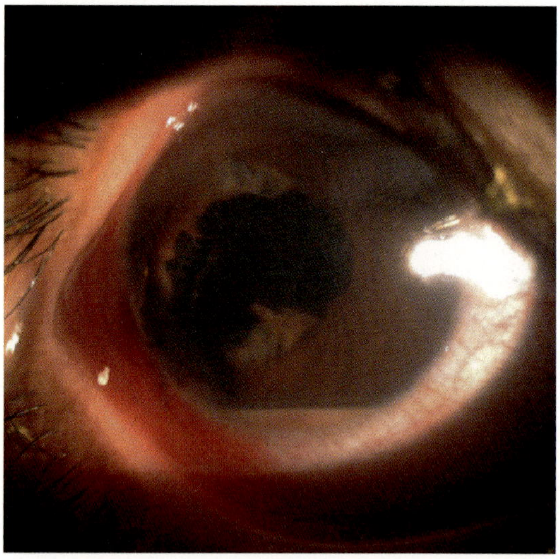

**Fig. 8.2** Slit lamp photo of endophthalmitis showing hypopyon, anterior chamber cells, and conjunctival injection

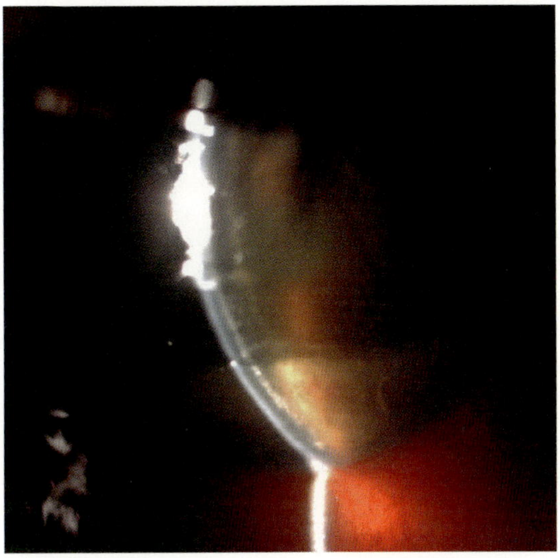

**Fig. 8.3** Endophthalmitis after complicated cataract surgery, with vitreous wick on the corneal incision

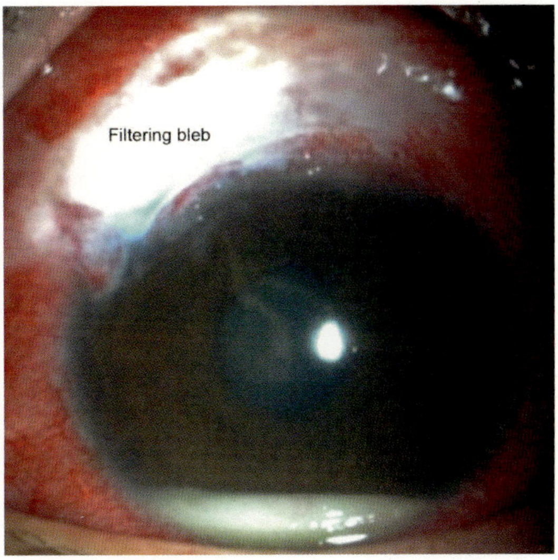


**Fig. 8.4** Filter-bleb-associated endophthalmitis with blebitis

## Clinical Features

Acute postsurgical endophthalmitis may present with progressive eye pain, conjunctival congestion, and decreased visual acuity. Examination would show anterior chamber inflammatory cells with fibrin formation, hypopyon (Fig. 8.3), vitreous cells, and fibrin [8].

Chronic post-cataract surgery endophthalmitis presents as a milder disease that causes loss of vision and mild eye pain. Presenting signs include cells in the anterior chamber, hypopyon, and a plaque on the posterior chamber capsule. Mild vitritis is also sometimes present.

Intravitreal injection of anti-vascular endothelial growth factor (anti-VEGF) into the vitreous cavity carries a small risk of postinjection endophthalmitis. Symptoms occur within 1–6 days after injection with around 80 % presenting with hypopyon [9].

A particular kind of postoperative endophthalmitis is filter-bleb-associated endophthalmitis. It is one of the long-term complications of trabeculectomy that has major implications for visual loss. It occurs as a sequela to blebitis. Presenting signs and symptoms are similar to other forms of infectious endophthalmitis, in addition to mucopurulent material seen in the filtering bleb [10] (Fig. 8.4).

## Microbiologic Isolates

The most common pathogen in postsurgical endophthalmitis is coagulase-negative *Staphylococcus*. The Early Vitrectomy Study (EVS) examined cases of post-cataract surgery endophthalmitis and found that infection caused by more virulent strains such as gram-negative organisms and gram-positive organisms other than coagulase-negative *Staphylococcus* presented within 2 days of surgery and with worse symptoms [11].

Chronic post-cataract endophthalmitis is caused by *Propionibacterium acne*.

## Treatment

The principal step in treating postsurgical endophthalmitis is with intravitreal injection of antibiotics (Table 8.3). The intravitreal antibiotics of choice are vancomycin (1 mg) for gram-positive coverage and amikacin (0.4 mg) or ceftazidime (2.25 mg) for gram-negative strains. A single dose is usually sufficient to control infection. Poor or none response to treatment may be due to infection with virulent organisms, like *Streptococci sp.* and *Pseudomonas*, and resistant organisms. In cases of poor clinical response, a second intravitreal

**Table 8.3** Suggested antibiotic treatment regimens for bacterial endophthalmitis

| Route of administration | Medication and suggested dose |
|---|---|
| Topical | Fortified antibiotics: vancomycin 50 mg/mL and cefazolin 50 mg/mL alternating q1–4H |
| | Gatifloxacin 0.5 % or moxifloxacin 0.5 % q1–2H |
| Intravitreal | Vancomycin 50 mg/mL, 1 mg/dose |
| | Amikacin 0.4 mg or ceftazidime 2.25 mg |
| Subconjunctival | Vancomycin 5 mg and |
| | Ceftazidime 100 mg or amikacin 25 mg |
| Intracameral | Cefuroxime 1 mg or |
| | Moxifloxacin 0.5 % 0.1 mL |
| Systemic | Vancomycin 1.0 g IV q 12 hand |
| | Ceftazidime 1–2 g IV q 8 h |
| | Ciprofloxacin 750 mg PO q 12 h or ofloxacin 400 mg PO q 12 h |
| | Prednisone 1 mg/kg/day PO |

injection is recommended after 48 h. Since repeated injections of these antibiotics suggest increased risk of retinal toxicity, this practice is not recommended unless necessary.

Vitrectomy helps to restore media clarity faster, obtain a better sample for culture, and remove bacterial toxins and inflammatory cells. The EVS remains to be the most extensive prospective trial that studied several aspects in management of post-cataract endophthalmitis. In their study to compare the benefit of performing vitrectomy over vitreous tap alone, they found that there was no apparent benefit to doing vitrectomy in patients with hand motion vision or better [12]. Still, vitrectomy is preferred by some surgeons in patients with severe visual loss or rapidly deteriorating vision and those where virulent bacteria has been isolated.

Fortified antibiotic eyedrops and/or fourth-generation fluoroquinolones may also be given, adjunctively, every 1–4 h as topical treatment. Subconjunctival antibiotics, likewise, may be injected to decrease bacterial load in aqueous although this is less often applied (Table 8.3).

Steroid use for infectious endophthalmitis is gaining acceptance with many clinicians as adjunctive therapy. It mitigates intraocular tissue damage by decreasing the inflammatory reaction to infection. When used systemically, prednisone 1 mg/kg/day is recommended. Topically, prednisolone acetate 1 % eyedrops may be given every 1–2 h. Dexamethasone is used for subconjunctival or intravitreal [13] injection.

In addition to antibiotic treatment, chronic post-cataract endophthalmitis is managed with intraocular lens removal or exchange to prevent relapse that occurs in up to 50 % [9].

Cycloplegic eyedrops are also given for pain control.

## Post-traumatic Endophthalmitis

### Risk Factors

The risk factors associated with post-traumatic endophthalmitis are summarized in Table 8.2.

Retained intraocular foreign body and delayed primary wound closure of more than 24 h can increase the likelihood of endophthalmitis. Lens rupture increases risk of infection by giving microorganisms direct access to the vitreous and impeding clearance by blocking aqueous clearance. Also, there is a higher incidence of soil contamination in a rural setting [1].

### Clinical Features

Post-traumatic endophthalmitis presents similarly with postsurgical endophthalmitis with the following additional signs and symptoms of open-globe injury: eyelid edema, hemorrhagic chemosis, flat anterior chamber, hyphema, corneal or scleral laceration with or without uveal prolapse, iris peaking, cataract, and central microbial keratitis.

### Microbiologic Isolates

Presence of multiple microorganisms is more frequent in post-traumatic endophthalmitis. The

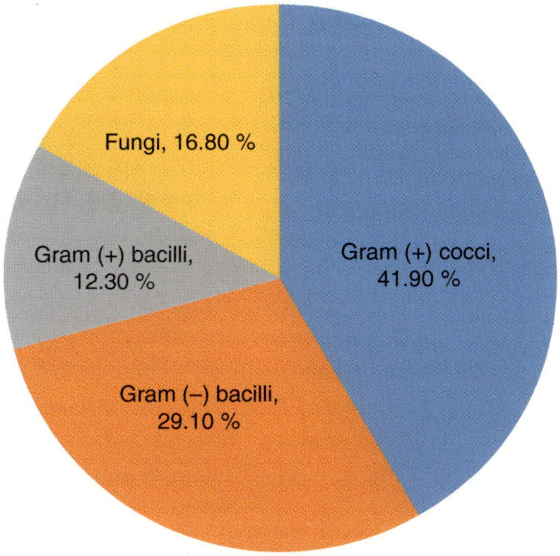


**Fig. 8.5** Culture-proven organisms

most commonly isolated organisms are from normal bacterial skin flora, likely because of direct contamination of the open wound. Fungal endophthalmitis should be suspected in the setting of organic matter-related injury such as wood and other plant products.

A 20-year retrospective study in China examined 912 post-traumatic endophthalmitis cases of which 347 were found to be culture positive [14]. The results are summarized in Fig. 8.5. The most common organism that was isolated was coagulase-negative *Staphylococcus*, followed respectively by *Staphylococcus saprophyticus*, *Bacillus subtilis*, and *Escherichia coli*. The most frequent fungal species was *Aspergillus*, followed by yeastlike fungi.

Bacillus cereus causes a fulminant infection and has been seen in post-traumatic endophthalmitis. It usually presents within 24 h and causes severe loss of vision and eye redness.

### Treatment

The most important step in managing open-globe injury to prevent post-traumatic endophthalmitis and its complications is to close the wound and restore globe integrity. Systemic prophylactic antibiotic should also be initiated promptly. Vitrectomy is sometimes indicated in this setting to decrease the load of vitreous toxins and microbial and inflammatory cells, to obtain a sample for microbiologic testing, and to administer intravitreal antibiotics. Removal of IOFB and repair of retinal detachment are also done, when necessary.

## Fungal Endophthalmitis

### Risks

Fungal endophthalmitis presents subacutely and may occur after trauma, as a complication of keratomycosis and, rarely, after intraocular surgery. Presence of contaminated organic matter increases the risk of infection.

### Clinical Features

Examination may reveal a hypopyon with white granulomatous cells in the anterior chamber, corneal filaments extending into the anterior chamber in keratomycosis, and vitritis.

### Diagnosis

As in bacterial endophthalmitis, diagnosis includes obtaining AC and vitreous taps for culture.

### Treatment

Treatment of fungal endophthalmitis includes surgery to clear the anterior chamber, vitrectomy, and intravitreal antifungal. Intravitreal amphotericin B is the drug of choice for initial empirical treatment (Table 8.3). Subsequent injection may be given at least 48 h apart. Intravitreal voriconazole is preferred for sensitive pathogens due to milder ocular side effects. IOL should be removed when present. Corneal transplantation is likewise indicated in cases caused by keratomycosis. Voriconazole is preferred for systemic treatment due to its high ocular bioavailability. Itraconazole and fluconazole are not recommended. Systemic amphotericin is reserved for adjunctive treatment in azole-resistant strains [9].

## Differential Diagnosis for Endophthalmitis

*Toxic anterior segment syndrome* (TASS) (Fig. 8.6) is a sterile exaggerated inflammatory reaction that occurs after intraocular surgery that mimics infectious endophthalmitis. It may be caused by complicated cataract surgery resulting in retained lens material, use of silk suture, and phacoanaphylaxis. This condition responds well to treatment with topical steroids.

*Infectious crystalline keratitis* (ICK) (Fig. 8.7) is a condition wherein crystal deposits are found on the corneal epithelium and/or stroma. It may arise from a de novo bacterial infection or as a complication of refractive and corneal transplant surgeries. ICK may present with eye pain, loss of vision, and photophobia. Examination would reveal branching crystalline corneal deposits and may have accompanying signs of inflammation. Microbiologic testing is helpful but may yield low. This condition is treated with fortified antibiotics (Table 8.3) for several weeks to months, depending on the response. In refractory cases, treatment with systemic antibiotics may help.

## Diagnostic Tools

*Microbiologic testing* helps to diagnose and treat endophthalmitis although up to 30 % of cases can yield a negative culture. Samples are obtained from aqueous and/or vitreous humor for microbiological analysis. Aqueous humor is aspirated from the anterior chamber (AC) using a needle (AC tap). Vitreous humor is obtained either by aspiration (vitreous tap) or vitrectomy.

Gram staining has up to 50 % detection rate for pathogen. Samples from vitrectomy have the highest yield for positive culture results (90 %) followed by vitreous tap (75 %) and then AC tap (40 %) [9].

*Polymerase chain reaction* (PCR) has been shown to be as sensitive as culture in detecting pathogens [15]. However, it has a higher sensitivity in subsequent samples owing to the fact that PCR cannot distinguish between live and dead microorganisms [9].

*Diagnostic imaging* is useful in the setting of trauma to localize IOFB or rule out retinal or choroidal detachment. Orbital computed tomography (CT) is most useful in locating IOFBs ≥5 mm, but it has limited use in locating organic, glass, and plastic materials. Plain film is inexpensive and fast but it can only detect 40 % of IOFB [16].

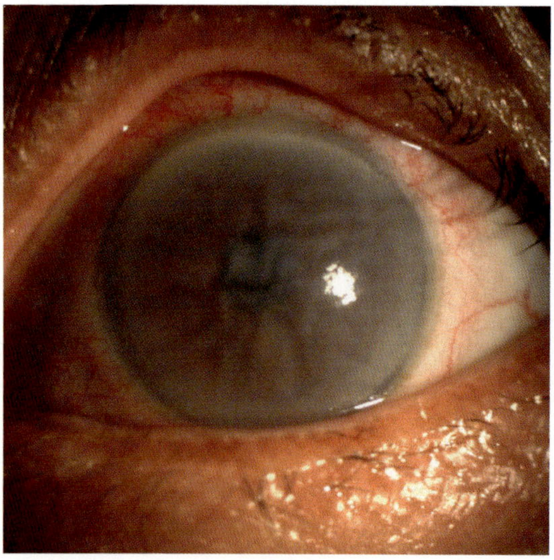

**Fig. 8.6** Toxic anterior segment syndrome

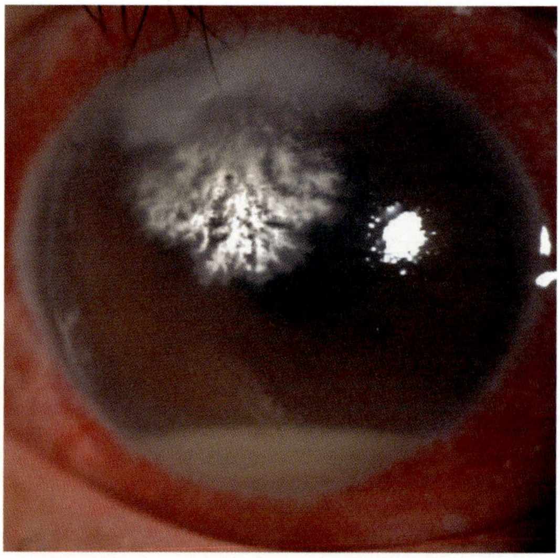

**Fig. 8.7** Infections crystalline keratitis

B-scan ultrasonography is likewise a useful tool in the setting of trauma. It can detect intraocular foreign body, degree of vitreous opacification, status of the posterior hyaloid phase, and presence of retinal or choroidal detachment. Its use in open-globe injury is, however, limited by the need to perform the examination under closed eyelids with minimal pressure over the compromised globe.

## Prognosis

Endophthalmitis that is culture negative or caused by coagulase-negative *Staphylococcus* has the best visual prognosis. Pathogens like *Streptococcus*, *Bacillus cereus*, and fungus that cause fulminant infection have the worst prognosis and often lead to loss of vision.

Delay in treatment can lead to spread of the infection throughout the entire globe causing panophthalmitis (Fig. 8.8).

## Prevention

The risk of infectious endophthalmitis is significantly decreased by practicing aseptic technique, treating any underlying periocular and periorbital infection or inflammation prior to surgery, and using clean drapes to exclude the eyelids and lashes which are potential sources of ocular pathogens. The surgical field is sterilized with 10 % povidone-iodine to clean the skin, and 5 % povidone-iodine may be applied topically to the conjunctiva prior to surgery. The use of 5 % povidone-iodine is clinically proven to reduce bacteria causing endophthalmitis. When used concurrently with preoperative topical antibiotics, its efficacy is further enhanced [17].

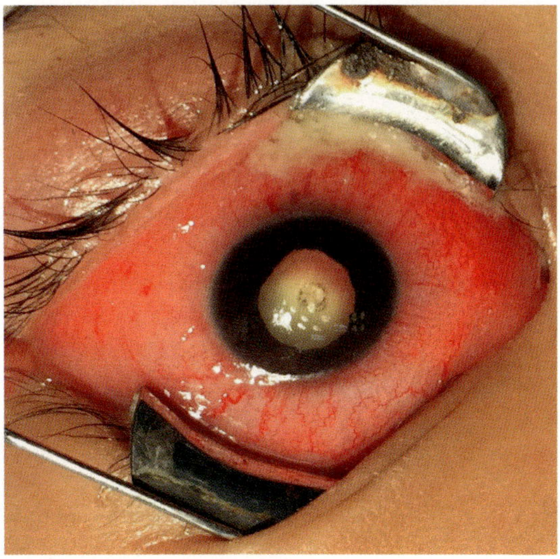

**Fig. 8.8** Panophthalmitis

Topical antibiotics are routinely given after intraocular surgery. Fourth-generation fluoroquinolones, such as moxifloxacin and gatifloxacin, are popular prophylactic pre- and postoperative agents. These prophylactic antibiotics may also be administered by intraoperative subconjunctival or intracameral [18] injections.

Initiating prompt antibiotic treatment and closing the wound in an open-globe injury best prevent post-traumatic endophthalmitis.

## Anophthalmic Surgery for Endophthalmitis

When medical treatment fails and vision has been lost but pain and signs of infection persist, anophthalmic surgery is the last resort for controlling infectious endophthalmitis. The dilemmas often attached to the peculiarities of endophthalmitis are (a) whether to perform evisceration or enucleation, (b) to place a primary implant or wait for inflammation to settle before implanting one secondarily, (c) what type of implant to use, and (d) identifying and managing complications common to endophthalmitis patients.

### Evisceration Versus Enucleation

Many perceived advantages and disadvantages have been cited when considering enucleation versus evisceration for anophthalmic surgery. Evisceration is associated with less operative time and dissection. There is less bleeding. The fornices are maintained leading to improved motility of the implant and prosthesis. There is less disruption of suspensory ligaments. Lastly, there is the purported decrease in risk of implant extrusion as both the sclera and Tenon's fascia serve as barriers.

On the other hand, advocates of enucleation cite a decreased risk of sympathetic ophthalmia with complete removal of the uvea. It requires removal of the sclera that is a potential nidus for persistence or recurrence of infection. Restoration of the orbital socket is optimized especially in cases where the globe has become phthisical.

Nakra et al. compared outcomes of evisceration and enucleation, for any indication including endophthalmitis, and revealed that while both had aesthetically similar outcomes, evisceration provided better motility and fewer complications [19]. Currently, there has been no reported large prospective study that has extensively reviewed the outcome of evisceration or enucleation when applied as treatment for endophthalmitis. Reports of retrospective case series have shown that evisceration for endophthalmitis has an acceptable outcome with complication rates ranging from 2.5 to 12 % [20–23]. On the other hand, enucleation for endophthalmitis had a 0–9 % complication rate [20, 24]. Many surgeons prefer evisceration as the procedure of choice for endophthalmitis-related anophthalmic surgery except when there is spread of the infection to the sclera or orbit, when enucleation is preferred.

## Primary Versus Secondary Implant

Before the discovery of the various effective antibiotic drugs that are available today, it was recommended not to place an orbital implant during evisceration or enucleation for endophthalmitis, to allow the infection and resultant inflammation to subside. Theoretically, the inflammatory reaction can delay wound healing and therefore increase the risk for complications. However, placing an implant during the initial surgery is less costly, affords faster recovery, obviates second surgery if there are no complications, and, consequently, decreases the anxiety of the patient in having to undergo another procedure. Placing a secondary implant potentially decreases postoperative extrusion from recurrent or persistent infection, but it necessitates a second procedure.

Small case series reports for both evisceration and enucleation for endophthalmitis with primary implant showed comparable rates to that reported for other indications [23, 24]. Since there is no apparent advantage for a secondary implant, placing one at the time of surgery is recommended. Providing adequate antibiotic treatment prior to surgery to prevent early and late postoperative wound breakdown and ensuring meticulous surgical technique decrease risks of complications. Secondary implants should be reserved for chronically inflamed eyes, aggressive pathogen, and purulent orbital infection refractory to antibiotic treatment.

## Type of Implant

There is no prospective clinical trial to date that compares outcomes among the various orbital implants used for endophthalmitis. Hui et al. reported a retrospective series of 54 eyes comparing porous and nonporous implants for various indications. They found that 2 out of 21 patients who underwent enucleation had extrusion of nonporous implant. These cases were culture positive for *Bacillus cereus* and *Streptococcus pneumoniae*. In the evisceration group, there was no reported extrusion [25]. Current literature suggests that the outcome is similar compared to when the implants are used for any other indication, including endophthalmitis. It is therefore up to the surgeon to decide which type of implant to use based on cost, experience, and specific circumstances of each case.

## References


1. Ahmed Y, Schimel AM, Pathengay A, Colyer MH, Flynn Jr HW. Endophthalmitis following open-globe injuries. Eye (London). 2012;26(2):212–7.
2. Thompson JT, Parver LM, Enger CL, Mieler WF, Liggett PE. Infectious endophthalmitis after penetrating injuries with retained intraocular foreign bodies. Ophthalmology. 1993;100(10):1468–74.
3. Cao H, Zhang L, Li L, Lo S. Risk factors for acute endophthalmitis following cataract surgery: a systematic review and meta-analysis. PLoS One. 2013;8(8):e71731.
4. Wejde G, Salomon B, Seregard S, et al. Risk factors for endophthalmitis following cataract surgery: a retrospective case-control study. J Hosp Infect. 2005; 61:251–6.
5. Parsons C, Jones DS, Gorman SP. The intraocular lens: challenges in the prevention and therapy of infectious endophthalmitis and posterior capsular opacification. Expert Rev Med Devices. 2005;2(2):161–73.
6. Kodjikian L, Beby F, Rabilloud M, Bruslea D, Halphen I, et al. Influence of intraocular lens material on the development of acute endophthalmitis after cataract surgery. Eye (London). 2008;22(2):184–93.
7. Colleaux KM, Hamilton WK. Effect of prophylactic antibiotics and incision type on the incidence of endophthalmitis after cataract surgery. Can J Ophthalmol. 2000;35:373–8.
8. Aaberg Jr TM, Flynn Jr HW, Schiffman J, Newton J. Nosocomial acute-onset postoperative endophthalmitis survey. A 10-year review of incidence and outcomes. Ophthalmology. 1998;105(6):1004–10.
9. Durand ML. Endophthalmitis. Clin Microbiol Infect. 2013;19(3):227–34.
10. Zahid S, Musch DC, Niziol LM, Lichter PR, Collaborative Initial Glaucoma Treatment Study Group. Risk of endophthalmitis and other long-term complications of trabeculectomy in the Collaborative Initial Glaucoma Treatment Study (CIGTS). Am J Ophthalmol. 2013;155(4):674–80.
11. Johnson MW, Doft BH, Kelsey SF, Barza M, Wilson LA, Barr CC, Wisniewski SR, The Endophthalmitis Vitrectomy Study. Relationship between clinical presentation and microbiologic spectrum. Ophthalmology. 1997;104(2):261–72.
12. Doft BH. The endophthalmitis vitrectomy study. Arch Ophthalmol. 1991;109(4):487–9.
13. Albrecht E, Richards JC, Pollock T, Cook C, Myers L. Adjunctive use of intravitreal dexamethasone in presumed bacterial endophthalmitis: a randomized trial. Br J Ophthalmol. 2011;95(10):1385–8.
14. Long C, Liu B, Xu C, Jing Y, Yuan Z, Lin X. Causative organisms of post-traumatic endophthalmitis: a 20-year retrospective study. BMC Ophthalmol. 2014;14:34.
15. Chiquet C, Cornut PL, Benito Y, et al. Eubacterial PCR for bacterial detection and identification in 100 acute post cataract surgery endophthalmitis. Invest Ophthalmol Vis Sci. 2008;49:1971–8.
16. Bryden FM, Pyott AA, Bailey M, McGhee CN. Real time ultrasound in the assessment of intraocular foreign bodies. Eye. 1990;4:727–31.
17. Coskun M, Altintas AG, Anayol MA, Raza S, Celikbilek N, Simsek S. Evaluation of efficacy of topical povidone-iodine and different types of fluoroquinolones in the sterilization of bacterial flora on the conjunctiva. J Ocul Pharmacol Ther. 2011;27(6):589–92.
18. Shorstein NH, Winthrop KL, Herrinton LJ. Decreased postoperative endophthalmitis rate after institution of intracameral antibiotics in a Northern California eye department. J Cataract Refract Surg. 2013;39(1):8–14.
19. Nakra T, Simon GJ, Douglas RS, Schwarcz RM, McCann JD, Goldberg RA. Comparing outcomes of enucleation and evisceration. Ophthalmology. 2006; 113(12):2270–5.
20. Ozgur OR, Levent A, Dogan OK. Primary implant placement with evisceration in patients with endophthalmitis. Am J Ophthalmol. 2007;143:902–4.
21. Tawfik HA, Budin H. Evisceration with primary implant placement in patients with endophthalmitis. Ophthalmology. 2007;114:1100–3.
22. Liu D. A comparison of implant extrusion rates and postoperative pain after evisceration with immediate or delayed implants and after enucleation with implants. Trans Am Ophthalmol Soc. 2005;103:568–91.
23. Dresner SC, Karesh JW. Primary implant placement with evisceration in patients with endophthalmitis. Ophthalmology. 2000;107:1661–5.
24. Abel AD, Meyer DR. Enucleation with primary implant insertion for treatment of recalcitrant endophthalmitis and panophthalmitis. OPRS. 2005;21(3):220–6.
25. Hui JI. Outcomes of orbital implants after evisceration and enucleation in patients with endophthalmitis. Curr Opin Ophthalmol. 2010;21(5):375–9.

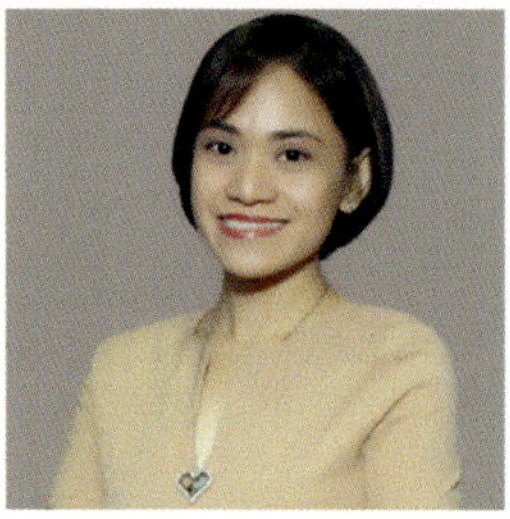

**Yvette Marie B. Santiago** Dr. Yvette Marie Santiago completed her clinical fellowship in Ophthalmic Plastic Surgery at Massachusetts Eye and Ear, Harvard Medical School in 2011. She is currently an active consultant at St. Luke's Medical Center Eye Institute-Quezon City, Philippines, and a Clinical Assistant Professor at St. Luke's College of Medicine.

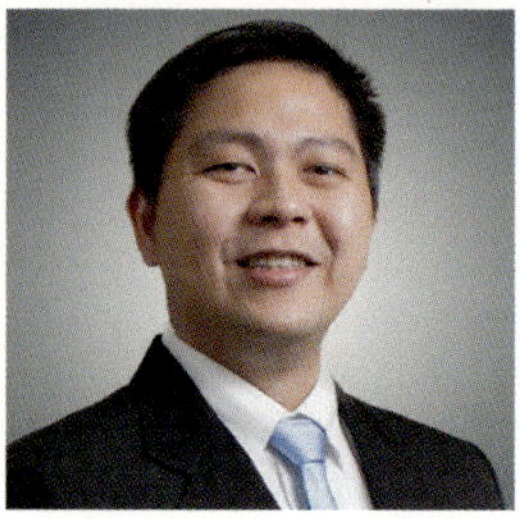

**Raymond Nelson C. Regalado** Dr. Raymond Nelson C. Regalado finished his clinical and surgical fellowship in External Disease and Cornea at the Philippine General Hospital in 2014. He is currently an associate active consultant at the St. Luke's Medical Center Eye Institute, Philippines.

# Eyelid Trauma: General Considerations

9

Ashok K. Grover, Saurbhi Khurana, and Shaloo Bageja

Eyelid injuries can occur due to a number of causes. In recent times, eyelid injuries are on the rise primarily because of the increasing incidence of road traffic accidents, industrial mishaps, and intentional assaults on the human body. Injury to the eyelids, lacrimal system, or orbital wall may be isolated or may occur in association with midfacial injuries.

It is important to look for associated systemic/facial injuries and address those before planning a repair of the eyelid. Moreover, any obvious/occult globe perforation should be carefully looked for and repaired first [1].

Every case of eyelid trauma is unique, and a thorough knowledge of anatomy and principles of repair is important for management of these cases. A meticulous planned repair is a must for achieving maximal functional and cosmetic outcome and preventing long-term complications.

A.K. Grover, MD, MNAMS, FRCS, FICO, FIMSA •
S. Bageja, DNB, MNAMS
Ophthalomology, Sir Ganga Ram Hospital,
New Delhi 110060, Delhi, India
e-mail: akgrover55@yahoo.com; bagejashaloo@yahoo.co.in

S. Khurana, MD, FICO (✉)
Ophthalmology, Medanta,
Gurgaon, Haryana 122001, India
e-mail: saurbhi.khurana@gmail.com

## History

A precise history is essential to assess the severity of injury. It is important to elicit the mode of injury, whether it is with sharp or blunt objects or due to thermal or chemical injury or due to dog bites. In cases of animal bites, a complete tetanus immunization history is obtained, and if required, proper immunization should be given. For chemical injuries, thorough irrigation of the eyes and adnexa is vital before any further intervention [2].

In some cases, an ophthalmologist can anticipate the extent and severity of injury from the mechanism of injury. Blunt trauma will lead to greater tissue edema and disruption. On the other hand, injury with sharp objects will usually create a direct cut.

In cases of penetrating injury, a suspicion of foreign body must be kept in mind.

## Examination of the Patient

Patient's injury must be dealt according to the priority. The basic "ABCs" (airway, breathing, circulation) must be evaluated, before proceeding to the management of localized injury. Repair of globe takes precedence over repair of eyelid laceration. In adnexal injury, the decision whether to repair the wound immediately or to delay repair depends on the degree of tissue edema or the presence of hematoma or infection.


B. Mukherjee, H. Yuen (eds.), *Emergencies of the Orbit and Adnexa*,
DOI 10.1007/978-81-322-1807-4_9

## Ophthalmological Examination

The ocular examination should be performed meticulously. Observation of ocular adnexa is done before manipulating the injured eye.

- Attempt should be made to determine the visual acuity. Conditions where in visual system evaluation is difficult, optic nerve and retinal functions may be tested by assessing the pupillary reactions. A confrontation visual field examination should also be done for any field loss, if possible.
- In the absence of signs of penetrating ocular injury, a thorough anterior segment examination, IOP measurement, and fundus evaluation must be performed [1].
- One should look for the presence of exophthalmos, since this may indicate a retrobulbar foreign body or hemorrhage [2].
- Subcutaneous emphysema, anesthesia of infraorbital skin, or bony step-offs of orbital rim all indicate orbital bone damage. Presence of marked lid edema may necessitate use of a Desmarres lid retractor [2].

## Evaluation of the Lid Injury

- *Duration*: The time lapsed since the patient acquired injury is important to decide the approach to wound repair. Eyelid wounds should be repaired within 24 h as primary repair gives best functional and cosmetic results. However, in case of life-threatening systemic injuries where the repair has to be postponed, a delayed primary repair can be done 3–5 days later. The wound should be kept clean during this period, and systemic antibiotics and anti-inflammatory drugs should be started. If a primary repair is not done, a secondary repair is usually done after 6 months after the scar has matured [3–5].
- *Mode of Injury*: Whether it is a blunt or penetrating injury. Penetrating injury will produce a clean cut where tissue apposition is easier. Blunt trauma may cause tissue edema and maceration. Identifying the wound edges and approximating in the correct anatomical position are important [3–5].
- *Site of Injury*: Whether the lid margin is intact or lacerated. Injuries in the region of the medial canthus may be associated with lacrimal injuries that should be repaired along with the primary repair.
- *Tissue Loss*: It is essential to note whether there has been any tissue loss because it may necessitate the mobilization of tissue or skin flaps from adjacent areas or free skin grafts (Fig. 9.1a–c).
- *Infection*: If infection is present, the wound repair may be postponed for a few days. During this time, antibiotic and anti-inflammatory drugs should be started. Once the infection has resolved, repair can be done after freshening the wound edges [3–5].
- *Injury to the Levator Aponeurosis*: Full-thickness lid defect or exposed orbital septum suggests injury to the levator muscle or aponeurosis. Inability to look up or absence of any wrinkling of the upper lid skin suggests injury to the levator complex (Fig. 9.2).

## Investigations

Complete blood count and necessary blood chemistry analysis are carried out. Radiologic evaluation is advised when indicated (see Chap. 2).

## Medicolegal Documentation

All injuries must be documented in detail with drawings and clinical photographs.

## Timing of Surgery

In patients presenting within 24 h of injury, primary repair of the wound is undertaken immediately. A delayed primary repair can be done up to 5–7 days provided the wound is not infected. In case of wound infection, the repair is postponed till the infection resolves. For patients with

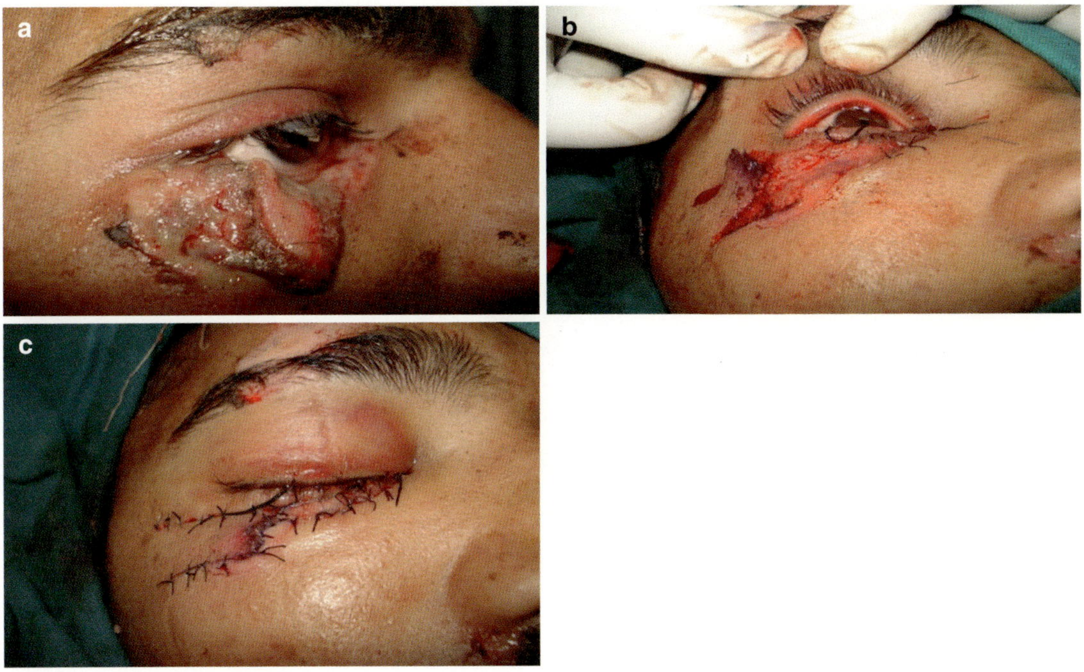


**Fig. 9.1** (**a**) Lower eyelid avulsion with tissue loss. (**b**) Approximation of eyelid margin. (**c**) Repair of the tissue defect done by raising a sliding flap

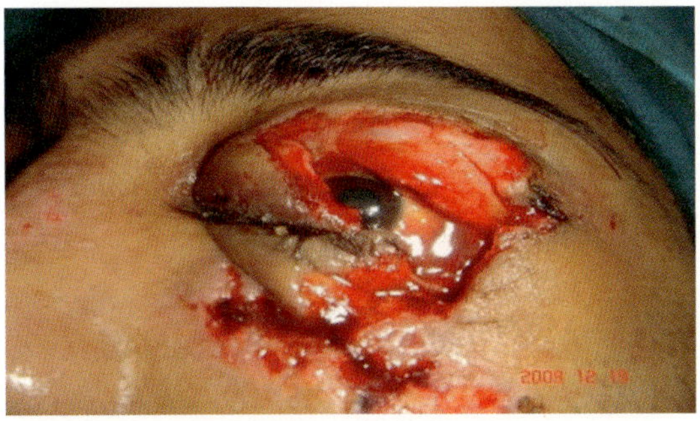

**Fig. 9.2** Eyelid laceration with exposed orbital septum and fat

delayed presentation, a secondary repair should be done 6 months after trauma [5].

## Goals of Eyelid Repair

- To reestablish anatomical configuration
- To restore physiological function
- To provide better cosmetic appearance

## Repair of Eyelid Injuries

Principles to be followed for repair:

- Local/general anesthesia: Most eyelid injuries can be repaired under local anesthesia. In uncooperative patients or children, general anesthesia is required.
- Sustained hemostasis with infiltration of 2 % Xylocaine with adrenaline with bupivacaine.
- Thorough examination (with a focus on the canaliculi, the canthal tendons, and the levator function).
- Cleansing of the wound.
- Removal of foreign material from the wound.
- Debridement of only that tissue that is conclusively devitalized. Due to a rich vascular supply, even tissues that may look ischemic can usually be saved in the periocular area.
- Repair of special structures like the canaliculi, canthal tendons, and levator aponeurosis.
- Closure in layers [4] (Fig. 9.3a, b).

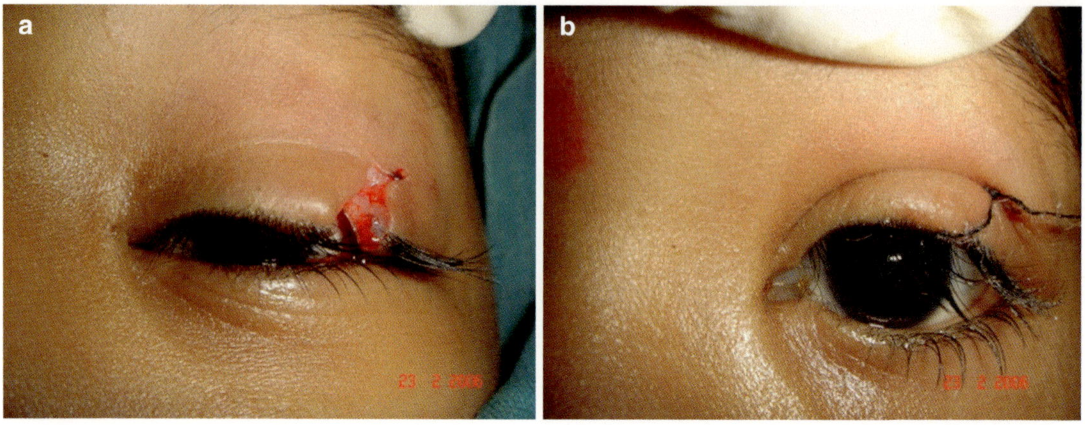


**Fig. 9.3** (**a**) Full-thickness eyelid laceration. (**b**) Full-thickness eyelid laceration repaired in layers

Some basic principles during reconstruction that should be kept in mind are:

- There should be no tension or vertical pulling effect on the lid margins.
- Wound is closed in layers:
  - Subcutaneous closure is done with 5-0 Vicryl.
  - Eyelid skin is usually sutured with 6-0 Nylon or Prolene suture.
  - Nonabsorbable skin sutures should be removed in about 5 days.
- Vertical linear wounds may be broken into multiple Z-plasty in order to improve the scar.
- If the laceration in the upper lid extends upward to involve the eyebrow, it is essential to align the eyebrow first [6].
- The lid margins should be freshened if devitalized tissue is present, to form straight, smooth surgical edges, sacrificing as little tarsus as possible. Meticulous closure of the eyelid margin is crucial. Inadequate closure can lead to lid notching, lagophthalmos, and exposure keratopathy [3, 5].
- Undue tension should be avoided on the marginal laceration as this may lead to wound dehiscence. Whenever there is tension on the wound, one can use the sliding or advancement flaps [7].
- Whenever the orbital fat is exposed, it indicates disruption of the orbital septum, and the wound should be adequately explored [4, 5].
- If the orbital septum has been opened due to injury, it should not be sutured since this could result in lagophthalmos.
- If the laceration is at the level of the lid fold, the eyelid crease is recreated by placing two to three sutures.
- If the lateral canthal tendon (LCT) is found to be severed, it is repaired. One should aim for overcorrection as the healing tends to shift the canthus inferiorly (Fig. 9.4a, b).
- Medial canthal injuries are usually associated with canalicular injury. Intubation of the canaliculus should be performed prior to canthal repair [4, 8].

Adequate primary repair of the lid injury gives the most satisfactory results, and meticulous repair is mandatory for lid injuries. However, where it becomes necessary, a secondary repair gives reasonably good correction, both functional and cosmetic.

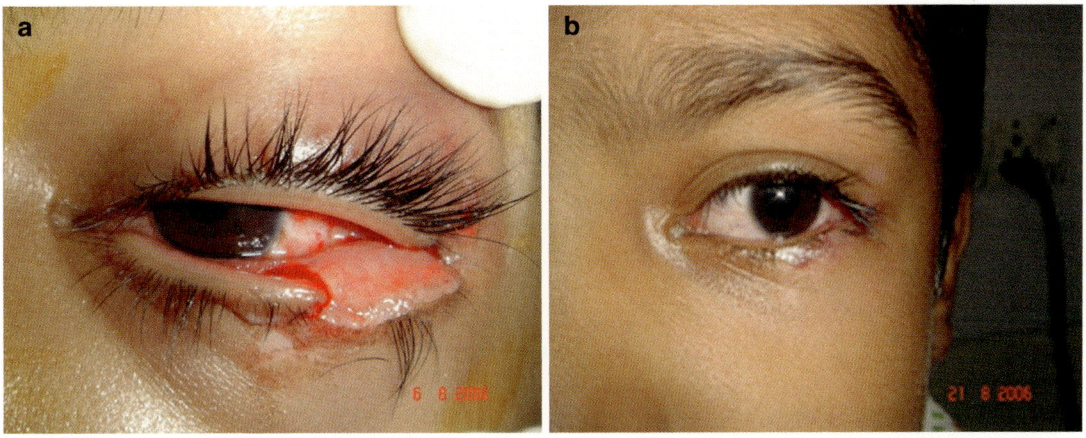


**Fig. 9.4** (**a**) Lower eyelid full-thickness laceration with lateral canthal injury. (**b**) After repair of lower eyelid full-thickness laceration with lateral canthal injury

## References


1. Goldberg MF, Tessler HH. Occult intra ocular perforations from brow and lid lacerations. Arch Ophthalmol. 1971:86;145.
2. Gossaman DM, Berlin JA. Management of acute adnexal trauma. In surgery of eye lid, orbit and lacrimal systems. Am Acad Ophthalmol. 1993;1:p20.
3. Grover AK, Kaur S. Principles of oculoplastic surgery: CME series no.5. AK Grover, editor. All India Ophthalmological Society CME series.
4. Grover AK, Bhatnagar A. Trauma to eyelids, canalicular lacerations and its management. JKSOS. 1991;3(2):135–46.
5. Gupta VP. Basic principles of eye lid reconstruction: CME series No.5. AK Grover, editor. All India Ophthalmological Society CME series.
6. Mustarde JC. Repair and reconstruction in the orbital region. Edinburgh: Churchill Living Stone; 1971. Chap 7–8.
7. Tenzel RR. Reconstruction of the central one half of an eyelid. Arch Ophthalmol. 1975;93:125–6.
8. Reifler DM. Management of canalicular laceration. Surv Ophthalmol. 1991;36:11.


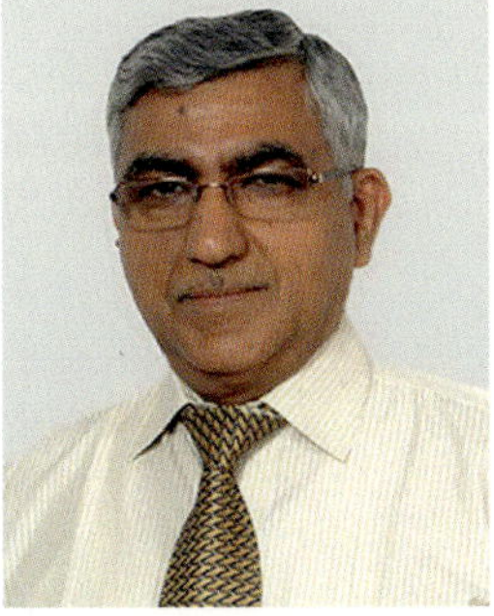

**Ashok K. Grover** Dr. A.K. Grover is recipient of Padmashri Award, one of the highest civilian awards by the President of India for his services to Ophthalmology. He is Chairman, Department of Ophthalmology at Sir Ganga Ram Hospital and Vision Eye Centre in New Delhi.

Dr. Grover is Chairman of Subspecialty Education Committee, International Council of Ophthalmologist (ICO), Councilor at large of the Asia Pacific Academy of Ophthalmology (APAO), Board Member of the Afro Asian Council of Ophthalmology (AACO), and Vice President of the Ocular Trauma Society of India (OTSI). He is Past President of the Asia Pacific Society of Ophthalmic Plastic and Reconstructive Surgery (APSOPRS), Oculoplastics Association of India (OPAI), and All India Ophthalmological Society (AIOS).

Dr. Grover serves on the Editorial Board of the *Asia Pacific Journal of Ophthalmology, Indian Journal of Ophthalmology, Nepalese Journal of Ophthalmology, Journal of International Medical Science Academy, Ocular Surgery News* (Asia Pacific Edition), and is a reviewer for several international/national journals. He is an examiner for FRCS (Glasgow).

Dr. Grover has received numerous prestigious Awards and Orations including the Distinguished Service Award from Asia Pacific Academy of Ophthalmology, Honorary FRCS, Honorary Fellowship of International Council of Ophthalmology (FICO), Col. Rangachari Award for the best paper from the All India Ophthalmological Society, and other numerous International and National Orations.

Dr. Grover has authored/edited 4 books, written over 60 chapters in textbooks, has over 75 publications, and over 1000 presentations at international and national levels. He has chaired sessions, been Guest Speaker, and done live surgery all over the globe including the World Congress, APAO, Afro Asian Academy, American Academy, APSOPRS, and National meetings.

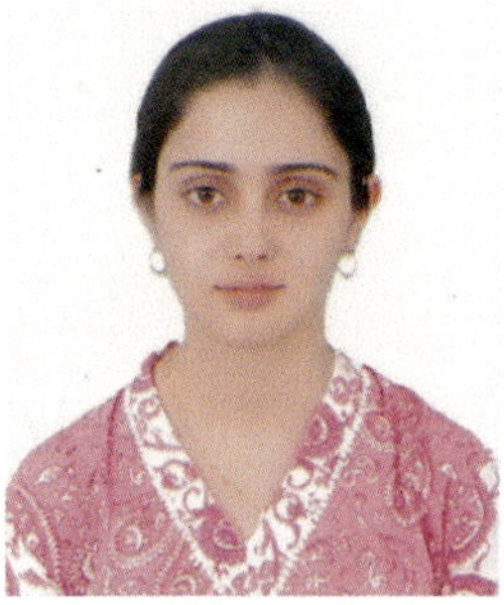

**Saurbhi Khurana** Dr. Saurbhi Khurana got her MBBS degree from the Maulana Azad Medical College in the year 2006. She did her MD in ophthalmology from Dr. Rajendra Prasad Centre for Ophthalmic Sciences, AIIMS, New Delhi in the year 2009. She was a senior resident at the same institute in the Department of Oculoplasty and Pediatric Ophthalmology till 2012. Following her senior residency, she did an oculoplasty fellowship at the Leicester University, UK. She has authored many peer-reviewed articles and is an invited faculty at various conferences. She is a skilled oculoplastic and aesthetic surgeon.

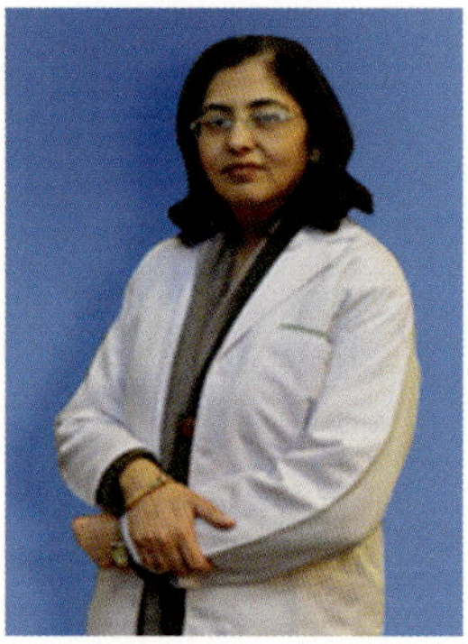

**Shaloo Bageja** Dr. Shaloo Bageja is working as a consultant in the Department of Ophthalmology at Sir Ganga Ram Hospital since January 2006. She is working as an anterior segment surgeon with special interest in Oculoplastics.

Dr. Shaloo Bageja is representing Ocular Trauma Society of India as North Zone representative. She has also served as joint secretary of the Ocular Trauma Society. She was the organizing secretary of the APSOPRS-OPAI meeting held in New Delhi in 2014.

Dr. Shaloo Bageja has written 38 chapters in textbooks, has over 15 publications in peer- and non-peer-reviewed journals. She has presented over 25 papers at the national level. She has won the best paper presentation in oculoplastic session in All India Ophthalmic Society meeting. She has chaired sessions and has been guest speaker in AIOS, OPAI, and DOS meetings.

# Investigation of Eyelid and Lacrimal Injuries

10

Marian Pauly and Bipasha Mukherjee

The number of investigations carried out in an emergency setting, in a patient of isolated lid and/or lacrimal trauma, is limited.

The primary aim of the treating consultant would be to rule out associated trauma to the globe or deeper orbital structures. Outlined below are the investigations that are useful in specific situations.

## Blood Tests

Routine blood examination and random blood sugar is sufficient before any surgical repair. Coagulation parameters are indicated if the patient is on anticoagulants or gives history of chronic liver disease. Test for viral markers like HIV/HbsAg/HCV, should be undertaken, with the patients' consent, before any major repair [1, 2].

M. Pauly, MBBS, MS, DNB
Orbit, Oculoplasty and Aesthetics,
Giridhar Eye Institute, Kochi 682020, Kerala, India
e-mail: marianpauly09@yahoo.com

B. Mukherjee, MS, DNB (Ophthalmology), FICO (✉)
Orbit, Oculoplasty, Reconstructive & Aesthetic Services, Sankara Nethralaya,
Chennai, Tamil Nadu 600006, India
e-mail: drbpm@snmail.org

## Imaging

Chest X-ray is indicated if the surgery is under general anaesthesia. Plain X-rays of the orbit and paranasal sinus (PNS) may be requested in suspected foreign bodies or orbital fractures where CT facility is unavailable (although blowout fractures maybe missed). After ruling out open globe injury, Ultrasound B scan is done if the fundus details are not visible, to rule out intraocular foreign body and/or posterior segment involvement.

Computed tomography (CT) [3, 4] scan is the investigation of choice in suspected orbital fractures, foreign bodies and extraocular injury to intracranial, nasal and sinus structures. High-resolution scan with 2–3 mm sections is obtained. The scan should be studied in both bone and soft tissue window settings. Reformatted coronal views [5] should be obtained.

Imaging of lacrimal system is often indicated in traumatic NLDO for proper assessment. CT-DCG is considered the gold standard for imaging of the nasolacrimal system.

Magnetic resonance imaging [6] may be useful to rule out organic or wooden foreign body, but it is contraindicated in the presence of metallic foreign bodies.


B. Mukherjee, H. Yuen (eds.), *Emergencies of the Orbit and Adnexa*,
DOI 10.1007/978-81-322-1807-4_10

## Further Investigations

A detailed ocular examination, preferably with the slit lamp, is mandatory in each and every patient, with special attention to medial canthal area so as not to overlook canalicular involvement.

Echocardiography may be needed in patients with cardiac disorders before proceeding to the repair under general anaesthesia.

Visual evoked potential (VEP) is helpful in documenting optic nerve function, especially in unconscious patients, pre-verbal children, and in cases of suspected optic neuropathy [7].

In conclusion, judicial use of various investigative modalities is helpful in attaining a satisfactory management outcome.

## References

1. McCord Jr CD. System of repair of full-thickness eyelid defects. In: McCord Jr CD, Tanenbaum M, editors. Oculoplastic surgery. 2nd ed. New York: Raven Press; 1987. p. 117–27.
2. Chang EL, Rubin PA. Management of complex eyelid lacerations. Int Ophthalmol Clin. 2002;42(3): 187–201.
3. Joseph DP, Pieramici DJ, Beauchamp NJ. Computed tomography in the diagnosis and prognosis of open globe injuries. Ophthalmology. 2000;107: 1899–906.
4. Lakets A, Prokesch R, Scholda C. Orbital helical computed tomography in the diagnosis and management of eye trauma. Ophthalmology. 1999;106: 2330–5.
5. Ho VH, Wilson MW, Fleming JC. Retained intraorbital metallic foreign bodies. Ophthal Plast Reconstr Surg. 2009;20:232–6.
6. Nasr AM, Hail BG, Fleming JC. Penetrating orbital injury with organic foreign bodies. Ophthalmology. 1999;106:523–32.
7. Cornelius CP, Altenmüller E, Ehrenfeld. The use of flash visual evoked potentials in the early diagnosis of suspected optic nerve lesions due to craniofacial trauma. J Craniomaxillofac Surg. 1996;24(1):1–11.

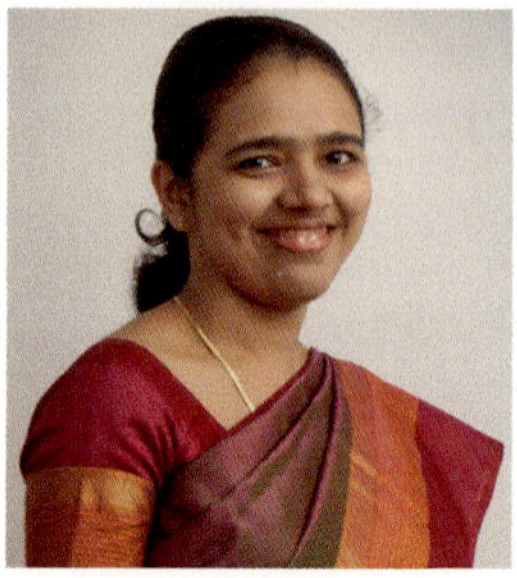

**Marian Pauly** Dr. Marian Pauly received her Master's Degree in Ophthalmology from University of Kerala, India and later she underwent for 2 years fellowship in Orbit and Oculoplasty from the prestigious Sankara Netralaya, Chennai, India. She is a life member of Oculoplastic Society of India. She is the recipient of Dr Gangadhara Sundar Award for young Oculoplastic Surgeon as well as Jayaben Chamanlal Shah Gold Medal for Best Outgoing Sub-Specialty Fellow. Currently she is practicing in Giridhar Eye Institute, Kerala, India

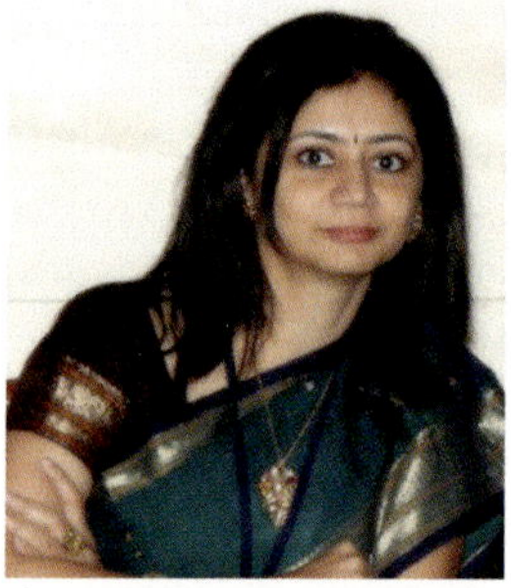

**Bipasha Mukherjee** Dr. Bipasha Mukherjee is a fellow in Orbit & Oculoplasty from Aravind Eye Hospitals, India, and ICO fellow from University Hospital of Limoges, France, under Prof. Jean-Paul Adenis. She has undergone clinical observerships with stalwarts like Jack Rootman, Richard Collins, Geoff Rose, Mark Duffy, and Robert Goldberg.

She currently heads the department of Orbit, Oculoplasty, Aesthetic & Reconstructive services in Medical Research Foundation, Chennai. She has numerous presentations in national and international conferences and publications in peer-reviewed journals and text books. Her areas of interest include diseases of the orbit and adnexa including tumors, lacrimal surgery, socket reconstruction, traumatic lid and adnexal injuries, training residents and fellows, and photography.

# Management of Eyelid Injuries

# 11

Marian Pauly

The most important function of the eyelid is to protect the globe. Therefore, eyelid trauma has to be managed in a very meticulous manner to avoid damage to eyeball.

## History

A thorough history is important as to the cause of injury. Road traffic accidents, machinery and intentional assaults can cause injury to the eyelid. History regarding the time, date and site of injury is important in deciding the management as well as medicolegal aspects. Injury to the surrounding structures should be ruled out by asking the history of epistaxis, double vision, decreased vision, numbness along infraorbital region and difficulty in opening the mouth.

## Examination

Before evaluating the localised injury to the eyelid, the general medical status of the patient has to be evaluated by looking at ABC (airway, breathing and circulation) [1, 2]. Patients with life-threatening emergencies have to be managed immediately by a specialised trauma team before proceeding to the management of eyelid.

Complete ophthalmological evaluation has to be done which includes visual acuity, pupillary reaction, applanation tonometry if the globe is intact and dilated fundus evaluation. In the absence of signs of intraocular injury/penetrating injury, management of eyelid injury can be planned.

Photograph and drawings of the injury are important chart documents.

## Examination of Eyelid Injury

Irrigate and explore (Fig. 11.1a, b): Irrigate the wound thoroughly with cold saline after putting the topical anaesthetic agent, and remove all foreign materials and blood clots and document the site, size and shape of injury.

Laceration involving the lid margin needs special attention. Injury near the medial and lateral canthus can have associated canthal tendon injury and canalicular injury.

Look for any loss of tissue. If tissue loss is present, tissue transfer/mobilisation has to be planned preoperatively.

Look for the presence of the fat in the wound. It indicates injury to the levator muscle/septum [3, 4]. Check the levator function by asking the patient to look up and down after occluding the frontalis action. Change in the lid contour also denotes levator injury/avulsion.

M. Pauly, MBBS, MS, DNB
Orbit, Oculoplasty and Aesthetics, Giridhar Eye Institute, Kochi, Kerala 682020, India
e-mail: marianpauly09@yahoo.com



B. Mukherjee, H. Yuen (eds.), *Emergencies of the Orbit and Adnexa*,
DOI 10.1007/978-81-322-1807-4_11

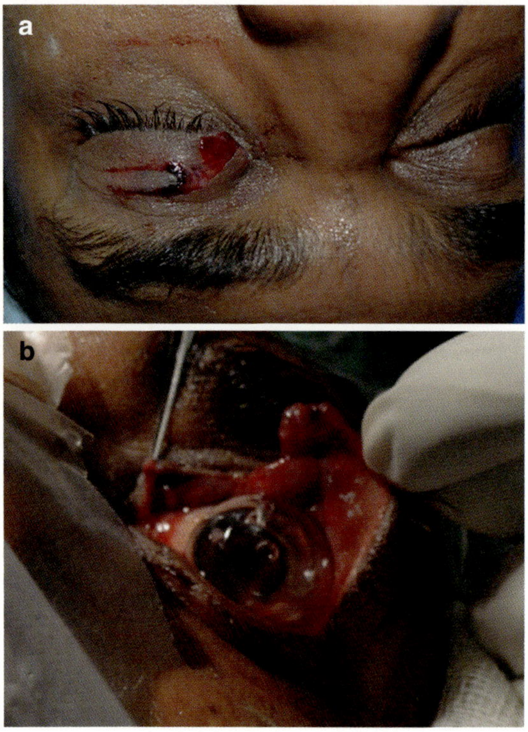

**Fig. 11.1** (**a**) On exploration, patient had levator and canalicular injury. (**b**) On exploration, patient had levator and canalicular injury

Look for any signs of infection. If infection is present, delay the wound repair till infection subsides.

## Laboratory and Radiologic Evaluation (See Sect. "Investigations" in Chap. 2)

### Timing of Repair

The timing of eyelid repair is flexible. In the toxicated or poorly cooperative patient, a prudent delay until the patient is fully manageable is often indicated. The delay may improve the overall chance of success and patient safety.

If the patient is presenting within 24 h of injury, primary repair can be done [4] which will improve the functional cosmetic results. Delayed primary repair is done when there is marked lid oedema or infection or when the patient presents after 24 h of injury [3, 5]. This is performed after 3–4 days. During this waiting time, cold compresses, systemic antibiotics and anti-inflammatory agents have to be administered.

### Basic Surgical Principles

1. Re-approximate the tissue as accurately as possible.
2. The closure should be done with minimal tension.
3. Obliteration of dead space.
4. Layered repair.
5. Good lighting and haemostasis.

### Anaesthesia

Local anaesthesia/general anaesthesia.

Sustained haemostasis with infiltration of 2 % Xylocaine with adrenaline.

Monitored anaesthetic care is preferred.

Regional anaesthesia is the most effective approach for laceration repair since it minimally distorts tissues and will provide profound anaesthesia to large areas [6]. Injection of the infraorbital, supraorbital, infratrochlear and supratrochlear nerves is adequate for the repair of most lacerations involving the eyelids, lacrimal drainage system and periorbital soft tissue.

## Common Clinical Scenarios

### Superficial/Deep Laceration Not Involving the Eyelid Margin (Fig. 11.2)

This can be managed by a simple closure/layered closure. 3-7 absorbable sutures are used for deeper tissues, and the skin is sutured with 3-7 silk/nylon/plain gut. Undermine the edges, if the wound is under tension. Rounded defects can be converted to elliptical defect before suturing, to avoid dog ears. The knots should be buried, and the suture is placed partially in the dermis to close the subcutaneous tissue.

Simple interrupted sutures are adequate, but horizontal/vertical mattress sutures are needed if the wound is under tension. The septum should be left unsutured both to avoid postoperative lagophthalmos and to lessen the effects of postoperative haemorrhage. It should not be closed or incorporated into deeper or superficial sutures. The skin sutures are removed in 5–7 days time.

Fibrin glue or cyanoacrylate glue can be used in dry clean wounds. The glue will disintegrate in 3–5 days time. Antibiotic ointments are avoided as it can facilitate the early disintegration of glue. It should not be used in ragged, stellate, contaminated and crush wounds [7–10].

Antitension taping (Fig. 11.3a, b) can be used in wounds involving only the skin which will approximate the skin edges and prevent the formation of a wide scar.

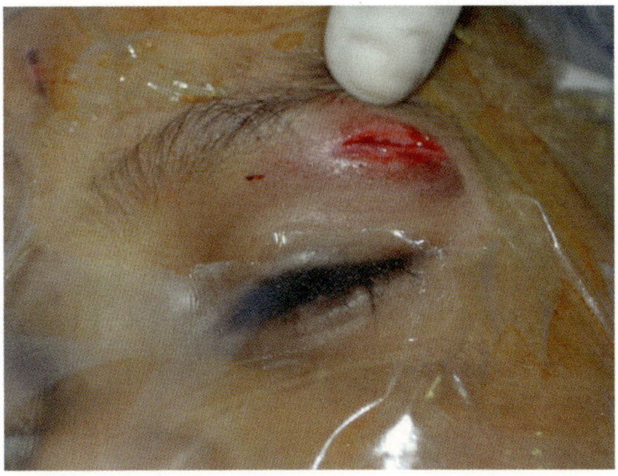

**Fig. 11.2** Deep laceration involving the eyebrow

## Lacerations Involving the Eyelid Margin

Exact repair of the lid margin is critical to avoid notching or margin discontinuity which can cause functional and cosmetic problems. The first step is to identify the tarsus and lid margin landmarks like the grey line, the meibomian gland orifices and the lash line. If the wound is ragged, freshening the edges with a scalpel blade may aid in structure recognition and wound apposition.

Using toothed forceps or skin hooks, the edges are brought together to allow assessment of tension on the wound. If the wound is tight, canthotomy or cantholysis is done to decrease the tension on the wound edges.

Margin is sutured by triple suture technique [11, 12]:

Meibomian gland orifice
Grey line
Lash line

First align the lid margin by passing a suture through the meibomian gland orifice on both edges of the cut 2 mm from the edge, and look for the alignment. If the alignment and wound tension is adequate, pass a vertical mattress suture [13] and keep the ends long. This long ends can be used as traction suture for further steps.

Align the tarsal plate with 5–0 Vicryl suture. The suture should pass through 90 % of the tar-

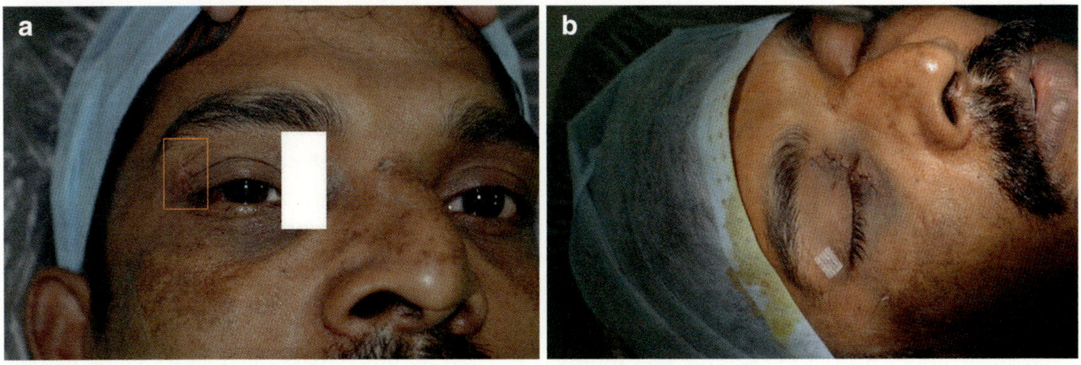


**Fig. 11.3** (**a**) Small superficial laceration involving only the skin managed with antitension taping (*before*). (**b**) Small superficial laceration involving only the skin managed with antitension taping (*after*)

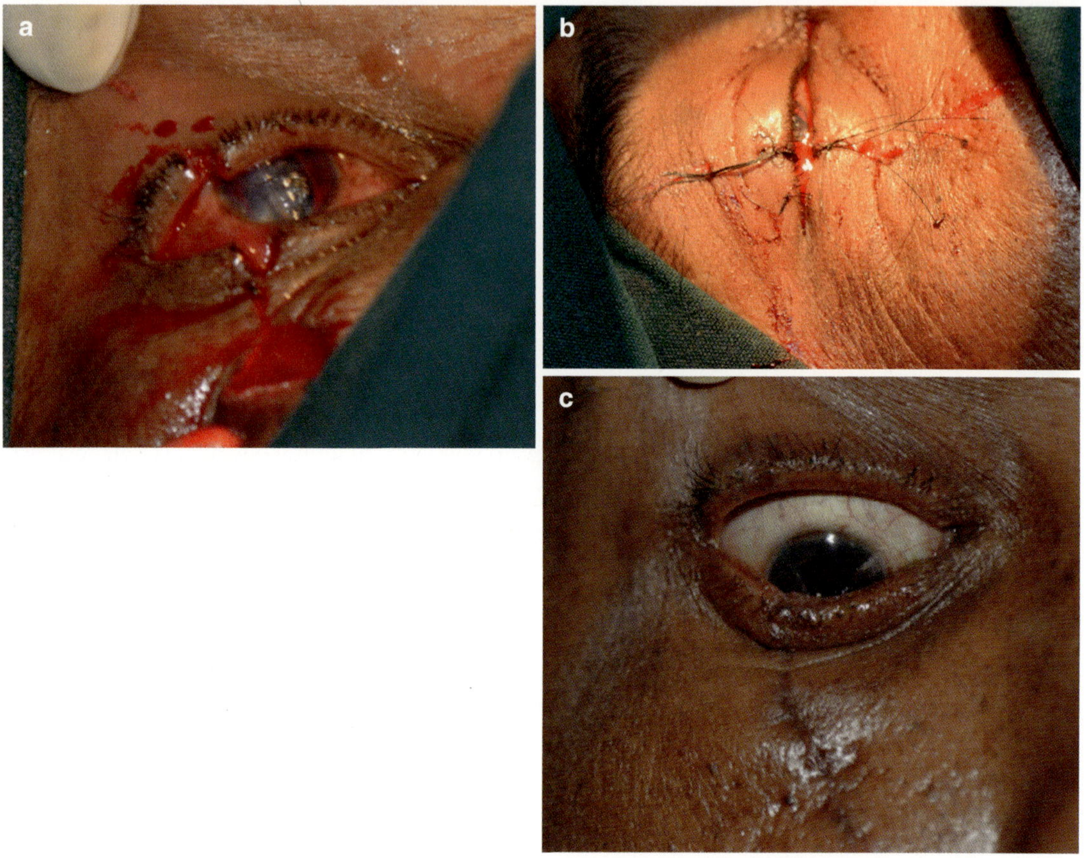


**Fig. 11.4** (**a**) Laceration involving eyelid margin of both the upper and lower lid. (**b**) Sutures are tied anteriorly. Long ends can be trimmed. The upper lid sutured with 6/0 silk, whereas the lower lid with 6/0 nylon. (**c**) Two weeks post-op view after suture removal

sal plate, and the knots should come on the anterior side [14]. Full-thickness tarsal sutures are avoided as it can erode the conjunctiva to cause suture keratopathy. Two sutures are taken in upper lid whereas single suture in the lower lid. These tarsal sutures support the lid and prevent a sag in the lid margin which may lead to a notch.

Complete the lid margin suturing by taking sutures along the grey line and lash line. All the knots should come anterior and tied in the skin suture so that the long ends will not irritate the ocular surface. The grey line suture can be an optional suture. The wound edges should be everted. Do not tie the margin sutures very tightly because tissue may die resulting in lid margin notch. The orbicularis and skin are sutured with simple interrupted sutures. The lid margin sutures are removed after 10 days (Fig. 11.4a–c).

In children (Fig. 11.5a, b), this can be done with 6–0 Vicryl sutures and can be left to dissolve spontaneously.

## Lacerations Associated with Canthal Tendon Injuries

Trauma to the medial and lateral canthal tendon is usually the result of horizontal traction on the eyelid leading to avulsion at the weakest part either medial or lateral canthus. Laceration near medial canthus is associated with canalicular and lacrimal sac injury in most of the cases. Assess the integrity of medial and lateral canthal tendon

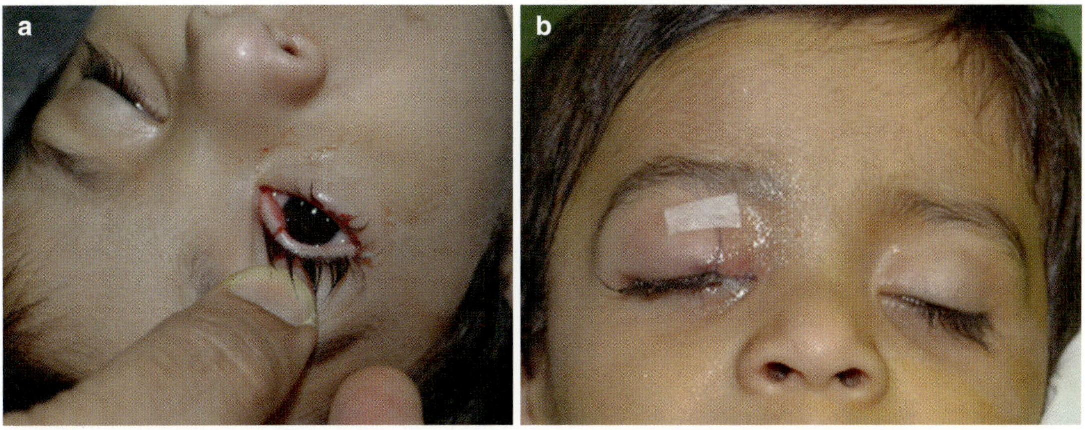

**Fig. 11.5** (**a**) Child with lid margin tear. (**b**) Lid margin tear sutured with Vicryl and long ends taped over the lid with Steri-Strip

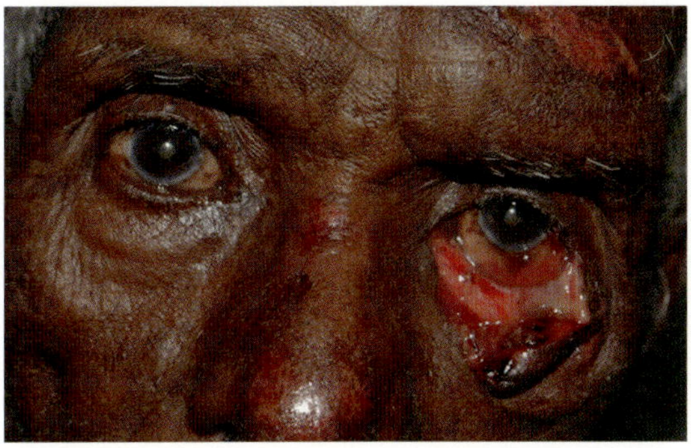

**Fig. 11.6** Photograph showing medial canthal avulsion with total displacement of the lid laterally

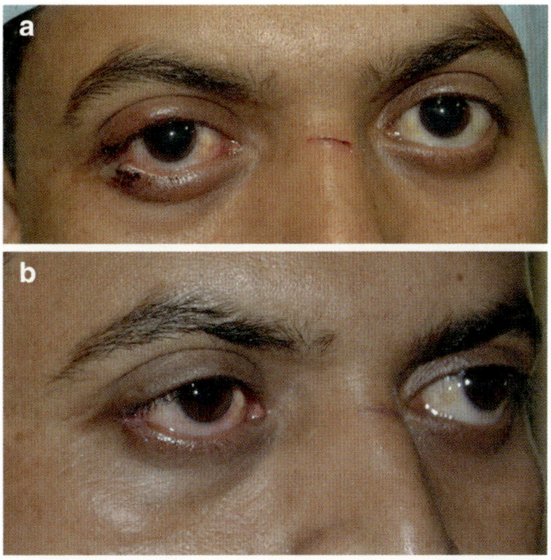

**Fig. 11.7** (**a**) The lower lid is detached from the lateral canthus involving the inferior limb of the lateral canthal tendon. (**b**) Direct suturing done and the lid is attached to the lateral canthus assuming the sharp contour

by grasping the lid with a toothed forceps and tugging away from the injury while palpating the tendon insertion. The surgeon should assess whether the anterior or posterior limb is avulsed. Repair of the posterior limb is more critical to achieve proper lid positioning.

One should assess whether there is soft tissue injury alone or bone is also fractured by taking a CT scan. There will be rounding of the medial canthus, lateral displacement of punctum and acquired telecanthus in medial canthal tendon injuries (Fig. 11.6), whereas the sharp contour of the lateral canthal angle will be lost (Fig. 11.7a, b) or distorted in lateral canthal injuries. Before proceeding to the repair, canalicular apparatus injury has to be managed.

## Injuries Involving the Medial Canthal Tendon

If the cut ends are identified, suture it with 5–0 or 4–0 Prolene or polyester suture in a horizontal mattress fashion. If the proximal part is not identified, suture the ends to the periorbita.

If the entire tendon is avulsed from the bone, including the posterior portion, but there is no naso-orbital fracture, the avulsed tendon should be wired through small drill holes in the ipsilateral posterior lacrimal crest [15].

If the entire tendon is avulsed and there is a naso-orbital fracture, transnasal wiring or plating is necessary after reduction of the fracture. A Y-shaped miniplate may be fixed anteriorly on the nasal bone, with posterior extension into the orbit [16]. The suture is sewn through the severed tendons and passed through the holes in the miniplate. This technique is particularly helpful when the bone of the posterior lacrimal crest is missing. If neither of these procedures can be utilised, it is necessary to reattach the tendon using transnasal wiring [17]. Special care should be taken to avoid damage to the lacrimal sac.

## Injuries Involving the Lateral Canthal Tendon [15]

If the cut ends are identified, it is sutured together with 4/0 Prolene in a horizontal mattress fashion.

If the cut ends are not identified, attach to the lateral orbital rim above the lateral tubercle using a drill hole and permanent large suture (2–0 nylon/28 gauge wire).

## Lacerations Involving Injury to the Levator Muscle or Aponeurosis

Levator injury is suspected when patient presents with ptosis (Fig. 11.8a, b) or fat in the wound. In case of ptosis alone without any external injuries, observe for 6–12 months before any surgical intervention, as spontaneous resolution can occur in this period [18].

If fat is present, the septum is injured, and there is a potential chance of injury to the levator also. Explore the wound and try to identify the levator. If patient is under general anaesthesia, the vertical orientation of levator fibres is helpful in contrast to the horizontal direction of orbicularis fibres. Under local anaesthesia, grasp the levator and ask the patient to look up and down. The muscle will move with the globe movement. To identify the septum, as patient looks down, we will get a tight feeling as it is attached to the orbital rim. If the levator aponeurosis is found detached, attach it the tarsal pate with 5/0 Vicryl suture. If the injury is at the level of the lid fold, recreate the lid fold by taking a bite through the levator while doing closure of the orbicularis muscle. Care should be taken to avoid suture of the septum or incorporating it in the other suture to avoid lagophthalmos and lid lag. Transient ptosis (Fig. 11.9a, b) can occur even after reattachment which will improve over a period of 1 year [18–21].

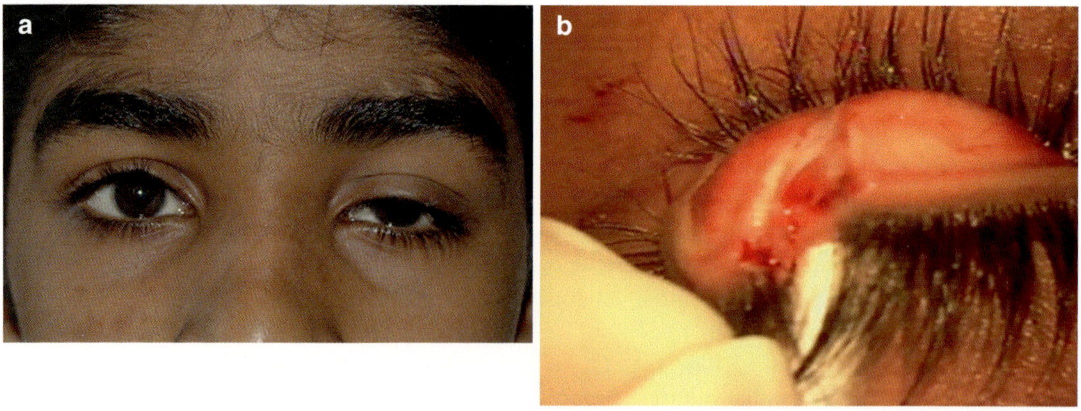


**Fig. 11.8** (**a**) A 12-year-old child presenting 5 days following trauma. Examination revealed mild ptosis with good levator function and healed lid margin tear. (**b**) On everting the lid, partial dehiscence of the levator along with the tarsal plate injury is noticed

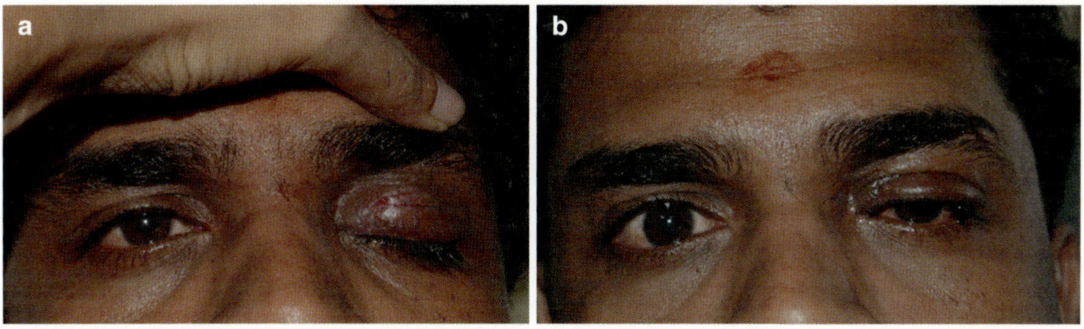


**Fig. 11.9** (**a**) Total ptosis following repair of the dehisced levator (1 week post-op). (**b**) Gradual recovery of ptosis over 2 months

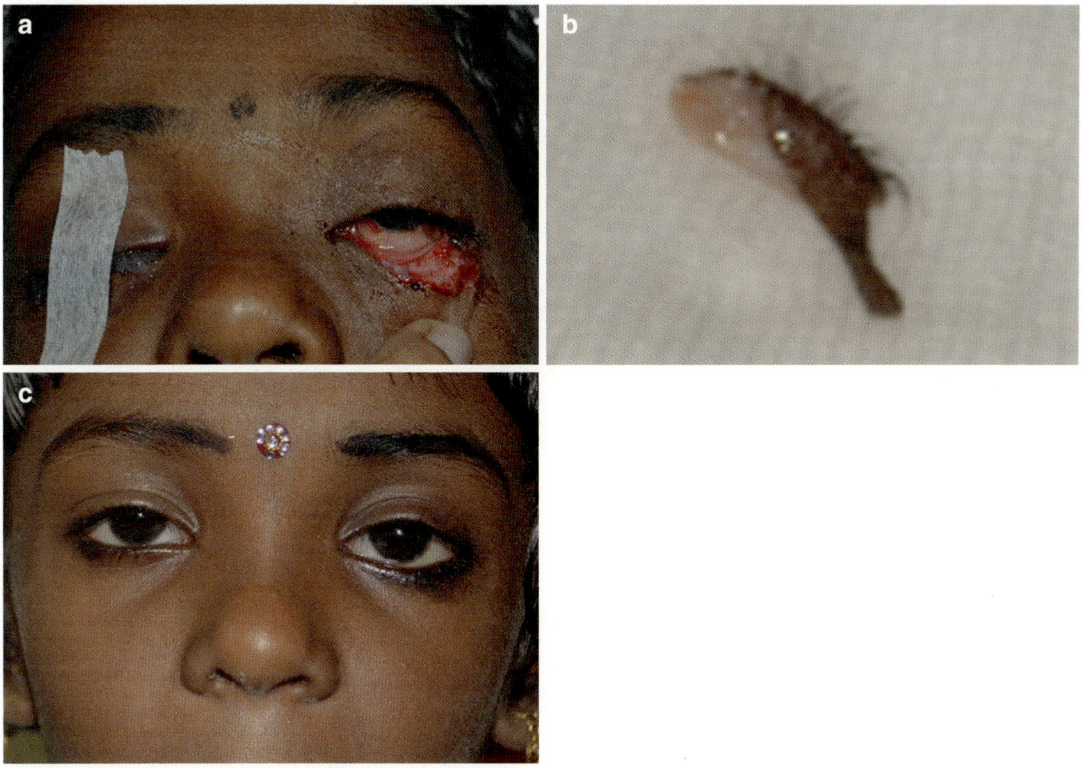


**Fig. 11.10** (**a**) Total lid avulsion following injury with bicycle. (**b**) The lost tissue retrieved from injury site after 2 h. (**c**) Replantation of the lid done after 6 h of injury with good graft take-up. Loss of cilia and lid retraction present

## **Total Lid Avulsion** (Fig. 11.10a–c)

In total avulsion, try to retrieve the lost tissues as early as possible [22, 23]. In isolated cases, examining the injury site will help in this regard. Once the tissue is retrieved, debride it and keep in wet gauze with gentamicin at 4 °C until the time of replantation. Even though there are chances of infection and tissue necrosis, excellent results are possible because of the rich blood supply of the lid. If the lost tissue cannot be retrieved, then the lid has to be reconstructed with various flaps and grafts.

## Postoperative Care

Small lacerations can be managed on an outpatient basis. Ice compresses should be used for 24–48 h to reduce postoperative oedema. Warm compresses can be used after that time period. Patients should be informed about the signs of wound infection. Postoperative pain management is done with nonsteroidal anti-inflammatory agent such as ibuprofen which is continued for 72 h, which will also help in reducing the tissue oedema. To reduce the incidence of postoperative oedema, it is helpful to have patients sleep with their head elevated and also try to sleep on the side opposite to the side of surgery.

Patients with severe trauma should be hospitalised for at least 24 h and possibly longer, depending on the extent of the trauma and the stability of the patient's condition. Postoperative ocular antibiotic ointments are applied twice daily to repair lacerations which will help in wound prophylaxis. It is usually not necessary to use oral or intravenous antibiotics in the postoperative period except in cases of "dirty" wounds or bite injuries. In these cases, intravenous clindamycin or cefazolin and oral amoxicillin-clavulanate are the antibiotics of choice to provide coverage for both resistant staphylococci and anaerobes.

Cutaneous sutures should generally be removed 5–7 days after placement. Skin sutures in areas under extensive tension such as the cheek and forehead may be left in place for 7 days. Silk sutures are associated with an inflammatory reaction and if left in place for too long will be associated with unsightly scarring. Nylon and polypropylene sutures do not have this problem. Eyelid margin sutures should be left for 10–14 days to prevent wound separation. After suture removal, if there appears to be some gaping of the wound or if the wound is still on some tension, Steri-Strips or adhesive tape can be used for support and to physically close the wound until adequate healing has taken place.

## Eyelid Contusion and Hematoma

Contusions are bruising injuries frequently associated with blunt trauma. The injured tissue becomes oedematous, and there may be an underlying hematoma or subconjunctival or orbital haemorrhage. Usually such injuries will resolve without the need for therapy beyond the use of cold compresses for 24–48 h. Warm compresses should be used after the initial 48 h. Imaging of the orbit is done to rule out underlying fractures. Dark glasses will help to further mask the presence of periorbital ecchymoses. Occasionally, the swelling may be severe and cause a dehiscence of the levator aponeurosis. However, this often cannot be determined until there has been resolution of the acute injury.

Significant hematomas of the eyelid and periorbital structures may not spontaneously resorb. If left untreated, this can provide a nidus for infection and result in significant scarring. A persistent hematoma (Fig. 11.11a, b) can be easily evacuated with a simple skin incision. This incision should be placed within the eyelid crease, a skinfold or a relaxed skin tension line to reduce the

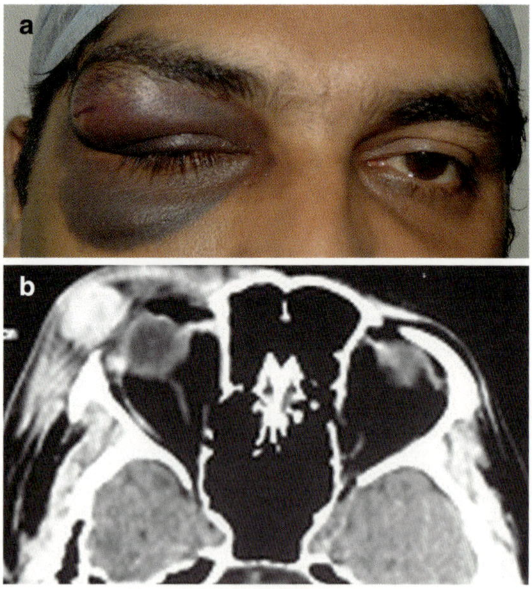


**Fig. 11.11** (**a**) A large hematoma involving the (R) eyebrow with mechanical ptosis and periorbital ecchymosis. (**b**) CT scan orbit showing organised hematoma

chance of postoperative scarring. When liquefied, the hematoma can be aspirated using a large-bore (16 or 18 gauge) needle. Loculated hematomas may require the aspiration needle to be inserted several times in different places. Patients should be warned that while initially unilateral, swelling and ecchymoses may spread to the uninjured side or to other portions of the face. The presence of proptosis indicates an associated orbital haemorrhage. Evaluation of the patient's vision, pupillary function and intraocular pressure for the first 24 h after injury is important for identifying the presence or occurrence of compressive optic neuropathy associated with orbital haemorrhage.

## Complications of Lid Repair

### Lid Margin Notching and Coloboma (Fig. 11.12)

Avoided by careful suturing. Small spontaneous improvement often occurs. However, a large notch requires full-thickness pentagonal wedge resection and repair.

### Lagophthalmos

Occurs from unrecognised tissue loss, scarring or incorporation of septum into the superficial wound. Prevention is the key, but once occurred, it can be corrected by vertical lid lengthening, lengthening of the skin and muscle with skin graft. Lower lid ectropion can occur resulting in lagophthalmos. Z-plasty and skin flap transpositions are often futile [24].

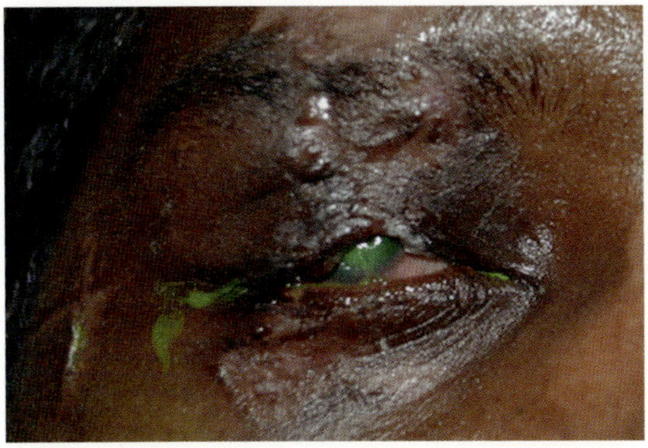

**Fig. 11.12** Lid coloboma with exposure keratopathy following lid repair

### Hypertrophic Scars

Various anti-scar creams and silicone gel sheet can be used to lighten the scar.

### Infections

Very rare. If it occurs, rule out unrecognised foreign body.

### Epiphora

Occurs due to various reasons like lid malposition, poor lacrimal pump and obstruction of drainage duct which has to be dealt individually.

### Traumatic Telecanthus and Canthal Dystopia (Fig 11.13)

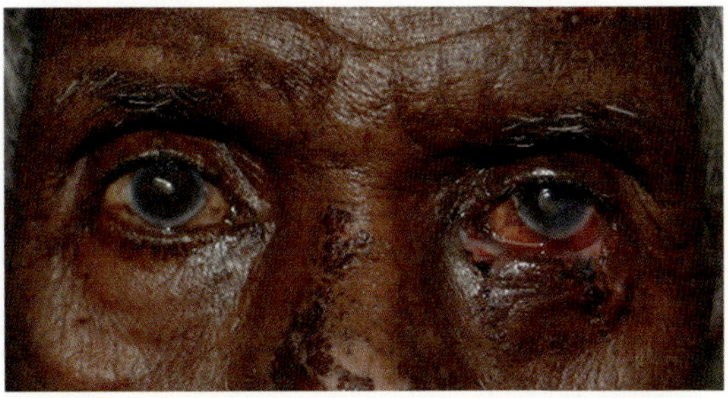

**Fig. 11.13** Failure to reattach the medial canthal tendon leading to canthal dystopia

**Conclusion**

Excellent functional and cosmetic results are possible with planned and meticulous surgical technique.

## References


1. Hartstein ME, Fink SR. Traumatic eyelid injuries. Int Ophthalmol Clin. 2002;42(2):123–34.
2. Beadles KA, Lessner AM. Management of traumatic eyelid lacerations. Semin Ophthalmol. 1994;9(3):145–51.
3. McCord Jr CD. System of repair of full-thickness eyelid defects. In: McCord Jr CD, Tanenbaum M, editors. Oculoplastic surgery. 2nd ed. New York: Raven Press; 1987. p. 117–27.
4. Nelson C. Management of eyelid trauma. Aust N Z J Ophthalmol. 1991;19:357–63.
5. Chang EL, Rubin PA. Management of complex eyelid lacerations. Int Ophthalmol Clin. 2002;42(3):187–201.
6. Ismail AR, Anthony T, Mordant DJ, MacLean H. Regional nerve block of the upper eyelid in oculoplastic surgery. Eur J Ophthalmol. 2006;16(4):509–13.
7. Lins RD, Gomes RC, Santos KS, Silva PV, Silva RT, Ramos IA. Use of cyanoacrylate in the coaptation of edges of surgical wounds. An Bras Dermatol. 2012;87(6):871–6.
8. Mattick A. Use of tissue adhesives in the management of paediatric lacerations. Emerg Med J. 2002;19(5):382–5.
9. Singer AJ, Quinn JV, Hollander JE. The cyanoacrylate topical skin adhesives. Am J Emerg Med. 2008;26(4):490–6.
10. Gilbert L, Pogorzalek N, Jounda G, Barreau E. Traumatic peri-ocular injuries: closing wounds using 2-octyl-cyanoacrylate medical glue. J Fr Ophtalmol. 2009;32(5):341–7.
11. Nerad JA. Techniques in ophthalmic plastic surgery: a personal tutorial. Chapter 13 eyelid and orbital trauma. USA: Saunders Elsevier; 2010. p. 355–87.
12. Kuhn F, Pieramici DJ. Ocular trauma: principles and practice: chapter 35 eyelid and lacrimal trauma. New York: Thieme Medical Publishers; 2002. p. 373–82.
13. Perry JD, Aguilar CL, Kuchtey R. Modified vertical mattress technique for eyelid margin repair. Dermatol Surg. 2004;30(12 Pt 2):1580–2.
14. Divine RD, Anderson RL. Techniques in eyelid wound closure. Ophthalmic Surg. 1982;13(4):283–7.
15. Black EH. Smith and Nesi's ophthalmic plastic and reconstructive surgery chapter 9 management of ocular adnexal trauma. 3rd ed. New York: Springer; 2012. p. 215–6.
16. Shore JW, Rubin PA, Bilyk JR. Repair of telecanthus by anterior fixation of cantilevered miniplates. Ophthalmology. 1992;99(7):1133–8.
17. Elbarbary AS, Ali A. Medial canthopexy of old unrepaired naso-orbito-ethmoidal (nose) traumatic telecanthus. J Craniomaxillofac Surg. 2014;42(2):106–12.
18. Betharia SM, Kumar S. Levator surgery in post traumatic ptosis. Indian J Ophthalmol. 1987;35(3):132–5.
19. Silkiss RZ, Baylis HI. Management of traumatic ptosis. Adv Ophthalmic Plast Reconstr Surg. 1987;7:149–55.
20. McCulley TJ, Kersten RC, Yip CC, Kulwin DR. Isolated unilateral neurogenic blepharoptosis secondary to eyelid trauma. Am J Ophthalmol. 2002;134(4):626–7.
21. Dinh Doan G, Noel D, Chassagne JF, Rodier C. Traumatic rupture of the levator tendon of the upper eyelid. Rev Stomatol Chir Maxillofac. 1992;93(3):154–7.
22. Yeatts RP, Hoopes Jr PC, Saunders SS. Eyelid replantation eight months after traumatic avulsion. Ophthal Plast Reconstr Surg. 2004;20(5):390–2.
23. Goldberg SH, Bullock JD, Connelly PJ. Eyelid avulsion: a clinical and experimental study. Ophthal Plast Reconstr Surg. 1992;8(4):256–61.
24. Shockley WW. Scar revision techniques: z-plasty, w-plasty, and geometric broken line closure. Facial Plast Surg Clin North Am. 2011;19(3):455–63.


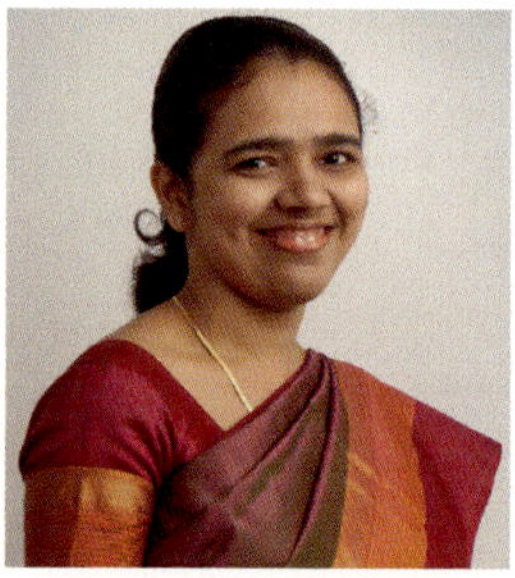

**Marian Pauly** Dr. Marian Pauly received her Master's Degree in Ophthalmology from University of Kerala, India and later she underwent for 2 years fellowship in Orbit and Oculoplasty from the prestigious Sankara Netralaya, Chennai, India. She is a life member of Oculoplastic Society of India. She is the recipient of Dr Gangadhara Sundar Award for young Oculoplastic Surgeon as well as Jayaben Chamanlal Shah Gold Medal for Best Outgoing Sub-Specialty Fellow. Currently she is practicing in Giridhar Eye Institute, Kerala, India

# 12 Management of Lacrimal System Trauma

Bipasha Mukherjee and Mangesh Dhobekar

## Introduction

Injuries to nasolacrimal system are common after blunt trauma to the periorbital region and usually damage the canaliculus, the lacrimal sac, or the nasolacrimal duct. Canalicular lacerations from blunt trauma likely result from lateral traction of the eyelid during trauma [1]. The dense fibrous tissue of the tarsus is much stronger than the medial canalicular portion of the eyelid; therefore, any tractional force along the eyelid margin can result in avulsion of the medial eyelid with canalicular involvement. The most common mechanism for canalicular laceration is blunt trauma from a fist punch, which accounts for 23 % of such injuries [2]. Dog bites account for 19 % of canalicular lacerations and are the most common cause of these lacerations in children [2, 3]. Lacerations of the inferior canaliculus occur more frequently than the superior canaliculus [3]. Concomitant medial canthal tendon injury has been reported to occur in 36 % of insults resulting in canalicular lacerations [4].

B. Mukherjee, MS, DNB(Ophthalmology), FICO (✉)
Orbit, Oculoplasty, Reconstructive and Aesthetic Services, Sankara Nethralaya,
Chennai, Tamil Nadu 600006, India
e-mail: drbpm@snmail.org

M. Dhobekar, MBBS, MS, FMRF
Orbit, Oculoplasty and Ocular Prosthetic Services, Shri Ganapati Netralaya, Jalna, Maharashtra, India
e-mail: eyeman1980@gmail.com

Midfacial trauma and the resultant facial fractures frequently involve the bone about the lacrimal sac fossa, and/or nasolacrimal ducts, leading to obstruction of the nasolacrimal system. Fractures involving the distal portions of the nasolacrimal duct include the midface fractures of naso-orbital, LeFort II, and LeFort III fractures [5]. Isolated naso-orbito-ethmoidal (NOE) fracture is an important cause of traumatic NLDO [6, 7]. The most frequent causes are high-energy traumas, such as motor vehicle accidents [8, 9]. Traumatic telecanthus has been reported to be the most common associated feature with traumatic NLDO [10] (Fig. 12.1). Hence, presence of this feature in a trauma patient can be a harbinger of NLDO. The incidence of posttraumatic persistent epiphora due to NLDO requiring DCR ranges from 5 % to 21 % [7, 11–13].

## **Relevant Anatomy** (Fig. 12.1)

The lacrimal system begins at the lacrimal punctum which starts at the myocutaneous junction of the medial aspect of the lid margin of upper and lower eyelids. The canaliculi extend from the punctum to the lacrimal sac. The canaliculus initially has a vertical path of 2 mm followed by a medial extension (8–10 mm) toward the lacrimal sac. As the canaliculi approach the lacrimal sac, they tend to combine to form the common canaliculus which enters the lateral wall of the lacri-


B. Mukherjee, H. Yuen (eds.), *Emergencies of the Orbit and Adnexa*,
DOI 10.1007/978-81-322-1807-4_12

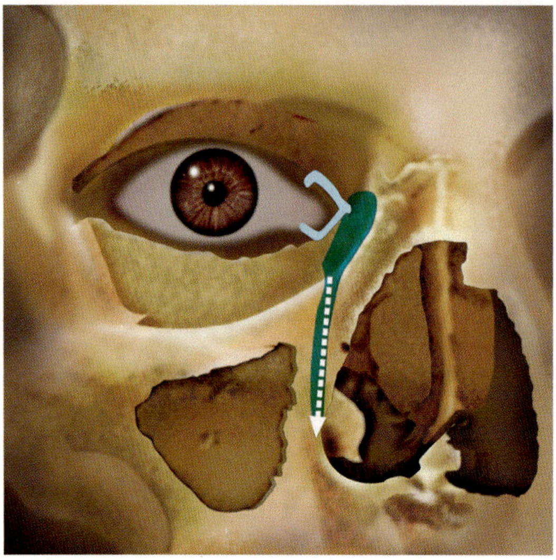

**Fig. 12.1** Anatomy of the lacrimal drainage system (the interosseous part is depicted by the interrupted line). Figure courtesy of Dr. Debmalya Das

mal sac. The lacrimal sac lies within the bony depression of the anteromedial orbital wall, called the fossa of the lacrimal sac. In an average adult, the sac measures 12 mm in height, 4–6 mm in depth, and 2 mm in width. The nasolacrimal duct measures 3–4 mm in diameter and extends inferiorly. The nasolacrimal duct has two parts: the intraosseous part, about 12 mm in length, within the nasolacrimal canal of the maxilla, and the membranous or meatal part, which is 5 mm long and runs beneath the nasal mucosa before ending at the inferior meatus. The flap of mucosa at this exit is referred to as the valve of Hasner.

## Diagnosis and Clinical Assessment

Patients with nasolacrimal injuries may present with significant concurrent facial wounds and multiple system injuries. It is essential to carefully check for any associated injuries such as neurological, thoracic, and abdominal trauma when significant facial trauma occurs. Such patients must be rapidly evaluated and stabilized first. The importance of meticulous history taking cannot be overemphasized. The physical examination should include an assessment of the soft tissues and bony involvement. Swelling, ecchymoses, and lacerations in periocular region are noted. Lacerations in the medial canthal region should be assessed to determine the integrity of the lacrimal drainage system and medial canthal tendon. A disruption of the medial canthal tendon can be assessed by a "traction test" [14, 15]. It is done by grasping the edge of the lower eyelid or upper eyelid laterally and pulling against the medial attachment. If the eyelid margin does not become taut and bowstring or you feel asymmetry in the two sides, then the medial portion of the tendon has likely been avulsed and disrupted. The other important structures in this area are the upper and lower canaliculi. Firstly, inspection of the lacrimal and canthal area should be done. A cotton tip can be used to gently palpate eyelid tissue. This can help define the location and extent of the injury. In addition, syringing and probing of the lacrimal system should be performed. Thorough lacrimal system evaluation including tear meniscus height, position and appearance of puncta and lids, regurgitation on pressure over lacrimal sac, irrigation of lacrimal system, fluorescein dye disappearance test, and whenever indicated diagnostic probing and nasal endoscopy should be carried out.

Inspection and physical examination of the patients with nasoethmoid–orbital injuries can help to predict the sites and extent of fractures prior to radiographical studies. The palpation over the bones onto the medial canthal tendon attachment may demonstrate bony crepitus or clicks depending on the degree of instability [16]. Bony fractures initiate an inflammatory and cicatrizing reaction that may result in NLDOs shortly or years after the injury [5]. Thorough clinical assessment of NLDO should be done 3–6 months after initial trauma or repair when resolution of edema and soft tissue injuries permit the definitive evaluation. The width and the symmetry of the medial canthi should be assessed for telecanthus. The normal inter-canthal width ranges from 30 to 35 mm in whites [14, 17, 18], or half of interpupillary distance [14, 19], which is a more reliable guide. The other obvious sign is saddle nose deformity which means loss of nasal skeletal support. Furthermore, typically, the medial aspect of the palpebral fissure may lose its sharpness and become rounded and slack with varying degrees of downward and outward displacement (Figs. 12.2 and 12.3). An ocular examination should be performed. Injuries in this area may be associated with ophthalmic emergency and problems such as ruptured globe or traumatic optic neuropathy especially when the principle fracture or displacement involves bones of the apex of the orbit [20–23]. A study by Holt et al. [24] found 59 % of nasal fractures showed concomitant eye injuries and 76 % of midfacial fractures were associated with eye injuries. Therefore, an initial ocular evaluation in midfacial fractures is necessary [25–27]. In conclusion, patients with naso-ethmoid–orbital injuries are evaluated in three ways. The bony involvement, such as nasoethmoid fracture or nasolacrimal, naso-orbital fractures, or complex fractures, should be considered. The soft tissue injuries are especially concerned in medial canthal tendon area and lacrimal drainage system which includes canaliculi and lacrimal sac. The third part is appropriate ocular examination and visual assessment.

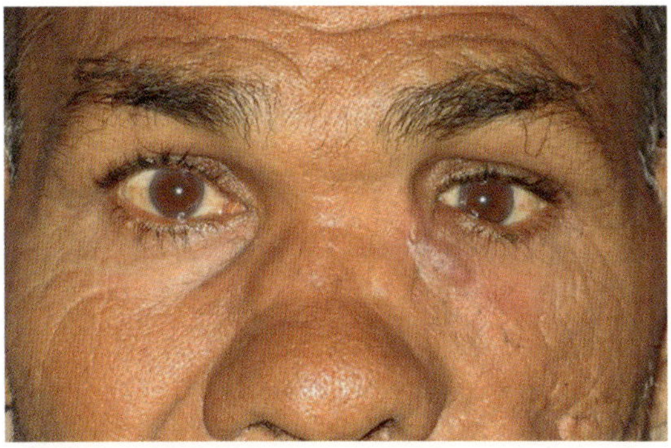

**Fig. 12.2** Traumatic NLDO [nasolacrimal duct obstruction] with telecanthus

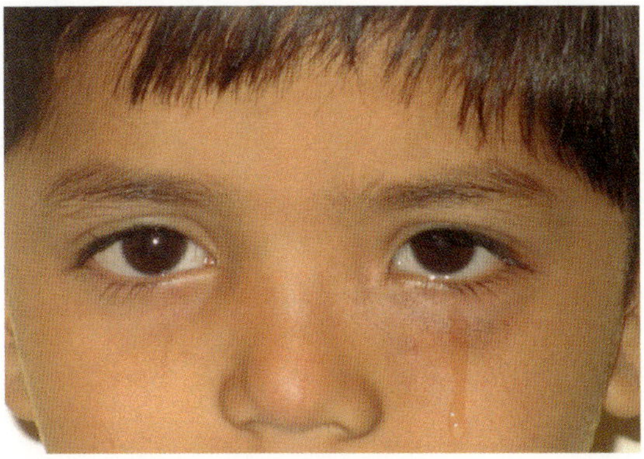

**Fig. 12.3** Displaced and rounded medial canthal angle in traumatic NLDO

A facial CT scan is required in any patients suspected of having nasoethmoid injuries. Axial and coronal images with bone windows, spaced at 1.5–2 mm, are most effective in evaluating and classifying nasoethmoid–orbital fractures [28] (Fig. 12.4). Imaging of lacrimal system is often indicated in complex situations such as traumatic NLDO for proper assessment. Although DCG is considered the gold standard for imaging of the nasolacrimal system, it does not allow for imaging of the soft tissue or bony structures surrounding the nasolacrimal sac or duct [29]. Plain CT alone, however, is unable to diagnose securely a point of obstruction in the nasolacrimal duct. The CT-DCG gives useful information about complexity of anatomical change after trauma and repair, exact localization of the lacrimal sac, associated fractures, and bone displacements. It also provides information about the location of previously placed miniplates and screws, wire, or silastic sheets, which helps in preoperative planning and intraoperative decision-making [30–34] (Fig. 12.5).

## Management

Definitive treatment of nasolacrimal injuries should be deferred until the patient has been stabilized regarding any concomitant, compromising, or life-threatening or vision-threatening trauma. Ocular contraindications include optic nerve injury and globe injury (e.g., hyphema, rupture, laceration). These injuries should be addressed and stabilized prior to surgical intervention, since osseous manipulation may exacerbate damage to the eye. Some injuries may not need correction, provided that the patient is satisfied with the appearance and function.

Once definitive diagnosis of nasolacrimal injuries has been made, based on clinical evaluation and lacrimal imaging, the patient should be

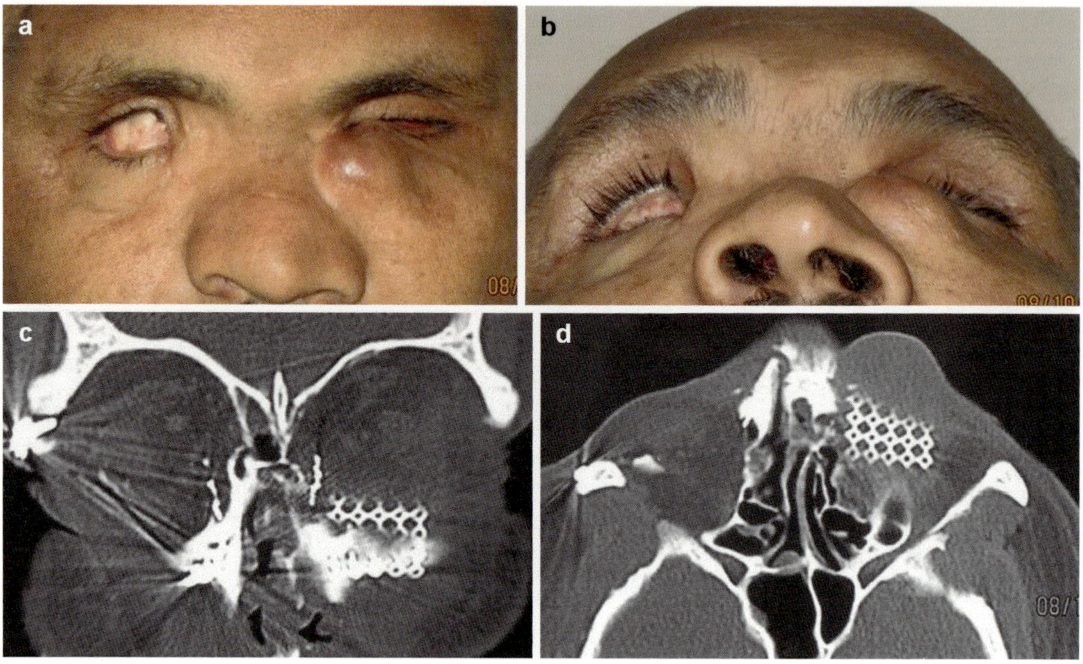


**Fig. 12.4** (**a**, **b**) external photographs showing left-sided traumatic NLDO with mucocele of lacrimal sac. Axial (**c**) and coronal (**d**) computed tomography scan showing left naso-orbito-ethmoidal fracture status post-primary repair in same patient

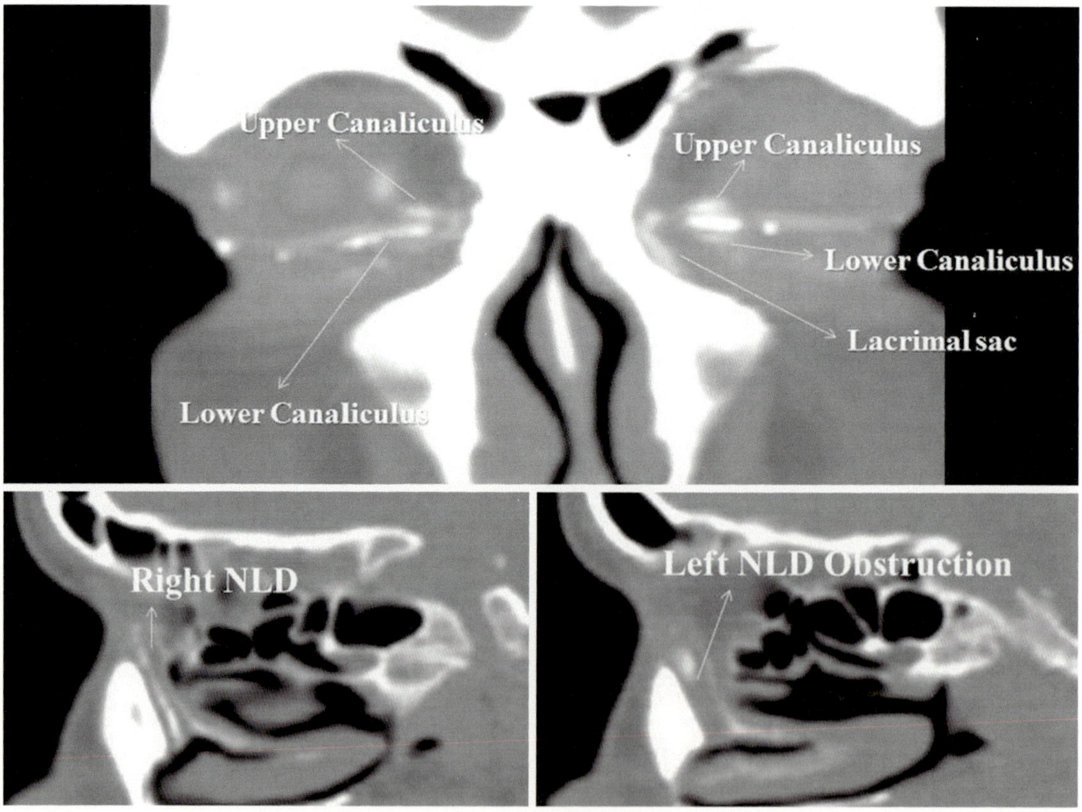


**Fig. 12.5** Computed tomography–dacryocystogram. *NLD* nasolacrimal duct

informed about their clinical condition, need for surgical intervention, types of surgery and anesthesia, and possible complications and success rate. Management for nasolacrimal injuries can be divided into two parts, bony fracture and soft tissue injuries which are divided into two subgroups, medial canthal tendon injuries, and lacrimal drainage system injuries which include canalicular lacerations.

Lacerations to the canaliculus and medial canthal injuries should be treated primarily, while injury to the lacrimal sac or nasolacrimal duct can be operated on later [35], because there is a chance of spontaneous improvement. Canalicular lacerations and medial canthal tendon injuries should be repaired within 72 h preferably to ensure the best possible outcome and to avoid scarring and epithelization of canalicular edges. Late repair is difficult, and patients often require conjunctivodacryocystorhinostomy (CDCR) to resolve their tearing problem.

Primary repair of maxillofacial and NOE injuries with open reduction and internal fixation of fractures should be performed early to provide optimal repair and minimize the incidence of late postoperative epiphora [7]. Lacrimal sac and nasolacrimal duct injuries should not be explored at the initial surgery if there is no obvious laceration. Studies showed spontaneous resolution of traumatic epiphora within 6 months after primary fracture repair [7, 13]. The incidence of late post-traumatic persistent epiphora due to NLDO requiring DCR ranges from 5 to 21 % [7, 11–13]. When DCR is necessary, it should be performed when the healing process is complete, which is 3–6 months after the primary repair.

## Anesthesia

Preexisting medical conditions need to be treated preoperatively to ensure that the patient is in the best possible health prior to surgery. General anesthesia is preferred in the setting of extensive nasoethmoidalorbital trauma, in more extensive injuries, and in pediatric population. There may be sclerosis and gross thickening of the bones after trauma, requiring drills or chisel–hammer to initiate the osteotomy [25]. Hence, it is preferable to operate cases of traumatic NLDO under general anesthesia whenever preoperative assessment predicts such intraoperative difficulty. Local anesthesia may be appropriate for adult patients with canalicular lacerations and medial canthal injuries and those with poor systemic health, particularly those with advanced cardiovascular or pulmonary disease.

## Canalicular Laceration

The traditional method for repair of mono- or bicanalicular lacerations involves repair of the eyelid defect after placement of a bicanalicular stent. The introduction of Mini Monoka© stents has allowed repair of simple monocanalicular lacerations under local anesthesia, avoiding intranasal manipulation and sedation.

The most difficult part of canalicular repair is locating the medial end of the severed canaliculus. Therefore, canalicular lacerations should be repaired within 24–48 h after injuries because the medial cut edge of canaliculus becomes progressively more difficult to identify as fibrin and granulation deposition occurs (Fig. 12.6). The medial cut edge of canaliculus is identified successfully by direct inspection. The cut canaliculus is identified as white mucosal tissue with wall and lumens. Careful inspection with gentle traction of the crowded tissue with cotton tips is often necessary. If discovery of the lumen remains difficult, injection of air into the uncut canaliculus while observing the medial cut area submerged in

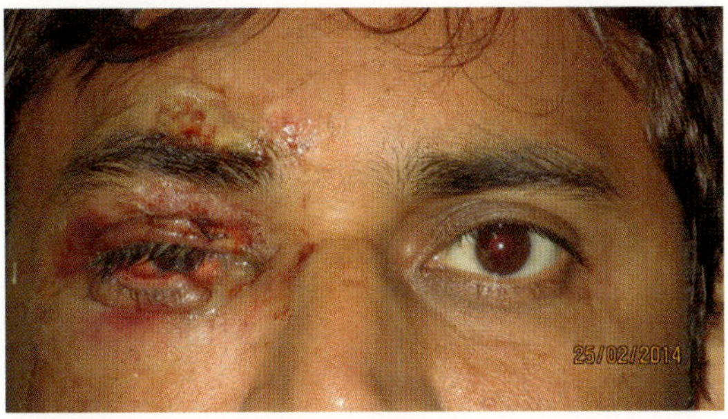


**Fig. 12.6** Fibrin and granulation tissue deposition in late canalicular injuries

saline may uncover its location with the appearance of air bubbles [36, 37].

Bicanalicular intubation is considered to be the gold standard for mono- or bicanalicular lacerations. This tube creates a "closed-loop" system that is unlikely to become dislodged. Placement of such tubes, however, does require intranasal packing with lidocaine and epinephrine; intravenous sedation or general anesthesia may be required.

Monocanalicular stent allows for placement under local anesthesia alone; however, these stents are less secure compared with the bicanalicular type and can be dislodged in children quite easily. Punctal injury precludes the use of a monocanalicular stent. The various types of stents are briefly described in Table 12.1.

## Bicanalicular Repair

After identification of the medial cut edge of the canaliculus, a Crawford bicanalicular tube is inserted into the proximal canaliculus, through the cut end of distal canaliculus, and then the lacrimal sac and duct. It is necessary to orient the probe to follow the anatomical course of the lacrimal system. The hook or grooved dissector is used to deliver the probe from beneath the inferior turbinate and out the nostril. When a bicanalicular system is used, the opposite canalicular system is inserted in a similar way and retrieved through the nostril. The canaliculus can be approximated by two to three absorbable 8-0 sutures placed in the mucosal wall of cut canaliculus in order to achieve an end-to-end anasto-

**Table 12.1** Lacrimal stents

| | Stent | Mono/bicanalicular | Intranasal manipulation | Comment |
|---|---|---|---|---|
| 1 | Mini Monoka/ Aurostent[a] | Mono | None | Self-retaining, securely anchored at the punctum |
| 2 | Masterka | Mono | None | Stent is "pushed" into the nasolacrimal duct and anchored at the punctum by the plug similar to Monoka |
| | | | | Needs disposable introducers and sizers |
| 3 | Mono-Crawford | Mono | Yes | Stent is "pulled" through the nasolacrimal duct transnasally and anchored at the punctum by the plug |
| | | | | Needs Crawford retrieval hook |
| 4 | Self-threading Monoka | Mono | Yes | Stent with thread as a guide which is pulled transnasally |
| | | | | Needs Ritleng probe and retrieval hook |
| 5 | Self-retaining bicanaliculus intubation set (SRS II) | Bicanalicular | None | Similar to no. 2, needs disposable introducers and sizers |
| 6 | Goldberg bicanaliculus cerclage | Bicanalicular | None | Creates bicanalicular "closed-loop" system |
| | | | | Needs pigtail probe |
| 7 | Bika – bicanalicular intubation stent | Bicanalicular | Yes | Stents with metallic nontraumatic guide with rounded tip |
| 8 | Crawford bicanalicular stent | Bicanalicular | Yes | Stents with metallic nontraumatic guide with an olive tip |
| | | | | Stent is "pulled" through transnasally and anchored at the punctum by the plug |
| 9 | Ritleng bicanalicular stent | Bicanalicular | Yes | Introduction similar to no. 4 |

Source: http://www.fci-ophthalmics.com/stents-tubes

[a]http://www.aurolab.com/canalicularlacerationtreatment.asp

mosis of the tube [38, 39]. Some authors [40, 41] used single-stitch repairs with 7-0 Vicryl horizontal mattress sutures, which passed in the plane directly anterior to the canaliculus. The results [40] are excellent, although 4 % still have epiphora and 13 % still have delay outflow with dye disappearance test.

With complete avulsion of the medial canthus from its origin at the anterior lacrimal crest, reapproximation can be done with a double armed suture. This suture should be placed through the lateral wound edge with a substantial bite followed by a deep medial bite which would ideally include periosteum of the anterior lacrimal crest. The sutures should be tied over the skin using bolsters of foam or rubber. If the punctum is lacerated, this should be sutured around the stent with 7-0 Vicryl sutures. The initial wound is closed with 6-0 Vicryl deep sutures, and the skin is closed with 6-0 silk sutures. Once both ends of the stent are brought out through the nose, the tubes should be placed on gentle traction and clamped with a small hemostat at the level of the nostril. This allows the tubes to provide traction on the canthal wound to aid in anatomic reapproximation. The distal tube ends are joined with five single throws of the silicone suture. The stent is sutured to the lateral wall of the nose at the mucocutaneous junction with a 6-0 Vicryl suture. This suture will dissolve by the time the tubes are removed in approximately 6 weeks.

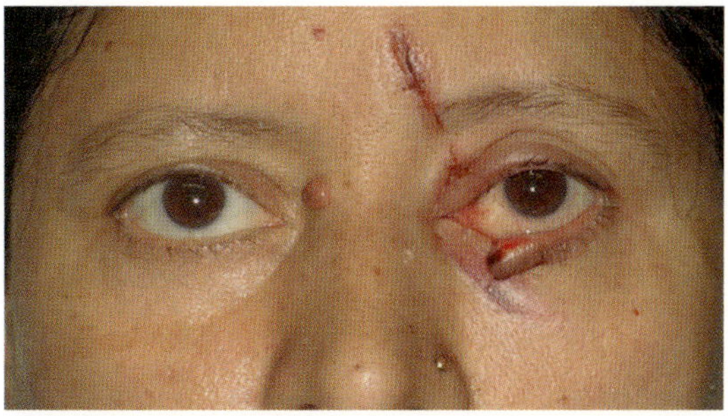

**Fig. 12.7** Preoperative external photo: lower canalicular laceration

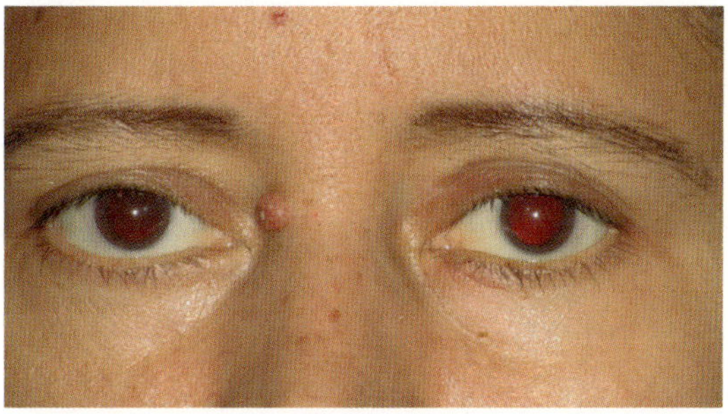

**Fig. 12.8** Postoperative external photo: lower canalicular repair with monocanalicular stent

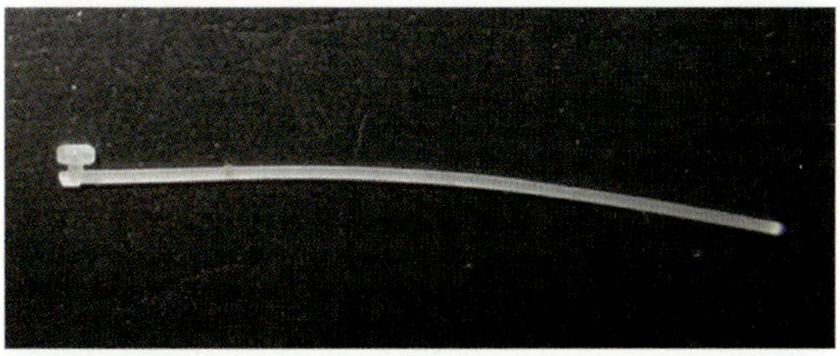

**Fig. 12.9** Monocanalicular stent

## Monocanalicular Repair

This is our preferred method (Figs. 12.7 and 12.8). The monocanalicular stent (Figs. 12.9 and 12.10) is a short silicone tube with a phalange at the proximal end. To insert the stent, the surgeon first passes Bowman's probe to identify the severed canaliculus (Fig. 12.11) and then passes distal end of the stent through the punctum and brings it out through the proximal end of the severed canaliculus. The phalange should be fixed securely in the punctum by gently pulling the distal end of the stent. When the distal canaliculus is identified, the stent can be threaded into it with forceps (Fig. 12.12). The monocanalicular stent cannot be used when a laceration to the punctum is present, because the proximal end cannot be fixed. Also, it should not be used with medial canthal avulsion, because the stent cannot provide the adequate inferior and posterior traction to close the wounds, as would a bicanalicular stent tied in the nose.

Following silicone tube intubation, the patient is given steroid–antibiotic eye drops four times a day for 4 weeks in a tapering manner. Tear supplements should be added as tube can irritate the cornea and conjunctiva. The patient is reevaluated at 1 week after surgery. Canalicular stents can usually be removed approximately 3–6 months after repair. Monocanalicular stents can be removed easily in office setting by holding phalange at the punctum with forceps. Bicanalicular stents are preferably removed from the nose after the loop between the puncta is cut. First ask the patient to forcefully exhale through the ipsilateral nare while compressing the other nare. Once nasal ends of the tubes come out through nose, surgeon holds ends of the tube with forceps in one hand and cut the loop between the puncta with other hand. An endoscope can aid in finding the nasal end of the stent. Silicone tubes are usually well tolerated; however, if the tube is tied too tightly "cheese wiring" through the puncta and canaliculi may occur, necessitating its removal. A pyogenic granuloma may develop near the punctum and these should be excised if present. If there is persistent keratoconjunctivitis, the tube should be removed earlier. The tube may prolapse and extrude in some cases (Fig. 12.13). Often the tube can be replaced into proper position with forceps; tube removal may be required in case of failed repositioning.

In some severe and extensive injuries, complete surgical repair of the lacrimal system may not be always possible. Orbital fracture and eyelids laceration should be repaired first [42], then conjunctivodacryocystorhinostomy with the insertion of bypass tube may be considered subsequently.

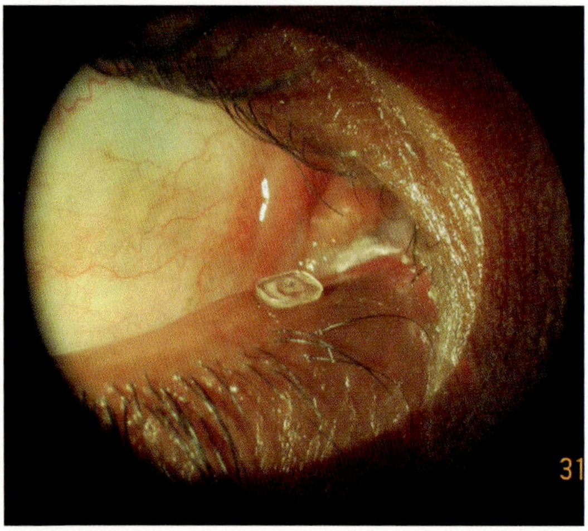

**Fig. 12.10** Monocanalicular stent in situ

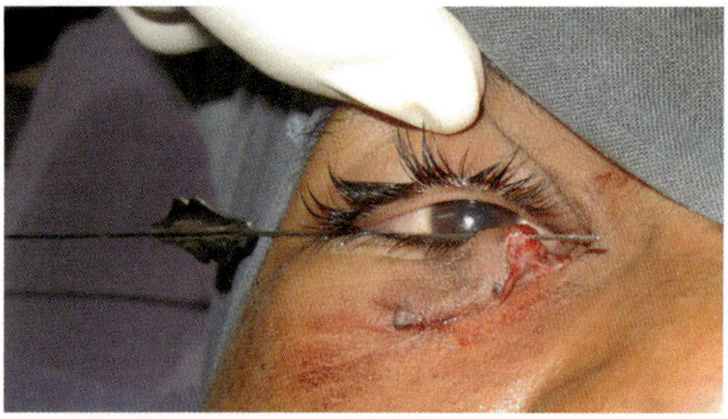

**Fig. 12.11** Bowman's probe is being inserted through punctum to identify proximal end of the severed canaliculus

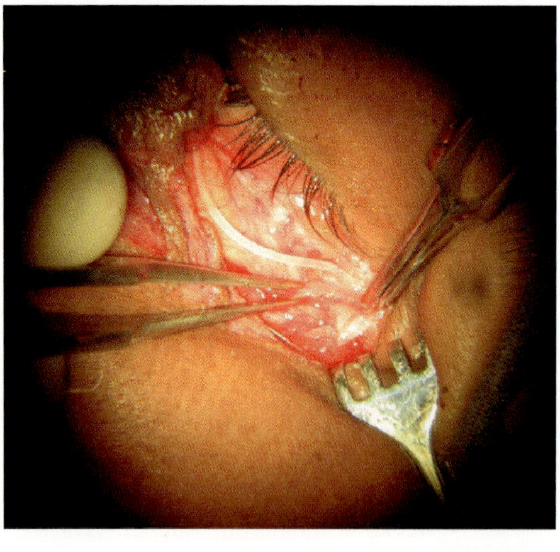

**Fig. 12.12** Monocanalicular stent is being threaded into the distal canaliculus with forceps

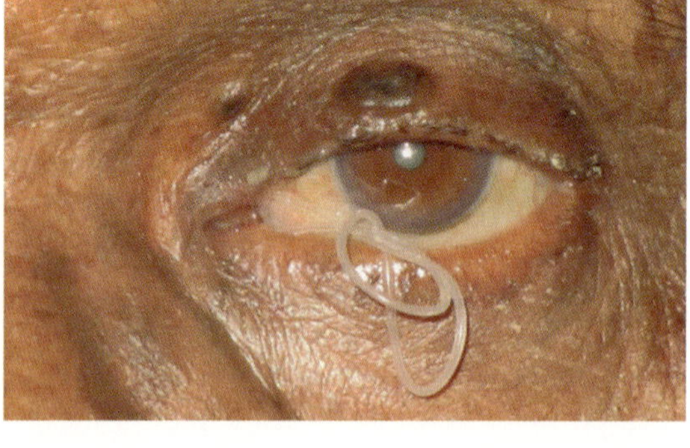

**Fig. 12.13** Prolapsed bicanalicular stent (spaghetti syndrome)

## Lacrimal Sac and Nasolacrimal Duct Injuries

As previously mentioned, when DCR is necessary, it should be performed when the healing process is complete, which is 3–6 months after the primary repair of maxillofacial and NOE fractures. As far as surgical management of traumatic NLDO is concerned, external DCR with a large rhinostomy gives satisfactory outcome with success rate of more than 90 % [13]. Nasolacrimal duct obstructions following maxillofacial trauma and subsequent surgeries are associated with significant scarring and fibrosis. Concomitant nasolacrimal intubation in such conditions is a safe and effective means of ensuring the establishment of a patent, functional drainage system [43].

Due to loss of bony anatomical landmarks after trauma and subsequent surgery, endoscopic, endonasal, or laser DCR is more difficult in traumatic NLDO. There may be sclerosis and gross thickening of the bones after trauma, requiring drills or chisel–hammer to initiate the osteotomy [44]. Hence, it is preferable to operate cases of traumatic NLDO under general anesthesia whenever preoperative assessment predicts such intraoperative difficulty. Adenis et al. studied 25 cases in which external DCR was performed for posttraumatic NLDO [45]. The success rate was 66 % when the delay from the time of primary repair was less than 6 months and 100 % in 21 cases when the delay was greater than 6 months. The overall success rate in the study (88 %) is similar to that obtained by performing a DCR in lacrimal stenosis of other etiologies. Hence, it is emphasized that DCR whenever necessary should be performed 3–6 months after primary injury or repair. Becelli et al. in a retrospective study of 58 consecutive NOE fractures observed 17 (34 %) cases of persistent traumatic NLDO [13]. External DCR with a large rhinostomy and silicone intubation achieved a success rate of 94 % in the reconstruction of lacrimal drainage. Such a technique proved to be effective in the treatment of posttraumatic dacryostenosis. Gruss et al. reported in a detailed review of 46 patients with severe NOE injury that 8 patients (17.4 %) required eventual DCR with good surgical outcome [7]. In our study [10], 26 out of 28 patients with traumatic NLDO underwent standard external DCR with or without silicone intubation. Absolute success with cessation of epiphora and patency on lacrimal irrigation was observed in 25 (96 %) patients. One patient had functional failure with diminished epiphora and patency on irrigation, and he did not require any additional surgical procedure. All patients were followed up regularly for at least 6 months. Mean follow-up period was 7.71 months.

In conclusion, a protocol-based approach for the management of traumatic NLDO is proposed:

- Early evaluation and management of primary trauma preferably with open reduction and internal fixation of midface fractures.
- Thorough initial evaluation of lacrimal system and reassessment at least 3–6 months after initial trauma or repair.
- Lacrimal imaging in the form of CT-DCG is useful in all cases of suspected traumatic NLDO.
- Proper preoperative counselling of patients regarding the clinical condition with discussion of complications and success rates.
- Conventional external approach for DCR remains the preferred approach rather than endonasal or endocanalicular DCR.
- Surgery should be carried out under general anesthesia if intraoperative difficulty is anticipated.
- Bone removal for rhinostomy may require drills or chisel–hammer. So additional instruments should be available.
- Silicone intubation for 3 months is a useful adjunct because of the presumed predisposition to inflammation after trauma.
- Dacryocystectomy or conjunctivodacryocystorhinostomy may be an alternative in difficult cases, and patients need to be counselled about the same beforehand.

## References

1. Wulc AE, Arterberry JF. The pathogenesis of canalicular laceration. Ophthalmology. 1991;98(8):1243–9.
2. Kennedy RH, May J, Dailey J, Flanagan JC. Canalicular laceration. An 11-year epidemiologic and clinical study. Ophthal Plast Reconstr Surg. 1990;6(1):46–53.

3. Reifler DM. Management of canalicular laceration. Surv Ophthalmol. 1991;36(2):113–32.
4. Dortzbach RK, Angrist RA. Silicone intubation for lacerated lacrimal canaliculi. Ophthalmic Surg. 1985;16(10):639–42.
5. Schaefer DP. Acquired etiologies of lacrimal system obstructions. The lacrimal system: diagnosis, management and surgery. New York: Springer; 2006. p. 43–65.
6. Uraloglu M, ErkinUnlü R, Ortak T, Sensöz O. Delayed assessment of the nasolacrimal system at naso-orbito-ethmoid fractures and a modified technique of dacryocystorhinostomy. J Craniofac Surg. 2006;17:184–9.
7. Gruss JS, Hurwitz JJ, Nik NA, Kassel EE. The pattern and incidence of nasolacrimal injury in naso-orbital-ethmoid fractures: the role of delayed assessment and dacryocystorhinostomy. Br J Plast Surg. 1985;38:116–21.
8. Epker BN. Open surgical management of naso-orbital-ethmoid facial fractures. Trans Int Conf Oral Surg. 1973;4:323–9.
9. Fedok FG. Comprehensive management of naso-ethmoidorbital injuries. J Craniomaxillofac Trauma. 1995;1:36–48. Osguthorpe JD, Hoang G. Nasolacrimal injuries. Evaluation and management. Otolaryngol Clin N Am. 1991;24:59–78.
10. Mukherjee B, Dhobekar M. Traumatic nasolacrimal duct obstruction: clinical profile, management, and outcome. Eur J Ophthalmol. 2013;23(5):615–22.
11. Osguthorpe JD, Hoang G. Nasolacrimal injuries. Evaluation and management. Otolaryngol Clin North Am. 1991;24:59–78.
12. Stranc MF. The pattern of lacrimal injuries in naso-ethmoid fractures. Br J Plast Surg. 1970;23:339–46.
13. Becelli R, Renzi G, Mannino G, Cerulli G, Iannetti G. Posttraumatic obstruction of lacrimal pathways: a retrospective analysis of 58 consecutive naso-orbito-ethmoid fractures. J Craniofac Surg. 2004;15:29–33.
14. Holt GR, Holt JE. Nasoethmoid complex injuries. Otolaryngol Clin N Am. 1985;18:87–98.
15. Harris GJ, Fuerste FH. Lacrimal intubation in the primary repair of midfacial fractures. Ophthalmology. 1987;94:242–7.
16. Paskert JP, Manson PN. The bimanual examination for assessing instability in naso-orbitoethmoidal injuries. Plast Reconstr Surg. 1989;83:165–7.
17. Hansman CF. Growth of interorbital distance and skull thickness as observed in roentgenographic measurements. Radiology. 1966;86:87–96.
18. Freihofer HP. Inner intercanthal and interorbital distances. J Maxillofac Surg. 1980;8:324–6.
19. Collin JRO, Tyers AG. Preoperative evaluation. In: Collin JRO, Tyers AG, editors. Colour atlas of ophthalmic plastic surgery. Oxford: Butterworth-Heinemann; 2001. p. 49–58.
20. Hooper RS. Orbital complication of head injury. Br J Surg. 1951;39:126.
21. King AB, Walsh FB. Trauma to the head with particular reference to the ocular signs. Part I injuries involving the cranial nerves. Am J Ophthalmol. 1949;32:191–205.
22. Milauskas AT, Fueger GF. Serious ocular complication associated with blow-out fractures of the orbit. Am J Ophthalmol. 1966;62:670–2.
23. Miller GR, Tenzel RR. Ocular complication of midfacial fractures. Plast Reconstr Surg. 1967;39:37–42. Oxford: Butterworth-Heinemann; 2001. p. 49–58.
24. Holt JE, Holt R, Blodgett JM. Ocular injuries sustained during blunt facial trauma. Ophthalmology. 1983;90:14–8.
25. Gossman MD, Roberts DM, Barr CC. Ophthalmic aspects of orbital injury: a comprehensive diagnostic and management approach. Clin Plast Surg. 1992;19:71–85.
26. Wessberg GA, Wolford LM, Zerdecki JW, et al. Ophthalmic consideration in maxillofacial trauma. Int J Oral Surg. 1981;10:236–46.
27. Pelletier CR, Jordan DR, Braga R, et al. Assessment of ocular trauma associated with head and neck injuries. J Trauma Injury Infect Crit Care. 1998;44:350–4.
28. Manson PN, Markowitz B, Mirvis S, et al. Toward CT-based facial fracture treatment. Plast Reconstr Surg. 1990;85:202.
29. Malik SRK, Gupta AK, Chaterjee S, Bhardwaj OP, Saha M. Dacryocystography of normal and pathological lacrimal passages. Br J Ophthalmol. 1969;53:174–9.
30. Udhay P, Noronha OV, Mohan RE. Helical computed tomographic dacryocystography and its role in the diagnosis and management of lacrimal drainage system blocks and medial canthal masses. Indian J Ophthalmol. 2008;56:31–7.
31. Ellis III E. Sequencing treatment for naso-orbito-ethmoid fractures. J Oral Maxillofac Surg. 1993;51:543–58.
32. Stranc MF, Bunce AH. Dacryo-cystography in midfacial fractures. Br J Plast Surg. 1972;25:269–75.
33. Unger JM. Fractures of the nasolacrimal fossa and canal: a CT study of appearance, associated injuries, and significance in 25 patients. Am J Radiol. 1992;158:1321–4.
34. Glatt HJ. Evaluation of lacrimal obstruction secondary to facial fractures using computed tomography or computed tomographic dacryocystography. Ophthal Plast Reconstr Surg. 1996;12:284–93.
35. Duvall AJ, Foster DA, Lyons DP, et al. Medial canthoplasty: early and delayed repair. Laryngoscope. 1981;91:173–83.
36. Lauring L. Silicone intubation of the lacrimal system: pitfalls, problems and complications. Ann Ophthalmol. 1976;8:489–98.
37. MacGillivray RF, Stevens MR. Primary surgical repair of traumatic lacerations of the lacrimal canaliculi. Oral Surg Oral Med Oral Pathol. 1996;81:157–63.
38. Leone CR. Periorbital trauma. Int Ophthalmol Clin. 1995;35:1–24.
39. Hawes MJ, Segrest DR. Effectiveness of bicanalicular silicone intubation in the repair of canalicular lacerations. Ophthalmic Plast Surg. 1985;1:185–90.

40. Kersten RC, Kulwin DR. "One stitch" canalicular repair: a simplified approach for repair of canalicular laceration. Ophthalmology. 1996;103:785–9.
41. Reed S, Lissner G. Clinical study on the effectiveness of tear drainage with a single canalicular system under environmental stress. Ophthal Plast Reconstr Surg. 1993;9:17–31.
42. Welham RA. The immediate management of injuries to the lacrimal drainage apparatus. Trans Ophthalmol Soc UK. 1982;102:216–7.
43. Spinelli HM, Shapiro MD, Wei LL, Elahi E, Hirmand H. The role of lacrimal intubation in the management of facial trauma and tumor resection. Plast Reconstr Surg. 2005;115:1871–6.
44. Della Rocca DA, Ahmad S, Schaefer SD. Atlas of lacrimal surgery: nasolacrimal system injuries. New York: Springer; 2007. p. 91–104.
45. Adenis JP, Mathon C, Franco JL, Lebraudo P. Dacryocystorhinostomy for post-traumatic lacrimal stenosis: a study of 25 cases. Orbit. 1987;6:135–7.

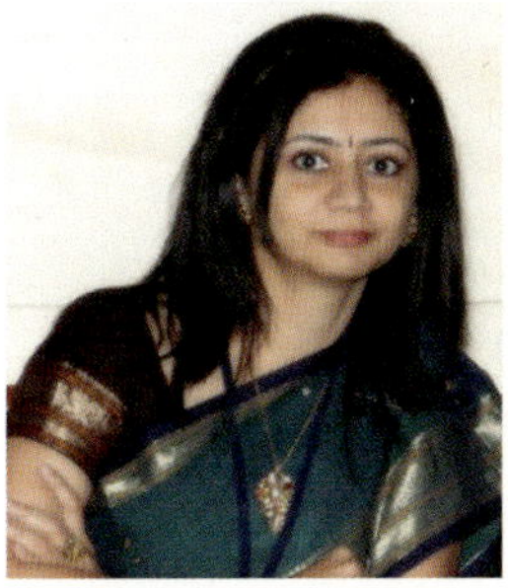

**Bipasha Mukherjee** Dr. Bipasha Mukherjee is a fellow in Orbit & Oculoplasty from Aravind Eye Hospitals, India, and ICO fellow from University Hospital of Limoges, France, under Prof. Jean-Paul Adenis. She has undergone clinical observerships with stalwarts like Jack Rootman, Richard Collins, Geoff Rose, Mark Duffy, and Robert Goldberg.

She currently heads the department of Orbit, Oculoplasty, Aesthetic & Reconstructive services in Medical Research Foundation, Chennai. She has numerous presentations in national and international conferences and publications in peer-reviewed journals and text books. Her areas of interest include diseases of the orbit and adnexa including tumors, lacrimal surgery, socket reconstruction, traumatic lid and adnexal injuries, training residents and fellows, and photography.

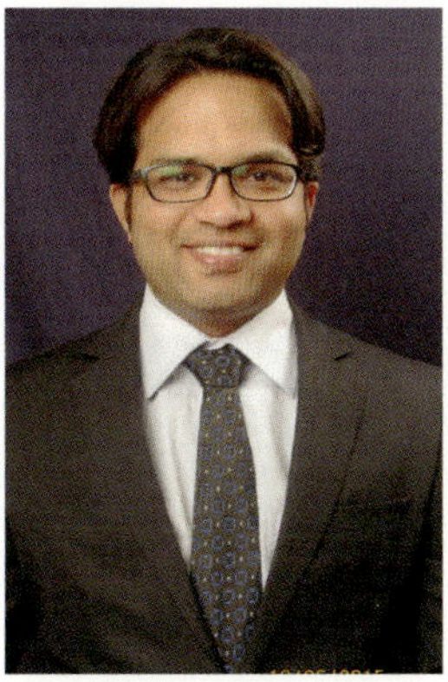

**Mangesh Dhobekar** Dr. Mangesh Dhobekar completed his postgraduate in Ophthalmology at Government Medical College, Ambejogai, Maharashtra, India. He then did his fellowship in Orbit and Oculoplasty from Sankara Nethralaya, Medical Research Foundation, Chennai, India, under the mentorship of Dr. Bipasha Mukherjee.

He presently heads the Department of Orbit, Oculoplasty and Ocular Prosthetic Services at Shri Ganapati Netralaya, Jalna, Maharashtra, India. He has numerous presentations in state and national conferences and publications in peer-reviewed journals. His areas of interest include eyelid and lacrimal surgery, socket reconstruction, and orbit and adnexal injuries and reconstructions. He has special interest in clinical photography and training of postgraduates and fellows.

# Orbital Trauma: Mechanisms and Investigations

# 13

Tomoyuki Kashima

## Introduction

The characteristic physiology and anatomy of the orbit must be understood before considering how to care for a patient of orbital trauma [1]. Orbits have a typical structure which is surrounded by facial bones, and the only open direction is anterior. In addition, there are the optic nerve and many motor nerves, arteries, and veins in the orbit. After blunt or penetrating trauma to the eyeball and/or its surrounding tissue, these structures are easily damaged by direct insult and/or compressive pressure, which leads to severe subjective symptoms [2]. Therefore, to treat orbital trauma, the orbital structure should be understood.

## Anatomy of the Orbit

The anatomy of the orbit is shown in Fig. 13.1. The structure has four walls, with the medial wall formed primarily by the orbital plate of ethmoid, as well as contributions from the frontal process of maxilla, the lacrimal bone, and a small part of the body of the sphenoid; the floor of the orbit (inferior wall) formed by the orbital surface of maxilla, the orbital surface of the zygomatic bone, and the minute orbital process of palatine bone; the lateral wall formed by the frontal process of zygomatic and more posteriorly by the orbital plate of the greater wing of sphenoid; and a roof (superior wall), formed primarily by the orbital plate frontal bone and also the lesser wing of sphenoid near the apex of the orbit. The medial wall and inferior wall of the orbit are located adjacent to the ethmoid and maxillary sinuses, respectively, and the two walls consist of very thin bones. Therefore, the medial and inferior walls are the most common sites of orbital fractures when blunt pressure is put on the orbit, causing injury to orbital contents, including not only bone, but also extraocular muscle and orbital fat extending into the sinus (Fig. 13.1). In contrast, the lateral wall, which consists of zygomatic, is very hard and thick and is more resistant to physical trauma [3]. Except as part of severe head trauma, the lateral wall is the least affected site in orbital blunt trauma. The ceiling of the orbit consists of the frontal bone. This bone is thin, but it is near the brain, and therefore, it is lined with thicker and harder tissue than the periosteum in other areas, including the maxillary or ethmoid sinus.

Roof fractures are commonly seen in young children because of the prominence of the frontal bone. Because pneumatization of the frontal sinus does not occur until the age of 5–8 years, frontal fractures tend to extend superiorly into the

T. Kashima, MD, PhD (✉)
Oculoplastic Service, Department of Ophthalmology, Gunma University,
Maebashi, Gunma 3710034, Japan
e-mail: kasimatomoyuki@yahoo.co.jp


B. Mukherjee, H. Yuen (eds.), *Emergencies of the Orbit and Adnexa*,
DOI 10.1007/978-81-322-1807-4_13

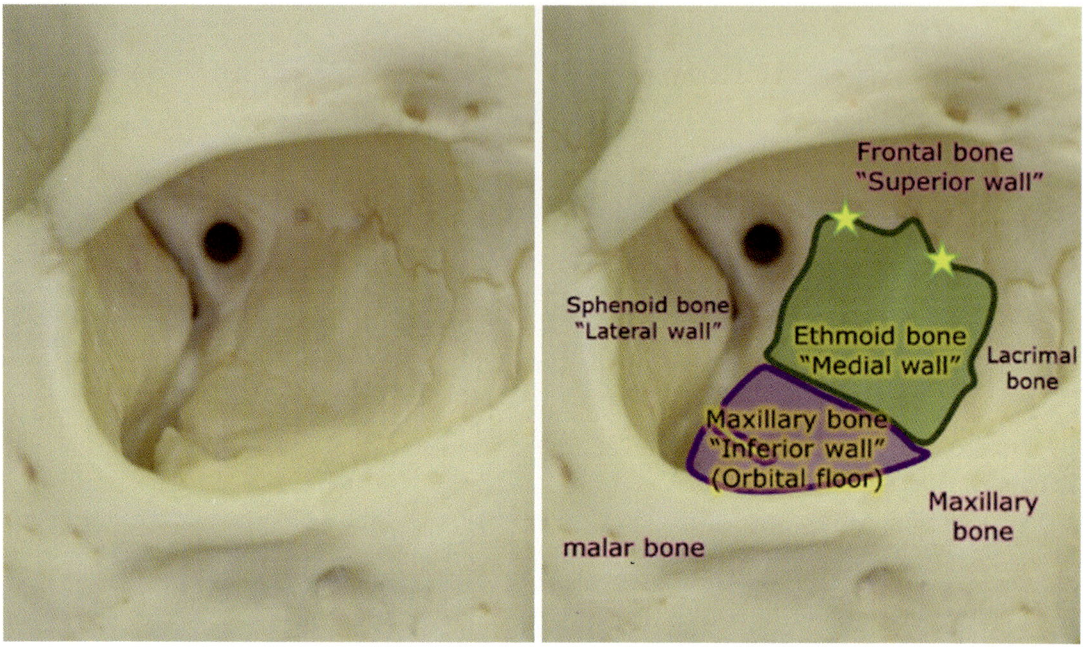


**Fig. 13.1** Bony anatomy of the orbit. *Left*, photograph of the right orbit in a skull model. *Right*, the same photo with the names of bones inserted. The orbit has four walls, with the medial wall formed primarily by the orbital plate of ethmoid, as well as contributions from the frontal process of maxilla, the lacrimal bone, and a small part of the body of the sphenoid; the floor of the orbit (inferior wall) formed by the orbital surface of maxilla, the orbital surface of zygomatic bone, and the minute orbital process of palatine bone; the lateral wall formed by the frontal process of zygomatic and more posteriorly by the orbital plate of the greater wing of sphenoid; and a roof (superior wall), formed primarily by the orbital plate frontal bone and also the lesser wing of sphenoid near the apex of the orbit. The colored fields show the sites which are susceptible to orbital blunt pressure. The *purple* bone shows the orbital floor and the *green* bone shows the orbital medial wall. *Yellow stars* indicate the anterior and posterior ethmoidal foramen, which are passed by anterior and posterior arteries, veins, and nerves

skull. These patients should have neurosurgeon consultation as there is a high incidence of associated intracranial lesions.

Within the orbit, this confined compartment has many important structures, and the physiological function of each will be discussed before considering orbital trauma [4, 5]. Orbital soft tissues are connected and support each other through connective tissue septa, which is a dense tissue in the orbit. Orbital fat is both a filler in orbital tissue and a supportive tissue of orbital connective tissue [6]. The extraocular recti and oblique muscles adhere to the orbital bone and move in an interconnected manner by connective tissue serving as a pivot for each muscle (Fig. 13.2) [7]. Orbital trauma, including both fracture and foreign body, affects these structures, through dislocation and fixation of the orbital tissue, leading to prevention of eye movement. Therefore, the orbital fat and surrounding

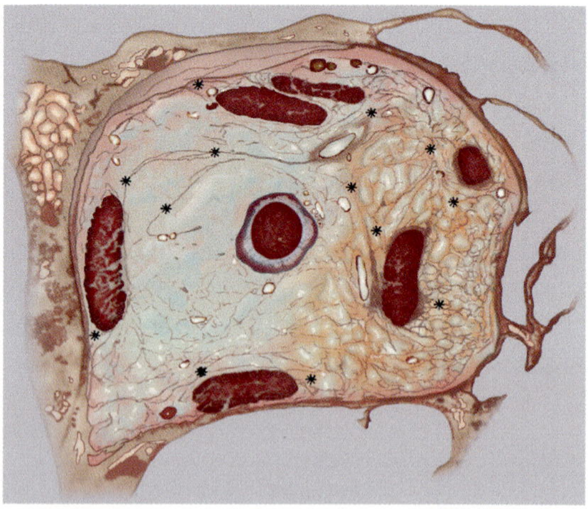

**Fig. 13.2** The schema of orbital contents. The cross section of the orbit. Orbital contents have several muscles, motor nerves, arteries, veins, and fat tissue. Fat tissue provides "filler" for the orbit, provides lubrication for eye movements, and is a supportive structure for connective tissue septa (Redrawn with permission from "Koornneef [9]")

connective tissue are also important in the physiopathology of orbital trauma.

## Aging Changes of the Bone

A graph of bone density throughout life is illustrated in Fig. 13.3. Bone density increases, year by year, until age 20 years [8], then remains almost the same until age 40 years. After reaching 40 years of age, the bone density gradually decreases. Before reaching 20 years of age, the bone is softer than in an adult, which causes different types of fractures, often called "green-stick fractures." This fracture occurs when the stress of physical force affects the immature bone, and instead of a bone breaking completely into pieces, it bends at the cracks. This condition, before 20 years of age, is observed in all systemic bones, including orbital bones.

Owing to their softness, younger orbital bones are usually restored to their original position, even if bent and fractured. The mature bone, however, will have a different pathology. The bones are hard enough to resist physical external forces, but this characteristic often precludes restoration to the original position. When the injury occurs, the mature orbital bone breaks completely and prolapses into the maxillary and/or ethmoid sinus.

When the fracture fragment is displaced inwards, it is called a blow-in fracture. Orbital blow-in fractures can present with proptosis indicating a decrease in orbital volume that may cause diffuse compression of orbital contents and ischemia.

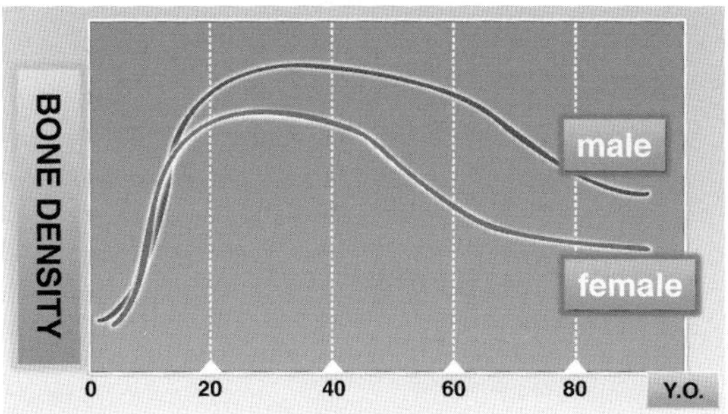


**Fig. 13.3** The aging changes of bone density throughout life. The bony density rises from birth to 20 years of age, during which bones are soft and usually do not break completely. From 20 to 40–50 years of age, the bone density does not change and bones are hard enough to usually resist minor physical trauma. However, in the latter one third of life, the bones become fragile and may break completely when exposed to even minor trauma (Redrawn with permission from "Orimo [10]")

## Investigations

Computed tomography is the best tool for the diagnosis of orbital trauma. It can identify orbital fractures, hemorrhage, globe rupture, and foreign bodies. However, there are several essential protocols to follow before using computed tomography images, including the medical history to differentiate orbital fracture from orbital foreign bodies. Similar to any trauma, it is important to identify the type of foreign body present in the patient's orbit and to determine how and when the trauma occurred. For example, a child who fell from the top of a wall into garden shrubs may have an orbital organic foreign body present, even though very little wound around the eyelids is noted (see Fig. 13.4 as an example). As another example, a patient who was hit by the hood of an automobile during an accident may not have any orbital foreign body present, but may also have orbital or facial bone fractures.

The next step would be to obtain information from the patient about their current subjective symptoms and symptoms immediately after the trauma. Orbital pain and nausea just after trauma is a symptom suggestive of entrapped orbital tissue by a trapdoor fracture. Diplopia is another subjective symptom for patients with open-type fracture. However, clinicians must examine the patient for epistaxis, which is the most reliable and subjective symptom of orbital fracture. In my experience, it is easier to find the susceptive orbital fracture before using images, by asking the patient if they are experiencing epistaxis. The orbital fracture frequently occurs on medial and inferior walls, which are lined by nasal mucosa. When the bone fracture occurs, it is often accompanied by breaks in the nasal mucosa, which leads to more or less degrees of epistaxis.

Patients who have mild orbital fractures do not have diplopia and orbital pain, but they have epistaxis even though the orbital region may have been hit, without the nose being affected. In that situation, the patient should undergo computed tomography (CT) of the orbit.

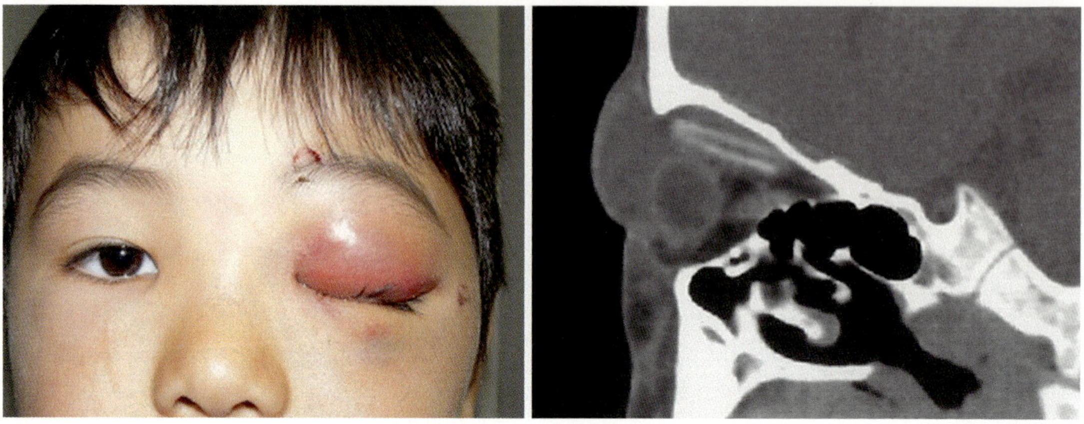

**Fig. 13.4** A young male with orbital foreign body trauma. *Left*, a frontal face photograph. The patient fell from the top of a wall into garden shrubs and had orbital organic foreign body trauma, even though very little damage was observed above the left eyebrow. *Right*, sagittal CT scan section of the patient's left orbit. The tube-shaped foreign body can be seen in the orbit

Before the use of CT scans, a diagnosis of orbital disease in coronal sections is essential. In some clinics, radiologists may not be trained in imaging of the orbital region for diagnosis, and they may only image axial sections, similar to when performing a whole brain CT scan with 5 mm slices. In our experience, thin-sliced CT scans, with reconstruction for coronal sections, are necessary. For an analysis of orbital foreign bodies, sagittal sections may provide superior results. Thus, an optimal procedure would be to perform an orbital CT scan using 1 mm slices, followed by reconstruction in three directions, axial, coronal, and sagittal.

Most current CT scanning devices have three-dimensional (3D) reconstruction capabilities for imaging. However, the orbital medial and inferior walls may be too thin to depict all structures in 3D CT.

We do not use 3D CT for newly diagnosed cases. Usually, we use 3D CT for previous patients because their damage has been repaired, and we may wish to explore the irregular orbital bones. The 3D CT is also useful to image the intraoperative orbital shape prior to surgery.

## References


1. Gentry LR. Anatomy of the orbit. Neuroimaging Clin N Am. 1998;8(1):171–94.
2. Lustrin ES, Brown JH, Novelline R, Weber AL. Radiologic assessment of trauma and foreign bodies of the eye and orbit. Neuroimaging Clin N Am. 1996; 6(1):219–37.
3. Winegar BA, Murillo H, Tantiwongkosi B. Spectrum of critical imaging findings in complex facial skeletal trauma. Radiographics: Rev Publ Radiol Soc N Am Inc. 2013;33(1):3–19.
4. Martins C, Costa ESIE, Campero A, Yasuda A, Aguiar LR, Tatagiba M, Rhoton Jr A. Microsurgical anatomy of the orbit: the rule of seven. Anat Res Int. 2011;2011:468727.
5. Ettl A, Zwrtek K, Daxer A, Salomonowitz E. Anatomy of the orbital apex and cavernous sinus on high-resolution magnetic resonance images. Surv Ophthalmol. 2000;44(4):303–23.
6. Ettl AR, Salomonowitz E, Koornneef L. Magnetic resonance imaging of the orbit: basic principles and anatomy. Orbit. 2000;19(4):211–37.
7. Zide BM, Jelks GW. Surgical anatomy of the orbit. Plast Reconstr Surg. 1984;74(2):301–5.
8. Liao EY, Wu XP, Deng XG, Huang G, Zhu XP, Long ZF, Wang WB, Tang WL, Zhang H. Age-related bone mineral density, accumulated bone loss rate and prevalence of osteoporosis at multiple skeletal sites in Chinese women. Osteoporos Int (A Journal Established as Result of Cooperation Between the European Foundation for Osteoporosis and the National Osteoporosis Foundation of the USA). 2002; 13(8):669–76.
9. Koornneef L. New insights in the human orbital connective tissue. Result of a new anatomical approach. Arch Ophthalmol. 1977;95:1269–73.
10. Orimo H. Bone change related to aging. In: Osteoporosis and prevention of bone fracture. Academic Press. Tokyo, Japan; 2005. pp. 3.

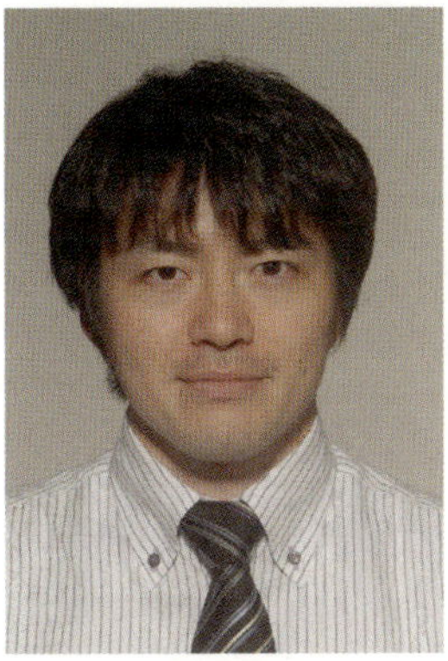

**Tomoyuki Kashima** Tomoyuki Kashima graduated from Medical school of Gunma University in 2002 and trained in general ophthalmology in Department of Ophthalmology in Gunma University. He achieved oculoplastic fellowship program in Seirei Hamamatsu Hospital, Shizuoka, Japan from 2005 to 2007. He became the chief of oculoplastic and orbit surgery in Gunma University from 2007, and also become council member of Asia Pacific Society of Ophthalmic Plastic and Reconstructive Surgery from 2010 to 2014. He achieved International fellowship program in UCLA Stein Eye Institute from 2015 to 2016.

# 14 Types and Management of Orbital Fractures

Tomoyuki Kashima

## Pathology of Fractures

Before treatment, clinicians must assess when and how the trauma occurred within the periorbital region. There are two possible mechanisms explaining orbital fractures, the hydraulic and the buckling theory [1]. When the intraorbital pressure rises suddenly, the indented force causes a deformity in the orbital floor and wall, which leads to bone fracture. A fracture could also be caused by direct dislocation of the globe to the walls [2]. As discussed in the previous chapter, age-related changes in bone hardness contribute to the dislocation of the fractured bone and orbital contents, which leads to subjective symptoms.

## Subjective Symptoms

Orbital fracture results in dislocation of bones and herniation of orbital contents. Due to these conditions, several symptoms could contribute to impaired quality of life for the patient. A dislocated bone may lead to the enlargement of the orbital cavity, and the globe could exhibit enophthalmos. Both the herniated orbital muscle and fat at the fracture site may cause impairment of ocular movements, because there are specific connections between orbital muscle and orbital fat [3]. A sharp edge fat of the bone could significantly impair EOM, and the patient could experience pain during eye movement. Another symptom of orbital fracture is nausea and vomiting from the oculocardiac reflex (Aschner phenomenon) [4]. The orbital tissues have sensory nerves which originate from the vagus nerve, a motor and sensory nerve of internal organs, which mainly controls the circulatory system, cardiovascular system, and gastrointestinal system. When the orbital tissues are herniated and tightly entrapped, they become congested and damaged, resulting in further damage to the orbital branch of the vagus nerves, causing nausea or vomiting via the oculocardiac reflex.

## Trapdoor-Type Fracture

Trapdoor fracture is the most common type of fracture in young patients, especially in those under 20 years of age [5]. As discussed in the previous chapter, because the bone is soft in young patients, clinical features and subjective symptoms differ from adults. When blunt trauma occurs, the adult orbital bone breaks. However, the young orbital bone is too soft to break and completely dislocates into the sinus, so that only a part of the orbital wall breaks. After an orbital bone break, the elevated intraorbital pressure

T. Kashima, MD,
Oculoplastic Service, Department of Ophthalmology, Gunma University,
Maebashi, Gunma 3710034, Japan
e-mail: kasimatomoyuki@yahoo.co.jp


B. Mukherjee, H. Yuen (eds.), *Emergencies of the Orbit and Adnexa*,
DOI 10.1007/978-81-322-1807-4_14

causes orbital tissue, such as muscle or orbital fat, to herniate into the adjacent sinus. Some orbital bones may not break completely and are thus able to return to their original position, causing entrapment of herniated orbital muscle and fat. In trapdoor fractures, retention of entrapped extraocular muscle may occur and cause irreversible damage due to congestion and lack of blood from venous occlusion, if surgical procedures to release the tissues are not performed within 24 h [6]. In these cases, the extraocular muscles not identified intraorbitally are referred to as "missing rectus" (Fig. 14.1) [7]. The density of extraocular muscle is the same as a hemorrhage in the sinus, thus, in those cases identification of herniated muscles are difficult. However, cases with only orbital fat entrapment present a different condition. Orbital fat exists both as a filler of the orbit and a lubricant for eye movement. Prolapsed orbital fat impairs extraocular motility, thus the release of prolapsed orbital fat should be considered in orbital fracture. However, surgical indications are not as emergent as with muscle herniation, but the surgery should be performed within several days.

## Open-Type Fracture

In the adult patient, open-type fracture is the most frequent and is a well-known result of periorbital blunt injury. In this type of fracture, the bones are dislocated and orbital tissues do not become entrapped. The patients' symptoms are therefore mild EOM impairment and enophthalmos [8]. To diagnose open-type fractures, coronal computed tomography (CT) scanning may be suitable. Coronal section CT scans can show both sides of the orbit, in the same section, to compare both orbital shapes (Figs. 14.2, 14.3, 14.4, 14.5, 14.6, and 14.7). During diagnosis, the clinician should see a soft tissue image, not a bone image. In cases with orbital fracture, the locations of the bones have less importance than understanding the degree of herniation of orbital contents. In a bone image, only the dislocation of bones and not the severity of the dislocation of orbital contents may be observable. However, in soft tissue

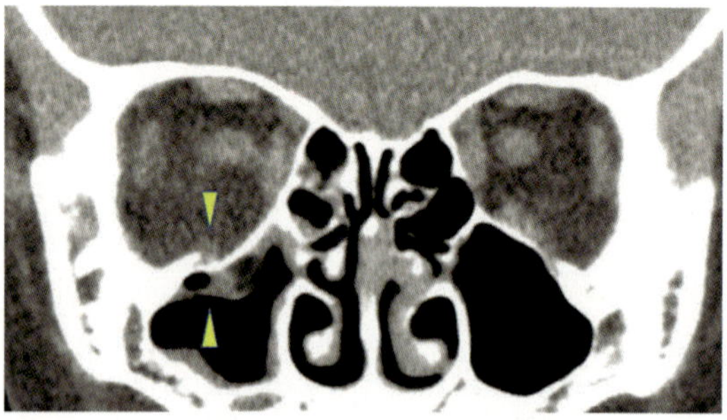

**Fig. 14.1** A case of "missing rectus" in the right orbit. The inferior rectus appears absent from the right orbit, but is actually dislocated into the maxillary sinus. Diagnosis using CT scans is misleading in this situation, because the density of the muscle is the same as the hemorrhage

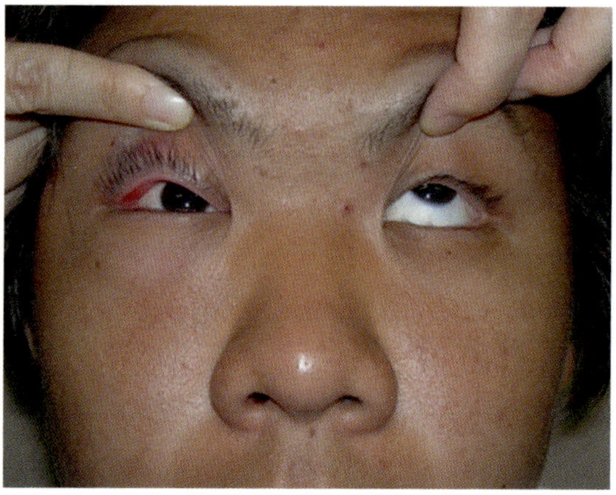

**Fig. 14.2** The trapdoor fracture on the orbital floor of the right eye. The inferior rectus and surrounding orbital fat herniated and caught in the sight, which leads to impairment of supraduction of the right eye

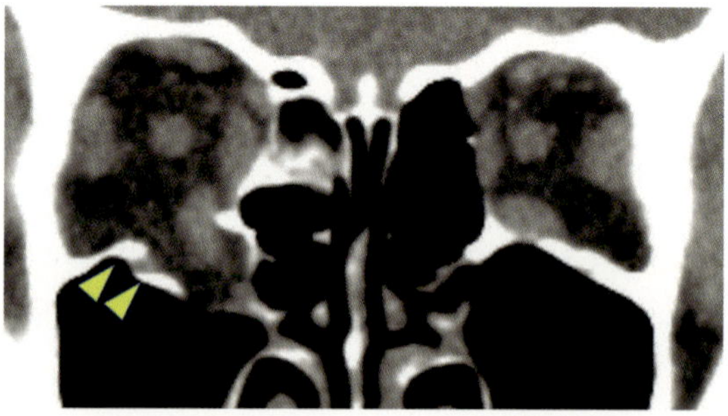

**Fig. 14.3** Right orbital fracture with lateral hinge in a coronal section. A common site of orbital floor fracture is the infraorbital canal, which is the thinnest area, due to the presence of the infraorbital nerve (*arrowheads*)

images, bones, rectus muscles, and orbital fat can be observed in the same scanned section, which is useful in diagnosing the severity of the orbital fracture. In these CT scans, the location of the fractured bones should be identified to determine if they can be reused to reconstruct an orbital wall defect. The surgeon must also identify which hinge of the fracture to approach during the dissection of the fracture in the periorbital region.

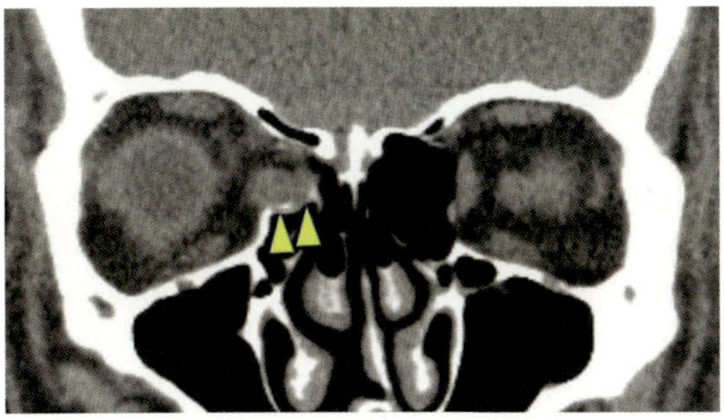

**Fig. 14.4** Right orbital wall fracture in the coronal section. The upper half of the medial wall is fractured and orbital contents are herniated into the ethmoidal sinus. The medial rectus appears swollen, due to retracted muscle (*arrowheads*)

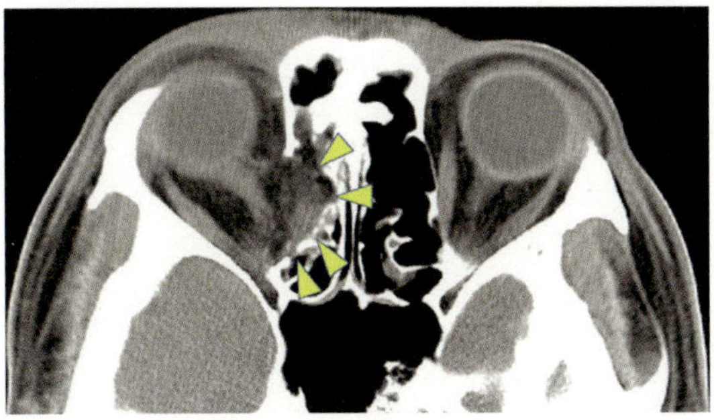

**Fig. 14.5** Medial wall fracture in an axial section. The image shows a medial wall fracture and disappearance of ethmoid sinus on the right side (*arrowheads*). The optic nerve is bent because of retraction from the herniated orbital contents

The orbital strut is one of the most important regions to analyze when diagnosing an open-type fracture, because misdiagnosis frequently occurs when examining this site. The orbital strut is a fundamental structure which provides support for the orbital inferior and medial walls. However, the fracture of an orbital strut may not be obvious in CT scans, when compared with medial and inferior fracture CT scans. If the orbital strut is displaced, it may cause severe enophthalmos. Therefore, the orbital strut should be examined in all fracture cases [9].

## Other Fractures

Other rarer types of orbital fractures are lateral wall and superior wall. Lateral wall is mainly

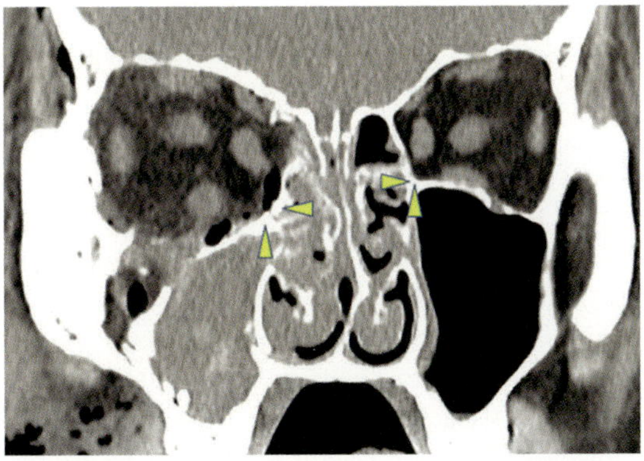

**Fig. 14.6** Medial and floor fracture with break of orbital strut. In cases with breaks of the orbital strut, the orbital shape appears to retain its original shape because it is round. However, this causes significant enophthalmos if the orbital strut is not reconstructed

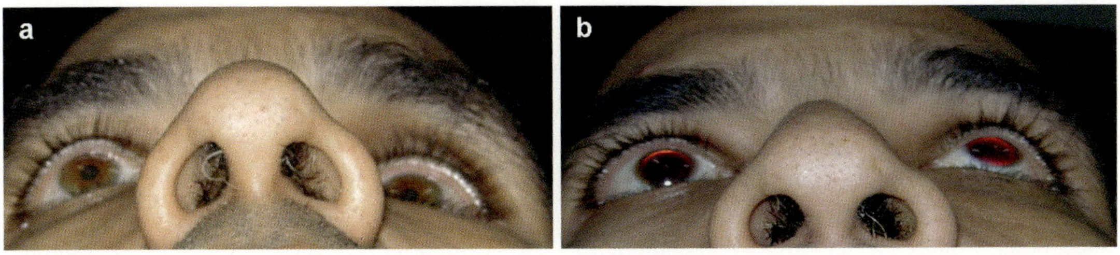


**Fig. 14.7** Significant right enophthalmos after surgery. A postoperative photo from Fig. 14.4 is shown. Because the surgeon did not reconstruct the orbital strut, the patient shows significant enophthalmos

constructed with zygomatic bone. Displacement of lateral wall causes the enlargement of orbital volume which leads to major enophthalmos. Zygomatic bone constructs the major part of orbital floor, and the middle part of orbital floor is the most fragile site of floor fracture due to the infraorbital canal. Because of this mechanism, lateral wall fracture usually accompanies floor fracture. EOM impairment is not frequent with the patients of lateral wall fractures. The orbital superior wall is consists mainly of frontal bone. A major part of orbital roof is lined by cranial dura mater which is harder than periosteum or nasal mucosa.

Due to this structure, orbital roof is harder to break than other orbital walls. In some patients who have protuberant frontal sinus, the anterior part of orbital roof is adjacent to the sinus. It sometimes leads roof fracture and herniation of orbital contents.

Orbital roof fractures associated with skull fractures are common in young children due to their higher cranium-to-facial skeleton ratios.

## Surgical Intervention

Surgical procedures for the two types of fractures are different, because the subjective symptoms are different. Open-type fracture surgery can be performed 1–2 weeks after the fracture, because there is no tissue damage prior to that time period. However, trapdoor fractures have to be treated within 24 h, because delayed surgical intervention may cause permanent tissue damage and a lifetime of diplopia [10].

There are two types of surgical approaches to the fracture site, transcutaneous and transconjunctival. Transcutaneous surgery uses a subciliary incision from the orbital floor and from the medial canthal cutaneous incision to the medial orbital wall. Transconjunctival surgery is from a lateral canthal incision with a palpebral conjunctival incision from the floor and from the lacrimal caruncle. Transcutaneous approaches can produce open wounds which are wide enough to observe the deepest part of the orbital fracture. However, the patient may have a scar that remains and is cosmetically unpleasant, especially for Asian skin. In contrast, the transconjunctival approach does not produce an obvious scar, because the wound is small. However, the surgical procedure requires experience and a more complete exploration and reconstruction of the orbital walls.

The surgical goals for each type of fracture are different. The clinician must first consider restoring normal orbital anatomy through surgical intervention before scarring of the orbital tissue occurs and becomes permanent.

For trapdoor-type fractures, repositioning of the displaced orbital contents should then be performed. The ophthalmologist should perform a diagnosis as soon as possible to avoid unnecessary examinations. Misdiagnosis of a rectus fracture could lead to prolonged nausea caused by the vasovagal reflex, which may result in patients in neurosurgery units being too conservatively treated with antiemetic drugs. Due to its structure, the fractured bone in a trapdoor fracture is not displaced very far; thus, surgical repair is not difficult. To release and restore the herniated orbital tissue, the fractured bone, which returns to its normal position and entraps orbital contents, may have to be fractured again without removing the bone. Then, the orbital tissues can be removed from the orbital wall. In our experience, replacing the original bone is sufficient to cover the defect, except when the bone is completely removed from the surgical site. If this is done, there will be a gap or microdefect around the bone edge to which the orbital contents will enter. In that situation, artificial materials like polycaprolactone or silicone sheets are required to prevent herniation.

Open-type fractures exhibit a different physical state. The main result of open-type fractures is the dislocation of orbital bone and contents. Therefore, one goal of open-type fracture surgery is to reposition the orbital wall to replace the herniated orbital contents. If the surgery is performed within 1–2 weeks after the injury, the dislocated orbital bones can be directly replaced. However, after that period, repositioning of bones is difficult, due to tissue adhesion and epithelialization of nasal mucosa, which may develop orbital mucocele, several years after the operation. As discussed above, the fractured bone tends to fragment, depending on the age of the patient. In our experience, if the fractured bone can be removed as a single plate, it can be used to patch the orbital defect. However, if the bones are fragmented, artificial materials should be used to repair the defect without reposition of bones. Once the orbital wall is reconstructed to its original position, the orbital contents may not return to the sinus, which suggests that the EOM and enophthalmos may be restored.

EOMs do not recover soon after an operation. Surgery causes swelling and scarring of orbital tissue, and it often requires 3–6 months to completely restore the orbital fracture. Moreover, if the extraocular muscles are entrapped in a trapdoor-type fracture, paralysis usually occurs, but may disappear 2–3 months after the surgical release of the tissue (Fig. 14.8).

## References


1. Warwar RE, Bullock JD, Ballal DR, Ballal RD. Mechanisms of orbital floor fractures: a clinical, experimental, and theoretical study. Ophthal Plast Reconstr Surg. 2000;16(3):188–200.
2. Erling BF, Iliff N, Robertson B, Manson PN. Footprints of the globe: a practical look at the mechanism of orbital blowout fractures, with a revisit to the work of Raymond Pfeiffer. Plast Reconstr Surg. 1999;103(4):1313–6. discussion 1317–1319.
3. Koornneef L. Orbital septa: anatomy and function. Ophthalmology. 1979;86(5):876–80.
4. Joseph JM, Rosenberg C, Zoumalan CI, Zoumalan RA, White WM, Lisman RD. Oculocardiac reflex associated with a large orbital floor fracture. Ophthal Plast Reconstr Surg. 2009;25(6):496–8.
5. Bansagi ZC, Meyer DR. Internal orbital fractures in the pediatric age group: characterization and management. Ophthalmology. 2000;107(5):829–36.
6. Gerbino G, Roccia F, Bianchi FA, Zavattero E. Surgical management of orbital trapdoor fracture in a pediatric population. J Oral Maxillofac Surg. 2010;68(6):1310–6.
7. Anda S, Elsas T, Harstad HK. The missing rectus: a CT observation from blow-out fracture of the orbital floor. J Comput Assist Tomogr. 1987;11(5):895–7.
8. Whitehouse RW, Batterbury M, Jackson A, Noble JL. Prediction of enophthalmos by computed tomography after 'blow out' orbital fracture. Br J Ophthalmol. 1994;78(8):618–20.
9. Kim JW, Goldberg RA, Shorr N. The inferomedial orbital strut: an anatomic and radiographic study. Ophthal Plast Reconstr Surg. 2002;18(5):355–64.
10. Hink EM, Wei LA, Durairaj VD. Clinical features and treatment of pediatric orbit fractures. Ophthal Plast Reconstr Surg. 2014;30:124–31.


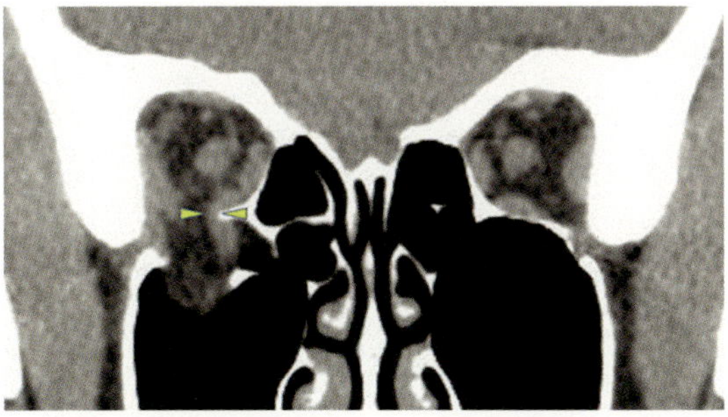

**Fig. 14.8** The impinged inferior rectus at the edge of a fractured bone. The inferior rectus is herniated into the maxillary sinus and is caught at the edge of the medial side of the fractured bone

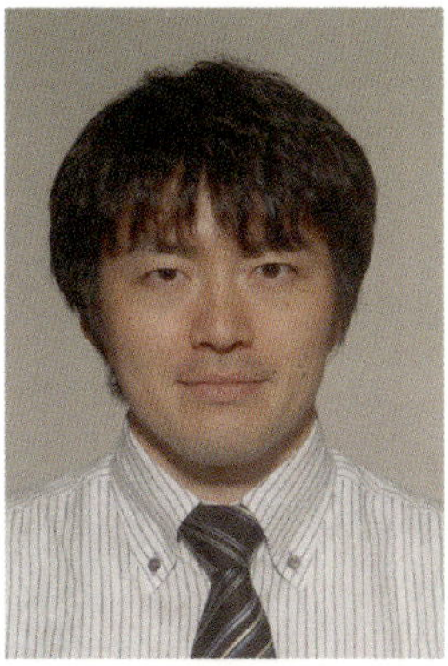


**Tomoyuki Kashima** Tomoyuki Kashima was graduated Medical school of Gunma University in 2002 and trained general ophthalmology in Department of Ophthalmology in Gunma University. He achieved oculoplastic fellowship program in Seirei Hamamatsu Hospital, Shizuoka, Japan from 2005 to 2007. He became the chief of oculoplastic and orbit surgery in Gunma University from 2007, and also become council member of Asia Pacific Society of Ophthalmic Plastic and Reconstructive Surgery from 2010 to 2014. He achieved International fellowship program in UCLA Stein Eye Institute from 2015 to 2016.

# Organic Foreign Bodies

# 15

Usha R. Kim, Priti Bhoutekar,
and Swapna Parekh-Chattopadhyay

## Introduction

Orbital and ocular traumas are important emergencies encountered by ophthalmologists. Orbital organic foreign bodies comprise one of the most common and serious sequelae following trauma. These incidents commonly occur in domestic, industrial, and agricultural life. The retention of wooden piece is among the most common organic foreign bodies following orbital trauma. Apart from the development of infection, another major concern related to these foreign bodies includes complications due to damage of important structures crowded in orbital cavity including the globe [1].

U.R. Kim, DO, DNB (✉) • P. Bhoutekar, MD
S. Parekh-Chattopadhyay, MS, DNB
Orbit, Oculoplasty & Ocular Oncology,
Aravind Eye Hospital, Madurai,
Madurai, Tamil Nadu 625 020, India
e-mail: usha@aravind.org; dr.priti.aiims@gmail.com;
swapna.parekh@gmail.com

## Etiologies

The types of organic foreign body which may be retained in orbit can be innumerable.

I. Vegetative materials
   - Wood piece
   - Thorn
   - Grains
II. Animal tissue
   - Insects
   - Fish

## Pathophysiology

Orbital cavity is formed by four bony walls and provides protection to the globe from major trauma. Owing to the presence of orbital wall on all sides except anteriorly, foreign bodies usually enter orbit from the anterior route penetrating the lid, canthus, conjunctiva, or globe. since the lateral aspect of the globe is more exposed it is susceptible to injuries and acts as a common entry for foreign bodies. It may be the ends of objects forced into the orbit and broken off and thus retained or flying particles which usually have sufficient energy to penetrate orbital tissue. Transorbital intracranial penetration of foreign bodies is highly unusual but carries a high risk of mortality owing to secondary intracranial infec-


B. Mukherjee, H. Yuen (eds.), *Emergencies of the Orbit and Adnexa*,
DOI 10.1007/978-81-322-1807-4_15

tions because of the contaminated nature of organic foreign bodies [2].

The organic foreign bodies tend to induce a granulomatous inflammatory reaction. The response of tissues is usually extremely slow and considerable time may elapse, before the granulomatous mass becomes clinically evident. Wood, with its porous consistency and organic nature, provides a good medium for microbial agents [3].

## Clinical Picture

Systematic and elaborate history taking is of utmost importance for diagnosis of any retained foreign body. The history of an accident involving lodgement of a foreign body in the orbit is usually definite, but may be absent or misleading. The diagnosis is often rendered more difficult if the entry wound of entry is not easily detected. However, usually the injury is associated with edema, ecchymosis, and proptosis, which can make the condition obvious. Clinical picture varies depending on the mode of injury and type and size of foreign body. Organic foreign bodies can have acute and/or delayed presentations.

- Acute presentation:
  1. Orbital cellulitis/abscess – It presents with painful proptosis, other signs of inflammation like chemosis and congestion, and loss of vision.
  2. Optic nerve injury causing loss of vision.
  3. Neurosensory disturbances – Trauma to orbital apex or superior orbital fissure leads to various sensory neurological deficits as well as motor paralytic strabismus. Anesthesia of the upper lid and eye following injury to first division of trigeminal nerve can occur.
  4. Extraocular muscle injury or adhesions causing diplopia.
  5. Ophthalmic vein thrombosis/cavernous sinus thrombosis.
  6. Injury to adjacent structure like intracranial or paranasal sinus injury.
- Delayed presentation:
  1. Discharging fistula – In less severe grade of infection, formation of chronic discharging fistula with constant drainage of purulent or serosanguinous discharge.
  2. Osteomyelitis and periostitis.
  3. Granulomatous tumor – Organic foreign body results in severe granulomatous reaction resulting in mass effect like proptosis, dystopia of globe, and movement restriction.
  4. Traumatic cyst – Sometimes traumatic cyst forms aroundw foreign body.
  5. Restrictive strabismus – The presence of severe fibrous tissue bands in orbit results in restricted ocular motility.

## Evaluation

The evaluation of patient begins with assessing general physical condition of the patient, as the trauma causing orbital injuries may be associated with severe life-threatening injuries which take precedence over orbital treatment. The spectrum of findings in orbital injuries is large, and injuries that appear to be trivial on external examination may be extensive. Lacerations or puncture wounds of the brow, lid, and face should be carefully inspected and gently probed to determine their direction and extent. Integrity of intraocular structures should be noted. Assessment of vision and pupillary reaction should be done.

## Investigation

1. Plain X-ray: Plain films cannot identify radiolucent foreign bodies such as wood.
2. Ultrasonography: It can detect radiolucent intraocular and anterior orbital foreign bodies but may be unable to find objects lying deep in the orbit.
3. CT scan: It can determine exact location of foreign body as well as any associated orbital wall fracture. But, CT may fail to delineate wooden foreign bodies since its radiodensity is similar to orbital tissue. An organic foreign body especially wood should be suspected if there is air on the scan, especially in a linear configuration [4] (Fig. 15.1a–c). Overall, CT appears to be diagnostic imaging of choice [5].
4. Magnetic Resonance Imaging: MRI provides better soft tissue delineation over that given by

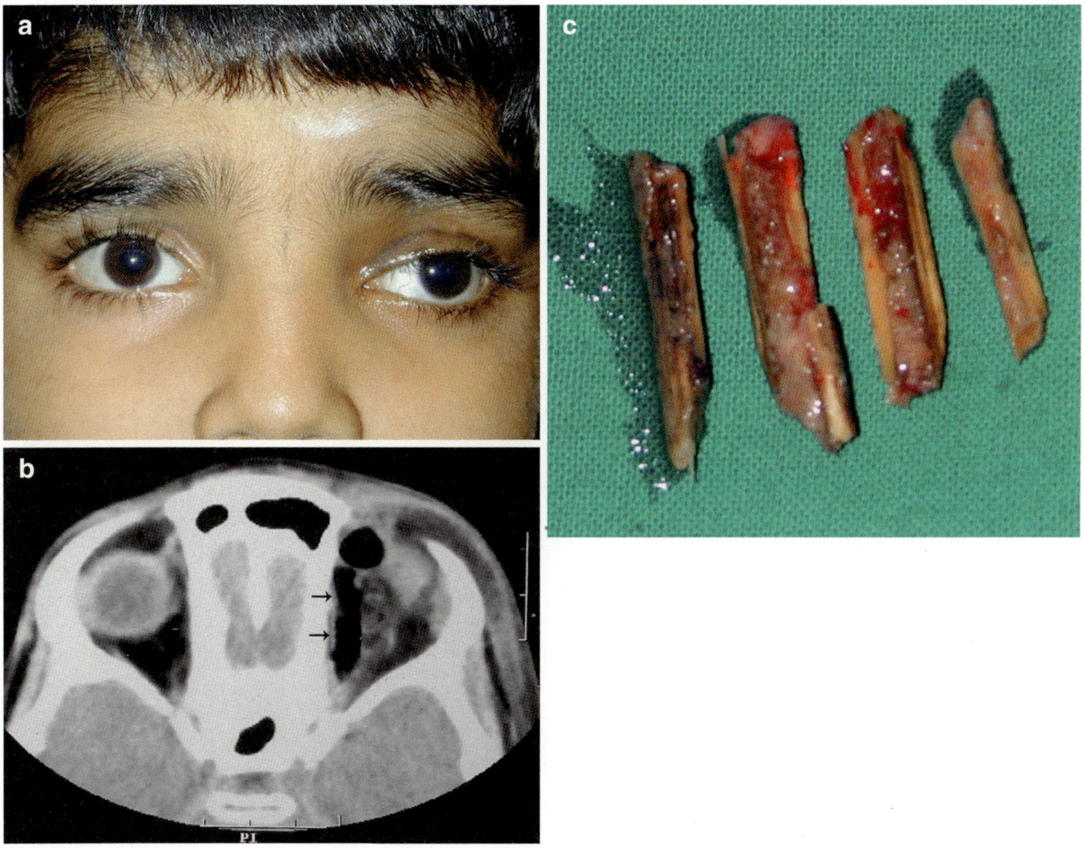

**Fig. 15.1** (**a**) Clinical picture of a 6-year-old boy with wooden stick injury to the left eye. (**b**) NECT axial view showing linear low-attenuation (air-isodense) foreign body. (**c**) Wooden foreign body removed in multiple pieces from orbit

CT. It provides better resolution of low-density objects such as organic matter and wooden foreign bodies.

## Management

The management of orbital foreign bodies is dependent upon the type of material and its location in the orbit. The foreign bodies which need to be removed include wood or any other vegetative material. The orbital foreign bodies that are causing impingement of the optic nerve or have penetrated adjacent structures, such as the cranial cavity or sinuses also need to be removed. The removal of foreign bodies is often through the entry wound, by following the wound track into the orbit, the foreign body can be found. Sometimes, orbitotomy may be required for deep lying foreign bodies. Organic and wooden foreign bodies may fragment easily during surgical removal leaving behind small splinters that can cause inflammation even after long intervals [6]. Any chronically infected orbit with or without a draining sinus must be suspected of harboring an intraorbital foreign body [7] (see Fig. 15.2a–c). At the time of exploration and foreign body removal, a culture should be obtained and the wound should be thoroughly irrigated with saline and a appropriate antibiotic solution [8]. In foreign bodies associated with orbital abscess, the placement of a drain and/or packing material may be needed. Proper antibiotic treatment is of utmost importance owing to the high risk of secondary infection. In all cases, development of tetanus should be kept in mind especially with organic

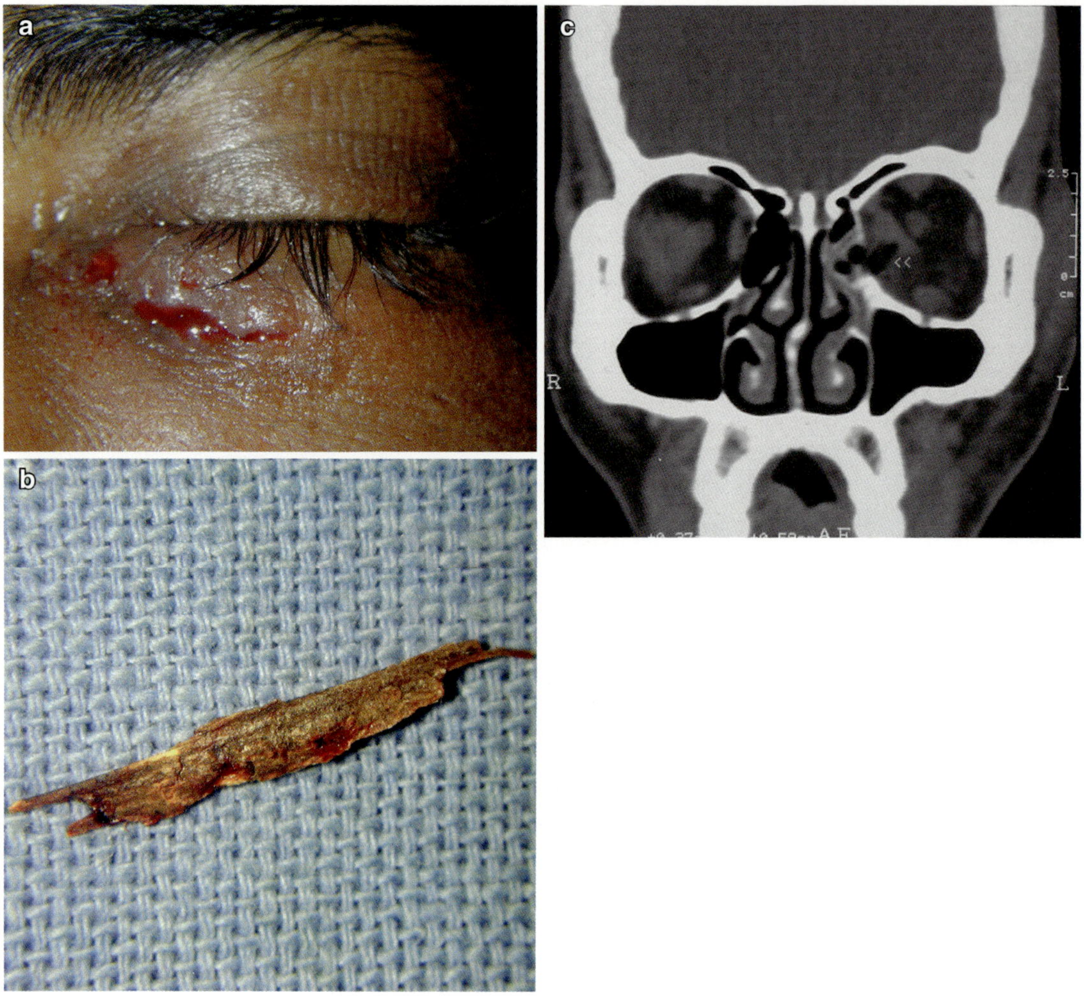


**Fig. 15.2** (**a**) Clinical picture of a 52-year-old male with trauma from the bark of tree. (**b**) NECT coronal view showing foreign body in medial quadrant of orbit and entering ethmoid sinus. (**c**) Wooden piece after removal

material and prophylactic tetanus toxoid administered in all appropriate cases.

To summarize, detection of orbital foreign bodies needs thorough history taking and evaluation. Most organic foreign bodies warrant removal for fear of infection.

## References

1. Henry Kimpton. Duke elder S. S. – Text Book of Ophthalmology. Vol VI. Mosby, St. Louis. London; 1954.
2. Lee JS, Lee JE, Oum BS, Cha SH. Orbitocranial injury caused by wood. Korean J Ophthalmol. 1999;13(2):128–32.
3. Zenter J, Hassler W, Petersen D. A wooden foreign body penetrating the superior orbital fissure. Neurochirurgia. 1991;34:188–90.
4. Ho VT, McGuckin Jr JF, Smergel EM. Intraorbital wooden foreign body: CT and MR appearance. AJNR Am J Neuroradiol. 1996;17(1):134–6.
5. Fulcher TP, McNab AA, Sullivan TJ. Clinical features and management of intraorbital foreign bodies. Ophthalmology. 2002;109(3):494–500.
6. Agarwal PK, Kumar H, Srivastava PK. Unusual orbital foreign bodies. Indian J Ophthalmol. 1993;41(3):125–7.
7. Michon J, Liu D. Intraorbital foreign bodies. Sem Ophthalmol. 1994;9(3):193–9.
8. Long JA, Tann TM. Ocular trauma. In: Kuhn F, Pieramici D, editors. Principles and practices. Chapter 36. Orbital trauma. Thieme. New York; 2002. p. 383–90.

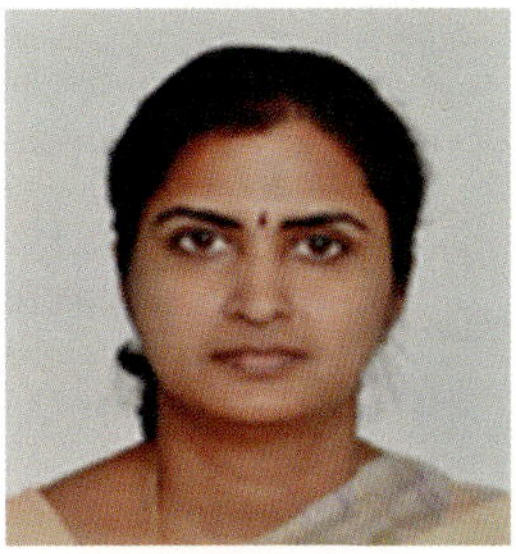

**Usha R. Kim** ***Current Position*** Head of the Department of Orbit, Oculoplasty and Ocular Oncology Services, Professor in Ophthalmology, Director of Mid-Level Ophthalmic Personnel, Head of Telemedicine-Supported Vision Centers Network at Aravind Eye Care System, Madurai.

***Qualification*** Dr. Usha Kim received her MBBS from Bharathiar University, Coimbatore, in 1991, Diploma in Ophthalmology and MNAMS (Oph), from Aravind Eye Hospital, Madurai, in the year 1994 and 1995 respectively. She completed her specialty training under the guidance of Dr. William B. Stewart at University of California, San Francisco, and at Salt Lake City, Utah, in the United States of America.

Dr. Usha Kim is heading the Department of Orbit, Oculoplasty and Ocular Oncology at Aravind Eye Hospital since 1998. Under her efficient leadership, the clinic has seen several innovations such as the addition of Ocular Oncology Services and an Ocular Prosthesis Center. She is actively involved in various teaching programs at Aravind Eye Hospital and Lions Institute of Community Ophthalmology (LAICO). She has trained nearly 55 national and 16 international candidates as fellows in the field of Orbit, Oculoplasty, and Ocular Oncology. She has also trained 41 ocularists both at the national and international level.

She has been a member of Aravind Research Committee since March 1998 and is a principal investigator for many studies conducted at Aravind Eye Care System. She is actively involved in various research activities and currently focuses on genetics of retinoblastoma.

She has presented papers, delivered lectures, and chaired various international, national, and state-level ophthalmic conferences.

**She has 43 publications to her credit – 23 international and 18 national**. She has also written chapters in many books and co-authored a book on Imaging in Orbit and Neuro-ophthalmology.

She established 'The Ring of Hope' in 2004, a program that provides free service to patients, children, and adults who have life-threatening cancers in the eye like retinoblastoma. The Ring of Hope Fund, since its inception, has supported 1600 ocular cancer patients, who would otherwise not have been able to receive treatment.

***Awards***

- **CP Gupta Award** for '**Best Paper**' from TNOA in 2002
- '**Best Orbital Photography**' **award** in Joint Meeting of the Oculoplastics Association of India & Asia Pacific Society of Ophthalmic Plastic and Reconstructive Surgery in 2007
- **'Best Poster' award for Prospective Evaluation of Contracted Anophthalmic Sockets** in the Indo Israel Meeting held in Chennai in 2005
- **'Vocational excellence Award'** from Rotary Club of Madurai in 2010 for her work in the community
- **International Women's day Excellence award** by the Lions Club of Madurai District 324-B3 March 8, 2015, for her work in the field of Ocular Oncology
- **PSG & Sons' Charities, Coimbatore Scroll of Honour awarded** for her an eminent expert in diagnosis, treatment, rehabilitation, and research in ophthalmology holding a key leadership position in a reputed Eye Care system, for having conducted a large number of cataract surgeries in addition to her widely acclaimed expertise in orbit oculoplasty, ocular prosthetic services, ocular oncology, and her personal involvement in the Ring of Hope initiative

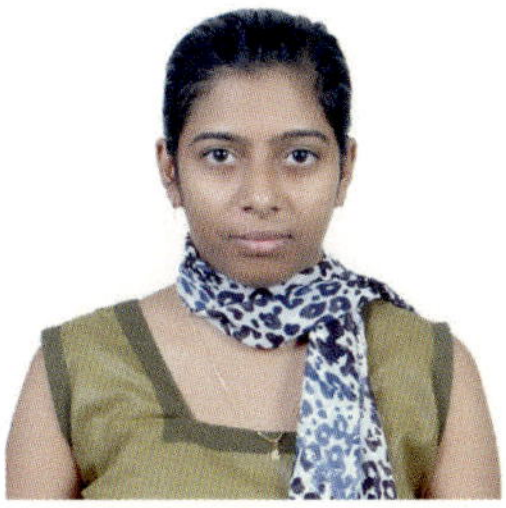

**Priti Bhoutekar** Dr. Priti Bhoutekar (Urade) is a dedicated medical professional with prior work and education experiences at renowned institutes in Delhi and South India. She works with sustained focus and interest in the field of Orbit and Oculoplasty. She completed her MBBS (2004 - 2010) from Government medical college, Nagpur. In 2013, she received M.D Ophthalmology from prestigious AIIMS, Delhi. She also received DNB Ophthalmology in 2015. During her fellowship in orbit and Oculoplasty (2013-2015), she worked and got trained under Dr. Usha Kim at Aravind eye hospital, Madurai. Currently works as consultant Orbit and Ophthalmic Plastic surgeon in central India. She has one international publication to her name. She presented a paper on "A novel approach for optic nerve sheath decompression; our experiences and outcomes" during APSOPRS-OPAI 2014, Delhi. Also, her poster on 'Large spot laser for treatment of retinopathy of prematurity' was presented in AAO, Chicago (Oct 2014).

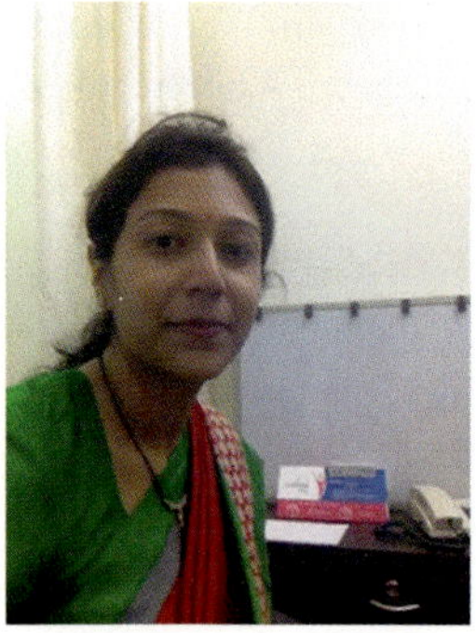

**Swapna Parekh-Chattopadhyay** Dr. Swapna has done her MBBS from Lokmanya Tilak Municipal Medical College and Sion Hospital, Mumbai, and postgraduation in Ophthalmology (M.S. Ophthalmology) from Topiwala National Medical Hospital and Nair Hospital, Mumbai, after which she joined Sir Ganga Ram Hospital, New Delhi, for 2 years as Senior Registrar, where she worked and trained under Dr. A. K. Grover and obtained extensive experience in orbit and oculoplasty surgeries. She then joined a long term fellowship program in Orbit, Oculoplasty and Ocular Oncology at Aravind Eye Hospital, Madurai, where she honed her technical skills under the guidance of Dr. Usha Kim, a stalwart in the field.

At present Dr. Swapna is a practicing orbit and oculoplasty consultant specializing in plastic surgery of the eyelids, eye socket reconstruction, lacrimal surgeries, pediatrics oculoplastics, cosmetic eyelid and brow surgery, and nonsurgical facial cosmetic treatments (Botox and fillers). Experience: 10 years.

# Inorganic Foreign Bodies

# 16

Usha R. Kim, Priti Bhoutekar, and Swapna Parekh-Chattopadhyay

## Introduction

Orbital foreign bodies comprise one of the most common and serious sequelae following trauma. They are often seen in patients with multiple trauma from traffic accidents, assault, fall from height, gunshot and warfare. Many orbital foreign bodies have been reported in the literature, including BB gun pellets, nails, pens, pencils, twigs, stone, glass. The clinical suspicion should be high as signs of trauma may be subtle.

## Aetiologies

Majority of inorganic foreign bodies can be classified into metallic and non-metallic foreign bodies.

1. Metallic
   - Iron
   - Copper
   - Steel
   - Aluminium
   - Lead
   - Gold
   - Silver
2. Non-metallic
   - Glass
   - Coal
   - Stone
   - Plastic

## Pathophysiology

Orbital bony frame and soft tissues provide a natural protection against foreign body penetration. The major factor determining severity of damage is the velocity of foreign body impact. Small-sized foreign bodies with high velocity can penetrate much deeper as compared to large-sized slow-velocity object. Depending upon the type, size and momentum of the foreign body, the after-effects are variable. Most metals, particularly iron, steel, aluminium, lead, gold and others, are inert and in the absence of infection cause no disturbance apart from their bulk. In fact, copper is the only badly tolerated metal causing severe purulent inflammation [1]. Other more common inert foreign bodies are glass and stone. Pieces of glass give rise to little reaction and may remain quiet for long periods. Stone pieces are also silent if infected usually develop low-grade infection.

U.R. Kim, DO, DNB (✉) • P. Bhoutekar, MD • S. Parekh-Chattopadhyay
Orbit, Oculoplasty & Ocular Oncology, Aravind Eye Hospital, Madurai,
Madurai, Tamil Nadu 625 020, India
e-mail: usha@aravind.org; dr.priti.aiims@gmail.com; swapna.parekh@gmail.com


B. Mukherjee, H. Yuen (eds.), *Emergencies of the Orbit and Adnexa*,
DOI 10.1007/978-81-322-1807-4_16

## Clinical Picture

Trauma causing orbital injuries is usually severe and may be associated with life-threatening complications. The effect of retention of metallic foreign body in orbit is usually much less dramatic and harmful than within the eye. Most of the metallic and non-metallic foreign bodies are inert in the orbit. Retained intraorbital metallic foreign bodies are well tolerated and typically have minimal adverse visual prognosis [2]. These inert metals will rarely be a nidus for infection or cause problems due to migration.

Clinical presentations are usually acute.

(a) Haemorrhage: Injury to major vessel usually a vein may result in severe haemorrhage into the orbital tissue. Most often they can be adequately treated with pressure bandaging. Sometimes, secondary haemorrhage can occur after a few days.
(b) Traumatic emphysema: This may be the immediate complication when there is an associated orbital wall is fracture and communication is established with an air-filled sinus. This may occur by impaction of flying stone causing orbital emphysema and cellulitis-like picture which can be readily treated by incision and release of air.
(c) Suppurative inflammation: It is the most feared complication, especially when it involves copper.
(d) Neurosensory disturbances: Foreign body impinging on the optic nerve will cause vision loss. Trauma to orbital apex or superior orbital fissure leads to various sensory neurological deficits.
(e) Others: Injury to neighbouring structures like paranasal sinuses and intracranial injuries should be considered.

## Evaluation

The spectrum of findings in orbital injuries is large, and injuries that appear to be trivial on external examination may be extensive. Lacerations or puncture wounds of the brow, lid and face should be carefully inspected and gently probed to determine their direction and extent. Integrity of intraocular structures should be noted (See Figs. 16.1a–c and 16.2a–c).

Elements of an orbital examination include:

- Visual acuity
- Pupillary reaction
- Hertel exophthalmometry
- Extraocular muscle movement evaluation
- Sensory examination in the distribution of the supra- and infraorbital nerves
- Palpation of the orbital rims
- Auscultation for bruits

## Investigation

Diagnostic imaging provides the ophthalmologist with a detailed anatomic view of the trauma site, surrounding structures, number and location of foreign bodies. Clinical judgement is necessary to determine the best diagnostic modality in each scenario.

I. Plain X-ray: They can document the presence and number of metallic foreign bodies but may not be able to definitively locate them.
II. Ultrasonography: It can detect intraocular and anterior orbital foreign bodies but may be unable to detect objects lying deep in the orbit. Metallic foreign bodies show a posterior reverberation artefact.
III. Computed tomography: CT allows detection of most radiolucent foreign bodies with great precision, including small pieces of stone, aluminium and lead-free glass (<1.5 mm), and copper and steel (minimum diameter of 0.06 mm). It can determine the exact location of foreign body as well as the presence orbital wall fracture. Overall, CT is considered to be the diagnostic imaging of choice.
IV. Magnetic resonance imaging: MRI provides better soft tissue resolution. MRI can be particularly useful in localising a non-metallic foreign body that appears similar to soft tissue on CT scan. But it cannot be used if there is suspicion of metallic foreign bodies and if the patient moves during the scan, which

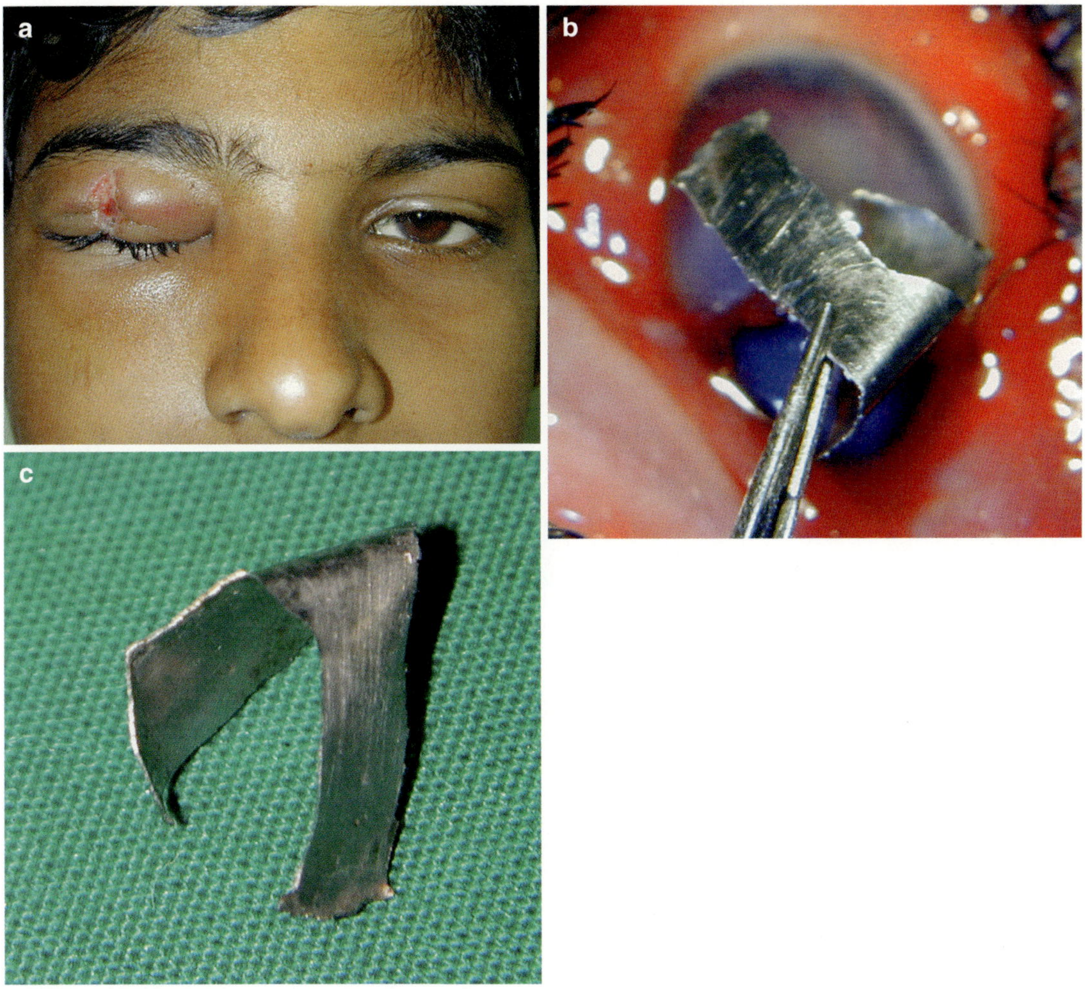


**Fig. 16.1** (**a**) Clinical picture of a 21-year-old male with injury with metal chip at workplace. (**b**) Metallic foreign body during removal. (**c**) After removal

may cause increased intraocular or intracranial injury.

## Management

The management of orbital foreign bodies is dependent upon the type of material, size and its location in the orbit. Depending upon size and location, metallic foreign bodies like steel, iron, gold and other inert metals can be allowed to remain in the orbit, if not causing intraorbital complication. The orbital foreign bodies that are causing impingement of the optic nerve or have penetrated adjacent structures, such as the cranial cavity or sinuses, need to be removed. Since most of the inorganic foreign bodies are inert may not indicate removal if present in non-dangerous position. But if copper is suspected, it forms an indication for exploration and removal. As a general rule, if the risk of removing the object is higher than the risk of leaving the object in place, surgery should be avoided. If vision is intact and the clinical situation is stable, surgery can be deferred. Inorganic orbital foreign bodies should be removed if it is causing complications or if located anteriorly only after discussion of potential surgical complications with the patient. Posteriorly located inorganic foreign bodies should be left alone, unless they are causing significant orbital complications [3].

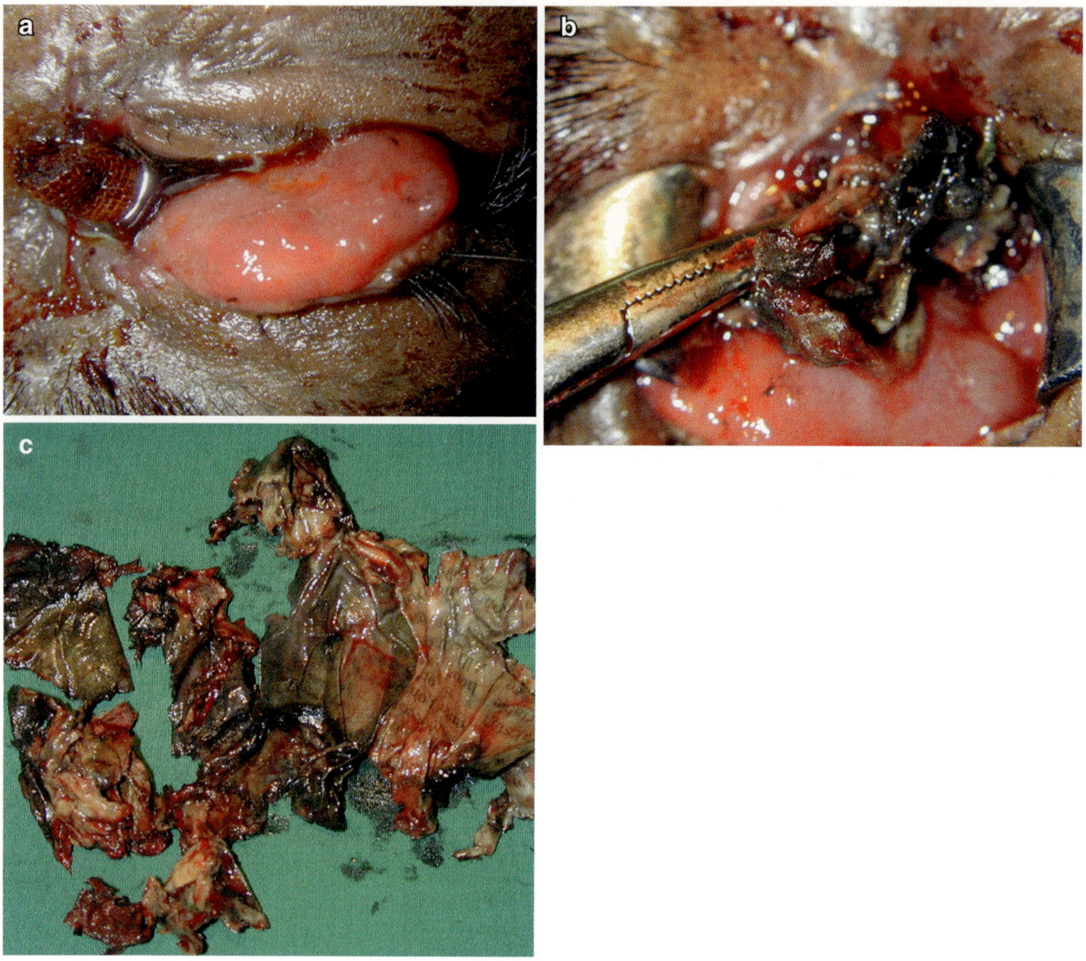

**Fig. 16.2** (**a**) Clinical picture of a 25-year-old male with firecracker injury with avulsion of the upper lid. (**b**) Foreign body (metal base and pieces of paper) during removal. (**c**) After removal

The indications for removal of foreign bodies are given in Table 16.1.

The removal of foreign bodies is usually done through the entry wound. Ferrous foreign body removal can be aided by strong electromagnets. A careful localisation of the foreign body is essential before attempting surgical removal, since there is risk of damage to important intraconal structures. Proper antibiotic treatment is of utmost importance to prevent secondary infection [3].

To summarise, orbital foreign bodies can pose diagnostic and management challenges. Most of the inert metallic foreign bodies can be left without any long-standing complications.

**Table 16.1** Indications of removal of orbital inorganic foreign bodies

| |
|---|
| 1. *Large size* – penetrating into adjacent structures like paranasal sinuses, intracranial space |
| 2. *Copper* [1] – potential to cause severe suppurative orbital inflammation |
| 3. *Contaminated foreign bodies* – causing orbital cellulitis or abscess formation |
| 4. *Superficial foreign bodies* – which are amenable to easy removal without any major orbital intervention or complication |
| 5. *Functional impairment* – any foreign body impinging on optic nerve or limiting ocular movements |

## References


1. Henry Kimpton. Duke elder S. S. – Text book of ophthalmology Vol VI. Mosby, St. Louis. London; 1954.
2. Ho VH, Wilson MW, Fleming JC, Haik BG. Retained intraorbital metallic foreign bodies. Ophthalmic Plast Reconstr Surg. 2004;20(3):232–6.
3. Fulcher TP, McNab AA, Sullivan TJ. Clinical features and management of intraorbital foreign bodies. Ophthalmology. 2002;109(3):494–500.


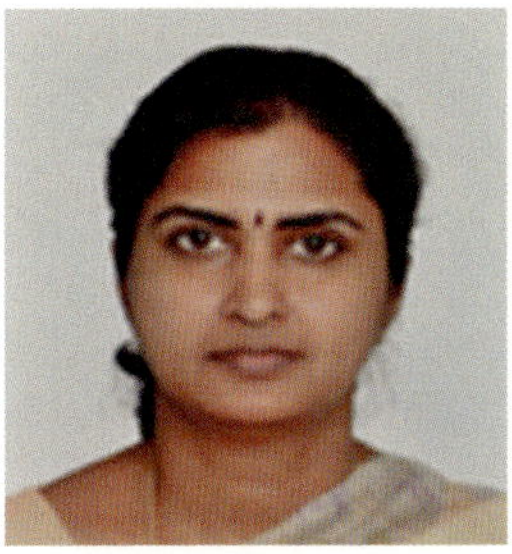

**Usha R. Kim** ***Current Position*** Head of the Department of Orbit, Oculoplasty and Ocular Oncology Services, Professor in Ophthalmology, Director of Mid-Level Ophthalmic Personnel, Head of Telemedicine-Supported Vision Centers Network at Aravind Eye Care System, Madurai.

***Qualification*** Dr. Usha Kim received her MBBS from Bharathiar University, Coimbatore, in 1991, Diploma in Ophthalmology and MNAMS (Oph), from Aravind Eye Hospital, Madurai, in the year 1994 and 1995 respectively. She completed her specialty training under the guidance of Dr. William B. Stewart at University of California, San Francisco, and at Salt Lake City, Utah, in the United States of America.

Dr. Usha Kim is heading the Department of Orbit, Oculoplasty and Ocular Oncology at Aravind Eye Hospital since 1998. Under her efficient leadership, the clinic has seen several innovations such as the addition of Ocular Oncology Services and an Ocular Prosthesis Center. She is actively involved in various teaching programs at Aravind Eye Hospital and Lions Institute of Community Ophthalmology (LAICO). She has trained nearly 55 national and 16 international candidates as fellows in the field of Orbit, Oculoplasty, and Ocular Oncology. She has also trained 41 ocularists both at the national and international level.

She has been a member of Aravind Research Committee since March 1998 and is a principal investigator for many studies conducted at Aravind Eye Care System. She is actively involved in various research activities and currently focuses on genetics of retinoblastoma.

She has presented papers, delivered lectures, and chaired various international, national, and state-level ophthalmic conferences.

**She has 43 publications to her credit – 23 international and 18 national.** She has also written chapters in many books and co-authored a book on Imaging in Orbit and Neuro-ophthalmology.

She established 'The Ring of Hope' in 2004, a program that provides free service to patients, children, and adults who have life-threatening cancers in the eye like retinoblastoma. The Ring of Hope Fund, since its inception, has supported 1600 ocular cancer patients, who would otherwise not have been able to receive treatment.

***Awards***

- **CP Gupta Award** for '**Best Paper**' from TNOA in 2002
- '**Best Orbital Photography**' **award** in Joint Meeting of the Oculoplastics Association of India & Asia Pacific Society of Ophthalmic Plastic and Reconstructive Surgery in 2007
- '**Best Poster**' **award for Prospective Evaluation of Contracted Anophthalmic Sockets** in the Indo Israel Meeting held in Chennai in 2005
- '**Vocational excellence Award**' from Rotary Club of Madurai in 2010 for her work in the community
- **International Women's day Excellence award** by the Lions Club of Madurai District 324-B3 March 8, 2015, for her work in the field of Ocular Oncology
- **PSG & Sons' Charities, Coimbatore Scroll of Honour awarded** for her an eminent expert in diagnosis, treatment, rehabilitation, and research in ophthalmology holding a key leadership position in a reputed Eye Care system, for having conducted a large number of cataract surgeries in addition to her widely acclaimed expertise in orbit oculoplasty, ocular prosthetic services, ocular oncology, and her personal involvement in the Ring of Hope initiative

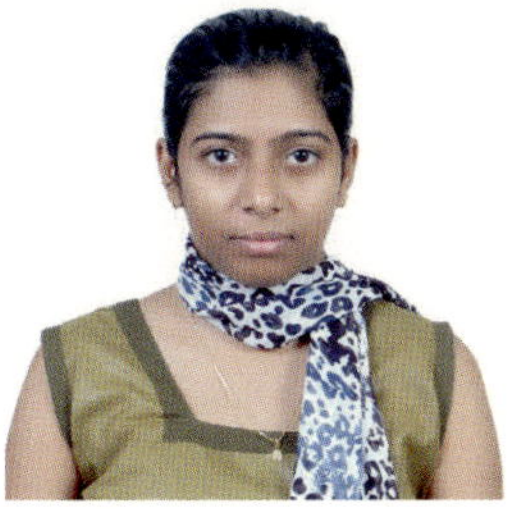

**Priti Bhoutekar** Dr. Priti Bhoutekar (Urade) is a dedicated medical professional with prior work and education experiences at renowned institutes in Delhi and South India. She works with sustained focus and interest in the field of Orbit and Oculoplasty. She completed her MBBS (2004 - 2010) from Government medical college, Nagpur. In 2013, she received M.D Ophthalmology from prestigious AIIMS, Delhi. She also received DNB Ophthalmology in 2015. During her fellowship in orbit and oculoplasty (2013-2015), she worked and got trained under Dr. Usha Kim at Aravind eye hospital, Madurai.

Currently works as consultant Orbit and Ophthalmic Plastic surgeon in central India. She has one international publication to her name. She presented a paper on "A novel approach for optic nerve sheath decompression; our experiences and outcomes" during APSOPRS-OPAI 2014, Delhi. Also, her poster on 'Large spot laser for treatment of retinopathy of prematurity' was presented in AAO, Chicago (Oct 2014).

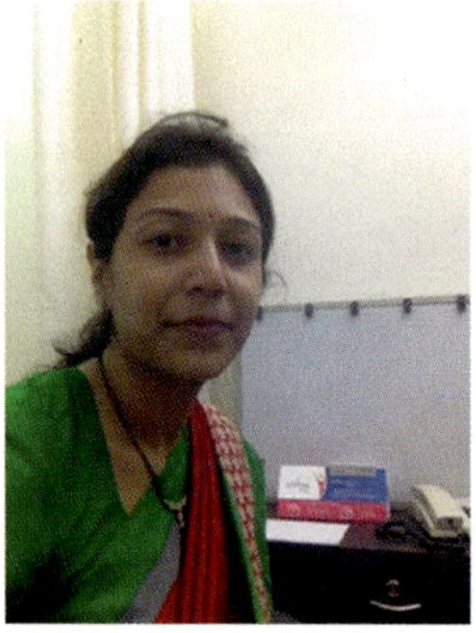

**Swapna Parekh-Chattopadhyay** Dr. Swapna has done her MBBS from Lokmanya Tilak Municipal Medical College and Sion Hospital, Mumbai, and postgraduation in Ophthalmology (M.S. Ophthalmology) from Topiwala National Medical Hospital and Nair Hospital, Mumbai, after which she joined Sir Ganga Ram Hospital, New Delhi, for 2 years as Senior Registrar, where she worked and trained under Dr. A. K. Grover and obtained extensive experience in orbit and oculoplasty surgeries. She then joined a long term fellowship program in Orbit, Oculoplasty and Ocular Oncology at Aravind Eye Hospital, Madurai, where she honed her technical skills under the guidance of Dr. Usha Kim, a stalwart in the field.

At present Dr. Swapna is a practicing orbit and oculoplasty consultant specializing in plastic surgery of the eyelids, eye socket reconstruction, lacrimal surgeries, pediatrics oculoplastics, cosmetic eyelid and brow surgery, and nonsurgical facial cosmetic treatments (Botox and fillers). Experience: 10 years

# Traumatic Optic Neuropathy

# 17

Jason N. Harris and Neil R. Miller

## Overview

Traumatic optic neuropathy (TON) is a paradox of superficial simplicity riddled with deep and hidden complexities. A host of different types of direct and indirect and primary and secondary injuries can affect different portions of the optic nerve(s). Thus, in the setting of penetrating as well as non-penetrating head or facial trauma, a high index of suspicion should be maintained for the possibility that TON is present.

TON is a clinical diagnosis, with imaging frequently adding clarification to the full nature/extent of the lesion(s) in question. Each pattern of injury carries its own unique prognosis and theoretical best treatment; however, the optimum management of patients with TON remains unclear. Indeed, further research is desperately needed to better understand TON. Observation, steroids, surgical measures, or a combination of these is the current cornerstones of management, but statistically significant evidence supporting any particular approach for TON is absent from the literature. To date, there has been one randomized placebo-controlled study investigating management of TON. It investigated high-dose corticosteroids vs. placebo in patients with traumatic optic neuropathy from non-penetrating trauma. No significant differences were seen in visual outcome among groups in this very small study. There have not been any randomized studies investigating surgical management. There exists the possibility that novel management strategies will emerge as more is understood about the converging pathways of various secondary and tertiary mechanisms of cell injury and death at play in TON.

Given our current deficiencies in knowledge regarding how to best manage TON, "primum non nocere" (first do no harm) is of utmost importance.

J.N. Harris, MD
Department of Neuro-Ophthalmology, Johns Hopkins, Baltimore, MD, USA
e-mail: jason.n.harris@gmail.com

N.R. Miller, MD (✉)
Department of Ophthalmology, Neurology and Neurosurgery, Johns Hopkins Hospital, Wilmer Eye Institute, Baltimore, MD, USA
e-mail: nrmiller@jhmi.edu

## Anatomy and Physiology of the Optic Nerve

In discussing traumatic optic neuropathy, it will be beneficial to first briefly discuss the anatomy of the optic nerve.

The term "optic nerve" is a misnomer. In fact, the optic nerve is anatomically and physiologically a white-matter tract of the brain [1]. Embryologically, it forms from the optic stalk, an outpouching of the diencephalon. It is myelinated by oligodendrocytes rather than Schwann cells. It


B. Mukherjee, H. Yuen (eds.), *Emergencies of the Orbit and Adnexa*,
DOI 10.1007/978-81-322-1807-4_17

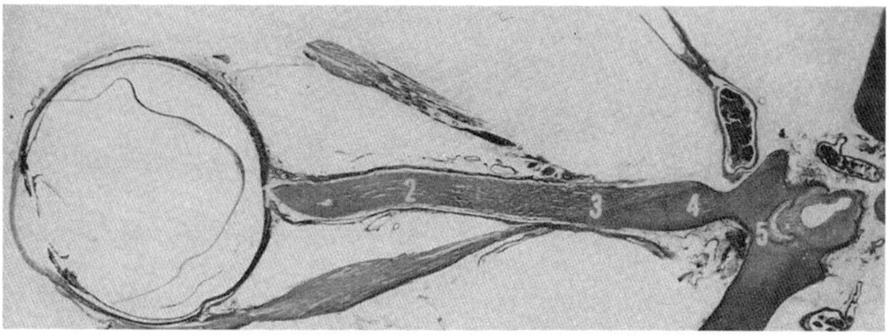


**Fig. 17.1** The optic nerve. Numbers refer to segments of the nerve. *1* intraocular segment, *2* orbital segment, *3* canalicular segment, *4* intracranial segment, *5* optic chiasm

has a blood-brain barrier identical with other portions of the brain (a possible exception being the optic nerve head or optic disc). It is nourished by pial vessels invested in pia mater and, like the rest of the brain, is surrounded by arachnoid and dura mater. Astrocytes support its axons, and fibroblasts also are present. As might be expected, the optic nerve does not behave as do other nerves (including the other cranial nerves) when injured. Given that the optic nerve is, in fact, part of the central nervous system (CNS), treatment paradigms for TON are largely extrapolated from traumatic spinal cord and to some extent traumatic brain injury literature [2].

The optic nerve can be described as having four anatomical sections: the intraocular, orbital, canalicular, and intracranial portions. It also can be divided more broadly clinically into anterior and posterior segments (Fig. 17.1) [3].

## The Intraocular Optic Nerve

The intraocular optic nerve is the shortest portion of the nerve. It can be divided into prelaminar and laminar segments. It is composed of about 1.2 million retinal ganglion cell (RGC) axons along with astrocytes, fibroblasts, and capillary-associated cells [4]. The prelaminar segment, also known as the optic nerve head or optic disc, is typically unmyelinated. At the optic disc, the RGC axons make an approximately 90° turn. They then pass through the 200–300 openings in the lamina cribrosa as the laminar segment of the nerve. The central retinal arteries and veins also travel through this portion of the nerve. The most superficial portions of the prelaminar portion of the nerve are supplied by small branches of the central retinal artery, whereas the remainder of the intraocular optic nerve is supplied mostly from the choroid, which in turn is supplied by short posterior ciliary arteries. The laminar portion usually is supplied more directly by several autoregulated posterior ciliary arteries (Fig. 17.2) [5–7].

The optic nerve is surrounded by blood-brain barrier throughout its entire course, although the prelaminar portion may be an exception [8, 9]. Venous drainage of this portion of the nerve is mainly via the central retinal vein.

## The Orbital Optic Nerve

The orbital portion of the optic nerve is approximately 30 mm in length (Fig. 17.3).

Collagenous tissue divides it into septae. It is surrounded by fat, the short and long posterior ciliary arteries, the short and long posterior ciliary nerves, and the rectus muscles. The distance from the posterior portion of the globe to the orbital apex is about 18 mm. This difference between the length of the nerve in the orbit and the distance from the posterior aspect of the globe to the orbital apex allows necessary eye movements and also provides a protective mechanism against optic nerve damage from proptosis unless it is extreme. The RGC axons usually become myelinated by oligodendrocytes after exiting the lamina cribrosa, resulting in enlargement of the nerve diameter from 3 to 4.5 mm. The nerve is encased by the optic sheath. The outer layer of this sheath, the dura mater, is 0.3–0.5 mm thick. The subarachnoid space of the nerve is contigu-

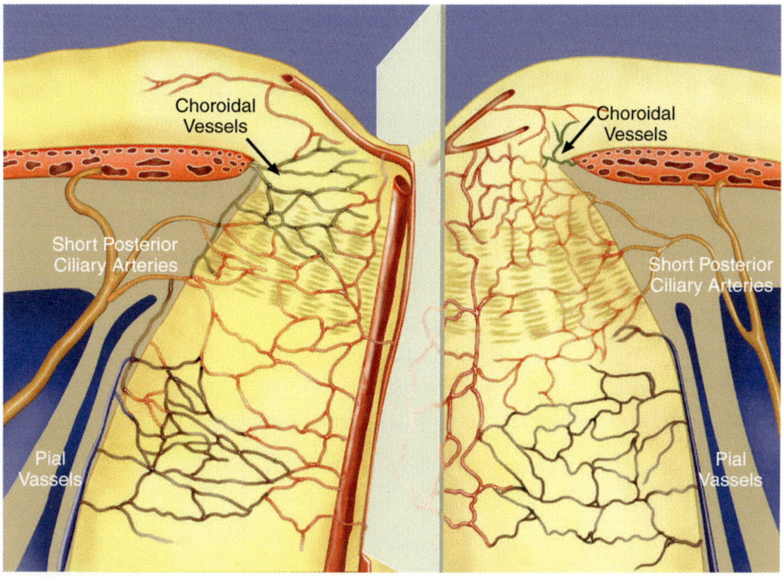


**Fig. 17.2** Blood supply of the intraocular optic nerve

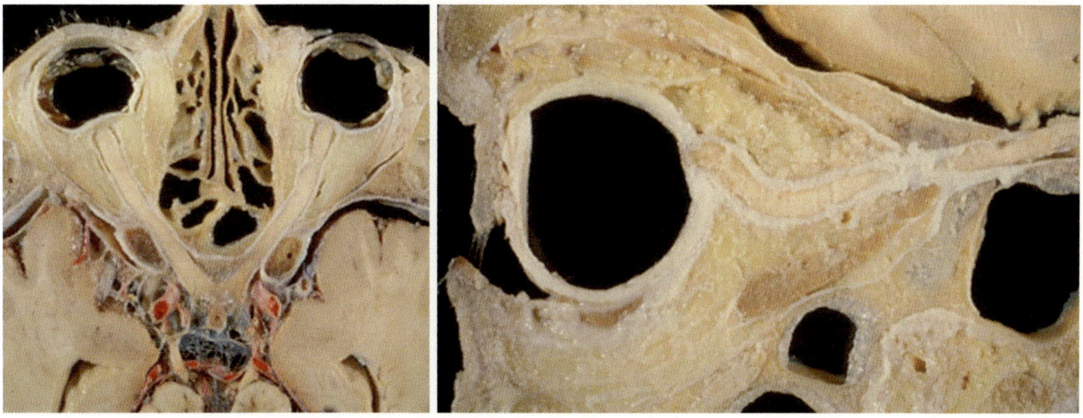

**Fig. 17.3** Anatomy of the optic nerve. The orbital portion of the nerve is approximately 30 mm in length. Note that the nerve is surrounded by orbital fat and covered by a dural sheath that extends through the optic canal

ous with the subarachnoid space of the brain. Pial layers, mostly supplied by posterior ciliary arteries, surround the nerve, carrying in them capillaries subserving the nerve. As is the case elsewhere in the brain, there is a blood-brain barrier. Approximately 10 mm posterior to the globe, the central retinal artery, a major branch of the ophthalmic artery, pierces the dura inferomedially to the nerve and travels within the nerve to exit at the optic disc where it divides into superior temporal, inferior temporal, superior nasal, and inferior nasal branches. The portion of the nerve anterior to where the central retinal artery pierces the dura is sometimes referred to as the "anterior" portion of the nerve, whereas the remainder of the nerve is referred to as the "posterior" optic nerve [10].

As the optic nerve continues to travel posteriorly, it traverses the annulus of Zinn prior to exiting the orbit. The annulus is a tendinous structure to which the four rectus muscles are attached. It overlies both the optic canal and a portion of the superior orbital fissure laterally. In this region, the ophthalmic artery is inferolateral to the optic nerve. Lateral to the optic nerve in the annulus as they traverse the superior orbital fissure are the superior division of the oculomotor nerve, the nasociliary nerve (a branch of V1), the abducens nerve, the inferior division of the oculomotor nerve, and the superior ophthalmic vein (Fig. 17.4a, b). Also lateral to the optic nerve but anterior to the annulus is the ciliary ganglion [2].

The blood supply of the orbital segment of the optic nerve is variable (Fig. 17.5). Centripetally penetrating pial vessels line the optic nerve throughout its extent; however, anteriorly, these vessels receive their blood supply primarily from posterior ciliary arteries, whereas posteriorly, their origin not only is from the posterior ciliary arteries but also directly from the ophthalmic artery. In addition, portions of the anterior nerve receive some blood supply from the central retinal artery and, in some cases, from the external carotid artery via branches from the middle meningeal, superficial temporal, and transverse facial arteries [2, 11]. Indeed, postmortem studies suggest a rich anastomotic network of blood vessels in this region, and this is perhaps one reason that this portion of the nerve seems more resistant to injury than other segments. However, there are in vivo animal studies that call into question the degree of anastomoses [12].

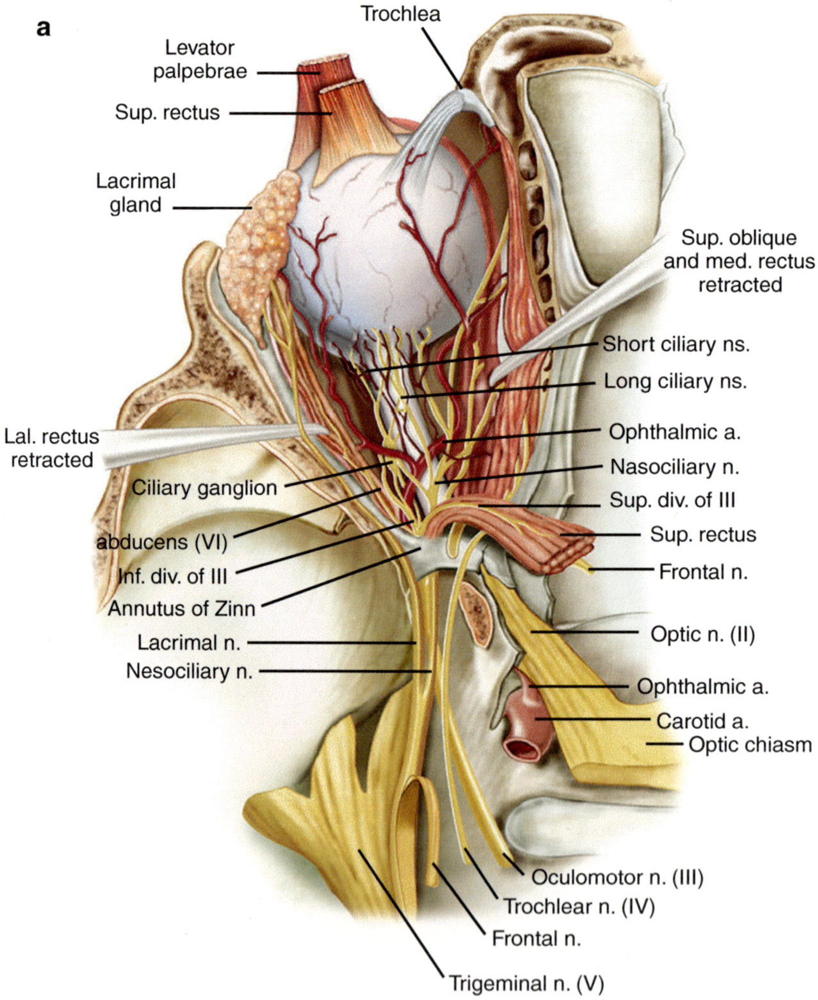


**Fig. 17.4** (**a**) Relationship of the orbital portion of the optic nerve to other orbital structures. (**b**) Relationship of the orbital portion of the optic nerve to other orbital structures

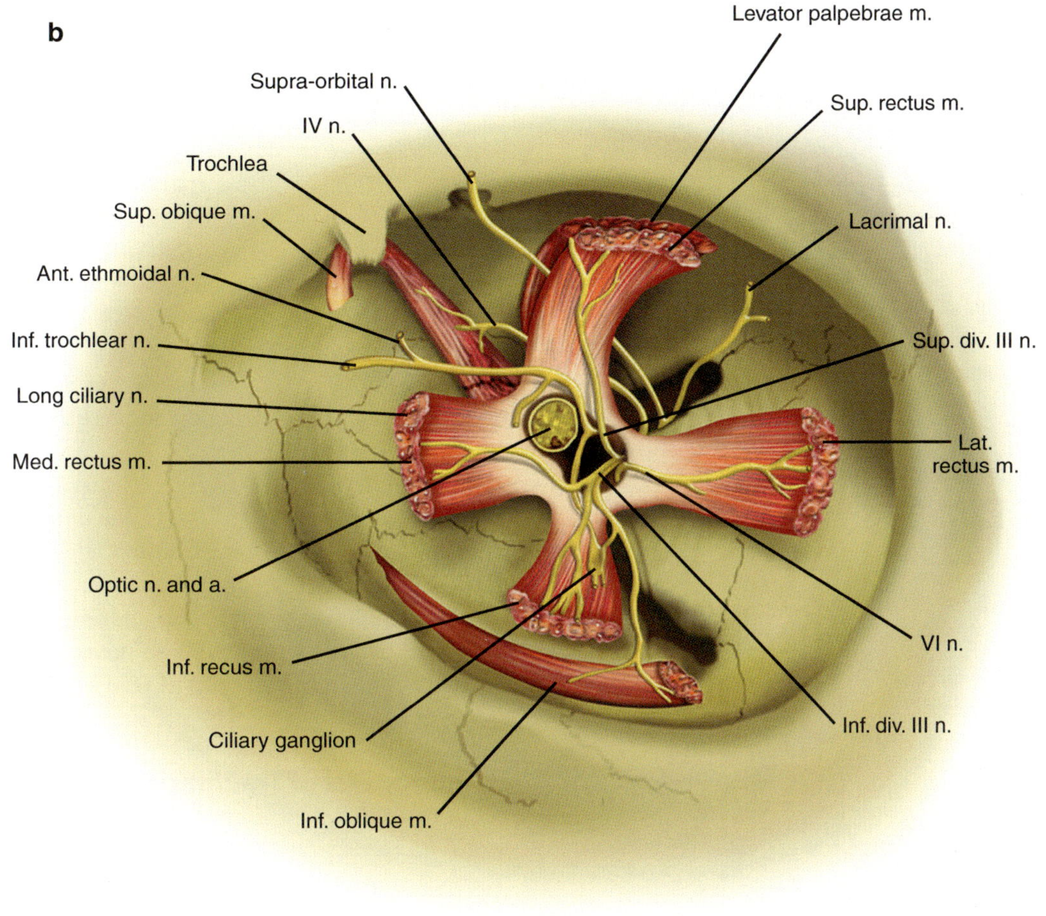


**Fig. 17.4** (continued)

## The Canalicular Optic Nerve

Immediately after the optic nerve traverses the annulus of Zinn, it enters the optic foramen to traverse the optic canal (Fig. 17.3). This canal runs posteromedially at an angle of about 35° with the mid-sagittal plane (Figs. 17.3 and 17.6).

The dura mater is contiguous with both structures, and the dura surrounding the nerve is tightly adherent to the periosteum of the canal, particularly superiorly (Figs. 17.3 and 17.7a, b).

The canal, which lies between the two roots of the lesser sphenoid wings, is 8–10 mm long and is wider at its intracranial end than at its orbital end [13]. The lateral wall of the canal is the optic strut, an important landmark that separates the canal from the superior orbital fissure. The thinnest portion of the canal is the medial wall, averaging 0.21 mm [14]. On the other side of this wall is the sphenoid sinus and, occasionally, a posterior ethmoid sinus. In 4% of patients, there is only membrane separating the canal and the sinus [15]. The roof of the optic canal is significantly thicker, 2 mm on average.

The canalicular optic nerve lies in a watershed zone. It is supplied anteriorly mainly by collateral branches of the ophthalmic artery and posteriorly by pial vessels from the superior hypophyseal arteries (Fig. 17.5) [16].

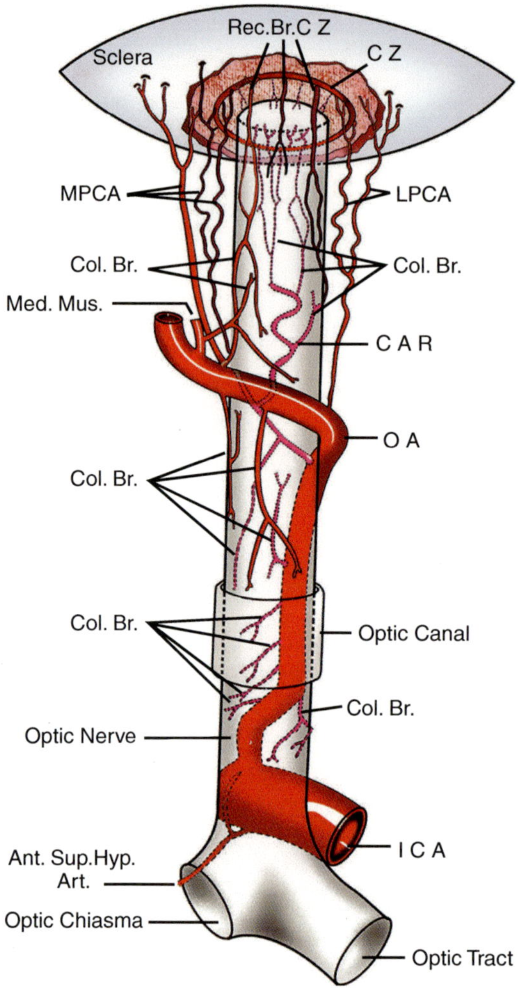


**Fig. 17.5** Blood supply of the optic nerve

## The Intracranial Optic Nerve

As the optic nerve exits the optic canal and enters the intracranial cavity, the dura that surrounds it peels away to line the skull base. Superiorly, however, it forms a sharp fold – the falciform fold – that overhangs the canal (Fig. 17.8).

Thus, the intracranial portion of the nerve is surrounded only by pia mater and arachnoid as it travels posteriorly, superiorly, and medially to merge with the opposite optic nerve to form the optic chiasm. The length of the intracranial optic nerve is highly variable, ranging from 4 to 15 mm [11].

The internal carotid artery is lateral to the optic nerve as is the anterior clinoid process (Fig. 17.8). The blood supply to the intracranial optic nerve comes from the internal carotid artery, the superior hypophyseal arteries, the A1 segment of the anterior cerebral artery and the anterior communicating artery (Fig. 17.5) [17].

## Pathogenesis of Traumatic Optic Neuropathy

The mechanism of injury is one important way of classifying TON, with most authors using the terms "primary" and "secondary" to describe the mechanisms by which the optic nerve can be damaged [10, 18].

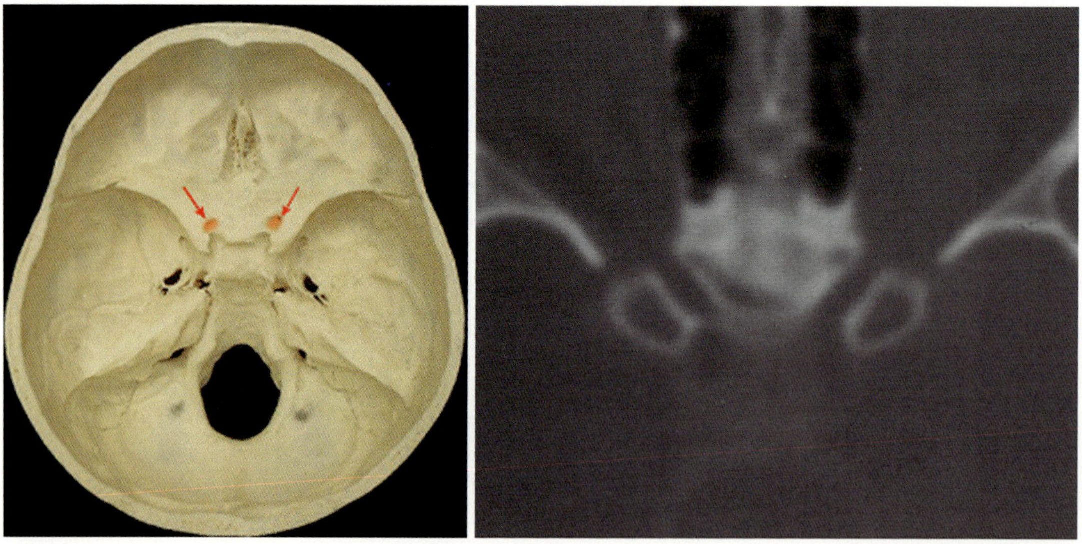

**Fig. 17.6** Orientation of the optic canals

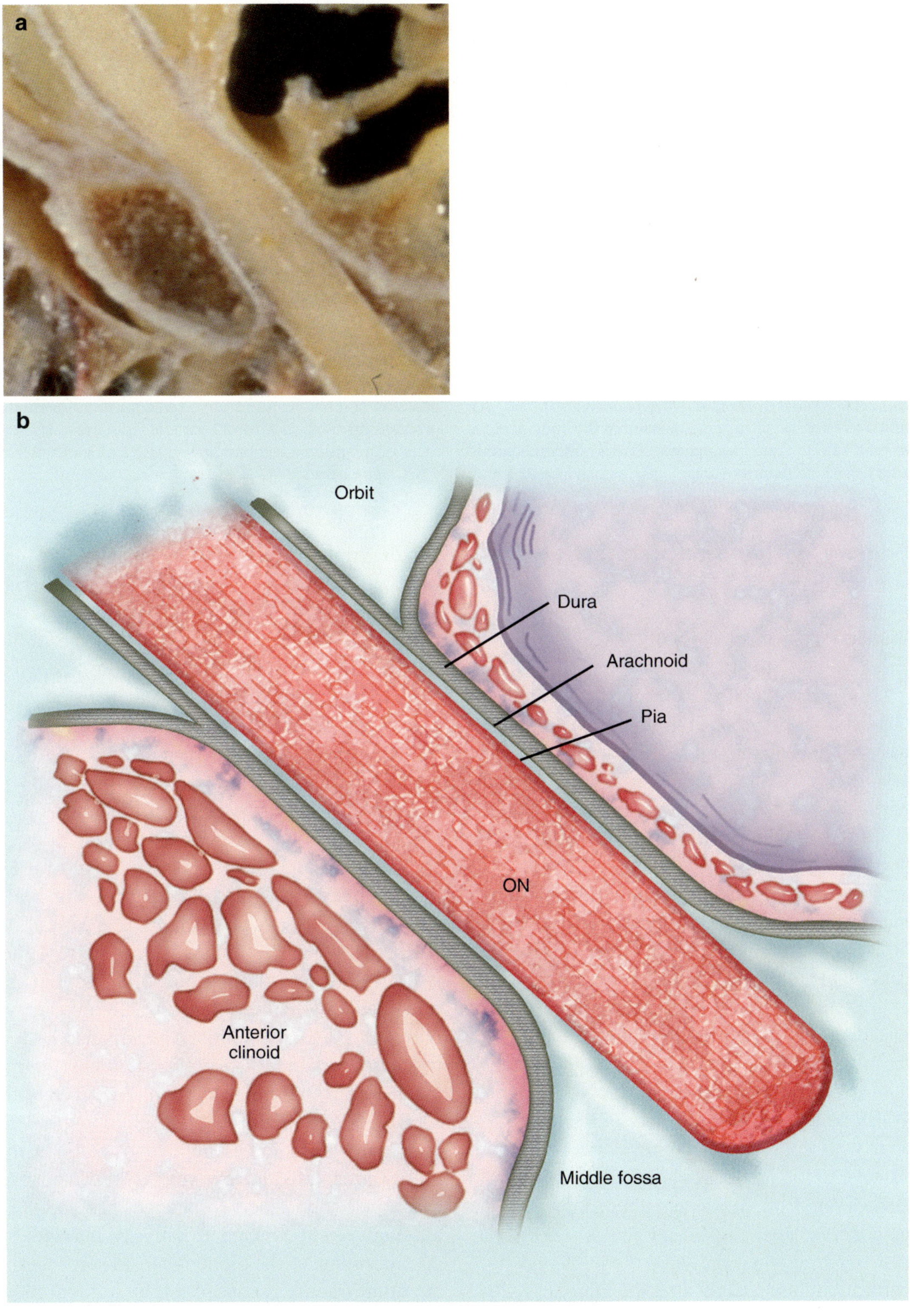


**Fig. 17.7** (**a**) The canalicular portion of the optic nerve, horizontal section. (**b**) The canalicular portion of the optic nerve, schematic drawing (note the tight attachment of the dura to the nerve within the canal)

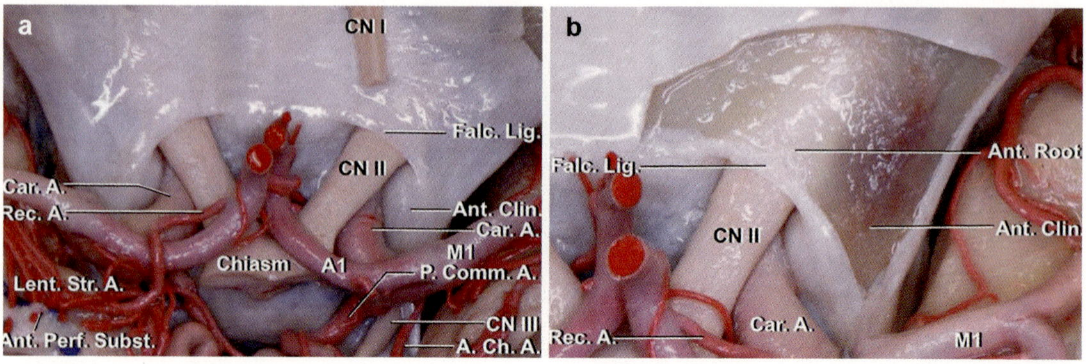


**Fig. 17.8** Anatomy of the intracranial portion of the optic nerves. Note the falciform ligament (or fold). (**a**) The ligament is intact. (**b**) The dura overlying the right optic canal has been removed, revealing the underlying bone. The fold overlying the intracranial portion of the optic nerve at its exit from the canal is apparent. *Car. A.* internal carotid artery, *Rec. A.* recurrent artery of Heubner, *Lent. Str. A.* lenticular striate arteries, *Ant. Per. Subst.* anterior perforated substances, *A1*, *A1* segment of the anterior cerebral artery, *A. Ch. A.* anterior choroidal artery, *P. Comm. Art.* posterior communicating artery, *Ant. Clin.* anterior clinoid process, *Falc. Lig.* falciform ligament (fold), *M1*, *M1* segment of the middle cerebral artery, *CN 1* olfactory nerve, *CN II* optic nerve

## Primary Mechanisms of Optic Nerve Damage

Primary mechanisms usually are described as either "direct" (penetrating) or "indirect" (blunt trauma). According to Steinsapir and Goldberg, "Direct injuries are open injuries where an external object penetrates the tissues to impact the optic nerve. Indirect optic nerve injuries occur when the force of collision is imparted into the skull and this energy is absorbed by the optic nerve" [10].

Direct injuries are less common than indirect injuries because of the protection offered by the orbit [2] and because a much larger surface area is available to receive the forces necessary for an indirect injury. Direct optic nerve injuries cause instantaneous and often irreversible damage to the portion of the nerve involved. Presumably, this is due to transection of the RGC axons. Walsh believed that immediate ischemia associated with contusion necrosis caused by direct damage to the microcirculation also plays a role [10]. Even with treatment, direct injury to the optic nerve carries a poor prognosis. This is particularly true when the injured eye has no light perception immediately after the injury [19, 20].

Indirect damage to the optic nerve occurs from a wide range of mechanisms [21–24]. In his descriptions of these mechanisms, Walsh included transient "concussion" of the nerve, more permanent "concussive" injuries, lacerations of some nerve fibers (but not the entire nerve), and immediate "contusion necrosis" [23]. Indeed, there are various manners in which forces can be transmitted to the optic nerve in indirect injury, ranging from transmission of concussive forces directly to the tightly adherent nerve in the optic canal to transmission of forces from attached structures farther away, such as may happen when rotational or translational forces are applied to the globe or brain (i.e., from a finger or a fall) [22, 23, 25–29]. In particular, when the forehead or temporal region is struck, forces travel posteriorly through the optic canal, potentially injuring the optic nerve within the canal [30]. This may explain why it is much more common for frontal blunt trauma than occipital trauma to cause indirect TON [22, 31, 32]. In addition to forces applied to the skull or facial bones, forces applied directly to the globe (both high- and low-velocity mechanisms) can cause optic nerve damage [29, 33–35], although such damage usually is masked by severe trauma to the globe itself. In some cases, the blunt trauma is caused not by a direct blow to the skull but by a distant effect such as a blast wave [36].

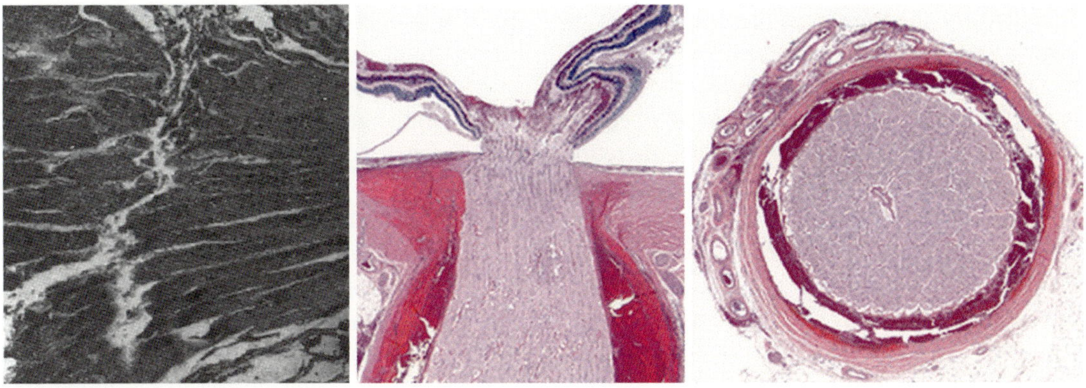

**Fig. 17.9** Direct injury to the optic nerve. *Left*, longitudinal section through the nerve shows full thickness laceration. *Right*, in another case, direct injury resulted in an extensive subdural hemorrhage surrounding the nerve

The distinction between direct and indirect mechanisms of injury can at times be blurred. For example, a fracture of the optic canal from an indirect injury that results in a transection of the optic nerve is considered an indirect injury by most authors, even though there may be little difference in outcome between this and a foreign body penetrating and lacerating the nerve [37], as either type of primary injury can cause tears in the dura or nerve sheath, hemorrhage into the nerve or sheath spaces, and compression necrosis (Fig. 17.9).

Unfortunately, by the time a patient with a direct or indirect injury to the optic nerve is evaluated by a physician, there usually is nothing that can be done to reverse the damage. All currently available therapies thus are aimed at preventing further – i.e., secondary – injury to the nerve, something about which we know even less than we do about primary mechanisms of injury.

## Secondary Mechanisms of Optic Nerve Damage

In addition to primary direct or indirect optic nerve damage, further injury/exacerbation of injury can be caused by secondary mechanisms that occur after the moment of impact. Usually, visual loss is immediate; however, delayed visual loss, presumably from secondary mechanisms, occurs in at least 10% of cases [8]. Hippocrates described this phenomenon over 2000 years ago, writing "Dimness of vision occurs in injuries to the brow and in those placed slightly above. It is less noticeable the more recent the wound, but as the scar becomes old, so the dimness increases" [39]. Proposed mechanisms of secondary injury include vasospasm, edema, hemorrhage, and local compression of vessels or systemic circulatory insufficiency/failure leading to necrosis of the nerve. There also is evidence of numerous cell death mechanisms at play, including but not limited to the generation of oxygen-free radicals, arachidonic acid release, triggering of bradykinin pathways, disturbances of intracellular calcium cascades, production of excitatory amino acids, and interference with TRP, NMDA, and AQP channels [10, 40–43]. An extensive discussion of these secondary mechanisms is beyond the scope of this chapter.

Perhaps the most important common element to remember with respect to the various secondary mechanisms of indirect injury to the optic nerve is the role that ischemia is believed to play in each of them, either as a causative or resultant factor. Given this role, optimum secondary injury prevention strategies generally are designed to decrease ischemia or the inflammatory and apoptotic cascades that lead to or are associated with it [44].

## Location of Injury

In addition to the mechanisms of injury, a description of TON should include the portion of the optic nerve that is injured [2, 3, 37].

Clinically, the injury can happen at either the anterior or posterior optic nerve (or both). As mentioned above, the anterior aspect of the nerve is that portion of the nerve anterior to where the central retinal artery enters and the central retinal vein exits the nerve, about 8–10 mm posterior to the globe [3, 21, 37, 44]. Both the anterior and posterior nerve can be injured by direct and indirect mechanisms as well as by one or more of the secondary mechanisms described above [10].

## Anterior Traumatic Optic Neuropathy

Anterior TON, whether of the direct or indirect variety, is characterized by optic disc swelling in the setting of other evidence of an optic neuropathy (e.g., decreased acuity, poor or absent color vision, a visual field defect, and a relative afferent pupillary defect if the injury is unilateral or asymmetric). It usually is accompanied by injury to associated vasculature. This, in turn, can lead to retinal ischemia or infarction, central retinal vein occlusion, anterior ischemic optic neuropathy, or a combination of these phenomena (Fig. 17.10) [45, 46].

Choroidal rupture can also be an accompanying feature [47]. Because of the severity of optic nerve and, often, intraocular damage that usually is associated with direct injury to the anterior optic nerve, the prognosis for anterior TON usually is poor in this setting, regardless of treatment [3]. The prognosis for anterior TON caused by indirect injury, however, is not as clear. Indirect anterior TON usually results from blunt forces applied to the globe. Rotational and translational forces as well as sudden shifts in intraocular pressure have all been implicated in the pathogenesis of the damage. In such instances, the main force to the optic nerve appears to be at the junction of the nerve and sclera, on the side opposite the impact [29]. Tangential glancing blows can cause a rotary avulsion with minimal globe disruption. More often, off-center impact to the globe may cause intraocular damage and also be associated with slower “rotational-rebound” evulsion of the nerve [48]. There thus are a variety of mechanisms by which forces on the globe can lead to partial or complete optic nerve avulsion [27, 28, 33, 49–51]. In milder cases, there may not be avulsion, but there still may be injury to the nerve and its vasculature. In most of these cases, regardless of the nature of the forces, no treatment is likely to be of benefit in limiting optic nerve damage, let alone restoring vision (Fig. 17.11).

The one exception to this rule is the presence of a hemorrhage in the subdural or subarachnoid space surrounding the anterior optic nerve. In such a setting, which can be suspected by the clinical findings and confirmed with computed tomographic (CT) scanning, magnetic resonance (MR) imaging, or ultrasonography, and urgent optic nerve sheath fenestration may be beneficial,

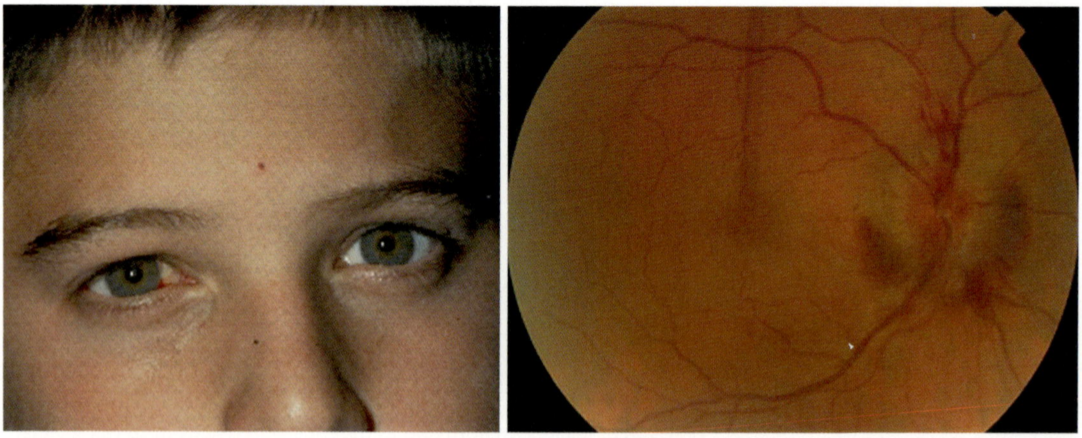

**Fig. 17.10** Anterior indirect traumatic optic neuropathy in a young boy who was hit in the right eye while playing soccer

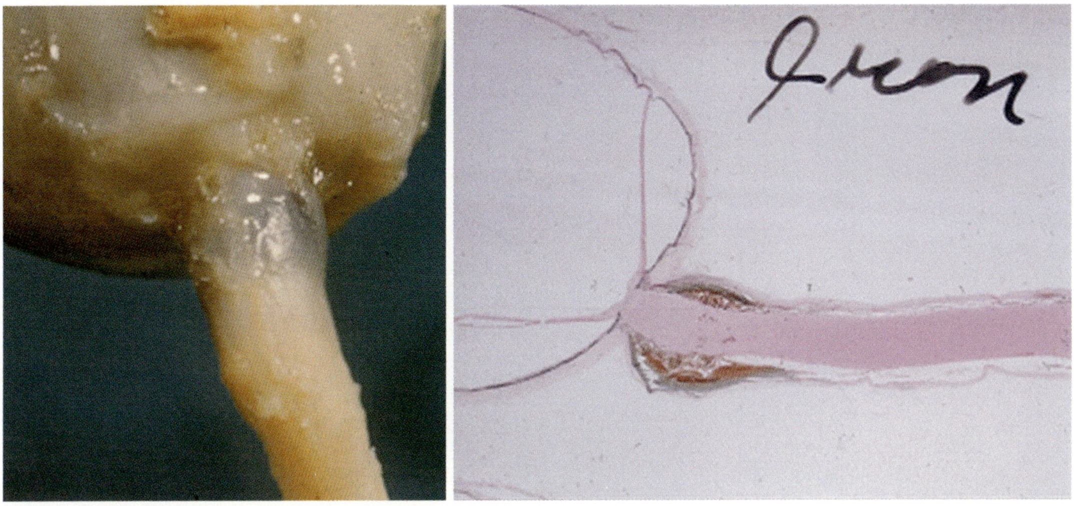

**Fig. 17.11** Fatal indirect anterior traumatic optic neuropathy. Note subdural hematoma at the junction of the optic nerve and globe

particularly if it is clear that the patient had vision immediately after the injury and/or had a normal-appearing optic disc but then experienced progressive visual loss associated with the development of optic disc swelling [52].

## Posterior Traumatic Optic Neuropathy

Posterior TON is much more common than anterior TON, with indirect trauma being much more common than direct trauma. As is the case with anterior TON, posterior TON caused by direct or penetrating trauma has a poor prognosis regardless of treatment; however, this is not necessarily the case with respect to posterior TON caused by indirect trauma.

In patients with posterior TON caused by indirect trauma, the canalicular portion of the optic nerve is most often the site of damage, with the next most common portion being the intracranial portion of the nerve as it passes beneath the falciform fold (Fig. 17.8) [21–23, 27, 28, 38, 45, 53, 54]. There are a number of reasons for this. First, as noted above, studies have shown that blunt trauma to the frontal region produces shock waves that travel posteriorly toward and often through the canal, at least in part because the conical shape of the orbit may funnel forces to this particular region (Fig. 17.12a, b) [30, 31].

This concussive force may or may not be associated with fractures of the optic canal that also can introduce a crushing or lacerating component to the initial trauma. In addition, the optic canal is the only location along the length of the optic nerve where the nerve is tightly tethered to a fixed structure – the bone of the canal (via the nerve sheath and periosteum) (Fig. 17.7a, b). Thus, not only are concussive forces more likely to be propagated via bone to this portion of the nerve than to any other portion, but this portion of the nerve has less ability to respond to even minor primary damage. Rotational or translational forces of the brain at the time of blunt head and/or facial trauma may play an important role with respect to injury to the portion of the optic nerve passing underneath the falciform fold [2, 10, 55, 56], whereas forces on the globe are less likely to play a significant factor to the tethered nerve given the generous laxity of the intraorbital nerve.

The above factors do not take into account the vulnerability of the canalicular portion of the optic nerve to subsequent secondary injury following the initial injury. The tight confines of the canal make this portion of the nerve particularly vulnerable to edema and hemorrhage, resulting in

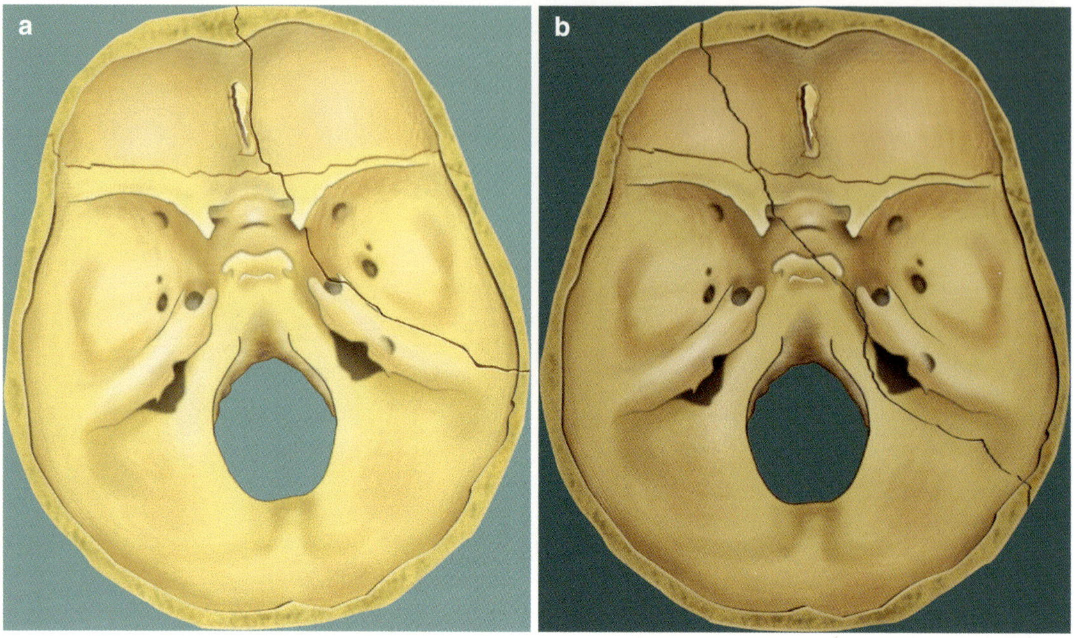


**Fig. 17.12** (**a**) Direction of concussive forces from blunt trauma to the forehead (note that the *lines* of force can traverse either the ipsilateral or contralateral optic canal). (**b**) Direction of concussive forces from blunt trauma to the forehead (note that the *lines* of force can traverse either the ipsilateral or contralateral optic canal)

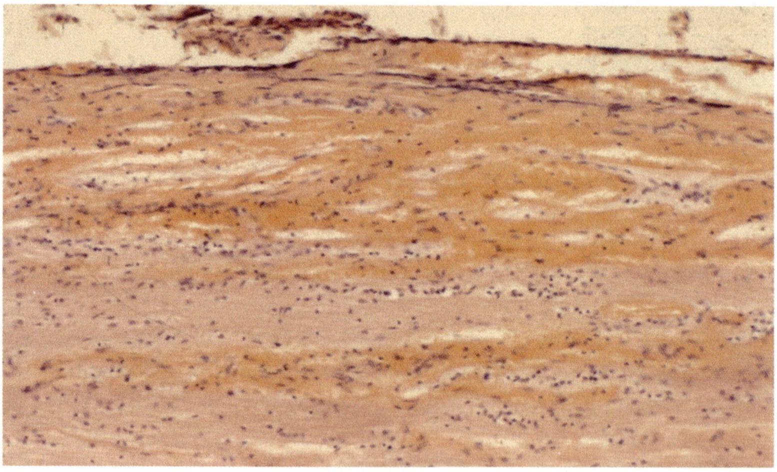

**Fig. 17.13** Subarachnoid, subdural, and intraneural hemorrhage of the optic nerve in a fatal case of posterior indirect traumatic optic neuropathy

a compartment syndrome causing further ischemia and secondary damage (Fig. 17.13) [23].

Additionally, as previously noted, this region of the nerve is a watershed zone, unlike other portions of the nerve that receive blood via rich anastomoses. It is not clear how – or if – this watershed component plays a role in the prevalence and evolution of secondary injury in posterior indirect TON to this region of the nerve, but it certainly may be a factor.

## Epidemiology of Traumatic Optic Neuropathy

A recent prospective surveillance in the UK found TON to affect 1 in 1,000,000 of the general population [57]. Series that have evaluated TON in the setting of both blunt and penetrating head and facial injuries have found that it is present in 0.7–2.5 % of cases [22, 58–60]. In most series, the vast majority of affected patients are young adult males [38, 57]. Motor vehicle accidents, bicycle accidents, falls, assaults, and sport injuries are common causes of injury [2, 38, 57]; however, other mechanisms of injury have been reported, including self-inflicted oedipism [51], diving accidents [33], and optic nerve massage [61]. Although seemingly trivial injuries can cause TON [44], the trauma usually is severe, with 34–75 % of cases in both prospective and retrospective series being associated with loss of consciousness and 36–82 % of affected eyes having no light perception [38, 57, 62]. The male prevalence and other presenting characteristics of TON are similar in pediatric and adult populations [63, 64].

Factors cited by various authors as portending a worse potential for recovery include age over 40, history of loss of consciousness or significant head injury, history of immediate visual loss, poor initial visual acuity, presence of blood in the posterior ethmoid air cells by imaging, presence of an orbital fracture or a fracture of the optic canal, and failure to recover after 48 h of steroid therapy (but see below) [20, 57, 65].

## Clinical Evaluation

TON is initially a clinical diagnosis, with imaging frequently adding clarification to the full nature and extent of the injury. As noted above, as up to 2.5 % of patients with head injury have TON, a high index of suspicion should be maintained for this condition in that setting. Obviously, the first priority in patient care needs to be ensuring and maintaining the patient's cardiorespiratory status and neurological stability. Given these requirements, initial assessments by the ophthalmologist may be limited or delayed. Indeed, it is not uncommon for head-injured patients, particularly those who have experienced loss of consciousness, to be diagnosed with TON weeks or even months after the injury when they are finally sufficiently alert and able to communicate with their physicians and families. Nevertheless, we believe that patients who have experienced head or facial trauma should be evaluated for the possibility of TON at the earliest opportunity.

### History

Once a patient who has experienced facial or head trauma is deemed stable from a cardiorespiratory and neurological standpoint, an in-depth ocular history and examination should be performed. If the patient is unconscious or confused (as is often the case), history from witnesses should be sought. It is important to elicit from the history when the trauma happened, what the mechanism(s) were, what associated factors may have been present (any exposure to chemicals, etc.), and the nature and progression (or lack thereof) of visual deficits since the incident. This latter point is particularly important as it may indicate a secondary injury amenable to therapy.

### Examination

The importance of the examination in the diagnosis of TON cannot be overemphasized, as patients often are unconscious or confused, with no witnesses available to provide an adequate history. General inspection of the eye and ocular adnexa is the first step. Any evidence of orbital or ocular penetrating injury should be noted, as should any periorbital swelling, ecchymosis, proptosis, and enophthalmos [10]. The orbital rim should be palpated gently for any fractures. When possible, a portable slit-lamp examination should be performed to determine if there is a hyphema or a lens dislocation, although the former often can be appreciated using a simple handlight.

If the patient is able to cooperate, his or her visual acuity should be assessed. It usually is significantly reduced, not infrequently to no light perception, light perception, or bare hand movements. For those eyes with better vision, delayed visual loss nevertheless may occur from secondary mechanisms (see above). Thus, serial assessments should be conducted in most settings [38, 57].

Despite the importance of visual acuity (and, occasionally, color vision testing), the most important examination finding to look for in patients in whom TON is being considered is a relative afferent pupillary defect (RAPD) [63], as it will *always* be present unless there is anatomically symmetric trauma to both optic nerves.

It is important to note, however, that an RAPD can be present in eyes with TON even when visual acuity is 20/20. Thus, although the finding of an RAPD in an eye without any visible retinal damage usually indicates TON, it does not necessarily correlate with the level of visual acuity. In addition, damage to the optic tract also can cause an RAPD. Thus, in a comatose or unresponsive patient, treatment, particularly surgical treatment, (see below) should not be initiated based solely on the presence of an RAPD. An RAPD can be detected by first simply assessing the pupillary reaction to light stimulation. In most cases, in the setting of isocoric pupils (i.e., both pupils are the same size), the failure of one pupil to constrict or the finding that one pupil constricts less briskly and more incompletely than the other suggests dysfunction of the afferent visual pathway. One next should perform a "swinging flashlight test" in which light is shined first in one eye for a few seconds and then in the other eye for the same length of time [66, 67]. In all cases, the light source should be bright and focused. In questionable cases, a 0.3 log unit neutral density filter can be used to clarify the presence or absence of the defect, but if it takes a filter to determine that an RAPD is present, it is unlikely that the patient has profound visual loss. In patients with TON, the presence and degree of an RAPD appears to have a high correlation with both the initial and final visual acuities [68]. The severity of an RAPD can be measured objectively using neutral density filters. Alford et al. found in a study of 19 consecutive patients with TON that no patients with an RAPD of 2.1 log units or greater had visual recovery better than hand motions, whereas all patients with an RAPD of 1.5 log units or less recovered vision to 20/30 or better [69].

Visual fields should also be tested when possible. In many cases of known or suspected TON, the fields will have to be tested at the bedside using confrontation measures such as finger counting, finger wiggling, or hand waving, with more "formal" testing reserved for ambulatory, cooperative patients. There are no field defects that are pathognomonic for TON; however, if testing suggests or demonstrates homonymous or bitemporal defects that respect the vertical meridian, a process involving the optic chiasm or postgeniculate pathway may be present instead of, or in addition to, a TON. In addition to helping quantify initial visual function, formal visual field testing also can be used to monitor the vision over time [22].

A fundoscopic examination should be performed in all patients with known or suspected TON. Unfortunately, it may be difficult for physicians, particularly non-ophthalmologists, to assess the ocular fundi, unless dilating agents are used. Given that a significant percentage of patients with head and/or facial injuries are unconscious or lethargic when they present to an emergency department, it may not be possible to use such agents. In such cases, an examination by an ophthalmologist may be crucial. In other cases, the use of a non-mydriatic camera to assess the ocular fundi may be helpful [70]. In all cases, it is important before instilling any dilating agents to coordinate this plan with other providers, as at times, such as when the patient is being serially monitored for evidence of impending herniation, dilation of the eyes may be contraindicated. When dilating agents are administered, both the agent and time instilled should be documented at the bedside and the information transmitted to both the physicians and the nurses caring for the patient. In addition, only short-acting agents should be used [10]. We have found it useful to place a sheet of paper over the patient's bed (and sometimes a piece of paper tape *on the patient's forehead!*) indicating the agents instilled and the time of instillation. In most cases, fundus examinations will be performed using a direct ophthalmoscope at the bedside; however, a handheld lens at the slitlamp or indirect ophthalmoscopy may be utilized in more stable patients.

In patients with anterior TON, there will always be changes on the fundoscopic examination. If there has been a partial or complete evulsion of the globe from the nerve at the juncture of the lamina cribrosa, a partial or complete ring of hemorrhage will be seen or there will be a deep pit [28, 49]. If the nerve has been injured between the globe and the entrance/exit of the central retinal artery/vein, evidence of a central retinal artery occlusion, central retinal vein occlusion, or both may be present. Disc swelling also may be seen acutely in patients with increased intracranial pressure, so this finding, particularly when bilateral, should be corroborated with other examination findings, such as the presence of an RAPD, before arriving at the diagnosis of anterior TON.

In fact, as the most common form of TON is posterior, due to indirect trauma, the vast majority of patients with TON have a normal fundoscopic exam and, specifically, a normal-appearing optic disc. In such cases, the presence of an RAPD will be the only objective sign of optic nerve injury in a patient complaining of decreased vision in one eye or in a comatose or lethargic patient unable to undergo testing of visual acuity, color vision, and/or visual field.

Visual evoked potentials (VEPs) theoretically are useful in establishing the presence or absence of TON; however, it has been our experience that it is rarely practical to obtain a VEP in the acute setting. Thus, from a diagnostic standpoint, we find them of little or no value.

## Imaging

Imaging may be a valuable adjunct in the assessment of a patient with known or suspected TON. CT scanning is superb at outlining bony anatomy (Fig. 17.14), whereas MR imaging is better for soft tissue structure, although in patients with penetrating trauma, the presence of intraocular or intraorbital metallic objects must be assessed with either CT scanning or plain x-rays before MR imaging is performed.

There is debate on whether or not to perform imaging in patients with TON, with some practitioners advocating imaging in nearly all cases and others only if the patient's clinical findings are worsening over time, implying potentially surgically correctable secondary mechanisms at play [71–73].

Although imaging may help influence treatment in some cases, such as when diffuse or focal orbital hematomas, optic nerve sheath hematomas, or orbital emphysema are present [74, 75], imaging is performed in most cases to assess the overall neurologic and orbital status of the patients and to determine if there is any evidence of structural damage to the brain. Surprisingly, there is no clear consensus on the significance of the presence of fractures or bony fragments in or near the optic canal or other areas of the orbit. Although some studies associate worse outcomes in patients with orbital fractures [20], others do not [68]. Thus, in our opinion, the clinical picture still must guide management.

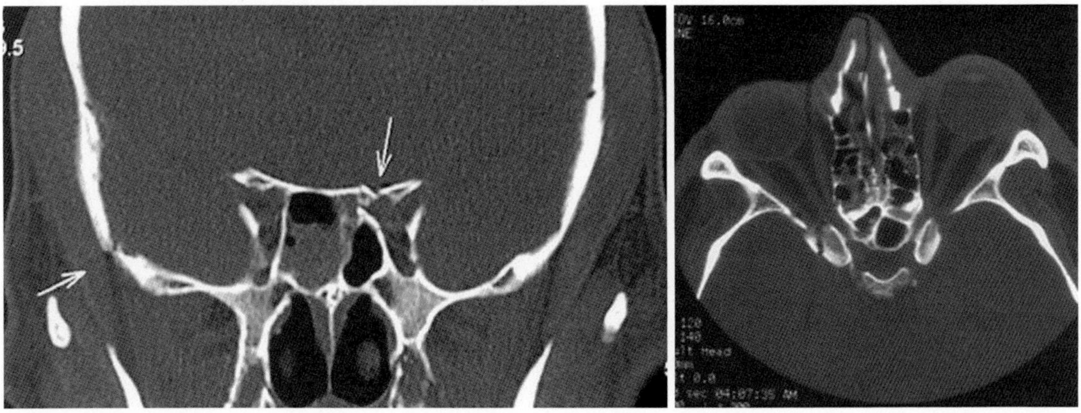

**Fig. 17.14** CT scans from two patients with indirect retrobulbar traumatic optic neuropathy. *Left*, patient has a fracture of the left anterior clinoid process (*long arrow*) as well as the right skull base (*short arrow*). Note that there is a soft tissue shadow in the right sphenoid sinus, probably representing blood. *Right*, there is a fracture of the right anterior clinoid process extending to the optic canal

## Management of Traumatic Optic Neuropathy

As has been repeatedly emphasized in this chapter, the treatment of TON is aimed at improving outcome by mitigating secondary rather than primary damage. Patients who experience direct trauma to the anterior and posterior optic nerve have a poor visual prognosis as do patients in whom there is indirect injury to the anterior optic nerve, regardless of the timing or type of intervention, although as noted above, a possible exception to this pessimistic prognosis is the association of an anterior TON with evidence of a subdural or subarachnoid hematoma adjacent to the orbital portion of the optic nerve. In such a setting, an urgent optic nerve sheath fenestration may be of benefit [52].

Current management paradigms for posterior TON due to blunt trauma (i.e., posterior indirect TON) include observation without intervention, use of oral or intravenous systemic corticosteroids of various doses, surgery, or a combination of surgery and steroid therapy [44]. None of these options has been studied in any large, prospective, randomized clinical trials [76, 77]. Thus, the optimum management of a patient with TON is unknown [40, 78, 79]. In the following sections, we will discuss the various management options in more detail.

### Observation

Observation without intervention is a valid management option for patients with TON. Many patients (>50 % in some series) improve spontaneously [38, 45, 57, 80], and even patients with well-documented no light perception may improve to useful vision without treatment [24, 45, 81, 82]. Indeed, there is no convincing evidence that any medical or surgical intervention is superior to observation. Observation without intervention is a particularly good choice when the patient is unconscious or unable to consent. Given that an RAPD can be present in the setting of 20/20 vision and that an RAPD need not be caused by optic nerve damage, even its presence does not necessarily indicate that a patient with a normal-appearing fundus has an optic neuropathy nor does it indicate the level of visual function unless the pupil is nonreactive to direct light but reacts normally consensually, in which case, one can be certain that the affected eye has no light perception. Studies investigating observation have mostly been small and retrospective or plagued by selection biases; i.e., patients with better initial visual acuities tended to be observed and also might be more likely to recover regardless of treatment [38, 57, 80, 82, 83].

### Corticosteroids

Corticosteroid therapy came into vogue for the treatment of posterior TON in the early 1980s as it was thought that it could reduce edema and secondary inflammation following the injury [84]. Since then, varying dosing regimens of steroids have been suggested, ranging from low-dose (1–2 mg/kg/day) oral or intravenous administration to "high-dose" (1000 mg/day) methylprednisolone in single or divided doses to "megadose" (30 mg/kg of methylprednisolone as a bolus, followed by 5.4 mg/kg/h for 24–48 h) [38, 80, 85, 86].

Almost all data regarding the potential efficacy of steroid therapy in patients with TON come not from studies of TON itself but from treatment trials in patients with acute injury to another CNS white-matter tract: the spinal cord [87]. The results of the first National Acute Spinal Cord Injury Study (NASCIS I), a prospective, randomized study designed to evaluate methylprednisolone in the treatment of acute spinal cord injury, were published in 1984 by Bracken et al., who compared the neurological effects of a 1000 mg bolus of methylprednisolone daily (i.e., "high-dose" steroids) with the effects of a dosage of 100 mg/day [88]. These investigators found no difference in neurological outcomes between the two groups of patients, and, in addition, there was a statistically significant higher rate of wound infections in patients who received the higher dose.

The Second National Acute Spinal Cord Injury Study (NASCIS II) was a prospective randomized placebo-controlled trial to evaluate the effects of methylprednisolone in the treatment of acute spinal cord injury [86]. In this study, patients were given either a bolus of 30 mg/kg of methylprednisolone within 8 h of spinal cord injury followed by infusion of 4 mg/kg/h for 23 h or placebo. The patients treated with so-called "megadose" methylprednisolone were found to have slightly better neurological outcomes at 6 months.

A third study (NASCIS III) also suggested benefit with megadose steroids in acute spinal cord injury, but it was not placebo controlled [89]. Despite the lack of a placebo group, many viewed this study as a further reinforcement and clarification of the use of megadose steroids in acute spinal cord injury (and by inference in traumatic optic neuropathy) [87].

After the results of the NASCIS trials were published, a number of authors reported individual cases and small retrospective case series indicating that steroids were efficacious in the treatment of TON. Unfortunately, these studies generally were not scientific and tended to be plagued with multiple forms of bias. To settle the question, the International Optic Nerve Trauma Study (IONTS) was conceived.

The IONTS was designed to be the largest study to investigate prospectively the treatment of TON, involving 76 investigators in 16 countries. The original study design was that there would be two arms: "high-dose" steroids (1000 mg/day) versus surgery consisting of optic nerve decompression by unroofing the optic canal. There was no control (i.e., observation) arm, because it was thought by the designers of the study that nonintervention would be unethical. Unfortunately, after 2 years, it became clear that enrollment of patients would not be sufficient to power the trial, even if it were to be continued for several more years. The study therefore was converted into an observational study of treatment paradigms of indirect posterior TON treated within 7 days of injury. One hundred thirty-three patients were included in the study, of whom 127 (95 %) had unilateral injuries. Of the 133 patients, 9 received no treatment, 85 were given steroids of varying doses, and 33 underwent optic canal decompression by several techniques, with 32 of these patients also receiving various doses of steroids. The primary outcome measure was last-measured visual acuity at least 1 month after treatment, with an improvement of at least three lines of acuity considered significant. One hundred and four patients (78 % of the cohort) were able to be assessed at least 1 month after treatment, at which time, the authors found no statistically significant difference in visual improvement among the three groups. Specifically with respect to steroid treatment, 52 % of patients who received steroids alone improved at three lines of acuity, whereas 57 % of patients who were observed showed such visual improvement [38].

A more recent surveillance study of patients with TON in the United Kingdom would appear to confirm the findings of the IONTS. Of the 121 patients with TON in this study, 20 % of those who received no treatment experienced improvement in visual acuity of at least three lines, compared with 24 % of those who received any form of treatment [57].

In 2000, shortly after the IONTS was published, the results of another prospective, randomized, placebo-controlled trial designed to compare treatment with "megadose" steroids with no treatment for patients with acute spinal cord injury were published by Pointillart et al. [90]. This trial, which enrolled 106 patients in France, reported no difference in neurological outcomes in those receiving megadose steroids (per NASCIS II guidelines) compared with patients who received no steroids. In addition, there was an increased rate of complications in the group of patients who received megadose steroids. The authors, therefore, suggested that the treatment of acute spinal cord injury with megadose steroids be revisited. At around the same time, increasing controversies regarding earlier reported results of the NASCIS trials were published. Concerns were expressed that statistical artifact retrospectively induced bias, and even withholding of data compromised the validity of the results of the trials, and it was recommended that steroids not be used to treat patients with acute spinal cord injury [91, 92].

Soon thereafter, the effects of megadose steroids (in this case, a loading dose of 2 g methylprednisolone vs. a placebo followed by a maintenance dose of 0.4 g methylprednisolone per hour for 48 h) were studied in the treatment of head trauma in the Corticosteroid Randomization After Significant Head Injury (CRASH) trial. This trial, the largest of its kind, enrolled 10,008 adults with head injury and a Glasgow coma scale of ≤14. All patients were randomly allocated to a 48-h treatment period, with treatment beginning within 8 h of injury. The initial goal was to recruit 20,000 patients, but the trial was stopped early when it became clear that the group receiving methylprednisolone had a significantly increased mortality, regardless of the severity of the injury [93, 94].

Due in part to the results of the study published by Pointillart et al. [90] and the CRASH trial results [93, 94], the Congress of Neurological Surgeons published in 2013 a statement decrying the use of steroids in traumatic spinal cord injury, downgrading much of the evidence presented in the trials supporting megadose steroids from class I to class III because of concerns of "omission of data from publication" and "retrospective post hoc analysis" [87]. The authors also cited concerns regarding data from these studies that showed a trend toward increased complications and mortality in those subjects who received higher doses of corticosteroids.

According to an exhaustive Cochrane review completed 21 May 2013 [76], there has been only one small trial investigating the effects of systemic corticosteroids vs. placebo in the treatment of TON in a prospective, randomized controlled fashion. This trial, performed by Entezari et al. [83], reported the visual outcome in 31 eyes of 31 patients with TON who were randomly assigned to either a treatment group (16 eyes) or a placebo group (15 eyes) within 7 days of initial injury. The treatment group received 250 mg of intravenously administered methylprednisolone every 6 h for 3 days followed by 1 mg/kg/day of oral prednisolone for 14 days. The placebo group received 50 ml of normal saline intravenously every 6 h for 3 days, followed by placebo for 14 days. An increase of at least 0.4 logMAR in final visual acuity measured at 3 months was considered visual improvement. Although both groups showed significant improvement in final visual acuity compared with initial visual acuity ($p<0.001$ and 0.010, respectively), there were no significant differences in final acuity between the two groups. Indeed, 68.8 % of the steroid-treated group had significant improvement in visual acuity compared with 53.3 % of the placebo group ($p=0.38$) [83].

Based on currently available evidence, we agree with Steinsapir and Goldberg [44] that there is no role for "megadose" steroids in the treatment of TON and there also is little evidence for the use of "high-dose" methylprednisolone.

## Surgical Measures

The results of surgery for TON have never been studied in a prospective, randomized, placebo-controlled fashion [77]. As noted above, visual loss from direct optic nerve trauma, in which the axons have been transected, cannot be reversed by any current surgical technique. Similarly, anterior indirect TON usually will not benefit from surgery, a possible exception being when there is compression of an otherwise intact optic nerve by a subdural or subarachnoid hematoma that can be evacuated via an optic nerve sheath fenestration [52].

Posterior indirect TON can be caused by a wide range of mechanisms. Diffuse orbital hemorrhage as well as more localized orbital or posterior optic sheath hematomas and orbital emphysema all are well recognized although being uncommon indirect mechanisms of injury to the optic nerve. Nevertheless, in such cases, particularly when there is evidence of delayed or progressive loss of vision, we agree with other authors that surgery, via nerve sheath fenestration, local evacuation of the blood or air, lateral canthotomy, or orbital decompression via a lateral or medial approach depending on the presumed mechanism of damage, should be performed [52, 74, 95].

In fact, the most common site of injury to the optic nerve in posterior indirect TON is within the optic canal. As already noted, the canalicular portion of the nerve is the most vulnerable region to trauma due to its being fixed via the dura to the periosteum of the canal. This portion of the nerve also is theoretically vulnerable to compressive and/or lacerating forces from fracture, hematoma expansion, swelling, etc. For this reason, optic canal decompression sometimes is advocated when a surgical lesion appears to be involving this portion of the nerve. If such surgery is thought to be appropriate, it probably should be performed immediately or no later than 48 h of the injury; [96] however, there are no convincing studies to date showing any clear benefit to optic canal decompression [38, 57]. The IONTS showed that 32 % of patients (33 of 127 patients) with unilateral TON who underwent optic canal decompression had improvement of visual acuity of three lines or more compared with 57 % in the untreated group and 52 % in the steroid-treated group [38]. The differences among groups were not significant. In addition, as this was not a randomized study, there almost certainly were intrinsic treatment biases, as patients with more severe visual loss and patients who were otherwise neurologically intact may have been more likely to receive surgery than patients with less severe visual loss and those who had other neurologic deficits. In a nonrandomized study, Fukado reported dramatic improvement in high percentages of individuals with TON who underwent optic canal decompression [97]; however, his results are not consistent with the results of most other authors. Similarly, other nonrandomized studies that have reported marked improvement in vision in patients with TON who have undergone decompression are likely less tenable given potential selection bias, timing bias, and other methodological errors [98–100].

Given the unclear benefit of optic canal decompression, it may be prudent to pursue this treatment only in instances in which the patient's vision is clearly normal immediately after the injury and then deteriorates or clearly is progressively worsening, the site of injury is clearly the optic canal, and, perhaps most importantly, the patient can consent to treatment even though he or she understands both the unproven benefit and the potential risks (e.g., further visual loss, damage to other neural or vascular structures) [101]. As noted above, unconscious patients should not be considered surgical candidates as they cannot give consent and there is no way to assess their vision. A possible exception may be when the affected pupil does not react at all to direct light but reacts consensually when light is shined in the opposite eye. Alternatively, however, one could argue that in such a setting, the vision is so poor that no surgical measures should be attempted. In addition, if surgery is performed in this setting and the patient awakens completely blind in the eye, the patient and family may question the appropriateness of the treatment even though consent was obtained from a relative. In such instances, a preoperative VEP may be of benefit in that a flat VEP in one eye with a normal VEP in the opposite eye would lend credence to the belief that the patient truly is blind in the affected eye.

There are a number of techniques by which the optic nerve can be decompressed within the optic canal, the most commonly used being the transethmoidal route [96, 102], usually either endonasally [103] or via an external ethmoidectomy or transcaruncular approach (Fig. 17.15a, b) [104].

Using this approach, the inferomedial wall of the canal is removed [105]. The advantage of this approach is that it is the least invasive of the surgical approaches. Another option is the supraorbital subfrontal approach. In this approach, the roof of the canal is removed. This approach is most useful when the anterior clinoid process is fractured and also allows opening of the falciform dural fold [2].

Sofferman [106, 107] provided criteria for adequate optic canal decompression, indicating that (1) at least 50 % of the circumference of the osseous canal should be removed, (2) bone along the entire length of the canal should be removed, and (3) there should be total longitudinal incision of the dural sheath including the annulus of Zinn. We do not necessarily endorse the third recommendation.

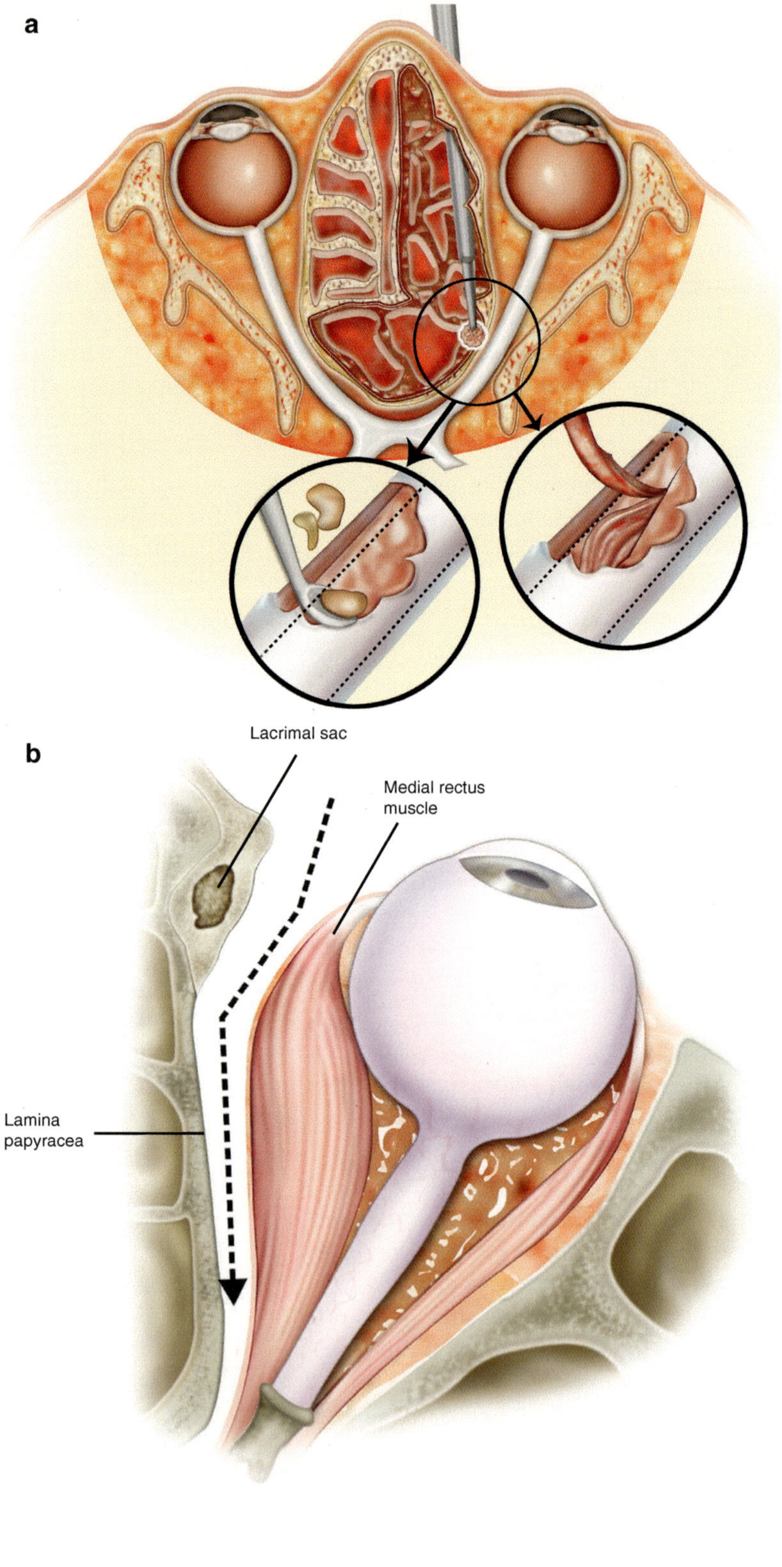


**Fig. 17.15** (**a**) One of the two routes by which the canalicular portion of the optic nerve can be decompressed: transnasal endoscopic. (**b**) One of the two routes by which the canalicular portion of the optic nerve can be decompressed: transcaruncular

## Recommendations

Given our current deficiencies in knowledge regarding how to best manage TON, we adhere to the dictum "primum non nocere" and emphasize that it is appropriate to observe any and all patients with TON, regardless of the level of vision in the affected eye. In addition, as noted above, we agree with Steinsapir and Goldberg [44] that it no longer is appropriate to argue that "steroids can't hurt," particularly "megadose" steroids. Although there is no evidence that "high-dose" steroids (e.g., 1000 mg/day of methylprednisolone) are harmful to visual recovery in human TON, there certainly is no evidence that they are helpful. As far as surgery is concerned, in rare cases of a clear-cut compartment syndrome within the orbit or optic nerve sheath, particularly when new and/or progressive, immediate optic nerve fenestration should be performed. In select cases of known or presumed injury to the canalicular optic nerve, particularly when there is clear-cut delayed visual loss or vision is worsening, immediate decompression of the optic nerve within the canal may be reasonable but only after a well-documented discussion with the patient and family. No treatment should be the default with unconscious patients with the possible exception of those in whom the pupil does not react directly but reacts consensually. In such cases, VEP may play a role as absence of any response from the affected eye with a normal response from the contralateral eye will indicate not only that the affected eye truly is blind but also that treatment is unlikely to improve vision [108–111].

## Future Outlook

The search for neuroprotective agents for various mechanisms of traumatic and ischemic CNS injury is the holy grail of the neurosciences. Unfortunately, despite decades of research and a better understanding of the pathways of apoptosis and cell death, there are no clinically proven neuroprotective or regenerative therapies for traumatic CNS lesions, including TON [3, 112]. In addition, different types of injury may respond to different types of treatment. Unfortunately, a large, prospective, randomized, placebo-controlled trial designed to determine optimum therapy for TON is unlikely to be forthcoming as demonstrated by the technical difficulties designing and conducting such a trial as evidenced by the failure of the IONTS. Nevertheless, we are hopeful that novel management strategies will emerge as more is understood about the converging pathways of various primary, secondary, and even tertiary mechanisms of cell injury and death at play in TON. Until then, the abiding theme in the treatment of traumatic optic neuropathy should be "primum non nocere."

## References

1. Newman NJ. The Cambridge symposium: September 2003. Eye (Lond). 2004;18(11):1025.
2. Steinsapir KD, Goldberg RA. Traumatic optic neuropathy. Surv Ophthalmol. 1994;38(6):487–518.
3. Levin L. Traumatic optic neuropathy. CME syllabus, adapted from Levin LA Traumatic optic neuropathy. In: Roy FH, Fraunfelder F, editors. Roy and Fraunfelder's current ocular therapy. 6th ed. Philadephia: Saunders; 2007. Available at: http://content.lib.utah.edu/utils/getfile/collection/ehsl-nam/id/83/filename/4.pdf.
4. Minckler DS, McLean IW, Tso MO. Distribution of axonal and glial elements in the rhesus optic nerve head studied by electron microscopy. Am J Ophthalmol. 1976;82(2):179–87.
5. Cioffi GA, Van Buskirk EM. Microvasculature of the anterior optic nerve. Surv Ophthalmol. 1994;38: S107–17.
6. Hayreh SS. Blood supply of the optic nerve head. Ophthalmologica. 1996;210(5):285–95.
7. Joos KM, Kay MD, Pillunat LE, et al. Effect of acute intraocular pressure changes on short posterior ciliary artery haemodynamics. Br J Ophthalmol. 1999;83(1): 33–8.
8. Tso MO, Shih CY, McLean IW. Is there a blood-brain barrier at the optic nerve head? Arch Ophthalmol. 1975;93(9):815–25.
9. Hofman P, Hoyng P, VanderWerf F, Vrensen GF, Schlingemann RO. Lack of blood-brain barrier properties in microvessels of the prelaminar optic nerve head. Invest Ophthalmol Vis Sci. 2001;42(5):895–901.

10. Steinsapir KD, Goldberg RA. Traumatic optic neuropathies. In: Miller NR, Newman NJ, editors. Walsh & Hoyt's clinical neuro-ophthalmology, vol. 1. 6th ed. Philadelphia: Lippincott Williams & Wilkins; 2005. p. 431–46.
11. Liu GT, Volpe NJ, Galetta SL. Neuro-ophthalmology. 2nd ed. New York: Saunders; 2010. p. 105–6.
12. Hayreh SS. Posterior ciliary artery circulation in health and disease: the Weisenfeld lecture. Invest Ophthalmol Vis Sci. 2004;45(3):748–57.
13. Slavin KV, Dujovny M, Soeira G, Ausman J. Optic canal: microanatomic study. Skull Base Surg. 1994;4(3):136–44.
14. Maniscalco JE, Habal MB. Microanatomy of the optic canal. J Neurosurg. 1978;48(3):402–6.
15. Renn WH, Rhoton Jr AL. Microsurgical anatomy of the sellar region. J Neurosurg. 1975;43(3):288–98.
16. Van Overbeeke JJ, Sekhar LN. Microanatomy of the blood supply to the optic nerve. Orbit. 2003;22(2):81–8.
17. Rizzo JF III. Embryology, anatomy, and physiology of the afferent visual pathway. In: Miller NR, Newman NJ, editors. Walsh and Hoyt's clinical neuro-ophthalmology, vol. 1. 6th ed. Philadelphia: Lippincott Williams & Wilkins; 2005. p. 24–35.
18. Levkovitch-Verbin H, Quigley HA, Martin KRG, et al. A model to study differences between primary and secondary degeneration of retinal ganglion cells in rats by partial optic nerve transection. Invest Ophthalmol Vis Sci. 2003;44(8):3388–93.
19. Feist RM, Kline LB, Morris RE, Witherspoon CD, Michelson MA. Recovery of vision after presumed direct optic nerve injury. Ophthalmology. 1987;94(12):1567–9.
20. Wang BH, Robertson BC, Girotto JA, et al. Traumatic optic neuropathy: a review of 61 patients. Plast Reconstr Surg. 2001;107(7):1655.
21. Kline LB, Morawetz RB, Swaid SN. Indirect injury of the optic nerve. Neurosurgery. 1984;14(6):756–64.
22. Turner J. Indirect injuries of the optic nerve. Brain. 1943;66:140–51.
23. Walsh FB. Pathological-clinical correlations. I. Indirect trauma to the optic nerves and chiasm. II. Certain cerebral involvements associated with defective blood supply. Invest Ophthalmol. 1966;5(5):433–49.
24. Lessell S. Indirect optic nerve trauma. Arch Ophthalmol. 1989;107(3):382.
25. Gross CE, DeKock JR, Panje WR, Hershkowitz N, Newman J. Evidence for orbital deformation that may contribute to monocular blindness following minor frontal head trauma. J Neurosurg. 1981;55(6):963–6.
26. Purvin V. Evidence of orbital deformation in indirect optic nerve injury. Weight lifter's optic neuropathy. J Neuroophthalmol. 1988;8(1):9–11.
27. Foster BSB, March GAG, Lucarelli MJM, Samiy NN, Lessell SS. Optic nerve avulsion. Arch Ophthalmol. 1997;115(5):623–30.
28. Tsopelas NV, Arvanitis PG. Avulsion of the optic nerve head after orbital trauma. Arch Ophthalmol. 1998;116(3):394–4.
29. Cirovic S, Bhola RM, Hose DR, et al. Computer modelling study of the mechanism of optic nerve injury in blunt trauma. Br J Ophthalmol. 2006;90(6):778–83.
30. Manson PN, Stanwix MG, Yaremchuk MJ, et al. Frontobasal fractures: anatomical classification and clinical significance. Plast Reconstr Surg. 2009;124(6):2096–106.
31. Spetzler RF, Spetzler H. Holographic interferometry applied to the study of the human skull. J Neurosurg. 1980;52(6):825–8.
32. Al-Sukhun J, Kontio R, Lindqvist C. Orbital stress analysis—part I: simulation of orbital deformation following blunt injury by finite element analysis method. J Oral Maxillofac Surg. 2006;64(3):434–42.
33. Fard AKA, Merbs SLS, Pieramici DJD. Optic nerve avulsion from a diving injury. Am J Ophthalmol. 1997;124(4):562–4.
34. Bellezza AJ, Hart RT, Burgoyne CF. The optic nerve head as a biomechanical structure: initial finite element modeling. Invest Ophthalmol Vis Sci. 2000;41(10):2991–3000.
35. Cirovic S, Bhola RM, Hose DR, et al. A computational study of the passive mechanisms of eye restraint during head impact trauma. Comput Methods Biomech Biomed Eng. 2005;8(1):1–6.
36. Weichel ED, Colyer MH, Ludlow SE, Bower KS, Eiseman AS. Combat ocular trauma visual outcomes during operations Iraqi and enduring freedom. Ophthalmology. 2008;115(12):2235–45.
37. Steinsapir KD, Goldberg RA. Traumatic optic neuropathy: a critical update. Compr Ophthalmol Update. 2005;6(1):11–21. Available at: http://www.medscape.com/viewarticle/501762.
38. Levin L, Beck RW, Joseph MP, Seiff S, Kraker R. The treatment of traumatic optic neuropathy. Ophthalmology. 1999;106(7):1268–77.
39. Chadwick J. The medical works of hippocrates: a new translation from the original Greek. Oxford: Blackwell; 1950. p. 264.
40. Arnold A. Symposium on the treatment of traumatic optic neuropathy resolved: corticosteroids should not be used. The 2nd World Congress on Controversies in Ophthalmology (COPHy), Barcelona. 3–6 March 2011. Available at: http://www.comtecmed.com/cophy/2011/Uploads/assets/arnold.pdf.
41. Maurer J, Hinni M, Mann W, Pfeiffer N. Optic nerve decompression in trauma and tumor patients. Eur Arch Otorhinolaryngol. 1999;256(7):341–5.

42. Unterberg AW, Stover J, Kress B, Kiening KL. Edema and brain trauma. Neuroscience. 2004; 129(4):1021–9.
43. Marmarou A. A review of progress in understanding the pathophysiology and treatment of brain edema. Neurosurg Focus. 2007;22(5):E1:1–10.
44. Steinsapir KD, Goldberg RA. Traumatic optic neuropathy: an evolving understanding. Am J Ophthalmol. 2011;151(6):928–33.
45. Hughes BB. Indirect injury of the optic nerves and chiasma. Bull Johns Hopkins Hosp. 1962;111:98–126.
46. Hedges 3rd TR, Gragoudas ES. Traumatic anterior ischemic optic neuropathy. Ann Ophthalmol. 1981;13(5):625–8.
47. Petrarca R, Saldana M. Choroidal rupture and optic nerve injury with equipment designated as 'child-safe'. BMJ Case Rep. 2012. doi:10.1136/bcr-2012-006476.
48. Sponsel WE, Gray W, Groth SL, Stern AR, Walker JD. Paintball trauma and mechanisms of optic nerve injury: rotational avulsion and rebound evulsion. Invest Ophthalmol Vis Sci. 2011;52(13):9624–8.
49. Hillman JS, Myska V, Nissim S. Complete avulsion of the optic nerve. A clinical, angiographic, and electrodiagnostic study. Br J Ophthalmol. 1975; 59(9):503–9.
50. Krauss HR, Yee RD, Foos RY. Autoenucleation. Surv Ophthalmol. 1984;29(3):179–87.
51. Leibovitch I, Pietris G, Casson R, Selva D. Oedipism: bilateral self-enucleation. Am J Emerg Med. 2006;24(1):127–8.
52. Mauriello JA, DeLuca J, Krieger A, Schulder M, Frohman L. Management of traumatic optic neuropathy – a study of 23 patients. Br J Ophthalmol. 1992;76(6):349–52.
53. Park JH, Frenkel M, Dobbie JG, Choromokos E. Evulsion of the optic nerve. Am J Ophthalmol. 1971;72(5):969–71.
54. Crowe NW, Nickles TP, Troost BT, Elster AD. Intrachiasmal hemorrhage: a cause of delayed post-traumatic blindness. Neurology. 1989;39(6):863–5.
55. McCann JD, Seiff S. Traumatic neuropathies of the optic nerve, optic chiasm, and ocular motor nerves. Curr Opin Ophthalmol. 1994;5(6):9.
56. Ott I, Schwager K, Hagen R, Baier G. Traumatic optic neuropathy: a review of the literature in the light of personal experiences. Laryngorhinootologie. 2010;89(11):647–52.
57. Lee V, Ford RL, Xing W, Bunce C, Foot B. Surveillance of traumatic optic neuropathy in the UK. Eye (Lond). 2010;24(2):240–50.
58. Edmund J, Godtfredsen E. Unilateral optic atrophy following head injury. Acta Ophthalmol (Copenh). 1963;41(6):693–7.
59. Nau HE, Gerhard L, Foerster M, et al. Optic nerve trauma: clinical, electrophysiological and histological remarks. Acta Neurochir (Wien). 1987;89(1–2):16–27.
60. Al-Qurainy IA, Dutton GN, Ilankobvan V, et al. Midfacial fractures and the eye: the development of a system for detecting patients at risk of eye injury-a prospective evaluation. Br J Oral Maxillofac Surg. 1991;29(6):368–9.
61. Borruat F-X, Kawasaki A. Optic nerve massaging: an extremely rare cause of self-inflicted blindness. Am J Ophthalmol. 2005;139(4):715–6.
62. Rajiniganth MG, Gupta AK, Gupta A, Bapuraj JR. Traumatic optic neuropathy: visual outcome following combined therapy protocol. Arch Otolaryngol Head Neck Surg. 2003;129(11):1203–6.
63. Goldenberg-Cohen N, Miller NR, Repka MX. Traumatic optic neuropathy in children and adolescents. J AAPOS. 2004;8(1):20–7.
64. Ford RL, Lee V, Xing W, Bunce C. A 2-year prospective surveillance of pediatric traumatic optic neuropathy in the United Kingdom. J AAPOS. 2012;16(5):413–7.
65. Carta A, Ferrigno L, Leaci R, et al. Long-term outcome after conservative treatment of indirect traumatic optic neuropathy. Eur J Ophthalmol. 2006;16(6):847–50.
66. Stanley JA, Baise GR. The swinging flashlight test to detect minimal optic neuropathy. Arch Ophthalmol. 1968;80(6):769–71.
67. Bell RA. Clinical grading of relative afferent pupillary defects. Arch Ophthalmol. 1993;111(7):938–42.
68. Tabatabaei SA, Soleimani M, Alizadeh M, et al. Predictive value of visual evoked potentials, relative afferent pupillary defect, and orbital fractures in patients with traumatic optic neuropathy. Clin Ophthalmol. 2011;5:1021–6.
69. Alford MA, Nerad JA, Carter KD. Predictive value of the initial quantified relative afferent pupillary defect in 19 consecutive patients with traumatic optic neuropathy. Ophthal Plast Reconstr Surg. 2001;17(5):323–7.
70. Bruce BB, Lamirel C, Wright DW, et al. Nonmydriatic ocular fundus photography in the emergency department. N Engl J Med. 2011;364(4):387–9.
71. Manfredi SJ, Raji MR, Sprinkle PM, et al. Computerized tomographic scan findings in facial fractures associated with blindness. Plast Reconstr Surg. 1981;68(4):479–90.
72. Seiff SR, Berger MS, Guyon J, Pitts LH. Computed tomographic evaluation of the optic canal in sudden traumatic blindness. Am J Ophthalmol. 1984;98(6):751–5.
73. Takehara S, Tanaka T, Uemura K, et al. Optic nerve injury demonstrated by MRI with STIR sequences. Neuroradiology. 1994;36(7):512–4.
74. Jordan DR, White GL, Anderson RL, Thiese SM. Orbital emphysema: a potentially blinding complication following orbital fractures. Ann Emerg Med. 1988;17(8):853–5.
75. Wood BJ, Mirvis SE, Shanmuganathan K. Tension pneumocephalus and tension orbital

emphysema following blunt trauma. Ann Emerg Med. 1996;28(4):446–9.
76. Yu-Wai-Man P, Griffiths PG. Steroids for traumatic optic neuropathy. Cochrane Database Syst Rev. 2013;(6):CD006032.
77. Yu-Wai-Man P, Griffiths PG. Surgery for traumatic optic neuropathy. Cochrane Database Syst Rev. 2013;(6):CD005024.
78. Berestka JS, Rizzo JFI. Controversy in the management of traumatic optic neuropathy. Int Ophthalmol Clin. 1994;34(3):87.
79. Volpe NJ, Levin L. How should patients with indirect traumatic optic neuropathy be treated? J Neuroophthalmol. 2011;31(2):169–74. Volpe NJ, Levin L, eds.
80. Yip CC, Chng NW, Eong KG, et al. Low-dose intravenous methylprednisolone or conservative treatment in the management of traumatic optic neuropathy. Eur J Ophthalmol. 2002;12(4):309–14.
81. Hooper RS. Orbital complications of head injury. Br J Surg. 1951;39(154):126–38.
82. Wolin MJ, Lavin PJ. Spontaneous visual recovery from traumatic optic neuropathy after blunt head injury. Am J Ophthalmol. 1990;109(4):430–5.
83. Entezari M, Rajavi Z, Sedighi N, Daftarian N, Sanagoo M. High-dose intravenous methylprednisolone in recent traumatic optic neuropathy; a randomized double-masked placebo-controlled clinical trial. Graefes Arch Clin Exp Ophthalmol. 2007;245(9):1267–71.
84. Anderson RL, Panje WR, Gross CE. Optic nerve blindness following blunt forehead trauma. Ophthalmology. 1982;89(5):445–55.
85. Seiff SR. High dose corticosteroids for treatment of vision loss due to indirect injury to the optic nerve. Ophthalmic Surg. 1990;21(6):389–95.
86. Bracken MB, Shepard MJ, Collins WF, et al. A randomized, controlled trial of methylprednisolone or naloxone in the treatment of acute spinal-cord injury. N Engl J Med. 1990;323(17):1207–9.
87. Hurlbert RJ, Hadley MN, Walters BC, et al. Pharmacological therapy for acute spinal cord injury. Neurosurgery. 2013;72:93–105.
88. Bracken MB, Collins WF, Freeman DF, et al. Efficacy of methylprednisolone in acute spinal cord injury. JAMA. 1984;251(1):45.
89. Bracken MB, Shepard MJ, Holford TR, et al. Administration of methylprednisolone for 24 or 48 hours or tirilazad mesylate for 48 hours in the treatment of acute spinal cord injury. Results of the third national acute spinal cord injury randomized controlled trial. National Acute Spinal Cord Injury Study. JAMA. 1997;277(20):1597–604.
90. Pointillart V, Petitjean ME, Wiart L, et al. Pharmacological therapy of spinal cord injury during the acute phase. Spinal Cord. 2000;38(2):71–6.
91. Coleman WP, Benzel E, Cahill DW, et al. A critical appraisal of the reporting of the National Acute Spinal Cord Injury Studies (II and III) of methylprednisolone in acute spinal cord injury. J Spinal Disord. 2000;13(3):185.
92. Hurlbert RJ. Methylprednisolone for acute spinal cord injury: an inappropriate standard of care. J Neurosurg. 2000;93(1 Suppl):1–7.
93. Roberts I, Yates D, Sandercock P, et al. Effect of intravenous corticosteroids on death within 14 days in 10008 adults with clinically significant head injury (MRC CRASH trial): randomised placebo-controlled trial. Lancet. 2004;364(9442):1321–8.
94. Edwards P, Arango M, Balica L, et al. Final results of MRC CRASH, a randomised placebo-controlled trial of intravenous corticosteroid in adults with head injury-outcomes at 6 months. Lancet. 2005;365(9475):1957–9.
95. Liu D. A simplified technique of orbital decompression for severe retrobulbar hemorrhage. Am J Ophthalmol. 1993;116(1):34–7.
96. Wohlrab T-M, Maas S, De Carpentier JP. Surgical decompression in traumatic optic neuropathy. Acta Ophthalmol Scand. 2002;80(3):287–93.
97. Fukado Y. Results in 400 cases of surgical decompression of the optic nerve. Mod Probl Ophthalmol. 1975;14:474–81.
98. Niho S, Niho M, Niho K. Decompression of the optic canal by the transethmoidal route and decompression of the superior orbital fissure. Can J Ophthalmol. 1970;5(1):22–40.
99. Matsuzaki H, Kunita M, Kawai K. Optic nerve damage in head trauma: clinical and experimental studies. Jpn J Ophthalmol. 1982;26(4):447–61.
100. Joseph MP. Extracranial optic nerve decompression for traumatic optic neuropathy. Arch Ophthalmol. 1990;108(8):1091.
101. Onofrey CB, Tse DT, Johnson TE, et al. Optic canal decompression: a cadaveric study of the effects of surgery. Ophthal Plast Reconstr Surg. 2007;23(4):261–6.
102. Goldberg RA, Steinsapir KD. Extracranial optic canal decompression: indications and technique. Ophthal Plast Reconstr Surg. 1996;12(3):163.
103. Horiguchi K, Murai H, Hasegawa Y, et al. Endoscopic endonasal trans-sphenoidal optic nerve decompression for traumatic optic neuropathy – technical note. Neurol Med Chir (Tokyo). 2010;50(6):518–22.
104. Sofferman RA. Transnasal approach to optic nerve decompression. Oper Tech Otolaryngol Head Neck Surg. 1991;2(3):150–6.
105. Levin LA, Joseph MP, Rizzo JF, Lessell S. Optic canal decompression in indirect optic nerve trauma. Ophthalmology. 1994;101(3):566–9.
106. Sofferman RA. An extracranial microsurgical approach to the optic nerve. J Microsurg. 1979;1(3):195–202.
107. Sofferman RA. Sphenoethmoid approach to the optic nerve. Laryngoscope. 1981;91(2):184–96.
108. Mahapatra AK, Bhatia R. Predictive value of visual evoked potentials in unilateral optic nerve injury. Surg Neurol. 1989;31(5):339–42.

109. Mahapatra AK. Visual evoked potentials in optic nerve injury. Does it merit a mention? Acta Neurochir (Wien). 1991;112(1–2):47–9.
110. Agarwal A, Mahapatra AK. Visual outcome in optic nerve injury patients without initial light perception. Indian J Ophthalmol. 1999;47(4):233–6.
111. Holmes MD, Sires BS. Flash visual evoked potentials predict visual outcome in traumatic optic neuropathy. Ophthal Plast Reconstr Surg. 2004;20(5):342–6.
112. Miller NR. Optic nerve protection, regeneration, and repair in the 21st century: LVIII Edward Jackson Memorial lecture. Am J Ophthalmol. 2001;132(6):811–8.

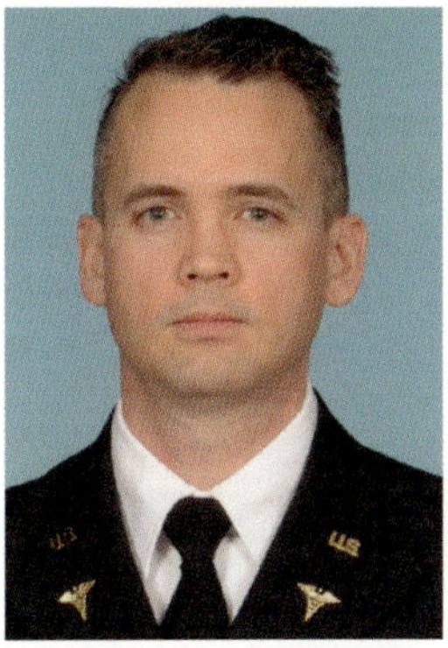

**MAJ Jason N. Harris, MD** practices neuro-ophthalmology and general neurology at the San Antonio Military Medical Center, TX, USA. He holds adjunct faculty appointments as an Assistant Professor of Neurology at the Uniformed Services University of the Health Sciences (USUHS), Bethesda, MD as well as UT Health Science Center, San Antonio, TX. He received a B.A. in Zoology from Idaho State University and subsequently attended the Uniformed Services University of the Health Sciences, Bethesda, MD where he graduated AOA in 2006. In 2010, he completed a neurology residency at Walter Reed Army Medical Center. He subsequently practiced general neurology at Tripler Army Medical Center, HI for three years and served in Afghanistan caring for patients with traumatic brain injuries. Dr. Harris completed a clinical fellowship in neuro-ophthalmology from The Wilmer Eye Institute at Johns Hopkins, Baltimore, MD in 2014.

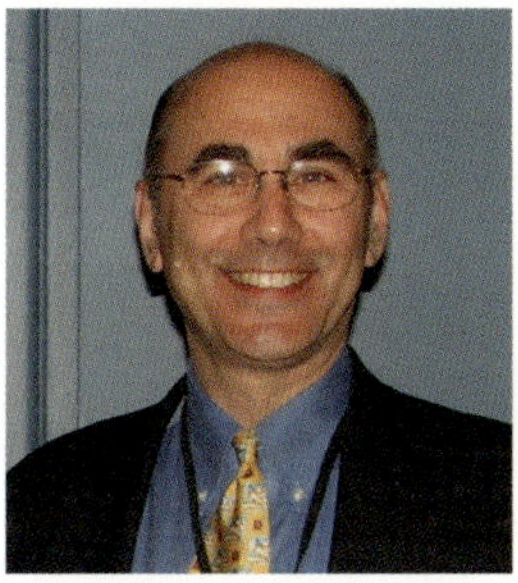

**Neil R. Miller** Dr. Neil Miller is currently Professor of Ophthalmology, Neurology, and Neurosurgery at the Johns Hopkins Medical Institutions and also the Frank B. Walsh Professor of Neuro-Ophthalmology. Dr. Miller was President of the North American Neuro-Ophthalmology Society from 2000 to 2002 and Chairman of its Executive Board from 2002 to 2004. He has been past President of the International Neuro-Ophthalmology Society on three occasions: in 1982, 1992, and 2008. He is also an emeritus member of the International Orbital Society. In 2009, he was given the Lifetime Achievement Award by the American Academy of Ophthalmology (AAO). He has authored or co-authored 500 articles, 90 chapters, and 13 books in the fields of neuro-ophthalmology and orbital disease. Many of Dr. Miller's previous fellows and residents hold faculty positions at major institutions throughout the United States and around the world.

# 18 Retrobulbar Hemorrhage: Etiology, Pathogenesis, Epidemiology, and Clinical Perspectives

Hatem A. Tawfik, Yousef Ahmed Fouad, and Yasmin Ashraf Hamza

## Introduction

*The only weapon with which the unconscious patient can immediately retaliate upon the incompetent surgeon is hemorrhage* (William Stewart Halsted, 1912)

On casual examination in a dried skull, the orbit looks like an open storage box, although in clinical practice, it behaves more like a watertight closed jewelry box [1]. Of the many nightmares any surgeon has after a busy day at surgery is a retrobulbar hemorrhage (RBH). Bleeding into the confined space of the orbit increases its internal pressure (orbital compartment syndrome or OCS) resulting in retinal ischemia and a subsequent irreversible loss of vision within 60–100 min [2]. However as we shall see, surgery is not the sole cause of a hematoma confined to the retrobulbar space.

The authors have no financial interest in the study.

H.A. Tawfik, MD (✉)
Ophthalmology, Ain Shams University Hospitals, 27705 Cairo, Egypt
e-mail: hatem35@gmail.com

Y.A. Fouad • Y.A. Hamza
Ain Shams University Hospitals, 1156 Cairo, Egypt
e-mail: yousef.a.fouad@gmail.com; YasminAshraf919@gmail.com

## Nomenclature

Orbital hemorrhage has been referred to by a number of terms in the literature, including orbital hemorrhage, orbital hematoma, hematic cyst, encysted hemorrhage, RBH, and OCS. Although the term OCS is gaining popularity in recent literature, we still prefer to use the term RBH because OCS may have a heterogeneous etiology and is not a term circumscribed to hemorrhages alone.

## Classification

Some authors have attempted a simple anatomical classification based on the location of hemorrhage into intraorbital hemorrhage and subperiosteal hemorrhage [3], while others have attempted a more elaborate classification systems into (1) diffuse intraorbital, (2) localized intraorbital (hematic cyst), (3) subperiosteal, (4) related to extraocular muscle (EOM), and (5) related to orbital floor implants [4]. Because of the inclusion of traumatic retrobulbar hemorrhage in the current discussion, an anatomical classification is not applicable because traumatic hemorrhage may not lend itself to specific anatomical location. In addition, it will be obvious after reading this chapter that there exists a significant overlap between nosological types of RBH, the


B. Mukherjee, H. Yuen (eds.), *Emergencies of the Orbit and Adnexa*, DOI 10.1007/978-81-322-1807-4_18

etiopathogenesis, and the anatomic location; therefore, we will adopt a simple etiological/anatomic classification solely for the purpose of the current discussion.

A. Traumatic hemorrhage
   I. Diffuse
   II. Localized
B. Surgical hemorrhage
   I. Diffuse
   II. Localized
C. Non-traumatic hemorrhage
   I. Diffuse
   II. Localized
D. Atypical forms
   (1) Subperiosteal hemorrhage
   (2) Hematic cyst
   (3) Beached whale hematoma

## Traumatic Hemorrhage

A traumatic RBH (Fig. 18.1) usually presents with an acute unilateral arterial bleed (infraorbital or ethmoidal arteries), which characteristically develops within a few hours following trauma, but may be delayed for days [2]. The incidence of traumatic RBH ranges from 0.45 to 12 % following blunt or penetrating trauma to the orbit or zygoma [5]. RBH is less likely to occur with displaced fractures of the orbit because of the sudden expansion of the tight orbital milieu, but it may still occur [2,6]. On the other hand, undisplaced, blow-in (Fig. 18.1a, b), or even small linear fractures of the orbital walls may cause minimal bleeding that cannot possibly drain into the paranasal sinuses [6]. Patients with displaced fractures however are not immune from developing a blinding RBH. The location of the hemorrhage/fracture is also important. In a recent study in eight patients with traumatic RBH presenting with vision loss, six out of the eight hemorrhages were superior [6].

## Surgical Hemorrhage

RBH may also develop as a complication of any surgery on or near the orbit or any anesthesia technique that violates the orbital septum (also referred to as iatrogenic RBH) [5]. Surgeries commonly associated with increased risk of RBH include:

### Blepharoplasty

The incidence of post-blepharoplasty orbital hemorrhage (Fig. 18.2a, f) was reported to be 1 in 2,000, with a 1 in 10,000 risk of development of permanent visual loss [7]. Most hemorrhages occur within the first 24 h, but delayed hemorrhage has been documented for as long as 9–15 days postoperatively [7]. Although Hass et al. put this figure at 6 h [7], in our experience the most critical period where close monitoring is mandatory is the first 3 h.

We usually avoid any form of orbital fat clamping to avoid tearing of deep orbital vessels. An important source of bleeding in lower eyelid blepharoplasty which manifests by a sudden gush during surgery and may be challenging to manage is hemorrhage due to injury of the inferior oblique muscle. The surgeon must outweigh the benefits of cauterizing the source of bleeding versus the risk of inducing fibrosis and subsequent diplopia with the cautery.

An often overlooked cause of bleeding in upper eyelid blepharoplasty is excessive dissection in and around medial orbital fat compartment which could result in inadvertent injury to the superior root of the superior ophthalmic vein (which represents the orbital continuation of the supraorbital and the supratrochlear veins) [8] or even the superior ophthalmic vein itself, with massive catastrophic bleeding.

### Endoscopic Sinus Surgery (ESS)

RBH is the most common orbital complication of ESS [9]. Inadvertent entry into the orbit through the lamina papyracea is the usual scenario [9].

### Endonasal Dacryocystorhinostomy (DCR)

A single case report (Fig. 18.2c) has been published detailing the occurrence of an RBH following an endonasal DCR and is probably related to hemorrhage [10].

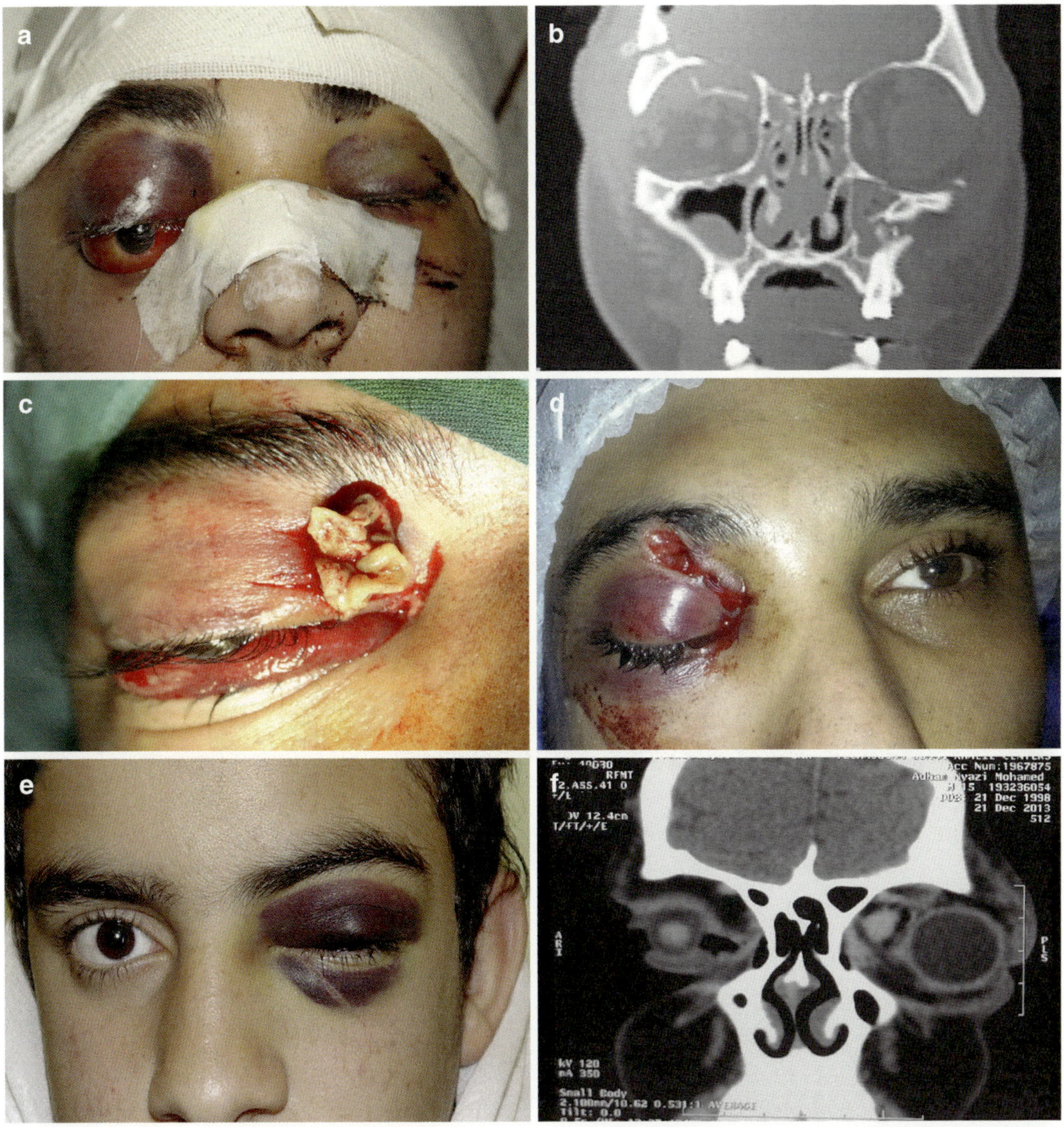


**Fig. 18.1** Traumatic hemorrhage. (**a**, **b**) Right frontal bone fracture, subdural hematoma, and massive right RBH with blow-in fracture of the orbital roof. The patient was unconscious on admission with right relative afferent pupillary defect. Urgent canthotomy, cantholysis, and inferior septal release resulted in complete recovery of vision. (**c**) Massive blow to the face with a high-velocity high-pressure pneumatic grease-gun at point-blank. Patient presented with light perception vision, stone-hard orbit, diffuse subconjunctival hemorrhage, diffuse intraconal RBH on CT, and greasy material coming out of a small superonasal eyelid wound. (**d**) Patient referred for repair of upper eyelid laceration and canalicular tear. On examination the orbit was stone hard with inability to open the eyelids even by force. Canthotomy/cantholysis under general anesthesia was complicated by persistent bleeding. The patient was finally diagnosed with mild hemophilia after three repeated factor VIII assays. (**e**, **f**) 17-year-old male patient presenting 1 week after a blow to the left orbit during a street fight. CT scan showed a well-circumscribed hematoma with layering of blood within it in the medial extraconal space. The right pupil was dilated irreactive with no light perception vision

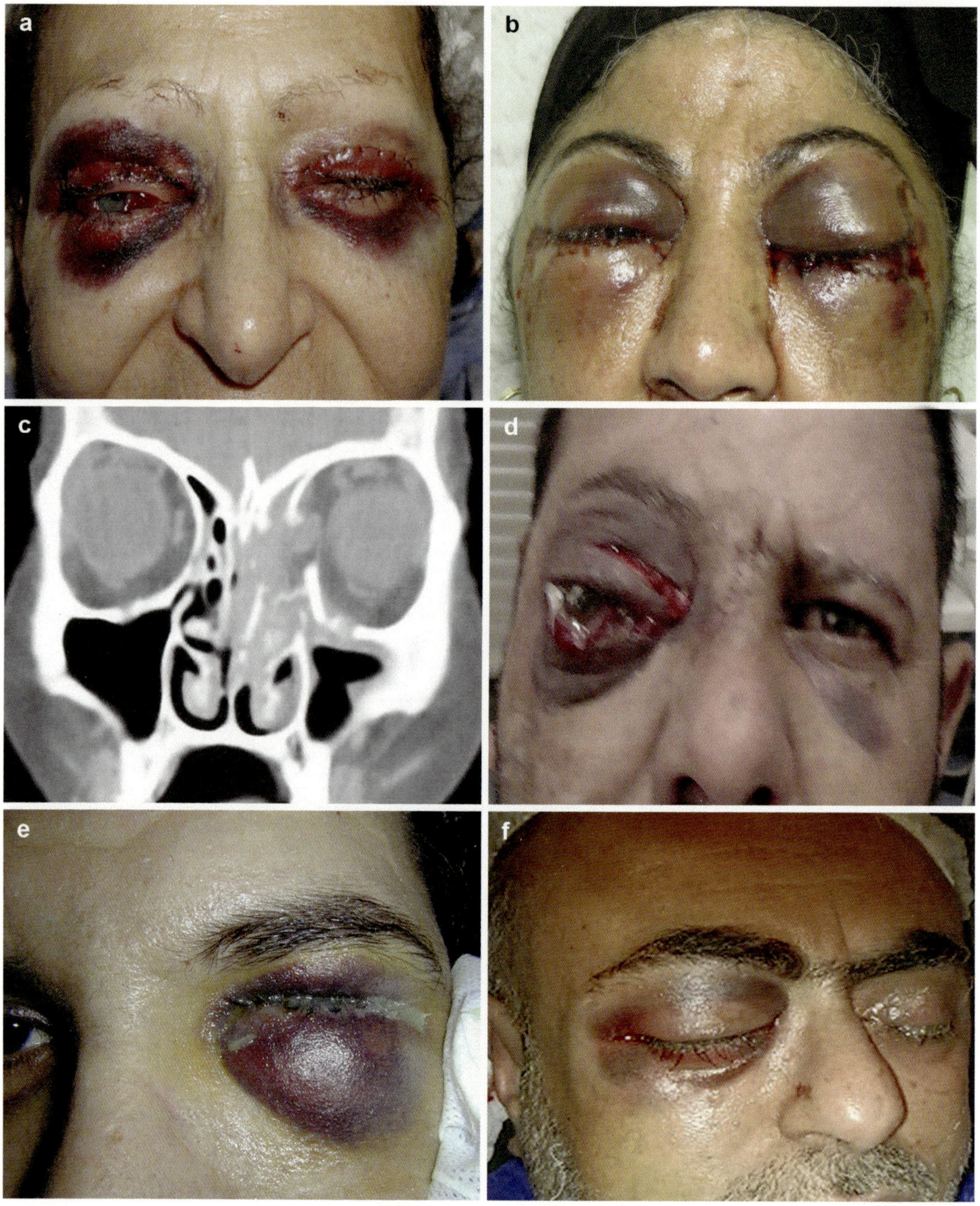


**Fig. 18.2** Surgical hemorrhage. (**a**) RBH in a patient who underwent upper and lower eyelid blepharoplasty. The patient later admitted she was abusing alprazolam for the past 2 months. (**b**) Bilateral RBH developing after balanced orbital decompression. (**c**) Unilateral RBH developing after bilateral endonasal nonendoscopic DCR in a 70-year-old female. (**d**) RBH developing immediately after debulking of hemangiopericytoma. Preoperative visual acuity was hand motion. Bleeding recurred despite immediate decompression through a lateral canthotomy and cantholysis. (**e**) *Periprosthetic bleeding*. Acute proptosis and delayed orbital hemorrhage due to prior fracture floor repair 6 years ago with a silicone sheet. (**f**) Severe unilateral RBH developing 3 h after transconjunctival blepharoplasty in a chronic Khat abuser with malignant hypertension. Patient was admitted to the ICU after canthotomy/cantholysis

### Orbital Surgery

Although fracture floor repair particularly with the use of solid implants (silicone, Teflon, Supramid) [11] is allegedly notorious for the development of RBH and is potentially the most serious complication of the surgery, with a reported incidence rate of 3.4 % [12], we have only encountered a single case so far (Fig. 18.2e).

Certain pathologies occasionally encountered during orbital removal of solid tumors may induce severe intraoperative or postoperative bleeding that may be challenging to manage. Hemangiopericytomas which are radiologically quite similar to venous malformations (previously called cavernous hemangioma) may present with life-threatening hemorrhage (Fig. 18.2d) that may only respond to ligation of the external carotid artery [13]. In our experience, even a simple biopsy for certain metastatic orbital lesions particularly hepatocellular carcinoma may be associated with severe uncontrolled RBH, and extreme care should be exercised if the primary is already well known [14].

Conventional wisdom would dictate that orbital decompression surgery for thyroid-associated orbitopathy should rarely be associated with RBH, and indeed this was the case in the era of inferomedial wall decompression because it created a huge communication with the sinuses. However, as more and more surgeons are moving toward lateral approaches, the risk of an RBH is becoming real regardless of whether the deep lateral wall is decompressed alone or with medial wall decompression (Fig. 18.2b). Because the orbit is divided into compartments and because of the proximity of the deep lateral wall to the orbital apex, a small collection of blood in this area may be critically close to the optic nerve and may rapidly impair vision [12] (Fig. 18.2b).

### Strabismus Surgery

Several case reports have appeared in the literature documenting RBH after strabismus surgery even without any predisposing factor [15].

### Anesthesia Techniques

Anesthesia techniques reported to be complicated with RBH include a retrobulbar block (0.44 % reported incidence rate) [16], a peribulbar block (0.74 % reported incidence rate) [17], sub-Tenon's anesthesia [18], and a frontal nerve block [19].

## Non-traumatic Hemorrhage

In the absence of trauma or surgery around the orbit, RBH is rare but is occasionally seen in clinical practice (Fig. 18.3). Absolutely spontaneous RBH is extremely rare, and usually a predisposing factor is encountered. In fact several case reports in the literature described as 'non-traumatic' are actually cases associated with an unusual form of trauma [20]. A survey of our own medical records as well as a review of the literature has revealed three different patterns of presentation of non-traumatic hemorrhage:

1. An elderly hypertensive patient presenting with an acute onset of unilateral proptosis or diplopia typically on waking up in the morning. This patient is usually on aspirin and may or may not recall a precipitating event such as severe coughing, severe straining, or vomiting [3,11,12]. These patients typically present with hemorrhage in the inferotemporal quadrant of the orbit with a "beached whale" configuration, although we have seen one patient with similar findings inferonasally (Fig. 18.3g, h) [12]. Prognosis for vision is usually excellent, but we have observed one such patient with complete amaurosis.
2. A young, probably muscular or athletic patient presenting with acute proptosis or diplopia following a severe bout of emesis, straining, or lifting weights. Location of hemorrhage is usually superior subperiosteal and prognosis for vision is usually excellent.
3. A pregnant woman developing an acute loss of vision during or immediately after labor (Fig. 18.3c, d). To the best of our knowledge, nine prior cases have been reported in the literature [3].

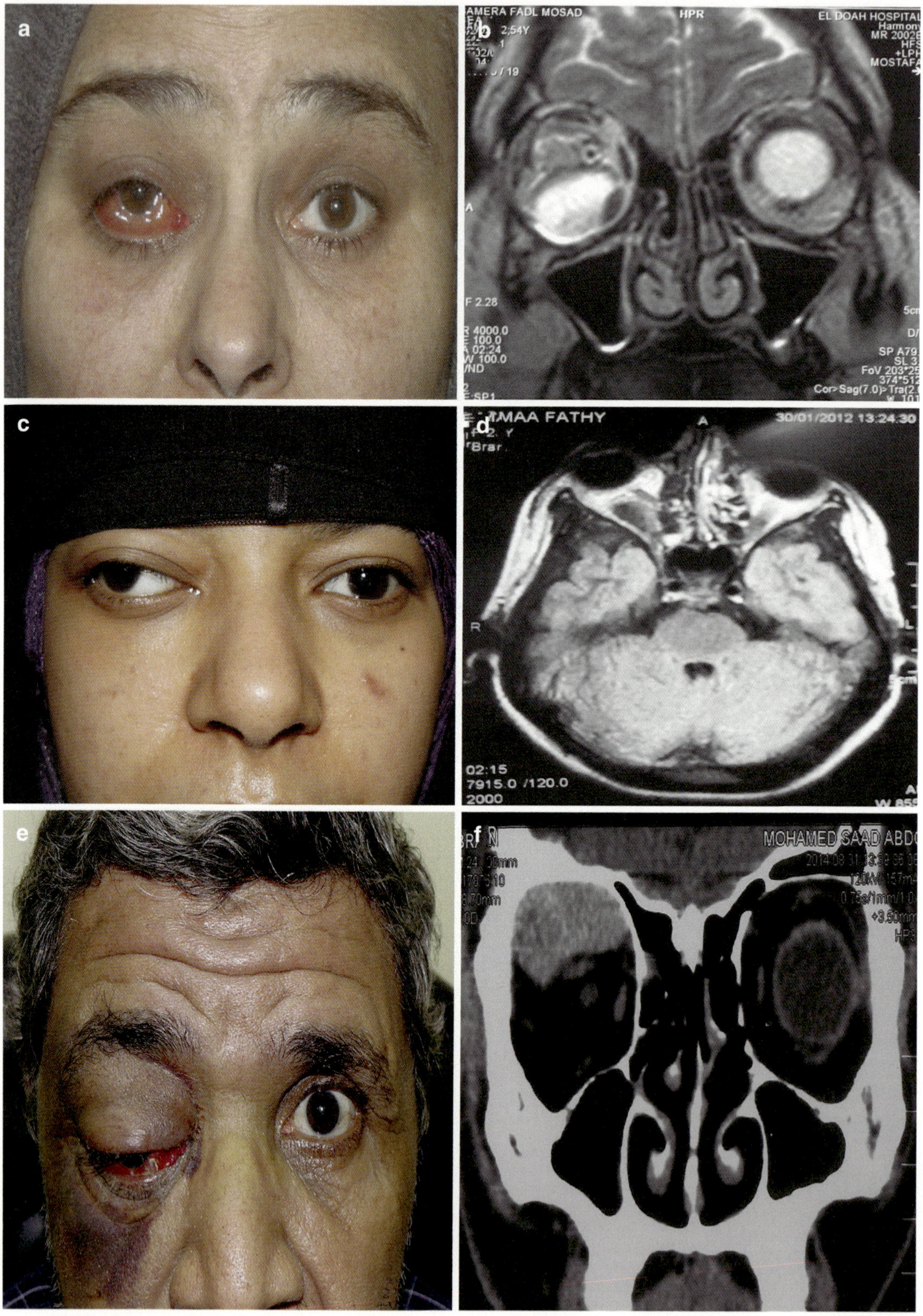
a
b
AMERA FADL MOSAD
HPR
EL DOAH HOSPITAL
c
d
TMAA FATHY
30/01/2012 13:24:30
02:15
7915.0 /120.0
2000
e
f
MOHAMED SAAD ABDO

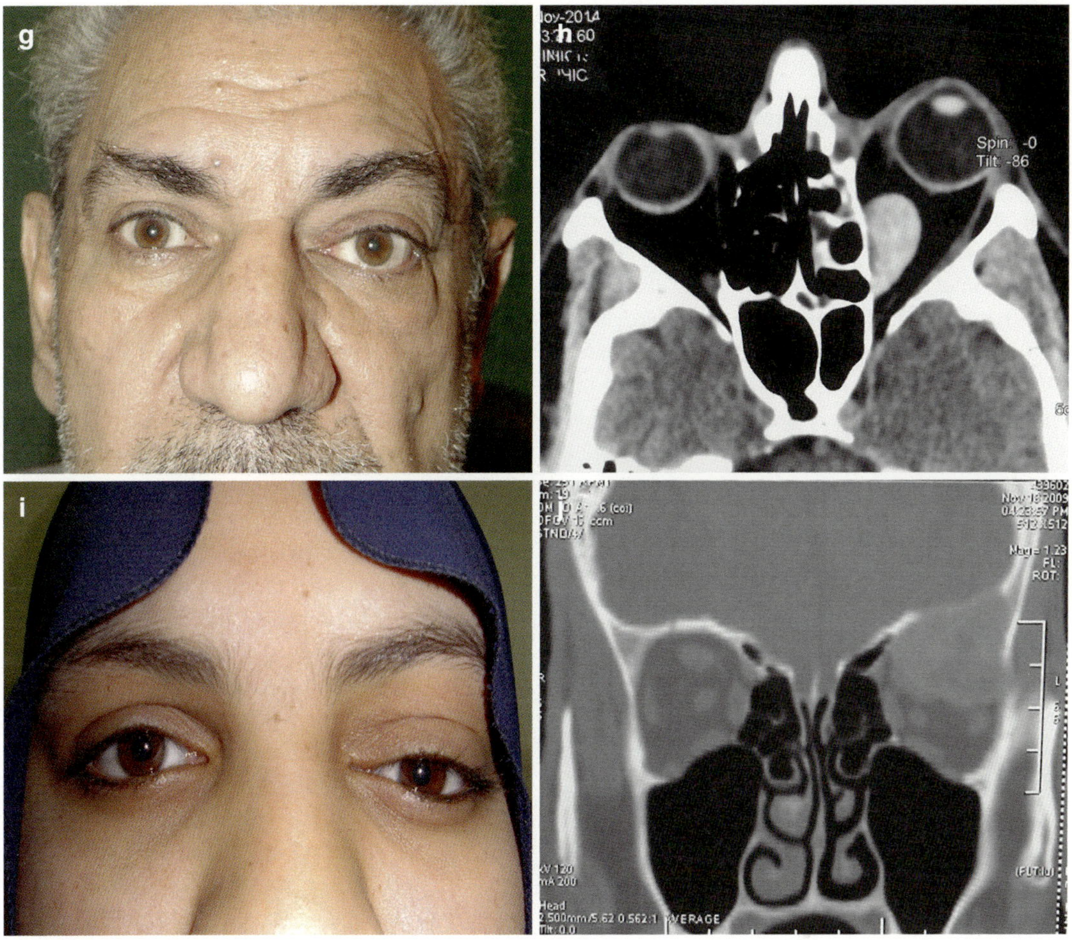


**Fig. 18.3** (continued)

**Fig. 18.3** Non-traumatic hemorrhage. (**a**, **b**) Subacute presentation of RBH in a patient with chronic liver disease. T2-weighted MRI showed a hyperintense inferior intraocular lesion not compressing the optic nerve. Vision was 20/20 (OU). (**c**, **d**) Complete loss of vision immediately following delivery in a multigravida female. Pregnancy was complicated by preeclampsia. A T1-weighted MRI performed at presentation 2 weeks after delivery shows a slightly hyperintensive intraconal collection of blood pushing the optic nerve medially. (**e**, **f**) A 73-year-old male on self-prescribed anticoagulants. On examination there was massive RBH, subconjunctival chemosis, and severe resistance to retropulsion. CT ordered at presentation (5 days following onset of symptoms) showed unilateral non-traumatic SOH superiorly with some globe compression. Vision loss was irreversible. (**g**, **h**) Inferonasal beached whale hematoma in a 71-year-old hypertensive male after severe bronchospasm. Patient was not anticoagulated. (**i**, **j**) Patient with a 4-month history of diplopia and 15-month history of slowly progressing painless proptosis. CT showed a relatively well-circumscribed lesion in the superotemporal quadrant with significant destruction of the frontal bone

## Hemorrhage in a Unique Anatomic Location

### Subperiosteal Hemorrhage

Subperiosteal hematomas (SOH) rarely occur in the orbit [4], as a rule develop superiorly near the roof of the orbit [4], and may be recurrent (Fig. 18.3e, f). They usually result from avulsion or rupture of subperiosteal blood vessels but may also be an extension of a subgaleal hematoma, and in such scenario, they may also be bilateral due to the fact that the subgaleal region is continuous with the orbital subperiosteal space [4]. CT usually shows a homogenous (occasionally heterogeneous due to blood layering) mass in the superior orbit with inferior displacement of orbital contents [11].

### Hematic Cyst

McNab strictly defined the term hematic cyst as an "intraorbital lesion characterized by a collection of blood and blood breakdown products within a cystlike structure without an epithelial lining and without an underlying vascular malformation" [11]. This specific terminology is used to differentiate it from the lymphangiomatous "chocolate cyst" which bears an epithelial lining [21]. Because these lesions are characteristically long standing, painless, and superior, with associated bone erosion, this has prompted some authors to theorize that they represent neglected SOH [4,21]. CT usually shows a soft tissue mass in the upper temporal quadrant with bone erosion that may simulate a malignant process in the lacrimal gland or a ruptured dermoid cyst (Fig. 18.3i, j). Pathological examination usually reveals a granulomatous or foreign body reaction to blood breakdown products with no epithelial or endothelial lining [21].

### Beached Whale Hematoma

To the best of our knowledge, Rose and Verity coined the term "beached whale" hematoma [12] and used it specifically to describe arterial hemorrhages that localize inferotemporally along the orbital floor in elderly patients with a fragile musculature. It is difficult to conclude whether the beached whale is a separate entity or simply a variation of SOH which attributes its specific shape on CT simply due to an inferior location (Fig. 18.3g, h).

## Risk Factors

## Drugs

### Antithrombotic Agents

As the use of antithrombotic therapy is expanding and evolving particularly among the elderly population, oculoplastic surgeons are more likely than ever to encounter patients on systemic anticoagulation and antiplatelet therapy. Generally the antithrombotics currently used in everyday practice fall into two groups: the antiplatelet agents, aspirin and clopidogrel (brand name, Plavix) that irreversibly inhibit platelets, and antithrombotic agents like warfarin (brand names, Marevan, Coumadin, and Uniwarfin) and heparin that interfere with thrombus formation. The literature is replete with extensive discussions about whether the prospective surgeon should or should not stop antithrombotic medications [22,23], and while this may indeed be permissible in elderly patients who self-medicate with antiplatelet agents, the real challenge however lies in patients receiving anticoagulants for secondary prevention of thromboembolic episodes, where the decision to withhold or continue the drug in question is not up to the patient or the oculoplastic surgeon but to the practitioner originally prescribing the medication and may involve a lawsuit if this rule is broken [24].

The management of a retrobulbar hematoma is beyond the realm of this chapter, but it suffices to point out that despite the emerging data that the interruption of anticoagulants results in a 40 % increase in the risk of ischemic episodes in cardiovascular patients [25], the decision should be individualized, and we are generally skeptical about the trend in recent literature to disregard stopping antithrombotic medications altogether because in contrast to surgery in other disciplines where bleeding might be inconsequential, bleeding in the confined space behind the eye could lead to the loss of vital organ function. This guarded outlook toward continuing anticoagulants may seem rather outdated but in fact has a strong foundation in everyday clinical practice because a drug like warfarin, for example, is on the top-ten list of drugs causing life-threatening emergencies in the USA with 29,000 unique yearly visits to the emergency room.

Another frequently overlooked issue is when to resume the anticoagulants after surgery. We generally advise the patients to wait 5 days after surgery; however again the cardiologist/neurologist in charge should be consulted.

### Other Medications, Vitamins, and Phytomedicines (Herbal Medications)

While the real concern with bleeding occurs with the antithrombotic agents described above, a long list of medications that could potentially cause bleeding is summarized in Table 18.1.

### Orbital Vascular Anomalies

In their comprehensive review on 115 patients with non-traumatic RBH, Timothy Sullivan and John Wright concluded that the majority of non-traumatic orbital bleeds occur in the setting of an orbital vascular anomaly [29]. They demonstrated an interesting bimodal pattern of presentation where 97 % of patients under the age of 20 years had an underlying orbital venous anomaly. RBH is more commonly encountered with low-flow venous or venous–lymphatic anomalies like lymphatic malformations or lymphatic–venous malformations (LVM) than with high-flow malformations or fistulae like arteriovenous fistulae (AVF) [12].

### Bleeding Disorders and Systemic Factors

Several endogenous bleeding disorders may lead to RBH, including Christmas disease, factor IX deficiency, thrombocytopenia, leukemia, aplastic anemia, sickle-cell disease, factor VII deficiency, and scurvy [30].

Spontaneous orbital hemorrhage can rarely occur during extreme Valsalva maneuvers causing an increase in central venous pressure, for example, during bouts of severe vomiting or coughing; delivery; extreme sports, such as powerlifting; or even strangulation [4,12,29]. As we mentioned earlier, the most likely candidates for such events are the elderly population with fragile microvasculature, but it may also occur in the younger population with "abnormal vasculature" (chronic hypertension or long-standing diabetes) [7,12] or even healthy young adults.

## Pathogenesis

### How a Hemorrhage Evolves?

Irrespective of the cause, the exact mechanism by which a RBH occurs may not be entirely clear. A thorough understanding of why RBH develops in postsurgical patients is of paramount importance because it is largely preventable. As a classic example, severe RBH may occur during or following blepharoplasty due to the following mechanisms:

1. Undue or excessive traction on orbital fat resulting in shearing of deep orbital vessels.
2. Rebound vasodilatation after the effect of epinephrine in local anesthetic wears off.
3. Increased venous pressure from Valsalva maneuvers especially if the patient coughs, strains, or forcefully vomits during recovery from general anesthesia; therefore we usually prefer local anesthesia whenever possible. Even if extubated prior to emergence to reduce coughing, patients may still experience significant hypertensive episodes during emergence which may result in significant bleeding. It is interesting to note that hypertensive episodes and raised intravascular pressure during recovery from general anesthesia may be severe enough even to lead to RBH in the unoperated contralateral eye [31] or after general anesthesia for procedures elsewhere in the body [32].

**Table 18.1** List of drugs causing bleeding alone or potentiating the effect of anticoagulants

| Drugs potentiating anticoagulants | Drugs that can cause bleeding | Phytomedicines and recreational drugs |
|---|---|---|
| Acetaminophen | Aceclofenac | Feverfew |
| Allopurinol | Acenocoumarol | Garlic in large amounts |
| Amiodarone | Alprazolam[a] | Ginger |
| Amoxicillin/clavulanate | Citalopram | Ginkgo biloba |
| Atorvastatin | Dexibuprofen | Ginseng |
| Azithromycin | Diclofenac | Khat (Catha edulis)[a] |
| Cefamandole | Dicoumarol | Marijuana (Cannabis sativa)[a] |
| Cefazolin | Escitalopram | Saw palmetto (Serenoa repens) |
| Chloramphenicol | Fluoxetine | Willow bark |
| Ciprofloxacin | Fluvoxamine | |
| Clarithromycin | Ibuprofen | |
| Clofibrate | Indomethacin | |
| Cotrimoxazole | Ketoprofen | |
| Dextropropoxyphene | Ketorolac | |
| Diltiazem | Lornoxicam | |
| Disopyramide | Meloxicam | |
| Doxycycline | Nabumetone | |
| Efavirenz | Naproxen | |
| Erythromycin | Paroxetine | |
| Etravirine | Phenprocoumon | |
| Ezetimibe | Piroxicam | |
| Fenofibrate | Sertraline | |
| Fluconazole | Sulindac | |
| Fluvastatin | Tenoxicam | |
| Gatifloxacin | Ticlopidine | |
| Gemfibrozil | Warfarin | |
| Glucagon | | |
| Indomethacin | | |
| Interferon | | |
| Isoniazid | | |
| Itraconazole | | |
| Leflunomide | | |
| Levofloxacin | | |
| Lovastatin | | |
| Methylprednisolone | | |
| Metolazone | | |
| Metronidazole | | |
| Moxifloxacin | | |
| Nabumetone | | |
| Nalidixic acid | | |
| Nevirapine | | |
| Norfloxacin | | |
| Phenylbutazone | | |
| Piroxicam | | |
| Propafenone | | |
| Propranolol | | |
| Quinidine | | |
| Saquinavir | | |
| Simvastatin | | |
| Sulfisoxazole | | |
| Sulindac | | |
| Terbinafine | | |
| Tetracycline | | |
| Tolmetin | | |
| Tramadol | | |

Modified from references [26–28]
[a]Authors' personal experience

4. Injury or excessive manipulation of muscles in and around the orbit, particularly the orbicularis oculi muscle.
5. The exclusive use of the electrosurgery unit (ESU) handpiece in cutting mode with low power settings could also tear blood vessels in the orbital fat/muscles without cauterizing them, and as counterintuitive as it might seem, this is an often overlooked source of unexplained bleeding during surgery particularly in procedures requiring frequent use of the ESU like blepharoplasty. Therefore we currently prefer the use of a bipolar handpiece and avoid monopolar electrosurgery if possible, but if a monopolar ESU is the only available option for hemostasis, we generally prefer the use of a cutting tip in coagulation mode over the use of a cutting mode or a combined cut/coagulation mode because electrode geometry is an overlooked factor influencing the final impact that an ESU has on tissues.
6. Improper use of epinephrine concentrations during local anesthetic injections. While a 1/200,000 concentration is standard dose in clinical practice and comparative studies have demonstrated that a 1/50,000 concentration provides a superior control of bleeding intraoperatively [33], in our experience a 1/200,000 may not provide sufficient hemostasis. A 1/50,000 concentration on the other hand should be used sparingly because it has resulted in a massive rebound bleeding at least in one of our patients.

### Pathogenesis of Visual Loss

The actual cause of visual loss in patients with RBH probably results when the raised retrobulbar pressure reaches a critical irreversible level [34] which could lead to occlusion of the central retinal artery and could also compromise the vascular supply to the optic nerve.

## Epidemiology

Any age or sex could be affected, but in general, the typical patient with a traumatic RBH is a young adult male [35]. This is attributed probably to the style of life in this particular age group and gender. There is however an explicable female preponderance in patients with an SOH [3], although other authors claim an equal sex distribution [11].

## Diagnosis

RBH is diagnosed based on the clinical picture, and unless life-threatening complications are suspected (such as intracranial hemorrhage), treatment should not be delayed waiting for imaging studies [2,5].

### History and Symptoms

Even before the patient arrives to the emergency ward, it is important to know what leading questions are to be asked on the phone to reach a tentative diagnosis. The most common presenting symptom is acute severe intolerable pain; however the pain is variable and may be moderately severe, although it is never mild or absent. Identifying the type of pain is also important because it may be simply related to a traumatic corneal abrasion. About 35 % of patients also present with worsening or fogging of vision if the patient is conscious [7,36]; therefore postoperative patching should be avoided to avoid a delay in diagnosis [7].

Acute onset of proptosis is also a typical presenting symptom, and if in doubt, a helpful tip on the phone is to ask whether the eyes could be easily opened to allow instillation of eyedrops or ointment. RBH patients typically find it almost impossible to open the eyes at will or even forcibly. Diplopia on the other hand is a relatively reassuring sign that all is not lost and optic nerve function is still preserved to some degree.

Constitutional symptoms in the form of severe pain, nausea, and vomiting may be mediated thorough the oculocardiac reflex [12]. Most importantly, particularly in post-traumatic RBH, symptoms suggestive of a subdural hematoma should be sought. Patients or kin should be specifically asked about confused speech, difficulty walking, loss of consciousness, headache, lethargy, nausea, vomiting, seizures, or slurred speech. Subgaleal hematomas on the other hand are less pernicious except in newborns. The presence of a bilateral orbital subperiosteal hematoma at any age should prompt suspicion of a subgaleal origin [4].

## Examination and Clinical Signs

At least three of the following criteria should be present in order to diagnose RBH: proptosis, pain, chemosis, decreasing visual acuity or diplopia, subconjunctival hemorrhage, increased intraocular pressure, resistance to retropulsion, loss of direct pupillary light reflex, or ophthalmoplegia [34]. A rock-hard or very tense orbit should be an alarming sign for immediate surgical intervention. Globe displacement in a non-axial direction could guide the surgeon as to the whereabouts of the hematoma.

A relative afferent pupillary defect is another sign of extreme clinical importance and is considered the most sensitive indicator for optic nerve affection and a detrimental factor in management, the absence of which should prompt observation alone. Severe restriction of ocular motility and marked resistance to retropulsion should also prompt immediate interference [12]. Chemosis, diffuse subconjunctival hemorrhage, and increased intraocular pressure are other recognized signs on examination, and fundus examination may reveal a pale optic disc, retinal edema, or retinal venous congestion [2]. However, the pathogenesis of RBH involves a dynamic process, and these features may not be initially present, and serial examinations are required for evaluation of symptom progression [2].

## Imaging

If indicated, imaging modalities can be utilized [5]. Ultrasonography aids the diagnosis of RBH by showing the characteristic "guitar pick" sign (deformation of the globe posteriorly) [37]. CT scan provides the definitive diagnosis but should not delay treatment if there are signs of worsening visual acuity. The role of orbital imaging in the setting of RBH is controversial and may be overstated. Ordering a CT or an MRI may be mandatory when an obvious cause cannot be elicited by history, but when the etiology is well known, treatment should be initiated immediately because the risk of deferring release of the raised orbital pressure far outweighs the risk of operating without radiological confirmation. However, radiology (CT not MRI) should be ordered if readily available not just to exclude simulating lesions like a retrobulbar edema but also to localize the blood and guide surgical intervention. The failure of the surgeon to find blood to evacuate during surgery may not always be attributed to an alternative etiology but may simply be due to the fact that blood has collected elsewhere, because extraconal blood in particular can collect anywhere. Therefore we believe that these two situations (a diagnosis in doubt or to localize the hematoma) are the situations where radiology is most needed [1].

In diffuse RBH CT usually shows a homogenous irregular mass that may or may not be associated with blood in the sinuses, globe laceration, an intraocular or retrobulbar foreign body, a blow-in or blow-out fracture, or bone fragments displaced inside the orbit, and it does not enhance with contrast. In SOH the mass is usually homogenous but may be heterogeneous due to layering of blood and is usually biconvex and located superiorly.

In 1993 Bradley [38] beautifully summarized the MRI findings of various stages of bleeding in the brain, and an identical staging could be applied to the orbit [11]. To summarize, the signal intensity of RBH depends upon the age of the lesion: A hyperacute hematoma is isointense on both T1 and T2; an acute hematoma is usually hypointense on T1 and may have a high signal on T2-weighted images. With progression of time (2–7 days) with accumulation of hemoglobin breakdown products, both T1 and T2 assume a high signal intensity. In the chronic stage, both have a low signal due to organization of the hematoma. We believe that these distinctions are academic, and the role of MRI in the setting of an RBH may be superfluous and time consuming.

## Differential Diagnosis

Proptosis following trauma, surgery, or occurring spontaneously may not always mean an RBH. It may occur due to massive edema (Fig. 18.4a, e), accumulation of air inside the orbit (Fig. 18.4f), displacement of pieces of bone after trauma, and intraconal herniation of brain tissue or CSF (Fig. 18.4d) [39], but the question that begs to be asked is if it really matters because the final common pathway is ischemia of the optic nerve or the retina with eventual loss of vision [1]. In fact we believe it does matter, because in some situations, the critical intraorbital pressure required for inhibition of tissue perfusion might never be reached with alternative etiologies. A classic example is shown in Fig. 18.44a where the patient maintained 20/20 vision, normal pupil responses, and a soft globe on retropulsion despite the presence of 11 mm of proptosis compared to the normal fellow eye. In addition the management approach may be entirely different. While a simple aspiration of air with a 25 gauge needle may suffice in cases of orbital emphysema, formal release of intraorbital pressure may be necessary in cases of an RBH. In a recent review article, up to half of the published cases of RBH following trauma, the diagnosis was questionable [39], and therefore the classically taught dictum that any proptosis following trauma or surgery is considered RBH should be revised but with caution. Differentiation between an RBH and the main simulating lesion (retrobulbar edema) may not be easy without radiology, but we believe the main differentiating point is that in RBH, proptosis is "tense," while in retrobulbar edema, it is relatively "softer" with lesser resistance to retropulsion. An orbital abscess and carotid–cavernous fistula are also on the differential diagnostic list, but they present relatively subacutely following trauma or surgery and therefore could be easily differentiated [34].

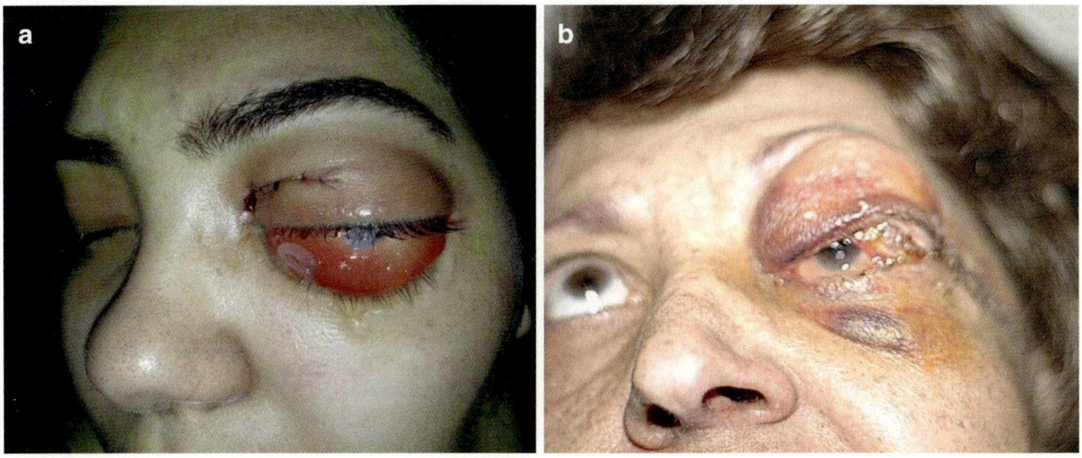


**Fig. 18.4** Simulating lesions. (**a**) Massive inflammation after piecemeal excision of a ruptured orbital dermoid cyst. The hallmarks of the case were absolute lack of pain, a soft orbit on palpation, and no resistance to retropulsion. Inflammation rapidly resolved with twice-daily injections of 100 mg hydrocortisone sodium succinate and alpha-chymotrypsin for 3 days. (**b**) Severe emphysema developing 6 h after a three-wall decompression. Air was aspirated with no long-term squeals on vision. (**c**) Acute onset of right massive proptosis developing 9 days after bilateral inferomedial decompression. The patient presented with severe pain, light perception vision, and severe restriction of motility. CT scan revealed a huge collection of pus in the maxillary sinus encroaching on the orbit. Immediate surgical drainage of the infected sinuses resulted in complete reversal of vision loss. (**d**) A 9-year-old child 3 weeks after massive trauma to the head with a CSF leak. Excluding RBH is usually easy, but the diagnosis may be acutely concealed acutely because of accompanying bleeding. (**e**) Massive unilateral proptosis 1 day after biopsy of an orbital mass that proved eventually to be an IgG4-related disease. An urgent canthotomy/cantholysis did not release any blood, and the patient was diagnosed with massive retrobulbar edema and responded very well to intravenous steroids. (**f**) A 68-year-old heavy smoker with chronic obstructive airway disease presenting 1 day following bilateral DCR with severe pain in the left eye. Surgery was complicated by orbital fat prolapse in both eyes. The swelling (air emphysema) was found in the left lower eyelid extending posteriorly, and the left eye was stone hard

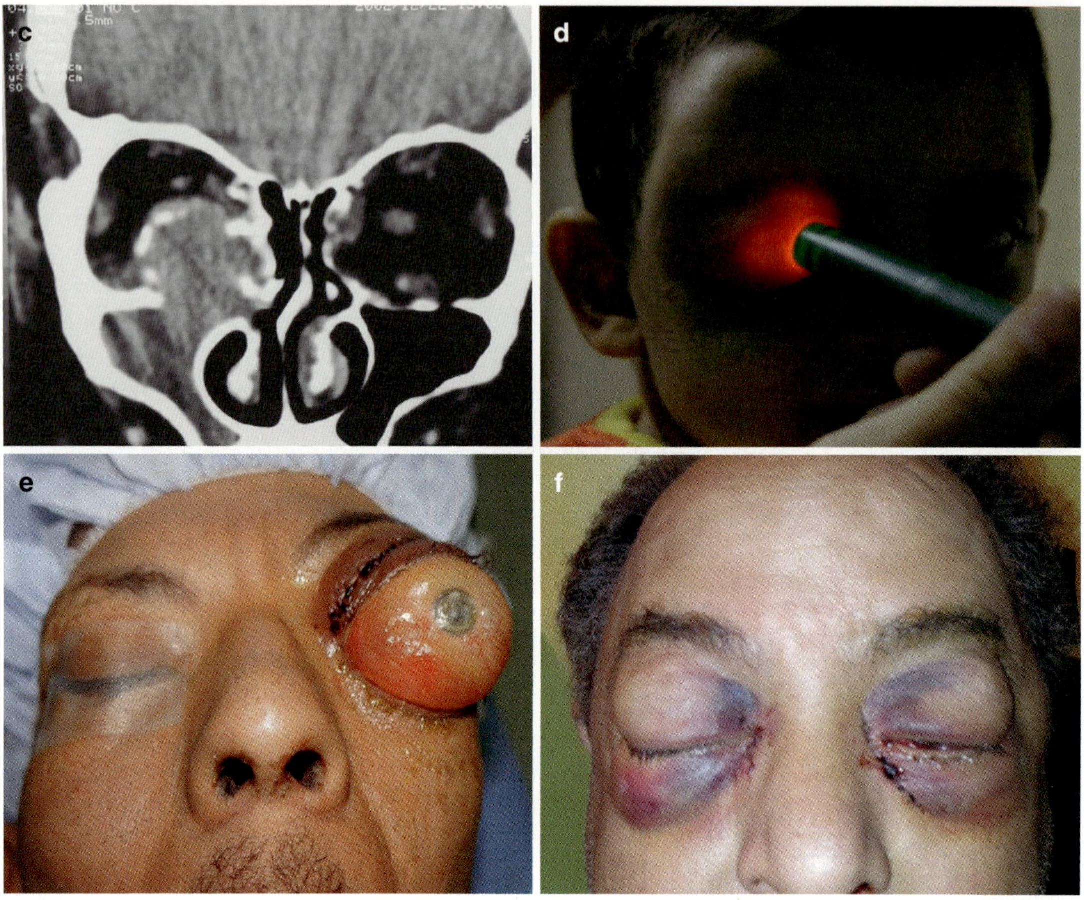


**Fig. 18.4** (continued)

## References

1. Perry M. Acute proptosis in trauma: retrobulbar hemorrhage or orbital compartment syndrome – does it really matter? J Oral Maxillofac Surg (Official Journal of the American Association of Oral and Maxillofacial Surgeons). 2008;66(9):1913–20.
2. Romaniuk VM. Ocular trauma and other catastrophes. Emerg Med Clin North Am. 2013;31(2):399–411.
3. Atalla ML, McNab AA, Sullivan TJ, Sloan B. Nontraumatic subperiosteal orbital hemorrhage. Ophthalmology. 2001;108(1):183–9.
4. Yazici B, Gonen T. Posttraumatic subperiosteal hematomas of the orbit in children. Ophthal Plast Reconstr Surg. 2011;27(1):33–7.
5. Colletti G, Valassina D, Rabbiosi D, et al. Traumatic and iatrogenic retrobulbar hemorrhage: an 8-patient series. J Oral Maxillofac Surg (Official Journal of the American Association of Oral and Maxillofacial Surgeons). 2012;70(8):e464–8.
6. Gerbino G, Ramieri G, Nasi A. Diagnosis and treatment of retrobulbar haematomas following blunt orbital trauma: a description of eight cases. Int J Oral Maxillofac Surg. 2005;34(2):127–31.
7. Hass AN, Penne RB, Stefanyszyn MA, Flanagan JC. Incidence of postblepharoplasty orbital hemorrhage and associated visual loss. Ophthalmic Plast Reconstr Surg. 2004;20(6):426–32.
8. Dutton JJ. The venous system of the orbit. In: Dutton JJ, editor. Atlas of clinical and surgical orbital anatomy. Philadelphia: W.B. Saunders Company; 1994. p. 81–93.
9. Bhatti MT. Neuro-ophthalmic complications of endoscopic sinus surgery. Curr Opin Ophthalmol. 2007;18(6):450–8.
10. Tawfik HA, Talib N, Elsamkary MA. Amaurosis as a complication of endonasal nonendoscopic dacryocystorhinostomy. Ophthalmic Plast Reconstr Surg. 2009;25(5):415. 410.1097/IOP.1090b1013e3181b1397df.
11. McNab AA. Nontraumatic orbital hemorrhage. Surv Ophthalmol. 2014;59(2):166–84.

12. Rose G, Verity D. Acute presentation of vascular disease within the orbit—a descriptive synopsis of mechanisms. Eye. 2013;27(3):299–307.
13. O'Driscoll D, O'Neill M. Progressive proptosis in a neonate. Postgrad Med J. 1998;74(875):559.
14. Eldesouky MA, Elbakary MA, Shalaby OE, Shareef MM. Orbital metastasis from hepatocellular carcinoma: report of 6 cases. Ophthal Plast Reconstr Surg. 2014;30(4):e78–82.
15. Todd B, Sullivan TJ, Gole GA. Delayed orbital hemorrhage after routine strabismus surgery. Am J Ophthalmol. 2001;131(6):818–9.
16. Edge KR, Nicoll JM. Retrobulbar hemorrhage after 12,500 retrobulbar blocks. Anesth Analg. 1993;76(5):1019–22.
17. Davis 2nd DB, Mandel MR. Efficacy and complication rate of 16,224 consecutive peribulbar blocks. A prospective multicenter study. J Cataract Refract Surg. 1994;20(3):327–37.
18. Rahman I, Ataullah S. Retrobulbar hemorrhage after sub-Tenon's anesthesia. J Cataract Refract Surg. 2004;30(12):2636–7.
19. Sierra CA, Gladstone GJ. Muller's muscle-conjunctival resection. In Complications in ophthalmic plastic surgery. New York: Springer; 2003. p. 91–102.
20. Woo D, Rogers S, Leong J, Clement CI, Kourt G. Non-traumatic subperiosteal orbital hemorrhage secondary to barotrauma. Orbit. 2012;31(5):347–9.
21. Bergin DJ, McCord CD, Dutton JJ, Garrett SN. Chronic hematic cyst of the orbit. Ophthalmic Plast Reconstr Surg. 1988;4(1):31–6.
22. Wahl M. Anticoagulants and antiplatelet drugs in dentistry: stop the interruption. 2013. http://www.rdh-mag.com/articles/print/volume-33/issue-8/ce-course/anticoagulants-and-antiplatelet-drugs-in-dentistry-stop-the-interruption.html. Accessed 15 Oct 2014.
23. Mingarro-de-León A, Chaveli-López B, Gavaldá-Esteve C. Dental management of patients receiving anticoagulant and/or antiplatelet treatment. J Clin Exp Dent. 2014;6(2):e155.
24. Alexander R. More nonsense. N Y State Dent J. 2003;69(4):11.
25. Rodríguez LAG, Soriano LC, Hill C, Johansson S. Increased risk of stroke after discontinuation of acetylsalicylic acid A UK primary care study. Neurology. 2011;76(8):740–6.
26. Sam Schulman. Drugs that can cause bleeding. http://www.wfh.org/en/page.aspx?pid=639. Accessed 24th Oct 2014.
27. Nutescu E, Chuatrisorn I, Hellenbart E. Drug and dietary interactions of warfarin and novel oral anticoagulants: an update. J Thromb Thrombolysis. 2011;31(3):326–43.
28. Al-Kholani AI. Influence of Khat Chewing on periodontal tissues and oral hygiene status among Yemenis. Dent Res J. 2010;7(1):1–6.
29. Sullivan TJ, Wright JE. Non-traumatic orbital haemorrhage. Clin Experiment Ophthalmol. 2000;28(1):26–31.
30. Goodall KL, Brahma A, Bates A, Leatherbarrow B. Lateral canthotomy and inferior cantholysis: an effective method of urgent orbital decompression for sight threatening acute retrobulbar haemorrhage. Injury. 1999;30(7):485–90.
31. Hunt KE, Ross JJ. Orbital hemorrhage in the nonoperated eye as a complication of general endotracheal anesthesia. Arch Ophthalmol. 1998;116(1):105–6.
32. Gunning K, Collett B. Spontaneous retrobulbar haemorrhage following anaesthesia. Anaesthesia. 1987;42(8):875–6.
33. Shoroghi M. Effect of different epinephrine concentrations on local bleeding and hemodynamics during dermatologic surgery. Acta Dermatovenerol Croat. 2008;16(4):0–0.
34. Rosdeutscher JD, Stadelmann WK. Diagnosis and treatment of retrobulbar hematoma resulting from blunt periorbital trauma. Ann Plast Surg. 1998;41(6):618–22.
35. Macfaul P. System of ophthalmology, vol. 14, injuries, part 1 mechanical injuries. London: Henry Kimpton; 1972.
36. Moser MH, DiPirro E, McCoy FJ. Sudden blindness following blepharoplasty: report of seven cases. Plast Reconstr Surg. 1973;51(4):364–70.
37. Theoret J, Sanz GE, Matero D, et al. The "guitar pick" sign: a novel sign of retrobulbar hemorrhage. CJEM. 2011;13(3):162–4.97. Bradley Jr WG. MR appearance of hemorrhage in the brain. Radiology. 1993;189(1):15–26.
38. Bradley Jr WG. MR appearance of hemorrhage in the brain. Radiology. 1993;189(1):15–26.
39. Allen M, Perry M, Burns F. When is a retrobulbar haemorrhage not a retrobulbar haemorrhage? Int J Oral Maxillofac Surg. 2010;39(11):1045–9.

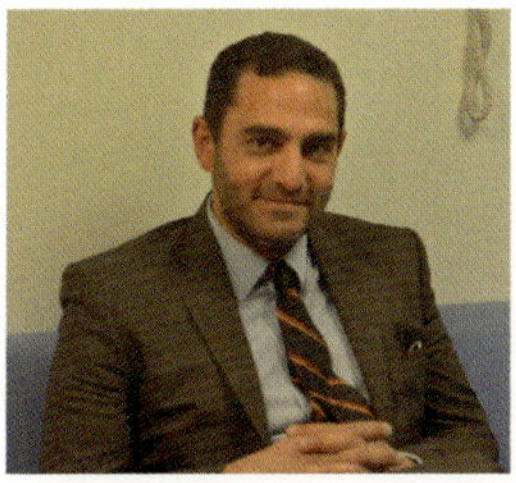

**Hatem A. Tawfik** Dr. Hatem A Tawfik, M.D., graduated from Ain Shams University School of medicine, Cairo, Egypt. He did his research fellowship at Duke University Eye center in 1998. He then served as a Lecturer in Ophthalmology at the University until his resignation in 2011. He is currently a Consultant Ophthalmic Plastic Surgeon at Watany Eye Hospital, and the Eye Subspecialty center in Cairo. He has 48 peer-reviewed international publications, 3 book chapters, and more than 200 oral and poster presentations in numerous international meetings. He is also a semi-professional photographer and a passionate art collector focusing specifically on contemporary Arab artists.

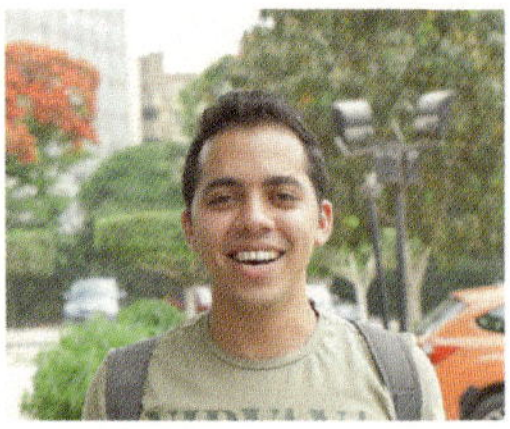

**Yousef Ahmed Fouad** graduated from the Faculty of Medicine, Ain Shams University, Cairo, Egypt. He then went on to study Cancer Biology and Therapeutics at Harvard Medical School. As a student, he worked as an assistant researcher on multiple projects, and even served as a principal investigator in one study. He has 7 peer-reviewed papers, 4 of which are related to ophthalmic plastic surgery. His fields of interest include Ophthalmic Plastic Surgery, Cancer Biology, and Medical Oncology.

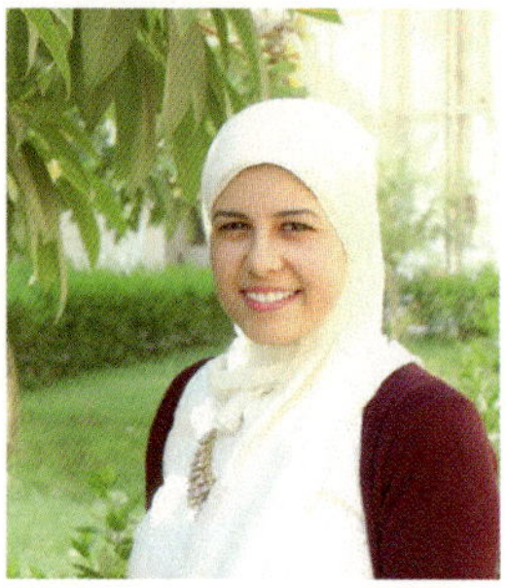

**Yasmin Ashraf Hamza** graduated from the Faculty of Medicine, Ain Shams University, Cairo, Egypt. She is currently halfway into her internship at Ain Shams University Hospitals. Yasmin chose to train in Ophthalmology as it has always been her passion since the start of medical school. She has assisted on multiple research projects and served leading positions in the Ain Shams Medical Students Research Association.

# 19 Orbital Compartment Syndromes

Andy C.O. Cheng

## Introduction

The orbit is a cone-shaped space confined by the four bony orbital walls posteriorly and bounded by the orbital septum and eyelid anteriorly. The eyelids are attached to the orbital rim by the medial and lateral canthal ligament, rendering it a fairly non-expansible boundary. An acute increase in volume within the orbit, for example, due to haemorrhage or swelling, may result in an acute rise in intra-orbital pressure.

The orbit is a complex anatomic region containing the globe, orbital fat, extraocular muscles, lacrimal gland, nerves and blood vessels [1]. Orbital compartment syndrome (OCS), due to an acute rise in orbital pressure, may compromise the perfusion of these important structures, which may result in devastating complications. For instances, permanent visual loss may result if the orbital pressure is larger than the perfusion pressure of the optic nerve or retina, resulting in ischaemic optic neuropathy or retinal artery occlusion [2]. Studies have suggested that 60–100 min of elevated orbital pressure may result in permanent visual loss [3]. Other mechanisms that may result in visual loss include direct optic nerve compression or stretching.

A.C.O. Cheng, MMedSc, FRCSEd
Ophthalmology, Hong Kong Sanatorium & Hospital, Hong Kong, Hong Kong SAR, China
e-mail: acocheng@gmail.com

## Aetiology

OCS can occur in any disease processes that result in an acute rise in orbital volume. Common causes include orbital haemorrhage due to head trauma, orbital or eyelid surgery, orbital injections, pre-existing vascular malformations and medical diseases resulting in bleeding tendency, accounting for about 64 % of the cases [2]. Other causes of OCS include fulminant orbital cellulitis, intra-orbital/subperiosteal abscess, orbital emphysema, inflammation, tumours, prolonged hypoxia with capillary leak, foreign material in the orbit, massive fluid resuscitation or position-dependent oedema [2].

## Diagnosis

OCS is mainly a clinical diagnosis based on history and physical examination [2]. The patient may complain of acute onset of pain, blurring, diplopia, periorbital oedema and proptosis. The symptoms may develop rapidly over a minutes or hours. A history of recent orbital or eyelid surgery, head injury, chronic sinusitis, pre-existing orbital diseases including tumours or bleeding tendency may also be elicited.

Examination may reveal decreased visual acuity, afferent pupillary defect, impaired colour vision, impaired ocular motility and proptosis. Extensive periorbital bruises and subconjunctival haemorrhage may be present in cases of orbital


B. Mukherjee, H. Yuen (eds.), *Emergencies of the Orbit and Adnexa*,
DOI 10.1007/978-81-322-1807-4_19

haemorrhage. The orbit is "tight" and resists retropulsion. The intraocular pressure may be grossly elevated. Fundus examination may reveal a swollen optic disc, retinal venous engorgement, the presence of central retinal artery pulsation or occlusion, central retinal vein occlusion or retinal oedema.

Investigations can be done to help confirming the diagnosis or elucidating the underlying cause for the OCS. This should, however, not delay the immediate treatment to decompress the orbit hoping to salvage vision. Orbital imaging including CT or MRI can be performed. Imaging sign of posterior globe tenting with posterior globe develops into a conical shape may be seen [4]. Studies have shown that posterior globe angle of less than 120° in the context of acute proptosis carries a poorer prognosis with higher risk of permanent visual loss [4]. MR angiogram or venogram may be used for selected cases where vascular lesions are suspected [2]. Blood test for coagulation studies should be performed in selected cases especially for spontaneous orbital haemorrhage.

## Management

Once the diagnosis of OCS is suspected, immediate treatment should be initiated even before performing investigation. Lateral canthotomy and inferior cantholysis (even at bedside) should be considered aiming to relieve the orbital pressure [2, 5]. In cases where orbital haemorrhage occurred after surgery, decompression through the surgical incision site and evacuation of blood clot with cauterization of the bleeder should be considered [2]. In cases where canthotomy and inferior cantholysis failed to relieve orbital pressure and restore perfusion, disinsertion of the superior limb of the lateral canthal tendon and division of the orbital septum from its attachment to the orbital rims can be considered [2]. Bony decompression of the medial, lateral or inferior walls of the orbit should also be considered in selected cases where the ocular perfusion could not be restored. Various medical management including pressure-lowering drops and acetazolamide for intraocular pressure control should also be initiated as necessary.

Further treatment should be directed to the underlying causes as necessary, e.g. draining of subperiorbital abscess, release of orbital emphysema, systemic antibiotics for orbital cellulitis, removal of orbital foreign material, correction of bleeding tendency or systemic steroid for orbital inflammatory disease. Many reported cases of OCS were treated adjunctively with high-dose systemic steroid. However, its effectiveness has not been systematically evaluated [2]. Other general measures that can be considered (but not scientifically proven) include elevation of the head of the patient, ice packs around the orbital region and systemic diuretic agents [2].

## References


1. Cheng AC, et al. Surgical anatomy of the Chinese orbit. Ophthal Plast Reconstr Surg. 2008;24(2):136–41.
2. Lima V, et al. Orbital compartment syndrome: the ophthalmic surgical emergency. Surv Ophthalmol. 2009;54(4):441–9.
3. Hayreh SS, Kolder HE, Weingeist TA. Central retinal artery occlusion and retinal tolerance time. Ophthalmology. 1980;87(1):75–8.
4. Dalley RW, Robertson WD, Rootman J. Globe tenting: a sign of increased orbital tension. AJNR Am J Neuroradiol. 1989;10(1):181–6.
5. Yung CW, et al. Efficacy of lateral canthotomy and cantholysis in orbital hemorrhage. Ophthal Plast Reconstr Surg. 1994;10(2):137–41.


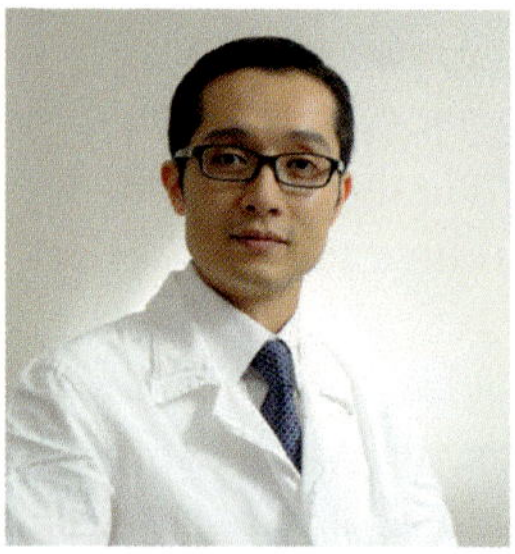

**Andy C.O. Cheng** Dr. Andy Cheng graduated from the Medical Faculty of the University of Hong Kong with honors and further attained the Master of Medical Science degree with distinction in HKU specializing in morphological science and neuroscience. He holds the Diploma in Practical Dermatology qualification from the Cardiff University. He is currently the Fellow of the Royal College of Surgeons of Edinburgh, College of Ophthalmologists of Hong Kong, and Hong Kong Academy of Medicine. Dr. Cheng is the Honorary Consultant Ophthalmologist of the Hong Kong Sanatorium & Hospital and the Honorary Clinical Assistant Professor of the Chinese University of Hong Kong. He has subspecialties interest in orbit & oculoplastic surgery and neuro-ophthalmology.

# Orbital Emphysema

# 20

Andy C.O. Cheng

## Introduction

Orbital emphysema is an uncommon condition, which is defined as the presence of air within the fascial layers of the orbit [1]. It occurs most commonly after orbital/facial trauma or surgery, e.g. dacryocystorhinostomy, orbital decompression and functional endoscopic sinus surgery. Rarely, it can occur with sinusitis (especially with gas-forming microorganisms), nose blowing, sneezing, during air travel with pressure changes or Valsalva manoeuvre [1–7].

Orbital emphysema occurs mostly from defects in the orbital walls, especially the medial lamina papyracea and orbital floor (Fig. 20.1). Air migrates from the ethmoid, the maxilla and, less commonly, the frontal sinus through the defect into the orbit. Air enters the orbit intermittently during episodes of acute rise in pressure in the respiratory passage, which can happen after nose blowing, coughing or sneezing [3]. Serious orbital emphysema may result from a small fracture site or when orbital tissues fall back to the defect acting as a one-way valve [3]. Subsequent pressure rise may build up within the orbit resulting in an orbital compartment syndrome (please see previous chapter). If not promptly identified and treated, it can result in severe and permanent visual loss. Fortunately, most cases of orbital emphysema are benign and self-limiting requiring only close monitoring and advice against nose blowing or deliberate Valsalva action [3].

## Diagnosis

Depending on the severity, orbital emphysema may present as an incidental finding in CT scan of the orbit in mild cases. In severe cases, it can present with symptoms and signs of orbital compartment syndrome, including acute proptosis, eyelid swelling, severe pain, diplopia with limited ocular motility and even severe visual loss. There may be associated eyelid emphysema with crepitus felt over the eyelids. The orbital pressure may be very high with "tightness" felt on retropulsion. The

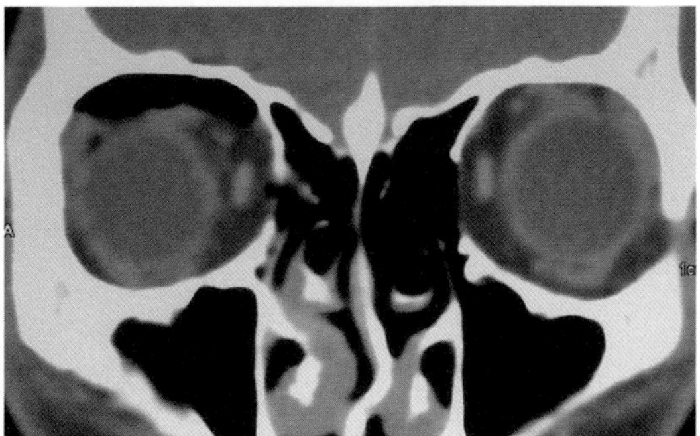

**Fig. 20.1** Axial CT scan of orbit showing right orbital emphysema due to fractured lamina papyracea

A.C.O. Cheng, MMedSc, FRCSEd
Ophthalmology, Hong Kong Sanatorium & Hospital, Hong Kong, Hong Kong SAR, China
e-mail: acocheng@gmail.com


B. Mukherjee, H. Yuen (eds.), *Emergencies of the Orbit and Adnexa*,
DOI 10.1007/978-81-322-1807-4_20

intraocular pressure may also be grossly elevated, documented to be >70 cm $H_2O$ in some cases [1]. CT scan of the orbit may show pneumo-orbitae and tenting of posterior globe of less than 120° [2] (please see chapter on orbital compartment syndrome). The acute rise in orbital pressure may cause ischaemic optic neuropathy, central retinal artery occlusion and stretch and compressive optic neuropathy, resulting in permanent visual loss.

## Management

Management of orbital emphysema depends on its severity and the underlying cause.

For mild cases of orbital emphysema without rise in orbital pressure or evidence of orbital compartment syndrome, conservative treatment with close monitoring may suffice. Some surgeons use nasal decongestant, systemic antibiotics and steroid as anecdotal treatment [3]. Most cases of orbital emphysema will resolve by itself within two to three weeks with no permanent visual sequel [1, 3].

For severe cases with clinically "tight" orbit, raised orbital or intraocular pressure, signs of ischaemic optic neuropathy, central retinal artery occlusion or severe proptosis, prompt treatment should be initiated even before further investigation. Initial management, as with orbital compartment syndrome, includes prompt lateral canthotomy and cantholysis to reduce the orbital pressure [1]. Immediate decompression can be achieved with needle aspiration using underwater drainage of air by a 24-gauge needle [8]. Bony decompression may be used in severe cases where needle aspiration fails to relieve the orbital compartment syndrome [1].

It is important to advise patients with orbital fractures to avoid manoeuvres that may result in an acute rise in respiratory passage pressure, including nose blowing. Air travel immediately after orbital fracture is best to be avoided. There is currently no consensus on the duration for these advices after orbital fracture. It has been reported that visual-threatening orbital emphysema can occur 5 months after an unrepaired orbital fracture after nose blowing [2]. In general, however, we advise such patients to avoid nose blowing for at least 1 month after orbital fracture.

It should be noted that orbital fracture repair itself does not create an airtight seal as the mucosa is not directly repaired. Time is required for healing of the mucosa. Hence, advice on avoidance of nose blowing should be given to all patients after orbital fracture repair [2].

## References


1. Tomasetti P, et al. Emergency decompression of tension retrobulbar emphysema secondary to orbital floor fracture. J Surg Care Rep. 2013;2013(3). doi:10.1093/jscr/rjt011.
2. Lee SL, et al. Orbital emphysema. Ophthalmology. 2006;113(11):2113 e1–2.
3. Sikarwar V, Bisht RS, Darbari A. Spontaneous orbital emphysema. IOSR J Pharm. 2012;2(2):225–7.
4. Castelnuovo P, Mauri S, Bignami M. Spontaneous compressive orbital emphysema of rhinogenic origin. Eur Arch Otorhinolaryngol. 2000;257(10):533–6.
5. Monaghan AM, Millar BG. Orbital emphysema during air travel: a case report. J Craniomaxillofac Surg. 2002;30(6):367–8.
6. Shah N. Spontaneous subcutaneous orbital emphysema following forceful nose blowing: treatment options. Indian J Ophthalmol. 2007;55(5):395.
7. Chiu WC, et al. Spontaneous orbital subcutaneous emphysema after sneezing. Am J Emerg Med. 2008;26(3):381 e1–2.
8. Benharbit M, et al. Emergency treatment of post-traumatic orbital emphysema: a case report. J Fr Ophtalmol. 2003;26(9):957–9.


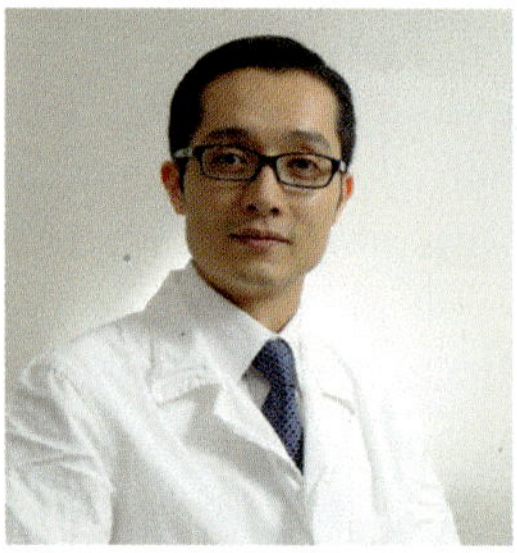

**Andy C.O. Cheng** Dr Andy Cheng graduated from the Medical Faculty of the University of Hong Kong with honours and further attained the Master of Medical Science degree with distinction in HKU specializing in morphological science and neuroscience. He holds the Diploma in Practical Dermatology qualification from the Cardiff University. He is currently the Fellow of the Royal College of Surgeons of Edinburgh, College of Ophthalmologists of Hong Kong and Hong Kong Academy of Medicine. Dr Cheng is the Honorary Consultant Ophthalmologist of the Hong Kong Sanatorium & Hospital and the Honorary Clinical Assistant Professor of the Chinese University of Hong Kong. He has subspecialties interest in Orbit & Oculoplastic surgery and Neuro-Ophthalmology.

# 21 Iatrogenic Visual Loss After Orbital and Eyelid Surgery

Andy C.O. Cheng

## Introduction

Perioperative visual loss (PVL) has been described in many types of surgery. The risk of PVL after any surgery in general was estimated to be about 0.002 % [1]. Not surprisingly, the risk of PVL is highest among patients undergoing cardiac, spinal or ophthalmic/neurologic surgeries, risk estimated to be about 0.086 %, 0.03 % and 0.05 %, respectively [1–3].

For most non-ophthalmic procedures, the face-down positioning (especially for spinal and neurosurgical procedures) has long been blamed as one of major causes for the visual loss, partly explained by the unintentional pressure over the periorbital region by the headrest in some cases, while some believe that compromise of orbital circulation due to raise in intra-orbital pressure caused by prone positioning itself may be a more important factor [4].

Visual loss after non-ocular ophthalmic procedures encompasses mainly orbital and eyelid surgeries. Though rare, it can result in major sequelae to both the patients and surgeons. A few studies have attempted to elucidate the incidence, aetiology, clinical course and optimal management of this devastating complication [4–7]. However, due to its rarity, different inclusion criteria and definition of visual loss used in various studies, this condition still remains not fully understood and unfamiliar to some practitioners.

A.C.O. Cheng, MMedSc, FRCSEd
Ophthalmology, Hong Kong Sanatorium & Hospital, Hong Kong, Hong Kong SAR, China
e-mail: acocheng@gmail.com

## Visual Loss After Orbital Surgery

The incidence of visual loss after orbital surgery in general was estimated to be about 0.44–0.6 % [4, 5]. In the study by Bonavolonta, which was one of the early studies on the incidence of visual loss after orbital surgery, all patients with preoperative visual acuity of <20/40 were excluded [5]. This may theoretically excluded those higher risk cases for visual loss, which resulted in a lower estimated risk of 0.44 % [5]. Moreover, the definition of visual loss was not standardized in various studies, which made comparison between studies not meaningful.

On the other hand, different procedures on different locations carry different risk. Orbital decompression was found to carry a lower risk of visual loss comparing to orbital exploration for tumour removal or biopsy [4]. In the study by Rose published in 2007, there was no case of visual loss after 1350 orbital decompression, whereas there were 14 cases of visual loss in 1150 orbital exploration (1.2 %) [4].


B. Mukherjee, H. Yuen (eds.), *Emergencies of the Orbit and Adnexa*,
DOI 10.1007/978-81-322-1807-4_21

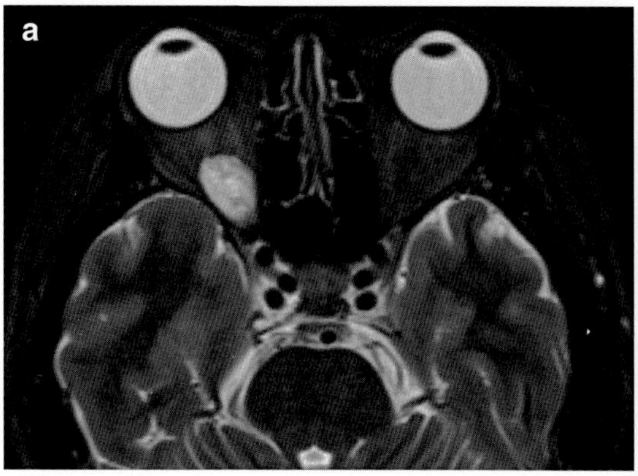


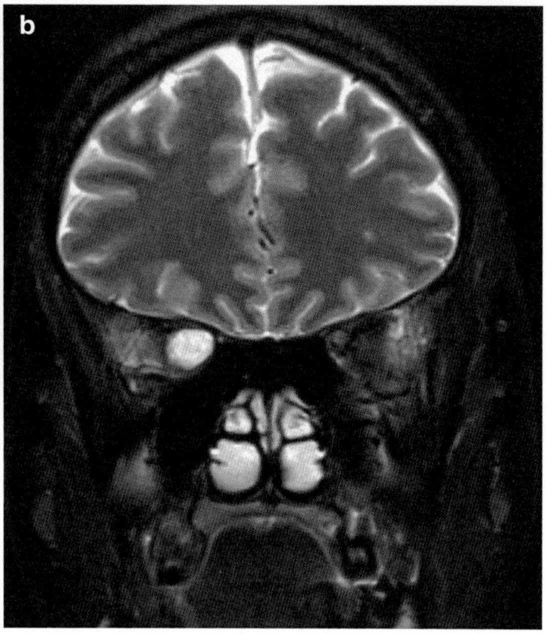


**Fig. 21.1** (**a**) MRI T2-weighted axial scan of patient with right optic apex cavernous venous malformation (cavernous haemangioma): axial scan. (**b**) MRI T2-weighted axial scan of patient with right optic apex cavernous venous malformation (cavernous haemangioma): coronal scan

Two major mechanisms were postulated to be the major causes of the post-operative visual loss after orbital surgery, namely, ischaemic optic neuropathy and retinal artery occlusion due to vasospasm [4, 5]. Manipulation around the posterior part of intra-orbital optic nerve is of particular risk since this part of the optic nerve has a sole blood supply from the perforating dural vessels [4]. Interruption of the blood supply due to vasospasm may cause irreversible ischaemic optic neuropathy, depending of the duration of ischaemia.

With the knowledge of the possible pathophysiology for visual loss after orbital surgery, it is not surprising that certain disease condition and patient characteristics carry a higher theoretical risk of post-operative visual loss.

## Risk Factors

It is thought that larger lesions, intraconal lesions, especially located around the orbital apex, and lesions that are in contact with/alongside the optic nerve or even displacing the middle and/or posterior third of the optic nerve are of higher risk [4]. The highest risk lesions are those "peanut" lesions wedged in the orbital apex and massive vascular malformations [4] (Fig. 21.1a, b). This may be related to the need for additional surgical manipulation around the optic nerve, which may induce reversible vasospasm of the perforating dural vessels or even transecting the vessels. Excessive bleeding (with free blood and inflammatory mediators) and use of bipolar cautery may also induce the vasospasm [4]. The former may also lead to an intraoperative "steal syndrome" compromising the blood supply to the optic nerve [4].

For patients with preoperative gaze-evoked visual obscuration, it is thought that the risk of post-operative visual loss due to cilio-retinal artery occlusion may be higher [4]. Rose postulated that the transient visual obscuration was due to a critical impairment of optic nerve head perfusion and this predisposed to post-operative vascular occlusion [4].

Delayed ischaemic optic neuropathy may also occur due to post-operative orbital swelling or haemorrhage compromising the blood supply or accumulation of inflammatory mediators which may induce arterial spasm [4, 5].

Other factors that might conjecturally increase the risk of visual loss include preoperative dehydration, intraoperative hypotension, atherosclerotic disease or other vascular risk factors including migraine [4, 5].

## Management

There is currently no universally accepted treatment for postorbital surgery visual loss. Treatments are mainly anecdotal and unproven.

For patients with visual loss due to retinal artery occlusion, traditional treatment for vasodilation including rebreathing bag, systemic acetazolamide or paracentesis may be considered, though all are not of any proven benefit. High-dose systemic steroid, one of the commonly anecdotal treatment prescribed, is also not of proven benefit [4, 5].

Several measures have been suggested to reduce the occurrence of post-operative visual loss. Avoiding prolonged globe and orbital retraction, prolonged surgery and extensive use of bipolar diathermy may reduce post-operative inflammatory debris and hence the risk of vasospasm; high-dose systemic steroid during and after surgery may also theoretically reduce the post-operative inflammation; placement of a vacuum drain to clear fluid from the operative site and positioning patient in a semi-recumbent position from immediately after surgery may help to reduce the intra-orbital venous pressure [4]. The use of lignocaine with adrenaline should be avoided for orbital surgeries as the adrenaline component may cause vasospasm of the central retinal artery potentially leading to retinal ischaemia. Checking of visual function and intraocular pressure should be done in the early post-operative for early detection of visual problem. Further workup including imaging with CT scan should be initiated if necessary.

## Visual Loss After Eyelid Surgery

Visual loss after eyelid surgery is a rare and even more unexpected complication as perceived by the patient. The most commonly described eyelid surgery with this complication in the literature is cosmetic blepharoplasty [8]. It is estimated to occur in about 0.0052 % blepharoplasty and permanent visual loss in about 0.0019 % [7].

The most common cause of the visual loss is retrobulbar haemorrhage. It is not surprising that this occurred mainly at two peaks: intraoperative to one post-operative hour and the second peak between 6 and 12 post-operative hour due to secondary haemorrhage [7]. Risk factors for retrobulbar haemorrhage include the use of anti-platelet or anticoagulating agents, use of certain herbal supplements (gingko biloba, ginseng, garlic), suboptimal controlled hypertension and suboptimal haemostasis during surgery [7]. Rarely, visual loss can be due to inadvertent corneal perforation during lid anaesthesia [6].

The most common presenting symptoms are pain, pressure sensation and proptosis [7]. If the patient is suspected to have retrobulbar haemorrhage and impending visual loss, treatment should be initiated immediately so as to prevent irreversible visual loss. Lateral canthotomy and inferior cantholysis to relieve the intra-orbital pressure should be considered. Orbital decompression can also be attempted in selected case. As in postorbital surgery visual loss, high-dose steroid is also used by some, but its use is again anecdotal and not well proven.

## References

1. Roth S. Perioperative visual loss: what do we know, what can we do? Br J Anaesth. 2009;103 Suppl 1:i31–40.

2. Zimmerer S, et al. Amaurosis after spine surgery: survey of the literature and discussion of one case. Eur Spine J. 2011;20(2):171–6.
3. Warner ME, et al. The frequency of perioperative vision loss. Anesth Analg. 2001;93(6):1417–21. table of contents.
4. Rose GE. The "devil's touch"; visual loss and orbital surgery. A synopsis of the Mustarde lecture, 2006. Orbit. 2007;26(3):147–58.
5. Bonavolonta G. Postoperative blindness following orbital surgery. Orbit. 2005;24(3):195–200.
6. Parikh M, Kwon YH. Vision loss after inadvertent corneal perforation during lid anesthesia. Ophthal Plast Reconstr Surg. 2011;27(5):e141–2.
7. Mejia JD, Egro FM, Nahai F. Visual loss after blepharoplasty: incidence, management, and preventive measures. Aesthet Surg J. 2011;31(1):21–9.
8. Svider PF, et al. In the eyes of the law: malpractice litigation in oculoplastic surgery. Ophthal Plast Reconstr Surg. 2014;30(2):119–23.


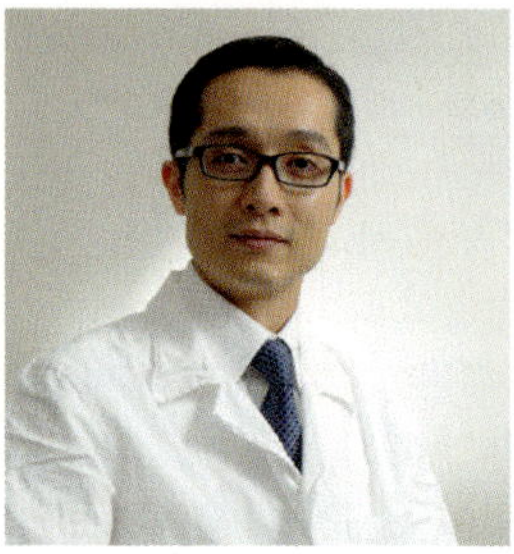

**Andy C.O. Cheng** Dr. Andy Cheng graduated from the Medical Faculty of the University of Hong Kong with honors and further attained the Master of Medical Science degree with distinction in HKU specializing in morphological science and neuroscience. He holds the Diploma in Practical Dermatology qualification from the Cardiff University. He is currently the Fellow of the Royal College of Surgeons of Edinburgh, College of Ophthalmologists of Hong Kong, and Hong Kong Academy of Medicine. Dr. Cheng is the Honorary Consultant Ophthalmologist of the Hong Kong Sanatorium & Hospital and the Honorary Clinical Assistant Professor of the Chinese University of Hong Kong. He has subspecialties interest in orbit & oculoplastic surgery and neuro-ophthalmology..

# General Considerations and Investigations for Inflammatory Orbital and Eyelid Disease

# 22

Geoffrey E. Rose and David H. Verity

Inflammation is the normal tissue response to any variety of noxious insults, and a mild degree of persistent inflammation is common in most tissues, especially those near the surface of the organism. With acute injury, there is typically vasodilatation and a protein-rich exudative inflammatory response, with rapid recruitment of neutrophils from the dilated neighbouring vasculature – this constituting the acute suppurative inflammation. Where the recruitment, degranulation and death of neutrophils occur in massive numbers, there is an excessive release of toxic cytokines and free radicals that will lead to destruction of neighbouring tissues and a spreading cytotoxic and ischaemic necrosis – as happens, for example, with the massive subcutaneous tissue death and purulence of necrotising fasciitis.

Where the neutrophil response is not overwhelming and the noxious inflammatory trigger(s) persists, the healing response starts almost simultaneously with the recruitment of cytotoxic inflammatory cells. This healing response includes the condensation of fibrin in and around the area of inflammation – the fibrin acting as a barrier to help limit spread of the inflammatory triggers, cytotoxic inflammatory cells and cytotoxic inflammatory mediators – and this fibrin "capsule" acts as a scaffold over which activated fibroblasts will migrate and secrete new collagen as a more permanent barrier (e.g. as in the "woody" wall of an abscess). Tissue debris accumulates rapidly during the acute inflammatory response, and part of the healing phase involves mechanisms to clear this undesirable debris that includes disabled invasive organisms, implanted foreign bodies and cellular debris due to the normal death of acute inflammatory cells (such as the neutrophil debris and proteins in pus) and from the unintentional death (necrosis) of "innocent-bystander" tissues in the vicinity of the inflammatory focus. Clearance of tissue debris occurs through the action of itinerant macrophages and starts a few days after inflammation is initiated. If the macrophages are unable to clear the debris – as, for example, with fine insoluble foreign bodies – then they may persist within coalescent macrophages, which are later manifest histologically as multinucleate foreign-body giant cells; very long-term persistence of this type of macrophage-predominant inflammation may lead to granulomas, with epithelioid macrophages – as seen with sarcoidosis or chronic tuberculosis.

With some inflammatory processes, there is a gradual shift from the neutrophil-predominant acute

G.E. Rose, MS, DSc, MRCP, FRCS, FRCOphth (✉)
Orbital, Lacrimal and Oculoplastic Service, Moorfields Eye Hospital NHS Trust, London EC1V 2PD, UK
e-mail: geoff.rose@moorfields.nhs.uk

D.H. Verity, MD, MA, FRCOphth
Adnexal Service, Moorfields Eye Hospital, EC1V 2PD London, UK


B. Mukherjee, H. Yuen (eds.), *Emergencies of the Orbit and Adnexa*,
DOI 10.1007/978-81-322-1807-4_22

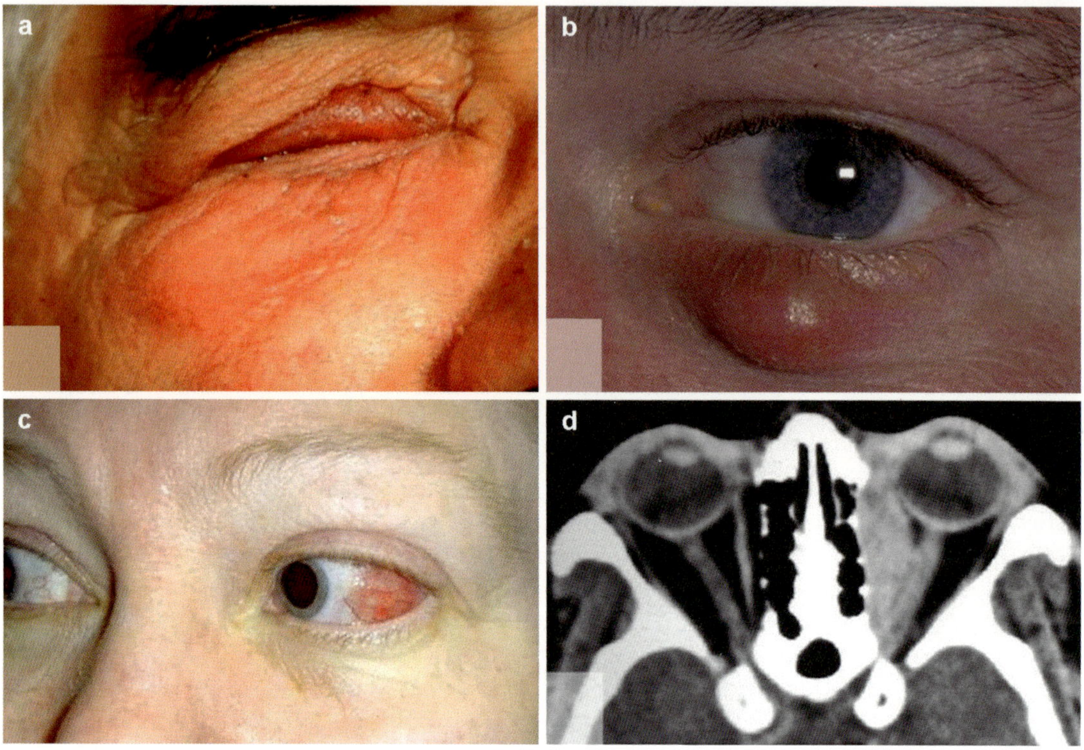

**Fig. 22.1** (**a**) Acute periocular eczema from allergy to neomycin eyedrops; the eczema is often most severe in the "spill-zone" of the lower eyelid. (**b**) Acute pretarsal abscess due to an infected Meibomian cyst erupting into the pretarsal space. (**c**) Left lateral rectus myositis presenting as pain, inflammation and localised redness developing over a few days. (**d**) Characteristic appearance of acute left medial rectus myositis, with marked swelling extending to the muscular insertion into the globe; the tendon is spared in most other causes of muscular enlargement

response to a lymphocyte-predominant chronic inflammation. Lymphocyte-predominant inflammation is often associated with the formation of characteristic follicles, with germinal centres and surrounding mantle zones, and these may rarely lead to the very late emergence of lymphomas.

When a patient presents with periocular inflammation, the most important caveat should be that this is *not* a specific diagnosis, but rather that is it a "normal" tissue response to some noxious stimulus [1]. The adage that "inflammation is a tissue response, and not a diagnosis" is extremely valuable as it should alert the clinician to remain ever vigilant for an emerging diagnosis in the patient with inflammation; this remains a key principle; otherwise, the cause of inflammation is easily missed, especially if anti-inflammatory drugs (particularly systemic corticosteroids) are used without establishing the underlying cause of inflammation. Anti-inflammatory drugs will not only mask the true state of the inflammatory process and lead to a delay in correct diagnosis, but also some of the unidentified causative agents will actually be worsened by use of these drugs.

The empirical use of anti-inflammatory drugs should be undertaken only if the clinical history, symptoms and signs are characteristic for a given disease. Such pathognomonic conditions include, for example, severe periocular eczema (Fig. 22.1a), an acute Meibomian abscess (Fig. 22.1b), acute orbital myositis (Fig. 22.1c, d) and the acute superior orbital fissure syndrome (Fig. 22.2). Although almost all of these characteristic inflammations will settle with treatment, if a "typical" condition does not respond as expected, the diagnosis should be reconsidered, and appropriate imaging and biopsy performed where appropriate.

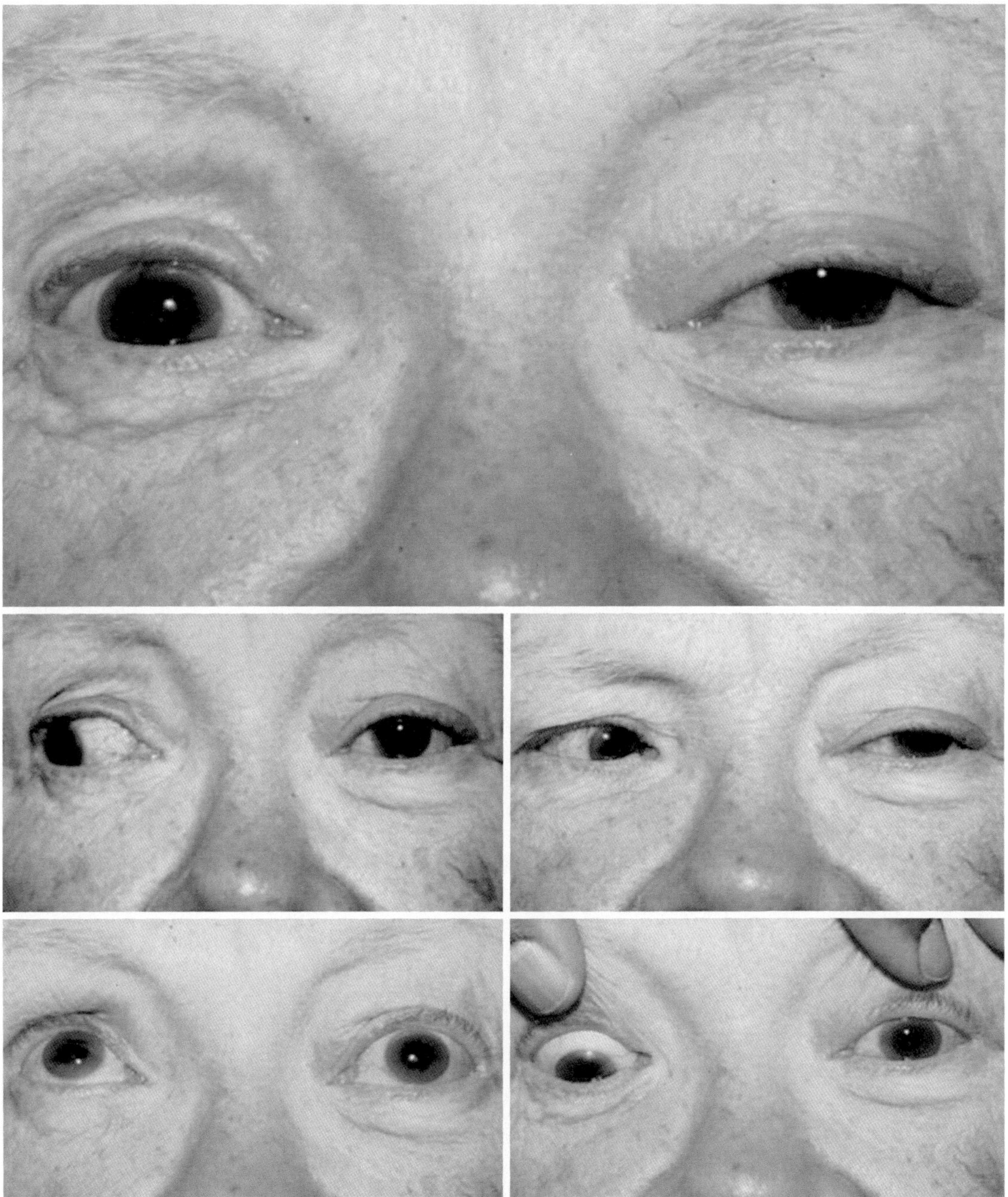

**Fig. 22.2** Acute inflammation of the orbital apex at presentation, with a one-day history of left retrobulbar ache and overnight onset of slight eyelid swelling with some ptosis, diplopia due to a marked reduction in all left ocular ductions and some hypoaesthesia of the left forehead and scalp. There was a mild reduction in left visual acuity

## Acute Inflammation of the Eyelid

Because of their external protective role and complexity, acute or subacute inflammation of the eyelids is most commonly due to infective causes – predominantly bacterial or viral – although trauma is another inflammatory cause. Localised and non-specific inflammation of the periocular skin often occurs due to collateral radiation damage during orbital radiotherapy or secondary to chemical or thermal injuries.

The location of an acute inflammation may be a guide as to the underlying infective cause: the inflamed tarsal nodule is almost always infection within a preceding Meibomian retention cyst, and this can erupt through the eyelid margin (Fig. 22.3a) or into the pretarsal space; rarely the tender eyelid nodule will be a harbinger of eyelid necrosis due to pyoderma gangrenosum [2]. Infection within the canaliculus is not uncommonly misinterpreted as an inflamed chalazion (Fig. 22.3b), but the defining feature is that canaliculitis occurs medially to the tarsus as defined by the presence of its lashes. Primary herpes simplex is the most common acute viral infection of the eyelid and usually has characteristic vesicles in an erythematous skin; recognition of this condition is important, as early treatment with topical antivirals may reduce the incidence of post-viral lacrimal canalicular obstruction. Low-grade infection within the frontal sinus tends, with time, to erupt into the preseptal tissues of the upper eyelid and present as erythematous swelling in the upper sulcus (Fig. 22.3c), and all such patients – in the absence of a tarsal inflammatory focus – should be imaged for underlying sinus disease, as it carries a risk of concomitant intracranial spread of infection [3].

Eczema is the most common non-infective eyelid inflammation, and a causative agent for this should be sought either locally (e.g. topical medications, this often being associated with a gross lower tarsal papillary response) (Fig. 22.1a) or a systemic agent – such as detergents or perfumes. Where there is persistent unilateral periocular inflammation in the absence of topical medications, particularly if the lower tarsal conjunctiva shows a chronic follicular inflammation, the astute physician will seek other local inflammatory stimuli – particular antigens being periocular *Molluscum* lesions (Fig. 22.3d), lacrimal gland *Actinomyces* ductulitis [4] or the overwhelming Staphylococcal load of giant fornix syndrome [5] (Fig. 22.3e).

Mild lid inflammation due to fluid retention within the lacrimal sac (and a secondary sterile, chronic dacryocystitis) can present as a tendency to white oedema of the medial part of the lower lid, often worse in the mornings. Very rarely, however, such mild inflammation may arise due to a tumour of the lacrimal sac. In contrast, infectious dacryocystitis tends to present as an acute, erythematous and tender mass just below the medial canthal tendon, with rapid spread of red oedema across the ipsilateral lower eyelid or, if severe, across the midface.

Whilst most eyelid inflammation will arise from an obvious cause and settle with treatment tailored to the presumed diagnosis, a poor response to treatment should prompt further investigation, imaging and biopsy as necessary. Pagetoid spread of sebaceous carcinoma, or the morphoeic spread of microcystic adnexal carcinoma [6], is an extremely rare and easily missed cause of persistent unilateral inflammation of the eyelids and conjunctiva (Fig. 22.3f). Biopsy should be considered for all patients with continued apparent inflammation of these tissues, and "chronic unilateral blepharitis" is a diagnosis that, in practical terms, should never be entertained.

## Acute Orbital Inflammation

In contrast to eyelids, orbital inflammation is most commonly due to non-infective processes, these being either associated with systemic diseases (such as sarcoidosis or systemic arteritides like granulomatous polyangiitis) or isolated to the orbit and without any known cause [7].

Acute infective orbital inflammation is normally clinically evident – commonly with a history of preceding sino-nasal infection, systemic malaise and pyrexia – and a diffuse orbital inflammation with chemosis, some proptosis and a reduction in extraocular movements (Fig. 22.4a).

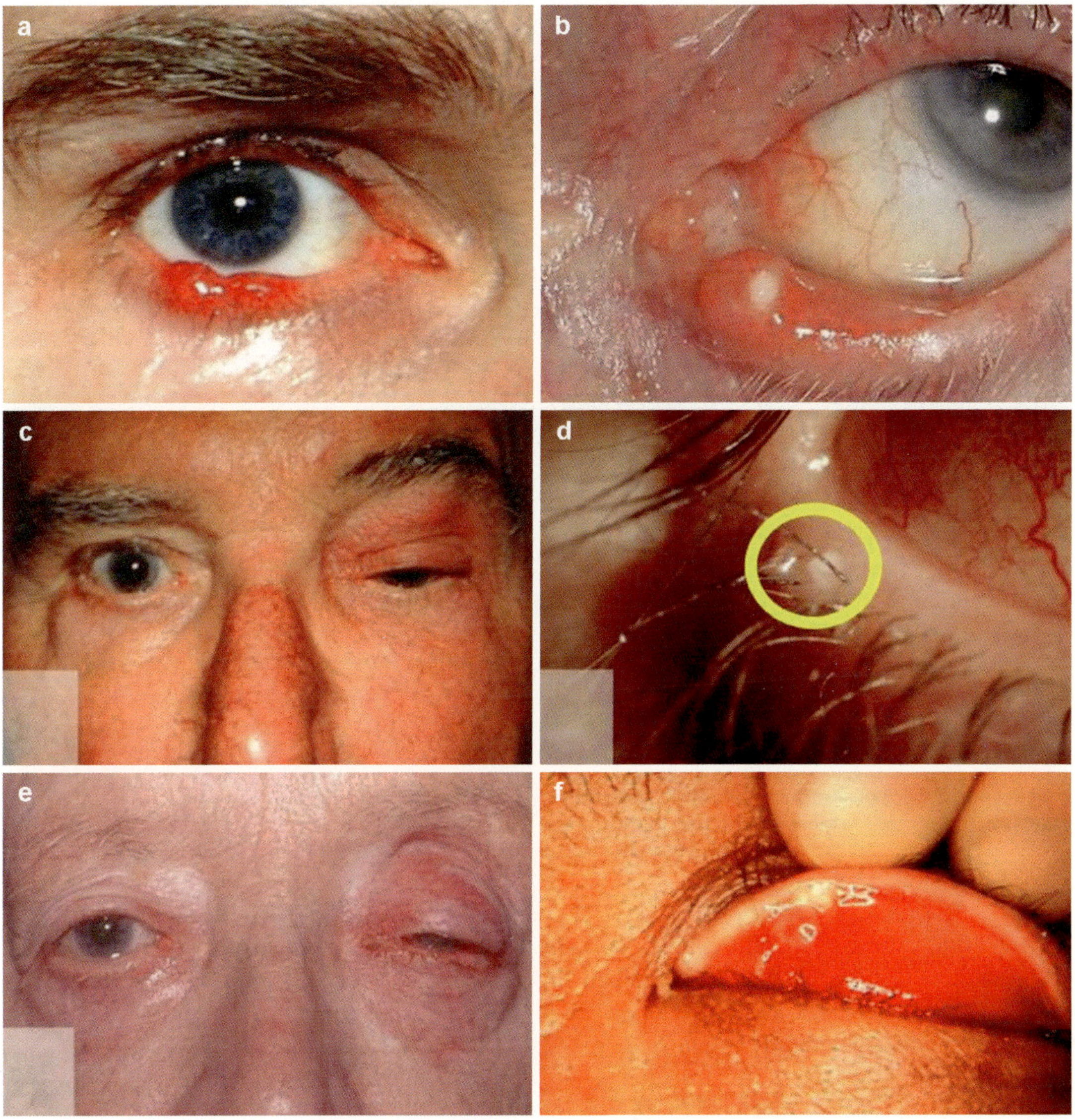


**Fig. 22.3** (**a**) Subacute infection of two Meibomian cysts, erupting through the eyelid margin and causing formation of granulation tissue. (**b**) Swelling due to *Actinomyces* canaliculitis is often mistaken for a Meibomian cyst, although there are no Meibomian glands medial to the lacrimal punctum. In this case, the affected left lower punctum is pouting with stringy, purulent mucus that is very hard to express from the affected canaliculus. (**c**) Chronic low-grade infection of the frontal sinus may rupture through to the orbit and lead to acute onset of upper eyelid erythema and swelling. (**d**) Inflammation of the eyelid margin and ocular surface may be due to a small, unobtrusive focus of molluscum contagiosum infection (ringed). (**e**) Severe ocular discharge and even a sight-threatening toxic kerato-conjunctivitis can result from the giant fornix syndrome. (**f**) Persistent unilateral severe ocular surface "inflammatory" signs may arise from ocular surface malignancy, and tarsoconjunctival biopsies should be considered in all such cases – as in this patient with widespread Pagetoid spread of sebaceous carcinoma

Prompt recognition and early treatment of presumed infective orbital cellulitis is essential, as this may prevent visual failure due to rising intraorbital pressures, intracranial or systemic infection with major morbidity and a significant risk of death [8]. Systemic antibiotics should be started *immediately* in any patient in whom a *clinical* diagnosis of orbital infection is entertained.

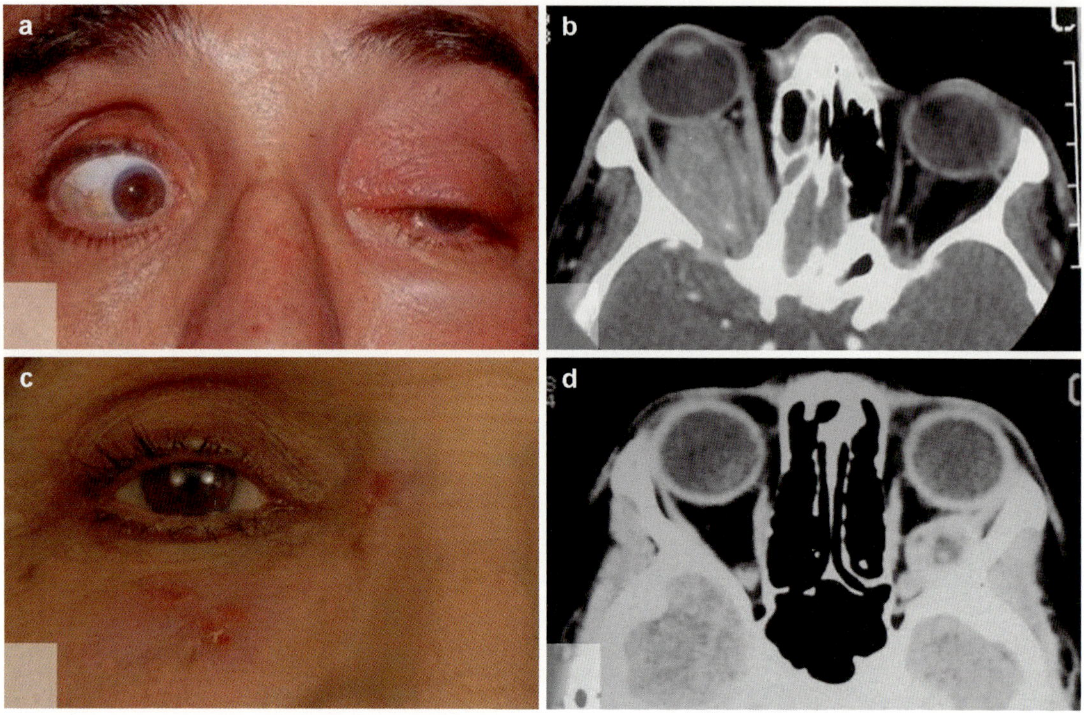


**Fig. 22.4** (**a**) Rapid onset of generalised left ophthalmoplegia, pain and mild proptosis due to acute infective orbital cellulitis. (**b**) Right orbital mass cloaking the optic nerve and extending into the superior orbital fissure, together with opacified sphenoid and posterior ethmoid sinuses in a patient with sino-orbital aspergillosis. (**c**) Persistent discharge from a dacryocystorhinostomy scar and from three small fistulae in the right lower eyelid in a patient referred with tuberculosis of the lacrimal sac and orbit. (**d**) Cystic mass in left lateral rectus due to *Taenia* infection

Where acute infective orbital cellulitis fails to respond rapidly to treatment, it is important to consider the possibility of multiresistant bacteria (e.g. community-acquired MRSA), missed orbital foreign bodies, orbital abscess formation or an unusual organism such as tuberculosis [9].

Rarer infective agents – such as fungi (in mucormycosis and invasive aspergillosis; Fig. 22.4b) or tuberculosis – tend to cause a more prolonged and modest inflammation, with a predominantly mass effect on orbital structures. The ischaemic orbit of mucormycosis is generally evident clinically and radiologically, as is the typical MRI appearance of aspergillosis, and these severe and life-threatening conditions require prompt medical and surgical treatment in the care of a multidisciplinary team. Orbital tuberculosis may be associated with formation of a chronically discharging sinus in the eyelid (Fig. 22.4c), and parasitic infestations, such as cysticercosis or histoplasmosis, may be associated with orbital cyst formation (Fig. 22.4d). Where unusual infective organisms are suspected, biopsied orbital tissues should be taken for microbiological culture and also the histopathologist alerted to search for appropriate organisms within the tissues. Likewise, where suspected, appropriate serum antibodies to the organism may be valuable, and various tests for systemic tuberculosis – such as chest X-ray and interferon-γ release assays – can be of value.

Non-infective orbital inflammation can be part of, or a harbinger to, systemic inflammatory conditions or may occur as part of tumour infiltration within the orbit. Biopsy should be considered wherever there is persistent or increasing inflammation and where an apparently inflammatory mass does not resolve when inflammation settles on treatment. There are three characteristic patterns of inflammation that do not require biopsy prior to systemic treatment: Orbital myositis typically has a rapid onset of eyelid and ocular redness after a short prodromal ache (Fig. 22.1c), pain on eye movement that is worse on stretching the affected muscle, imaging that usually shows a muscle enlarged up to its insertion (Fig. 22.1d) and a rapid response to systemic corticosteroids – with pain relief often within hours of the first dose. As with any inflammation, a failure of appropriate response to treatment should prompt further imaging and probably biopsy to exclude underlying tumour or a specific type of inflammation. Secondly, the risks of biopsy in orbital apex inflammation greatly outweigh the benefits in patients with acute orbital apex inflammation ("Tolosa-Hunt syndrome"). Patients with this condition should have a sudden and simultaneous onset of pain, loss of eye movements, ptosis, reduced periocular sensation and optic neuropathy (Fig. 22.2) – and, like myositis, the condition should very rapidly respond to systemic corticosteroids; if the apex signs occur sequentially over days to weeks, the presence of a slowly infiltrative malignancy or infection should be considered and biopsy undertaken at an early stage. Lastly, acute dacryoadenitis is the most common orbital inflammation not dictating early biopsy: a prodromal headache is associated with red swelling of the upper eyelid and enlargement of the lacrimal gland, with secondary ptosis – the gland often being exquisitely tender. Dacryoadenitis should settle over days to weeks with non-steroidal anti-inflammatory drugs, and if it does not do so – or if the lacrimal gland mass persists for more than 3 months – biopsy is advisable (being intact incision if imaging reveals a pleomorphic adenoma). As the palpebral lobe is often spared the underlying pathology, incisional biopsy is best harvested from the orbital lobe of the lacrimal gland.

Tests for underlying diseases should include urine analysis and chest X-ray. Serum tests are useful where non-specific orbital inflammation is present and should include a full blood count, non-specific inflammatory markers (such as C-reactive protein or ESR), liver and renal function tests, titres of serum angiotensin conversion enzyme (sACE), anti-nuclear cytoplasmic antibodies (ANCAs) and, in some cases, anti-proteinase 3 (anti-PR3) antibodies. Serum immunoglobulin-G (IgG) assays are valuable where sclerosing lymphocytic inflammation is present, with specific assays of Ig-G4 levels. Immunoglobulin-G4 disease is a recently recognised variant of inflammatory disease that is commonly associated with many systemic illnesses – such as pancreatitis, cholangitis, malabsorption syndromes, retroperitoneal fibrosis and other tissue fibroses; [10] identification of IgG4 sclerosing disease is important, as it has a propensity to later formation of lymphoma. In all patients, serum should be harvested (preferably on at least two occasions) prior to starting systemic corticosteroids, as many of the tests – such as ANCA and IgG4 titres – will usually revert to normal within days of starting such immunosuppression.

## References


1. Rose GE. A personal view: probability in medicine, levels of (Un)certainty, and the diagnosis of orbital disease (with particular reference to orbital "pseudotumor"). Arch Ophthalmol. 2007;125:1711–2.
2. Rose GE, Barnes EA, Uddin JM. Pyoderma gangrenosum of the ocular adnexa: a rare condition with characteristic clinical appearances. Ophthalmology. 2003;110:801–5.
3. Rossman D, Verity DH, Lund VJ, Rose GE. Eyelid fistula: a feature of occult sinus disease. Orbit. 2007; 26:159–63.
4. Hay-Smith G, Rose GE. Lacrimal gland ductulitis caused by probable Actinomyces infection. Ophthalmology. 2012;119:193–6.
5. Rose GE. The giant fornix syndrome: an unrecognized cause of chronic, relapsing, grossly purulent conjunctivitis. Ophthalmology. 2004;111:1539–45.
6. Liyanage SE, Saleh GM, Rose GE, Luthert PJ, Beaconsfield M, Verity DH. Delayed diagnosis of microcystic adnexal carcinoma in progressive eyelid distortion. Arch Ophthalmol. 2010;128:132–5.
7. Tan LT, Davagnanam I, Isa H, Taylor SJ, Rose GE, Verity DH, Pusey CD, Lightman S. Clinical and imaging features predictive of orbital granulomatosis with polyangiitis (previously Wegener's granulomatosis) and the risk of systemic involvement. Ophthalmology. 2014;121:1304–9.
8. Rose GE. Suspicion, speed, sufficiency and surgery: keys to the management of orbital infection. Orbit. 1998;17:223–6.
9. Salam T, Uddin JM, Collin JRO, Beaconsfield M, Rose GE. Periocular tuberculous disease; experience from a UK eye hospital. Brit J Ophthalmol. 2015; 99:582–5.
10. Berry-Brincat A, Rose GE. Idiopathic orbital inflammation – a new dimension with discovery of IgG4-related disease. Curr Opin Ophthalmol. 2012;23:415–9.

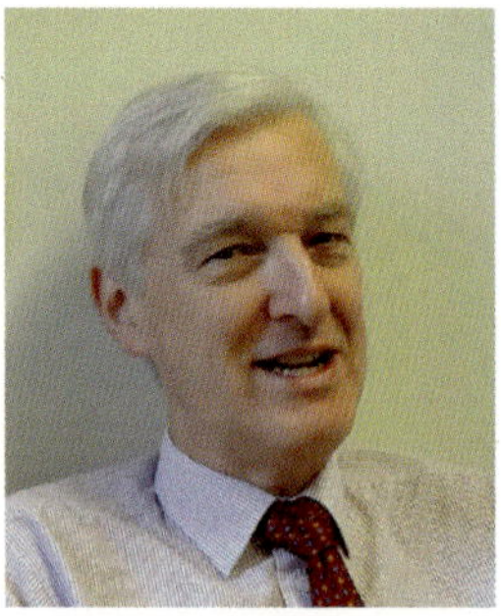

**Geoffrey E. Rose** Geoffrey Rose graduated BSc Pharmacology, MBBS, and MRCP. His postgraduate ophthalmic training culminated in award of FRCS in 1985 and FRCOphth at its foundation in 1988. In 1990, the University of London granted an MS doctorate for corneal research and, in 2004, a Doctor of Science in Ophthalmology and Ophthalmic Surgery.

Professor Rose was appointed consultant to Moorfields Eye Hospital, London, in 1990 and is also a Senior Research Fellow of the NIHR Biomedical Research Centre of the Institute of Ophthalmology. He served as the British Council member of the European Society of Ophthalmic Plastic and Reconstructive, is a Past-President of the British Oculoplastic Surgical Society, and is President of the European Society of Oculoplastic and Reconstructive Surgeons.

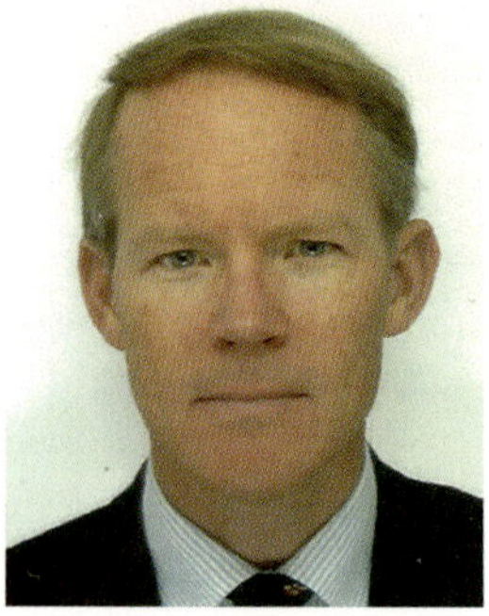

**David H. Verity** Dr. Verity is a Consultant Ophthalmic Surgeon, and Adnexal Service Director, Moorfields Eye Hospital, London.

He is a Honorary Senior Clinical Lecturer, University College London.

Trained in ophthalmology in the UK, Dr. Verity undertook two Fellowships in ophthalmic adnexal disease before joining the Consultant staff at Moorfields Eye Hospital in 2004.

He is a Full Member of the British Oculoplastic Surgery Society (current Treasurer), Treasurer Elect for the European Society of Ophthalmic Plastic and Reconstructive Surgery, and Full Member of the International Society of Ocular Oncology.

In 2009, he was elected to the Orbital Society, in 2010 became Editor-in Chief of the journal ORBIT, and in 2016 became Oculoplastic Section Editor for the Journal of Ophthalmic and Vision Research.

His medical publications in peer-reviewed journals and books include 90(+) publications, and with a wide range of research interests, he is an active national and international teacher and surgical trainer.

Dr. Verity also has a life-long interest in the charitable work of the St John Eye Hospital Group. In 2014, he was invested in the Order of St John, and in 2016 he joined the Board as Trustee of the Hospital Group.

# 23 Management of Fulminant Thyroid Eye Disease

Geoffrey E. Rose and David H. Verity

Thyroid eye disease (TED) is an idiopathic lymphocytic orbital inflammation that usually occurs in patients with autoimmune thyrotoxicosis (Graves' disease), but can occur in hypothyroid patients or those without any measured abnormality of thyroid gland function. The underlying autoimmune mechanisms remain uncertain, but activation of orbital fibroblasts is thought to be central – with these cells displaying TSH receptors and producing inflammatory molecules, orbital adipocytes and extracellular matrix [1, 2].

The acute inflammatory phase of TED mainly affects the extraocular muscles and orbital adipose tissue, with increasing accruement of tissue oedema, pro-inflammatory cytokines and lymphocytes. Expansion of the extraocular muscles and fat within the rigid confines of the bony orbit – together with deposition of glycosaminoglycans and other extracellular matrix – leads to rising intraorbital pressures, particularly in the orbital apex. The effect of this escalation in hydrostatic pressure is a projection of the soft tissues from within the socket (exophthalmos) and, where eyelid and septum laxity permit gross exophthalmos, ocular surface exposure which can rapidly progress to severe keratopathy and even corneal perforation. The risk of corneal perforation is exacerbated by the upper eyelid retraction and lagophthalmos that typically accompany TED (Fig. 23.1). Where the anterior orbital tissues no longer permit progression of exophthalmos – this being most problematic in patients with healthy septal collagen – there will be an acute rise in intraorbital pressure, with embarrassment of arteriolar perfusion and tissue ischaemia, this being manifest as loss of optic nerve function and visual failure.

Although severe disease is rare (fewer than 5 % of patients), in a small minority, the condition accelerates rapidly due to marked venous congestion, this causing corneal exposure, orbital congestion and optic neuropathy (Fig. 23.2a). Such patients with fulminant TED should be treated

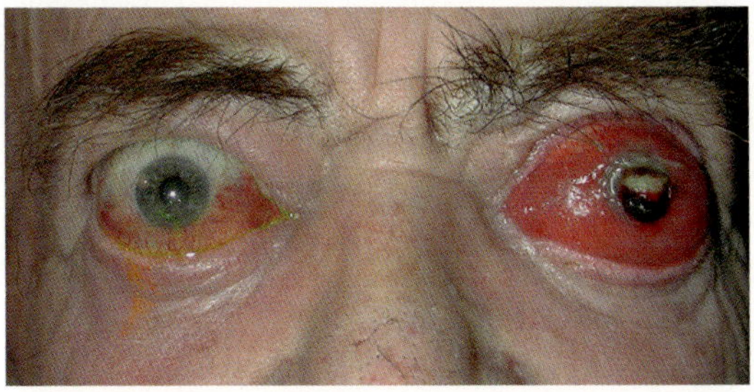

**Fig. 23.1** Patient with fulminant thyroid eye disease, having marked bilateral orbital inflammation causing gross proptosis, and spontaneous left corneal perforation due to untreated exposure keratopathy

G.E. Rose, MS, DSc, MRCP, FRCS, FRCOphth
Orbital, Lacrimal and Oculoplastic Service, Moorfields Eye Hospital NHS Trust, London, UK, EC1V 2PD
e-mail: geoff.rose@moorfields.nhs.uk

D.H. Verity, MD, MA, FRCOphth (✉)
Adnexal Service, Moorfields Eye Hospital, London, UK, EC1V 2PD
e-mail: david.verity@moorfields.nhs.uk


B. Mukherjee, H. Yuen (eds.), *Emergencies of the Orbit and Adnexa*,
DOI 10.1007/978-81-322-1807-4_23

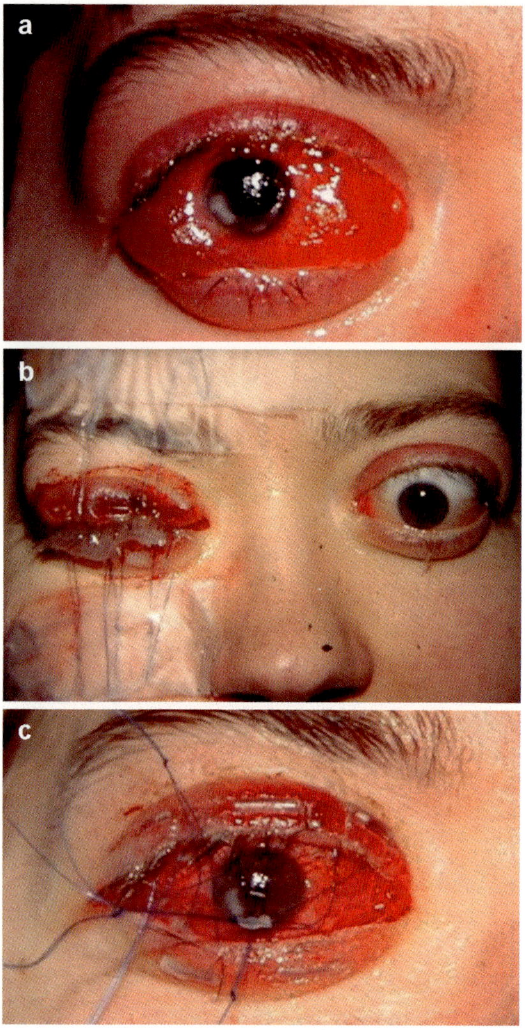

**Fig. 23.2** (**a**) Untreated severe active thyroid eye disease leading to complete corneal dessication and keratitis; view with attempted eye closure. (**b**) Placement of multiple bolstered traction sutures in both the upper and lower eyelids allows complete closure of the eyelids whilst intravenous immunosuppression is started. (**c**) Marked improvement in the cornea after 24 h of occlusion, with complete corneal rehydration and reduced stromal keratitis

urgently to avoid irreversible visual impairment due to corneal scarring or optic neuropathy.

## Treatment of Fulminant Thyroid Eye Disease

The vast majority of patients with TED experience only mild symptoms and signs, these being mainly upper eyelid retraction and altered blink pattern. Such symptoms are treated with ocular protection (from wind and bright lights), topical lubricants, oral selenium, cessation of smoking and late upper lid repositioning. Likewise, most patients with moderate disease – that is, those with proptosis, diplopia, orbital congestion and more marked inflammatory signs – will generally respond well to systemic immunosuppression and later rehabilitative surgery. Although low-dose orbital radiotherapy is an effective steroid-sparing agent in the treatment of moderate TED (where there is a recognised response to systemic steroids), treatment is given in fractions over 2–3 weeks, and this, together with the delay to maximum response, precludes its use as a primary therapy in patients with severe TED.

Most patients with mild or moderate disease do not progress to severe and fulminant TED. However, men, elderly patients, smokers and those with poorly controlled disease are at risk of more severe orbital inflammation, and among smokers the risk of disease progression is estimated to be 8- to 14-fold greater than for non-smokers [3–5]. Furthermore, in patients with TED who continue to smoke, immunosuppressive therapy – the mainstay of treatment for fulminant disease – is generally less effective at controlling disease, and such patients are also at significantly increased risk of requiring rehabilitative squint surgery [6]. Thus, cessation of smoking and urgent control of thyroid gland function are of paramount importance in the care of patients with fulminant TED.

## Suppression of Severe Inflammation in Fulminant TED

For decades, systemic corticosteroids have formed the mainstay of treatment for TED (Table 23.1), with a trend towards parenteral treatment in recent years. Typically, patients with fulminant disease respond well to systemic immunosuppression: parenteral corticosteroids have a higher efficacy (83 % response, compared with 64 % on oral steroids) [7] and fewer side effects (56 % and 85 %, respectively) [8] than oral steroids. In practical terms, 500 mg intravenous methylprednisolone once-weekly

**Table 23.1** Typical corticosteroid regimes for treating active thyroid eye disease

| |
|---|
| *Oral prednisolone* |
| Start with 1 mg/kg body weight to a maximum of 80 mg daily |
| Review at 1 week and taper dosage over 2–3 weeks towards 20 mg prednisolone daily (dependent on clinical response) |
| Consider low-dose orbital radiotherapy if an objective clinical response to the steroids |
| After radiotherapy completed, tail off the dosage from 20 mg daily over about 3 months |
| If persistent optic neuropathy at 1 week after starting high-dose prednisolone, consider early orbital decompression |
| Consider oral calcium and vitamin D supplements and/or biphosphonates where steroid courses are prolonged or in patients at risk of osteopaenia |
| *Intravenous methylprednisolone* |
| Many: a well-established and convenient regime with relatively few side effects is that of 500 mg weekly for 6 weeks and then 250 mg weekly for 6 weeks |
| If severe optic neuropathy, consider 1 g methylprednisolone on alternate days to a total of 3 g in the first week; continue with 500 mg weekly for 6 weeks and then 250 mg weekly for 6 weeks |
| Careful systemic monitoring required during the slow intravenous infusion of methylprednisolone |
| Avoid doses of >500 mg daily for three or more consecutive days or >3 g in the first week |
| Consider low-dose orbital radiotherapy if an objective clinical response to the steroids |
| If persistent optic neuropathy at 1 week after starting high-dose prednisolone, consider early orbital decompression |
| Major cardiac and hepatic morbidity, and even deaths, have been associated with total dosages of >8 g methylprednisolone; total doses above 8 g should therefore be avoided |
| Consider oral calcium and vitamin D supplements and/or biphosphonates where steroid courses are prolonged or in patients at risk of osteopaenia |

for 6 weeks and then 250 mg once-weekly for 6 weeks provides a useful regime, with a good response in three-quarters of patients with severe active TED [9].

Parenteral steroids are, however, recognised to cause major morbidity – or even death with total doses of >8 g methylprednisolone – and are best avoided in patients with a history of major hepatic, cardiovascular or renal disease, uncontrolled hypertension or severe diabetes [10–12].

Steroid-sparing medications and other 'biologic' immunosuppressants can be effective in treating steroid-resistant disease or reducing steroid side effects. However, because most steroid-sparing medications (in common with low-dose orbital radiotherapy, as discussed above) have a slow onset, they have no practical use in the acute phase of patients with fulminant disease.

The use of biological agents in TED remains limited to case reports and small studies, although rituximab (RTX), which causes a sustained depletion of B-cell lymphocytes, has shown encouraging results and appears to have fewer side effects than prolonged systemic steroids [13–15]. Although the optimum dosage for RTX has yet to be established, the drug appears to be effective at infusions of both 0.5 g and 1 g, with some reports suggesting that lower doses might be equally effective for mild to moderate disease. The depletive effect of RTX on B-lymphocytes is associated with sustained clinical remission for up to 2 years after treatment, this being in marked contrast to systemic steroid treatment where orbital inflammation can rebound within weeks of cessation of treatment.

Whilst B-cell depletion is becoming well-established in the treatment of refractory disease – and, indeed, might become first-line therapy in due course – the use of anti-TNF-α antibodies (such as infliximab) has also been used for TED [16–18]; raised levels of serum TNF-α are seen with more severe TED.

## Corneal Protection in Fulminant TED

Severe exposure keratopathy can be a major concern with fulminant TED (Figs. 23.1 and 23.2a), this being due to impaired blink dynamics and exophthalmos with resultant corneal desiccation (Fig. 23.2a), the latter leading to epithelial sloughing and secondary bacterial infections of the corneal stroma or frank endophthalmitis (Fig. 23.1). Thus, the 'first-aid' treatment for fulminant TED includes corneal rehydration with frequent and copious applications of ophthalmic gel by day and night – this containing an antibiotic where infective keratitis or endophthalmitis is suspected. Treatment can be enhanced by the

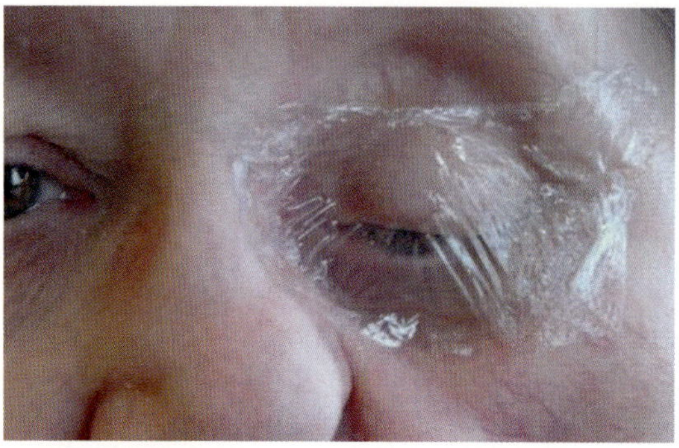

**Fig. 23.3** Ophthalmic ointment placed under a patch of cellophane food-wrapping (or similar soft and impervious material) provides a valuable 'first-aid' protection for any cornea with severe exposure keratopathy due to lagophthalmos

formation of a watertight humidity chamber over the cornea and by mechanical closure of the eyelids. An 'in the field' humidity chamber can be formed – over the gel-laden eye – by adhering a clean cellophane or polythene membrane across the orbit (Fig. 23.3), by the sealing of an eyeshield using a non-porous adhesive tape or by other similar means. As gross swelling and watering in these patients can preclude taping the eyelids closed, in some such patients mechanical closure will be needed and is achieved by placing interlacing 4-0 nylon traction sutures in the upper and lower eyelids, these sutures allowing both corneal examination and instillation of drops as often as necessary. The sutures – usefully two in the upper eyelid and three in the lower – should be placed under local anaesthesia and on bolsters (Fig. 23.2b); if required, these can be left for up to 3 weeks, until the cornea has healed and the orbital swelling subsided. Even 24–36 h of protection and rehydration will markedly improve the corneal integrity (Fig. 23.2c), with subsequent treatment tailored to each particular case. Infective endophthalmitis obviously requires immediate investigation, with vitreous biopsy where possible and appropriate intraocular and systemic antibiotic therapy.

Botulinum toxin has little value in lowering the upper eyelid in patients with severe keratopathy due to fulminant TED, as its effect is limited, unpredictable and of delayed onset. Indeed, the keratopathy might be increased if any residual protective Bell's phenomenon is reduced by a drug-induced paresis of the neighbouring superior rectus – and the risk of jeopardising the Bell's phenomenon is even higher if upgaze is already poor due to a tight inferior rectus.

Early surgery to lower the upper lid, with or without a temporary suture tarsorrhaphy, should be considered in the presence of severe eyelid retraction with exposure keratopathy, until medical therapy becomes effective. The high orbital pressure in TED probably exacerbates tissue ischaemia, and in cases where medical treatment is inadequate, extreme proptosis (e.g. >27 mm exophthalmos) is present; consideration should be given to early decompression and upper lid lowering; with marked proptosis and 'hydraulic stasis', there is no real chance of overcorrection with early decompression. Levator weakening is readily performed through a skin crease incision or, where retraction is mild, through a conjunctival approach. In all cases, the levator complex should be recessed adequately: upper lid retraction to 8 mm above the corneal limbus is not uncommon in severe cases, and extensive release of the central aponeurosis, lateral horn and Muller's muscle from the tarsus and conjunctiva is usually required. Recession of the medial retractors should be graded to reduce contour abnormalities, particularly medial kinks or a flat post-operative contour. Patients undergoing lid lowering during the fulminant disease phase should understand that this is an emergency 'first-aid' procedure and that further eyelid adjustment might be required later when the inflammatory phase has completely settled.

## Orbital Decompression for Fulminant TED

Orbital decompression should be considered within 1–2 weeks for patients with fulminant TED that progresses despite adequate medical treatment, as decompression disrupts the cycle of increased orbital congestion, vascular engorgement and further inflammation. Impaired vision

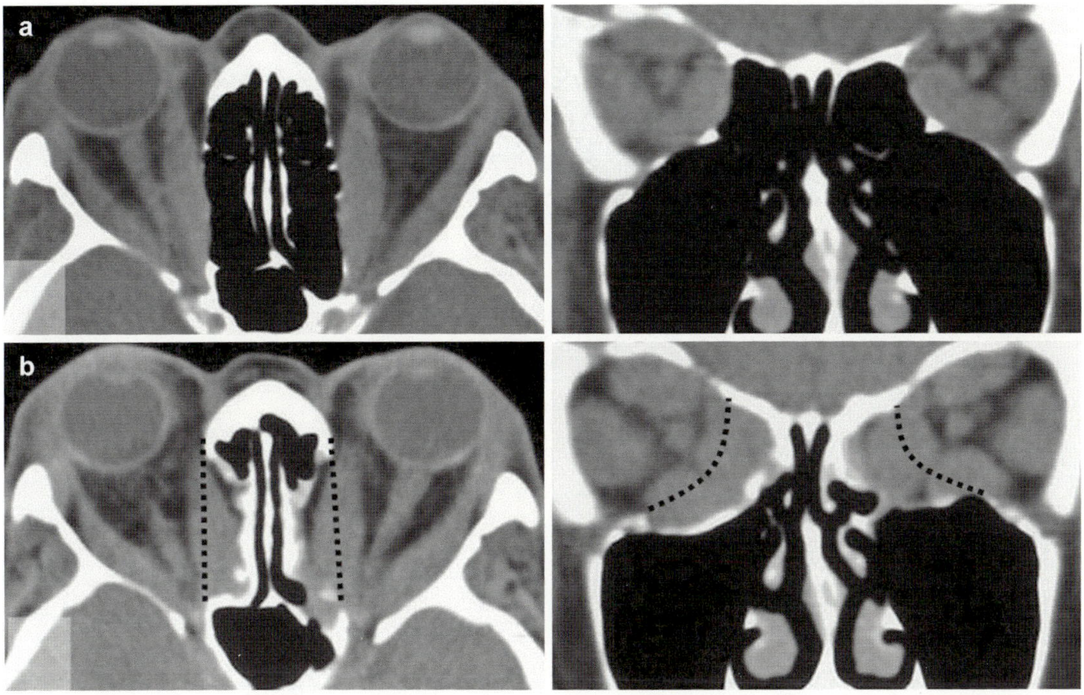


**Fig. 23.4** (**a**) Axial and coronal CT images of patient with bilateral proptosis and severe thyroid optic neuropathy, these showing crowding of the optic nerves particularly at the orbital apices. (**b**) After infero-medial orbital decompressions, there is clear prolapse of the tissues into the extra space with relief of optic neuropathy; the *dotted lines* indicate the site of orbital walls prior to decompression

that is uncorrected by lid closure or topical lubricants, impaired colour appreciation and/or visual field defects are all indicative of dysthyroid optic neuropathy (DON). As noted, DON can be accompanied by a paucity of overt inflammatory signs, and, in such cases, patients can present with severe neuropathy but without other manifest signs of inflammation – objective findings limited to a firm orbit, neuropathy with or without optic disc swelling and orbital apex crowding on imaging (Fig. 23.4a).

Where DON occurs without significant exophthalmos, decompression should address all removable bone closest to the orbital apex (Fig. 23.4b), with a good infero-medial decompression typically having a rapidly beneficial effect on vision [19, 20]. In practical terms, apical decompression for optic neuropathy should entail removal of the medial wall back to the annulus of Zinn, most of the medial floor (excluding the palatine plate) and the posterior half of the infero-medial maxillo-ethmoidal bone strut (Fig. 23.5). This decompression is

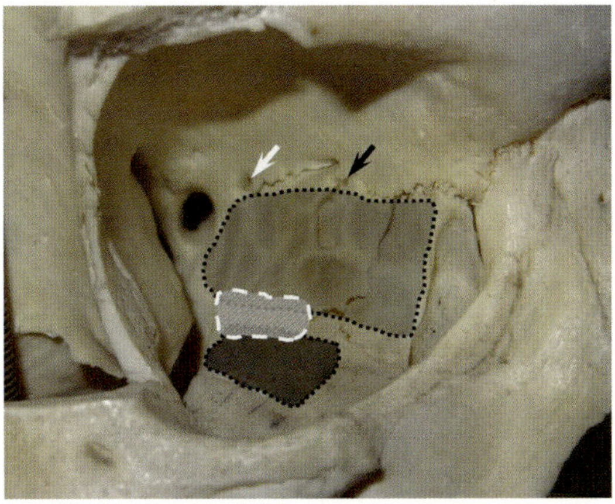

**Fig. 23.5** Sites of bone removal during infero-medial decompression for optimum relief of a right-sided optic neuropathy: (**a**) complete ethmoidectomy should be performed (*light grey area*), then (**b**) removal of the orbital floor, medial to the infraorbital nerve (*dark grey area*), and finally (**c**) removal of the posterior half of the infero-medial (maxillo-ethmoidal) bone strut (*white hatched area*). Removal of the maxillo-ethmoidal strut joins the first two areas and effectively decompresses the orbital apex and annulus of Zinn over about 180°

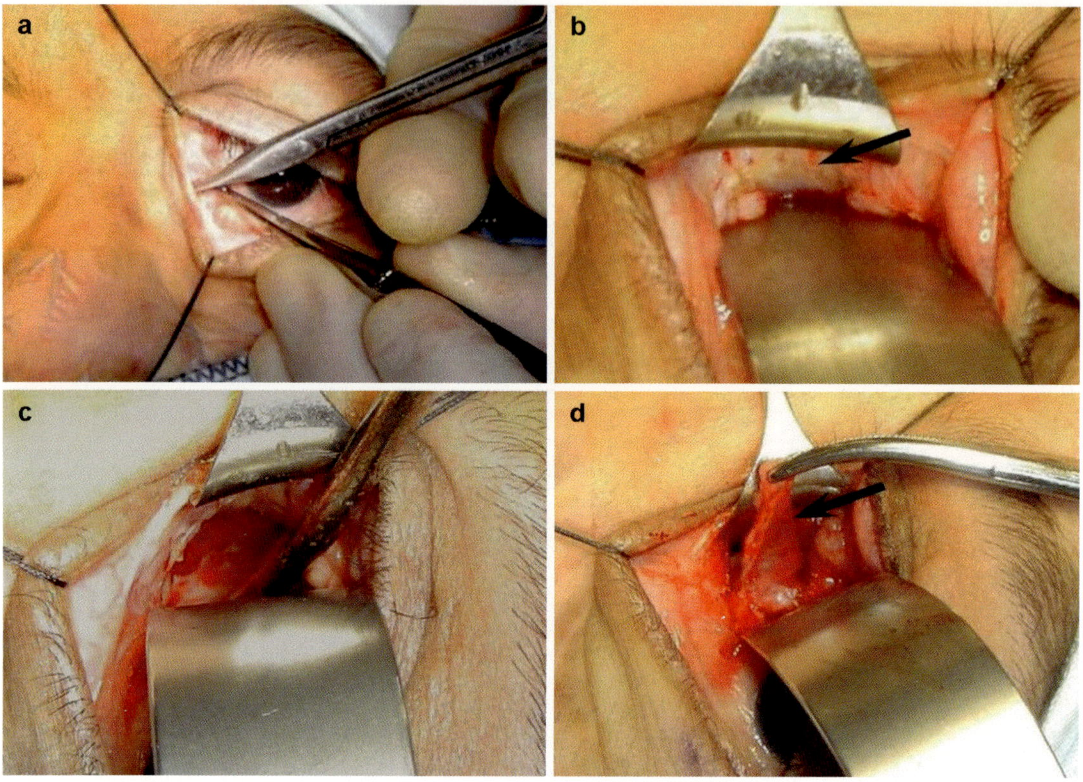


**Fig. 23.6** Infero-medial decompression is very readily performed through the retrocaruncular approach. (**a**) Retrocaruncular incision after placement of lid traction sutures. (**b**) Blunt dissection postero-medially behind the lacrimal sac fascia reveals the posterior lacrimal crest (*arrow*). (**c**) Opening of the periosteum of the medial wall can be difficult, but exposes the lamina papyracea of the ethmoid air cells. (**d**) After complete ethmoidectomy and removal of the medial orbital floor, in many cases, it is possible to mobilise and excise the neighbouring periosteum (*arrow*), thereby releasing the orbital contents for prolapse into the extra space provided by decompression

readily performed through a retrocaruncular incision – this giving a wide, 'open-sky' view of the entire area that is better than the endonasal view and leaving no visible scar. The lids are more conveniently held open with traction sutures than a speculum (Fig. 23.6a) and the retrocaruncular incision extended by blunt dissection postero-medially to the posterior lacrimal crest (Fig. 23.6b). The extraconal orbital fat is then displaced laterally with a 16 mm malleable retractor, and the medial periosteum opened just behind the posterior lacrimal crest to expose the lamina papyracea as far posteriorly as the annulus of Zinn (Fig. 23.6c). The mid-ethmoidal air cells are then entered, and all of the mid and posterior ethmoid complexes (both bone and soft tissue) are removed back to the orbital apex, using upward cutting rongeurs and Tilley's ethmoidectomy forceps; care should be taken not to work above the level of the anterior and posterior ethmoidal vessels, these usefully indicating the height of the anterior cranial fossa. After raising the periosteum across the orbital floor, the middle of the floor is perforated with an artery clip medial to the infraorbital nerve, and the bone of the floor removed using up-cutting and end-cutting rongeurs. Finally, the posterior half of the infero-medial (maxillo-ethmoidal) bone strut is removed to join up the posterior ethmoidectomy and the floor defect, the periosteum opened widely back to the apex and the periosteum removed if possible (Fig. 23.6d), or at least opened widely to permit maximal soft tissue release. Two 7-0 absorbable sutures closing the conjunctival incision prevent local prolapse of orbital fat and the patient can be double padded, nursed semi-recumbent and advised against blowing the nose for 2 weeks.

Infero-medial decompression as described typically leads to a very rapid recovery of vision, often with a return of absent colour perception within 12 h of surgery, but also carries a significant risk of diplopia about which the patient should be warned. If a greater reduction in proptosis is required, infero-medial decompression can be combined with lateral wall fenestration and removal of the orbital floor lateral to, and from around, the infraorbital nerve.

## References


1. Bahn RS, Heufelder AE. Pathogenesis of Graves' ophthalmopathy. N Engl J Med. 1993;329:1468–75.
2. Douglas RS, Gupta S. The pathophysiology of thyroid eye disease: implications for immunotherapy. Curr Opin Ophthalmol. 2011;22:385–90.
3. Bartalena L, Marcocci C, Tanda ML, et al. Cigarette smoking and treatment outcomes in Graves' ophthalmopathy. Ann Intern Med. 1998;129:632–5.
4. Thornton JKS, Harrison RA, Edwards R. Cigarette smoking and thyroid eye disease: a systematic review. Eye. 2007;21:1135–45.
5. Cawood TJ, Moriarty P, O'Farrelly C, O'Shea D. Smoking and thyroid-associated ophthalmopathy: a novel explanation of the biological link. J Clin Endocrinol Metab. 2007;92:59–64.
6. Rajendram R, Bunce C, Adams GGW, Dayan CM, Rose GE. Smoking and strabismus surgery in patients with thyroid eye disease. Ophthalmology. 2011;118:2493–7.
7. Zang S, Ponto KA, Kahaly GJ. Clinical review: intravenous glucocorticoids for Graves' orbitopathy: efficacy and morbidity. J Clin Endocrinol Metab. 2011;96:320–32.
8. Marcocci C, Bartalena L, Tanda ML, Manetti L, Dell'Unto E, Rocchi R, Barbesino G, Mazzi B, Bartolomei MP, Lepri P, Cartei F, Nardi M, Pinchera A. Comparison of the effectiveness and tolerability of intravenous or oral glucocorticoids associated with orbital radiotherapy in the management of severe Graves' ophthalmopathy: results of a prospective, single-blind, randomized study. J Clin Endocrinol Metab. 2001;86:3562–7.
9. Kahaly GJ, Pitz S, Hommel G, Dittmar M. Randomized, single blind trial of intravenous versus oral glucocorticoid monotherapy in Graves' orbitopathy. J Clin Endocrinol Metab. 2005;90:5234–40.
10. Gursoy A, Cesur M, Erdogan MF, Corapcioglu D, Kamel N. New-onset acute heart failure after intravenous glucocorticoid pulse therapy in a patient with Graves' ophthalmopathy. Endocrine. 2006;29:513–6.
11. Marinó M, Morabito E, Brunetto MR, Bartalena L, Pinchera A, Marocci C. Acute and severe liver damage associated with intravenous glucocorticoid pulse therapy in patients with Graves' ophthalmopathy. Thyroid. 2004;14:403–6.
12. Wichary H, Gasińska T. Methylprednisolone and hepatotoxicity in Graves' ophthalmopathy. Thyroid. 2012;22:64–9.
13. Nielsen CH, El Fassi D, Hasselbalch HC, Bendtzen K, Hegedüs L. B-cell depletion with rituximab in the treatment of autoimmune diseases. Graves' ophthalmopathy the latest addition to an expanding family. Expert Opin Biol Ther. 2007;7:1061–78.
14. Salvi M, Vannucchi G, Campi I, Currò N, Beck-Peccoz P. New immunomodulators in the treatment of Graves' ophthalmopathy. Ann Endocrinol (Paris). 2008;69:153–6.
15. Bonara P, Vannucchi G, Campi I, Rossi S, Cantoni F, Frugoni C, Sbrozzi F, Guastella C, Avignone S, Beck-Peccoz P, Salvi M. Rituximab induces distinct intraorbital and intrathyroidal effects in one patient satisfactorily treated for Graves' ophthalmopathy. Clin Rev Allergy Immunol. 2008;34:118–23.
16. Durrani OM, Reuser TQ, Murray PI. Infliximab: a novel treatment for sight-threatening thyroid associated ophthalmopathy. Orbit. 2005;24:117–9.
17. Paridaens D, van den Bosch WA, van der Loos TL, Krenning EP, van Hagen PM. The effect of etanercept on Graves' ophthalmopathy: a pilot study. Eye. 2005;19:1286–9.
18. Komorowski J, Jankiewicz-Wika J, Siejka A, Lawnicka H, Klysik A, Gos R, Majos A, Stefanczyk L, Stepien H. Monoclonal anti-TNFalpha antibody (infliximab) in the treatment of patient with thyroid associated ophthalmopathy. Klin Oczna. 2007;109:457–60.
19. Liao SL, Chang TC, Lin LL. Transcaruncular orbital decompression: an alternate procedure for Graves ophthalmopathy with compressive optic neuropathy. Am J Ophthalmol. 2006;141:810–8.
20. McCann JD, Goldberg RA, Anderson RL, Burroughs JR, Ben Simon GJ. Medial wall decompression for optic neuropathy but lateral wall decompression with fat removal for non vision-threatening indications. Am J Ophthalmol. 2006;141:916–7.

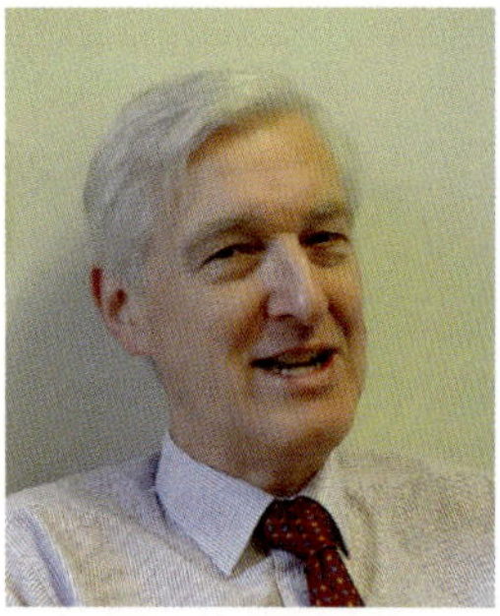

**Geoffrey E. Rose** Geoffrey Rose graduated BSc Pharmacology, MBBS, and MRCP. His postgraduate ophthalmic training culminated in award of FRCS in 1985 and FRCOphth at its foundation in 1988. In 1990, the University of London granted an MS doctorate for corneal research and, in 2004, a Doctor of Science in Ophthalmology and Ophthalmic Surgery.

Professor Rose was appointed consultant to Moorfields Eye Hospital, London, in 1990 and is also a Senior Research Fellow of the NIHR Biomedical Research Centre of the Institute of Ophthalmology. He served as the British Council member of the European Society of Ophthalmic Plastic and Reconstructive, is a Past-President of the British Oculoplastic Surgical Society, and is President of the European Society of Oculoplastic and Reconstructive Surgeons.

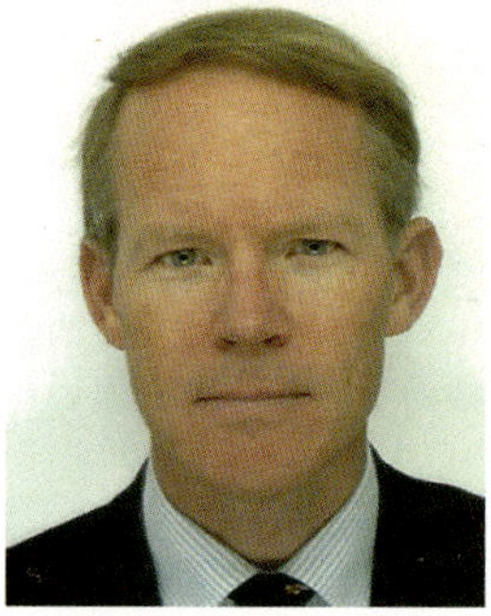

**David H. Verity** Dr. Verity is a Consultant Ophthalmic Surgeon, and Adnexal Service Director, Moorfields Eye Hospital, London.

He is a Honorary Senior Clinical Lecturer, University College London.

Trained in ophthalmology in the UK, Dr. Verity undertook two Fellowships in ophthalmic adnexal disease before joining the Consultant staff at Moorfields Eye Hospital in 2004.

He is a Full Member of the British Oculoplastic Surgery Society (current Treasurer), Treasurer Elect for the European Society of Ophthalmic Plastic and Reconstructive Surgery, and Full Member of the International Society of Ocular Oncology.

In 2009, he was elected to the Orbital Society, in 2010 became Editor-in Chief of the journal ORBIT, and in 2016 became Oculoplastic Section Editor for the Journal of Ophthalmic and Vision Research.

His medical publications in peer-reviewed journals and books include 90(+) publications, and with a wide range of research interests, he is an active national and international teacher and surgical trainer.

Dr. Verity also has a life-long interest in the charitable work of the St John Eye Hospital Group. In 2014, he was invested in the Order of St John, and in 2016 he joined the Board as Trustee of the Hospital Group.

# 24 Orbital Apex Inflammation

Bokkwan Jun and Neil R. Miller

A wide variety of pathologic processes can involve the structures located at the apex of the orbit. In this chapter, we will discuss only those due to inflammation.

## Introduction

The osseous anatomy of the orbital apex may be difficult to conceptualize because of the different shapes and orientations of the optic canal, superior and inferior orbital fissures, and foramen rotundum; however, understanding the anatomy is crucial in the understanding of the clinical manifestations produced by the pathologic processes that affect the orbital apex.

The orbits are conical or four-sided pyramidal cavities, each consisting of a base, an apex, and four walls. There are three main bony openings at the orbital apex: the optic canal, the superior orbital fissure, and the inferior orbital fissure (Fig. 24.1).

B. Jun, MD
Neuro-Ophthalmology, University of Missouri, Columbia, MO 65212, USA
e-mail: junbo@health.missouri.edu

N.R. Miller, MD (✉)
Ophthalmology, Neurology and Neurosurgery, Johns Hopkins Hospital, Baltimore, MD 21287, USA
e-mail: nrmiller@jhmi.edu

The optic canal is formed by the two roots of the lesser wing of the sphenoid bone. If projected forwards, its axis passes about through the middle of the inferolateral quadrant of the orbital opening. Through the canal pass the optic nerve and the ophthalmic artery [1]. Thus, it connects the orbit with the subarachnoid intracranial space (Figs. 24.2 and 24.3).

The superior orbital fissure, a gap between the greater and lesser wings of the sphenoid bone, is located inferolateral to the optic canal and contains the superior and inferior divisions of the oculomotor nerve, the trochlear nerve, the ophthalmic division of the trigeminal nerve, the abducens nerve, the superior and, when present, inferior divisions of the ophthalmic vein, and the sympathetic fibers (Figs. 24.1 and 24.4). It connects the orbit with the cavernous sinus.

The inferior orbital fissure is located between the lateral wall and the floor of the orbit. It is bounded anteriorly by the maxilla and the orbital process of the palatine bone and posteriorly by the entire lower margin of the orbital surface of the greater wing of the sphenoid (Fig. 24.1). It connects the orbit with the pterygopalatine and infratemporal fossae.

In addition to the structures described above, the orbital apex contains the origins of the four rectus muscles, the superior oblique muscle, and the levator palpebrae superioris (Figs. 24.4 and 24.5).


B. Mukherjee, H. Yuen (eds.), *Emergencies of the Orbit and Adnexa*,
DOI 10.1007/978-81-322-1807-4_24

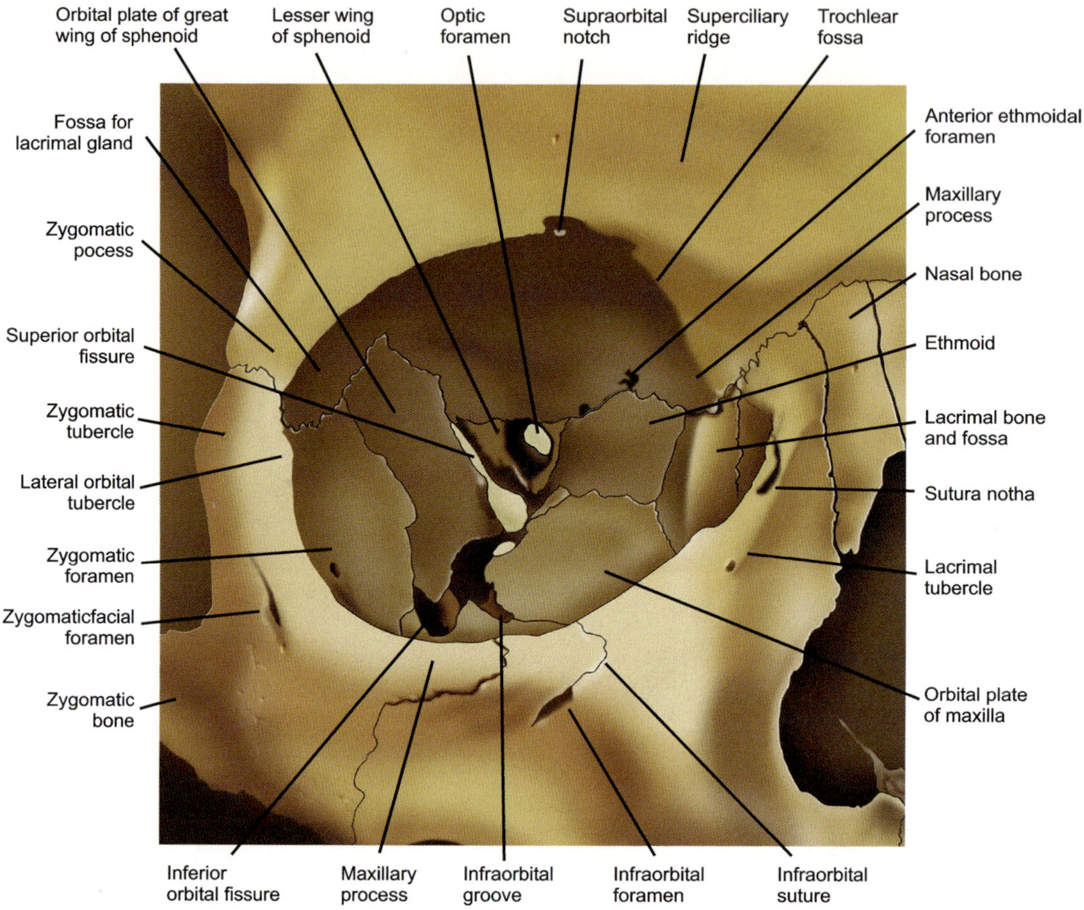


**Fig. 24.1** Bony anatomy of the orbit. Note locations of the superior and inferior orbital fissures and the optic canal

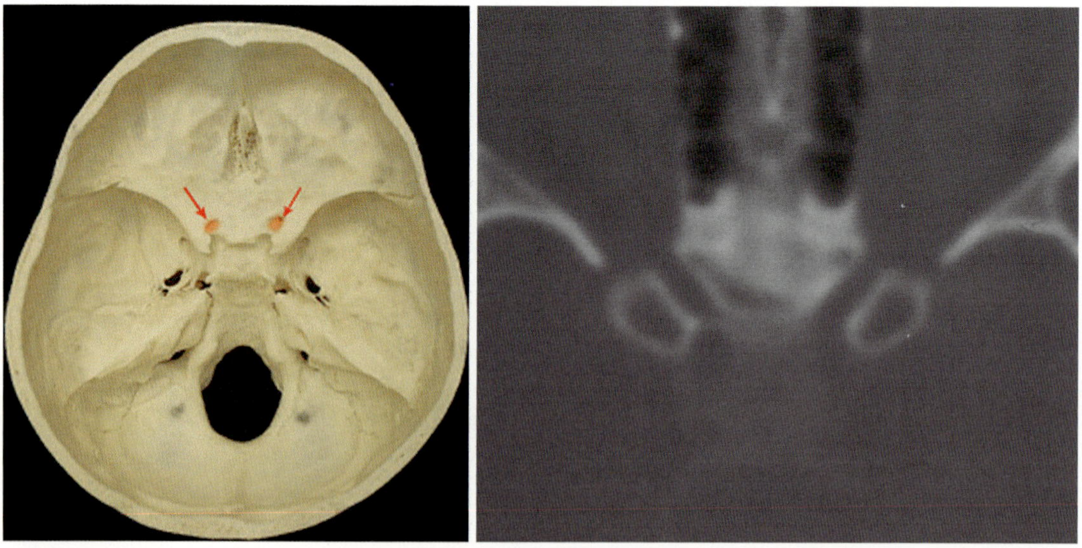

**Fig. 24.2** Anatomy of the optic canals. *Left*, direction of the canals from anterolateral to posteromedial. *Right*, axial CT scan showing the canals

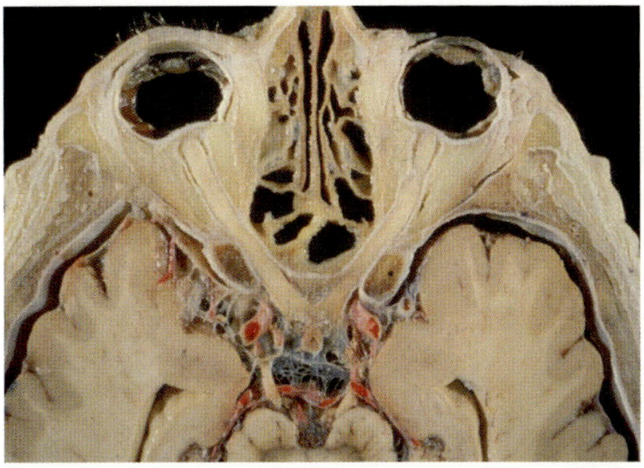

**Fig. 24.3** Axial view of the brain at the level of the optic canals showing the path of the optic nerves through the canals

The four rectus muscles are attached posteriorly by a short tendinous ring that encloses the optic foramen and the inferomedial end of the superior orbital fissure (Fig. 24.5). The origin of the superior oblique muscle is located just superior and medial to the orbital end of the optic canal. The origin of the levator muscle is located just superior to the annulus. Thus, structures at the orbital apex include the optic nerve, the ocular motor nerves, the origins of all but one of the extraocular muscles, and the branches of the first and second divisions of the trigeminal nerve.

In view of the neural and muscular structures in close proximity at the orbital apex, it

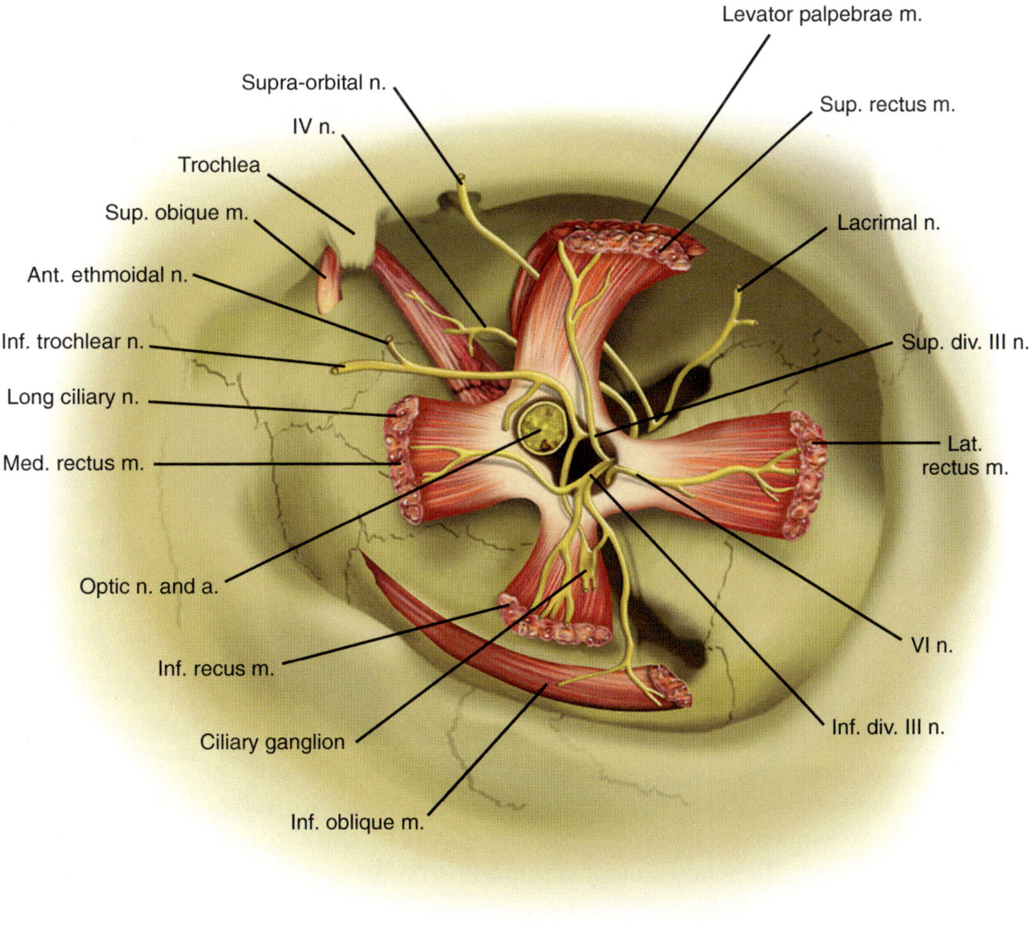


**Fig. 24.4** The structures at the apex of the orbit showing the location of the ocular motor nerves as they pass through the superior orbital fissure

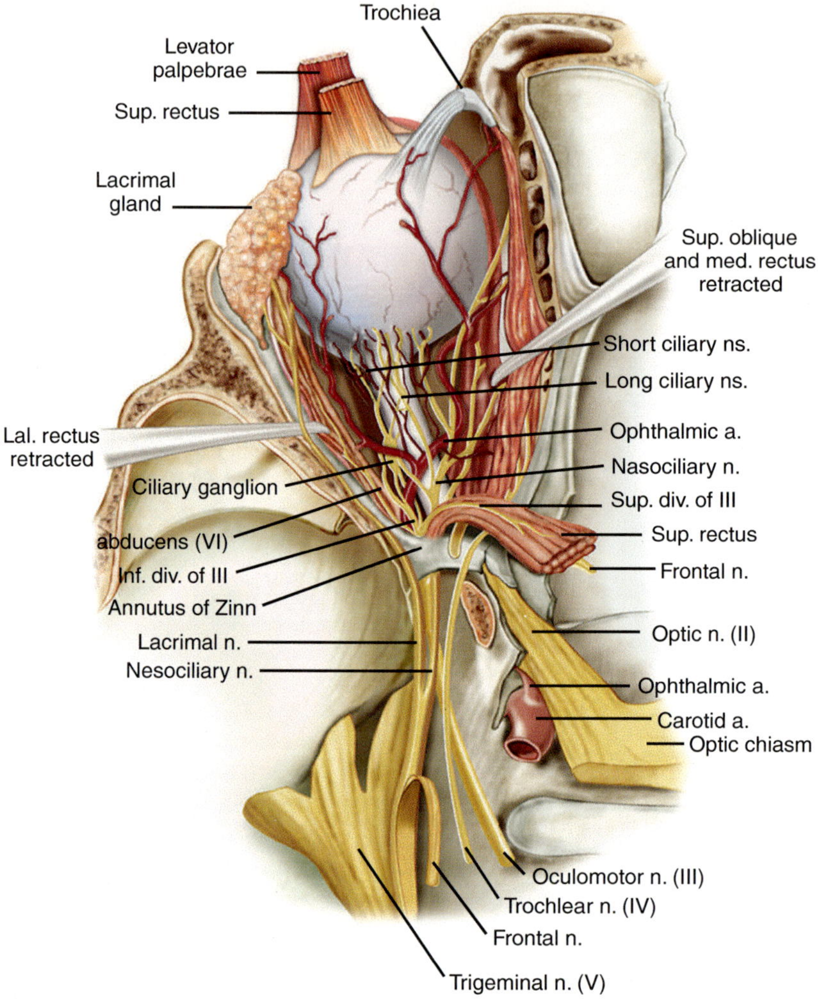


**Fig. 24.5** Drawing of the structures at the orbital apex

should not be surprising that lesions at the orbital apex typically cause a combination of visual loss and ocular motor dysfunction. The visual loss usually results from damage to the optic nerve, whereas the ocular motor dysfunction may result from damage to one or more ocular motor nerves, the extraocular muscles they innervate, or both. In addition, depending on the nature and extent of the process, there will be variable proptosis and pain in and around the orbit. In general, numbness in the territory of the ophthalmic (first) division of the trigeminal nerve is not present in the orbital apex syndrome. Indeed, patients in whom there is corneal anesthesia or hypesthesia and anesthesia or hypesthesia in the cutaneous distribution of the ophthalmic division of the trigeminal nerve are considered to have either a "sphenocavernous" syndrome or a pure cavernous sinus syndrome, particularly if there is no evidence of an optic neuropathy.

## General Approach to and Management of Specific Causes of the Orbital Apex Syndrome

An orbital apex lesion should be considered in all patients who present with unilateral blurred vision, ophthalmoplegia, and proptosis (Fig. 24.6).

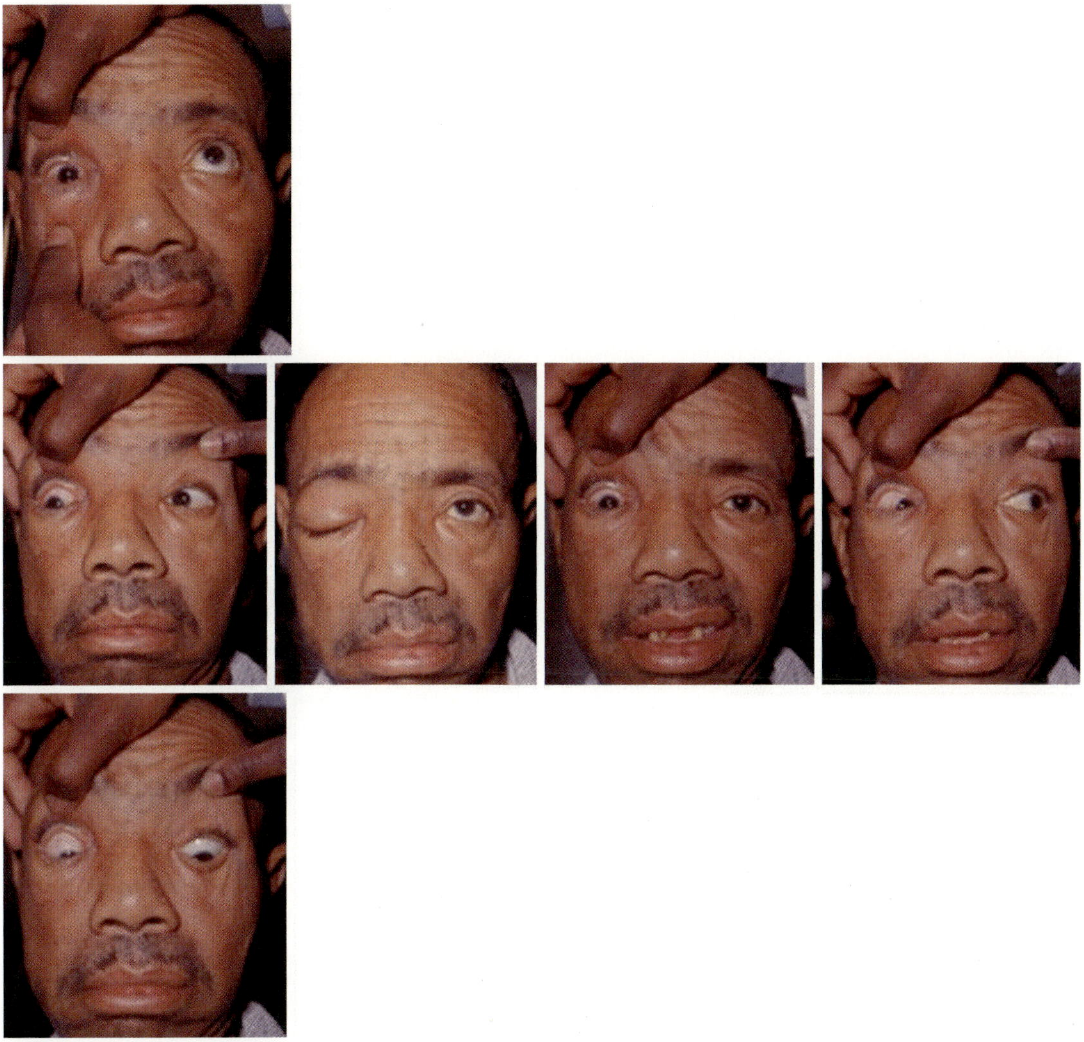

**Fig. 24.6** Patient with right orbital apex syndrome. Note ptosis, ophthalmoplegia, and proptosis. The patient also had right-sided visual loss due to an optic neuropathy

When the presentation is acute and associated with pain, an infectious or inflammatory process should be suspected, even though other processes such as primary or metastatic tumors can cause a similar or identical presentation.

In patients suspected of harboring an infectious or noninfectious inflammatory process in the orbital apex, urgent laboratory studies and neuroimaging need to be performed as may a biopsy of any abnormal tissue identified by the imaging.

Laboratory tests that may be performed in patients with known or suspected inflammation at the orbital apex include a complete blood count with differential, serum chemistry, erythrocyte sedimentation rate (ESR), C-reactive protein (CRP), hemoglobin A1c, rapid plasma reagin, microhemagglutination assay for antibody to *Treponema pallidum*, fluorescent treponemal antibody test, antinuclear, anti-double-stranded DNA antibody, and anti-smooth muscle antibody assays, serum protein electrophoresis, antineutrophil cytoplasmic antibody assays (both p-ANCA and c-ANCA), angiotensin-converting enzyme, and human immunodeficiency virus assessment. A lumbar puncture is appropriate if a generalized central nervous system (CNS) process is suspected, with the cerebrospinal fluid

(CSF) assessed for cell count and differential as well as protein and glucose concentration. Depending on the presentation, culture of the CSF for bacterial, fungal, or mycobacterial disease may be performed.

Neuroimaging should be performed on all patients with a known or suspected orbital apex syndrome. Both computed tomographic (CT) scanning and magnetic resonance (MR) imaging have pros and cons. CT scanning is superior to MR imaging for the depiction of bony anatomy and is especially helpful in determining if there is bone destruction from inflammation or infection is suspected clinically (Fig. 24.7) [2].

In addition, by obtaining both axial and direct coronal views, one can identify any extension of the process to (or from) the adjacent paranasal sinuses or the cavernous sinus. Indeed, abnormal material in the paranasal sinuses often can be seen with CT scanning when it is not evident on MR imaging. On the other hand, MR imaging usually provides excellent detail of soft tissue in the orbit and shows the cavernous sinus much better than CT scanning, particularly when appropriate sequences such as T1-weighted images with fat suppression and contrast are included (Fig. 24.8).

3-Tesla (3-T) MR machines have been found to be superior to the standard 1- and 1.5-T machines in defining parasellar anatomy and identifying invasion of the cavernous sinus by infections, inflammation, and tumors [3]. To rule out and investigate a vascular lesion of the cavernous sinus, MR or CT angiography may be helpful. If the index of suspicion remains high despite negative neuroimaging studies, conventional diagnostic cerebral angiography can be considered. Although orbital apex inflammation

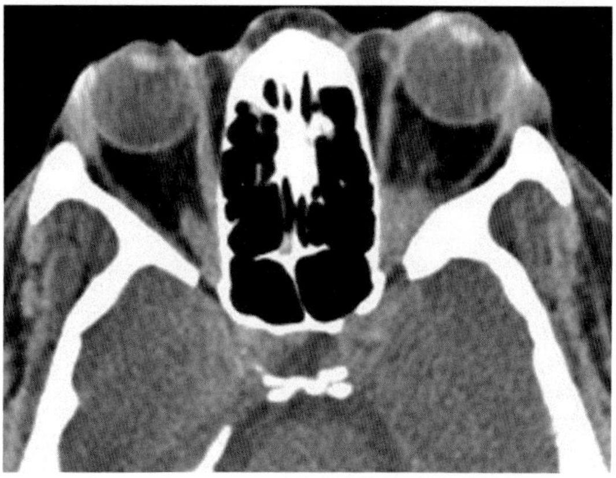

**Fig. 24.7** Axial CT scan showing lesion of the left orbital apex. Note absence of bony destruction

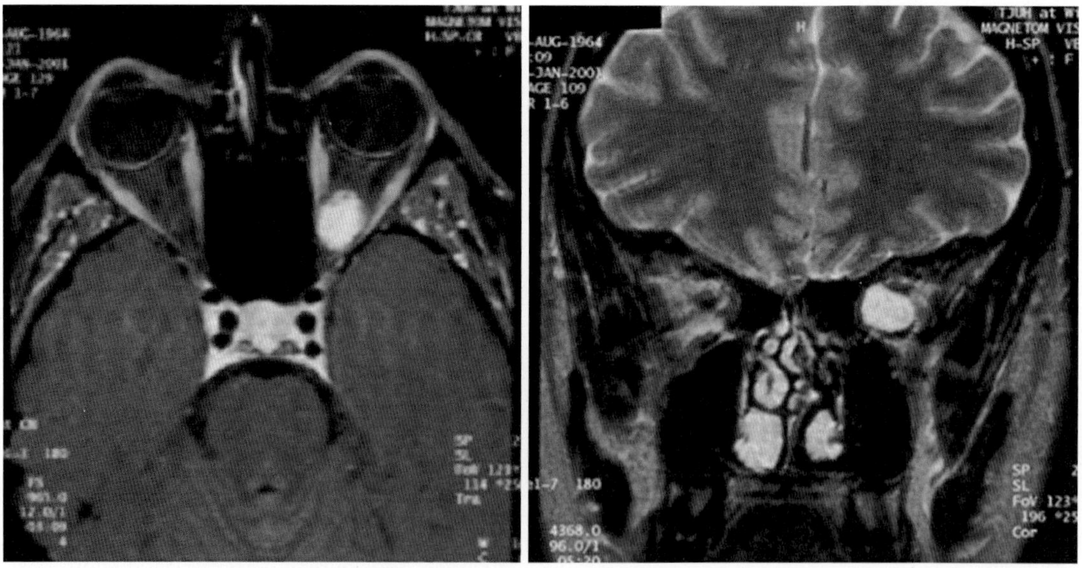

**Fig. 24.8** MR imaging, axial (*left*) and coronal (*right*) views, shows a well-circumscribed mass at the left orbital apex

or infection may be suspected on the basis of the results of laboratory studies and neuroimaging, a culture or biopsy of abnormal material for pathologic confirmation may be required to determine the correct diagnosis and direct treatment. A variety of surgical techniques can be used to reach the orbital apex with relative safety, including both transcaruncular and endoscopic endonasal approaches.

The management of patients with orbital apex inflammation is aimed at the underlying etiology. If a specific etiology cannot be determined, the primary management options may include close observation, an empiric trial of systemic corticosteroids, antibiotics, or both, and biopsy and/or culture of abnormal material. The distinction between inflammation, infection, and other etiologies, especially neoplasms, can be difficult, particularly as all may respond – at least initially – to corticosteroids. However, in patients with occult infections, particularly those caused by fungi, systemic corticosteroids may result in severe morbidity or mortality. Thus, if symptoms and signs progress despite steroid treatment, one must consider repeat neuroimaging and obtaining tissue for culture or biopsy. In many cases, neurosurgical and otolaryngological consultations are warranted, particularly if a cavernous sinus or paranasal sinus lesion is accessible for biopsy [4]. Consultations with a specialist in internal medicine, infectious diseases, rheumatology, and/or neurology may be appropriate.

## Inflammatory Conditions That Can Cause an Orbital Apex Syndrome

Inflammatory conditions that can cause an orbital apex syndrome may be infectious or noninfectious (Table 24.1). Noninfectious inflammatory etiologies include sarcoidosis, vasculitis (e.g., Wegener's granulomatosis, Churg-Strauss syndrome, giant cell arteritis (GCA), and systemic lupus erythematosus (SLE), Tolosa-Hunt syndrome, and both idiopathic and IgG4-related orbital inflammations [5].

**Table 24.1** Differential diagnosis of inflammatory orbital apex syndromes

| |
|---|
| *Noninfectious* |
| Sarcoidosis |
| Vasculitis |
| Wegener's granulomatosis |
| Churg-Strauss syndrome |
| Polyarteritis nodosa |
| Giant cell arteritis |
| Systemic lupus erythematosus |
| Tolosa-Hunt syndrome |
| Idiopathic and immunoglobulin G4 (IgG4)-related orbital inflammation |
| *Infectious* |
| Fungal infections |
| Mucormycosis |
| Aspergillosis |
| Bacterial infection |
| *Staphylococcus aureus, Streptococcus pneumonia, Actinomyces israelii, Pseudomonas aeruginosa* |
| Viral infection |
| Herpes zoster |
| Spirochetal infection |
| Syphilis |
| Lyme disease |
| Mycobacterial infection |
| Tuberculosis |
| Parasitic infection |
| Gnathostomiasis |

## Noninfectious

### Sarcoidosis

Sarcoidosis is a multisystem disorder of unknown etiology that is characterized histologically by granulomatous inflammation in the affected organs (Fig. 24.9).

Ocular involvement is seen in approximately 25 % of patients with sarcoidosis [6]. Anterior uveitis is the most common ocular manifestation, but sarcoidosis may involve any part of the eye, orbit, or lacrimal system. Orbital and adnexal manifestations of sarcoid are less common than ocular involvement with conflicting data on incidence due to the different diagnostic criteria for sarcoidosis employed in various studies [7–9]. Nevertheless, both orbital apex and cavernous

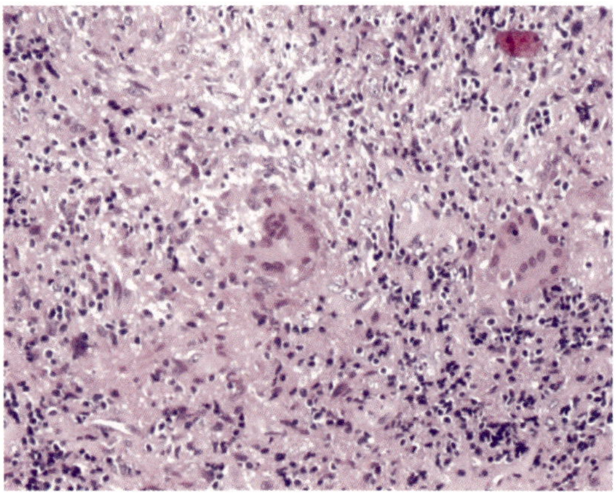

**Fig. 24.9** Histology of orbital sarcoidosis. Note noncaseating granulomatous inflammation with multiple multinucleated giant cells

sinus syndromes have been reported as presenting manifestations of sarcoidosis [10, 11]. Orbital involvement is most commonly seen in the fifth to seventh decades and is more frequent in women [12].

The diagnosis of sarcoidosis can be determined by biopsy demonstrating noncaseating granulomas; a constellation of typical clinical features such as restrictive lung disease, erythema nodosum/lupus pernio, and uveitis; chest imaging demonstrating hilar lymphadenopathy and/or parenchymal infiltrates; or a combination of these findings. In addition, lymphocytosis with a CD4/CD8 ratio >5 on bronchoalveolar lavage strongly suggests the diagnosis of sarcoidosis [13]. Although both serum and CSF angiotensin-converting enzyme levels often are elevated in patients with systemic sarcoidosis, normal values do not eliminate the diagnosis.

The management of patients with sarcoidosis involving the orbital apex depends on the extent of disease, degree of functional impairment, and presence or absence of active systemic disease. Although up to two-thirds of cases of systemic sarcoidosis show spontaneous remission [14], there are insufficient data on the natural history of orbital and adnexal disease to recommend observation as a plan of management. Oral steroids are the mainstay of treatment in these patients, and most reported cases show a good response. In cases without active systemic disease, a short course of oral prednisolone (starting at 1 mg/kg and tapering over 3 months) may be considered for initial therapy. In those patients who fail to respond or are steroid intolerant, cytotoxic agents such as methotrexate may be used. In localized orbital disease, periocular steroids (1-mL injection of triamcinolone acetonide 40 mg/ml) may be considered [15]. Unfortunately, although treatment with corticosteroids often results in significant improvement in patients with sarcoidosis, nearly 50 % of patients subsequently experience a recurrence of the disease when steroids are tapered, in which case they may require a prolonged course of treatment with a very slow taper.

## Vasculitis

Noninfectious vasculitis may be classified based on the pathologic findings and size of vessels involved in the pathologic process as large-vessel vasculitis (e.g., giant cell arteritis), medium-vessel vasculitis (e.g., polyarteritis nodosa (PAN)), and small-vessel vasculitis. Small-vessel vasculitis may be divided into ANCA-associated small-vessel vasculitis (e.g., Wegener's granulomatosis, Churg-Strauss syndrome) and non-ANCA-associated small-vessel vasculitis (e.g., lupus vasculitis).

Although rare, a number of different noninfectious systemic vasculitides can cause orbital inflammation [16]. These include Wegener's granulomatosis, Churg-Strauss syndrome, polyarteritis nodosa, giant cell arteritis, and systemic lupus erythematosus.

## Wegener's Granulomatosis

Wegener's granulomatosis, also called "granulomatosis with polyangiitis," is the most common noninfectious vasculitis causing orbital inflammation. It thus must be considered in patients presenting with an orbital apex syndrome. It is an autoimmune disease characterized by inflammation involving small blood vessels, most often of the upper respiratory tract, lungs, kidneys, and skin. The vasculitis and associated granulomatous inflammation lead to vascular occlusion, tissue ischemia, and localized necrosis (Fig. 24.10).

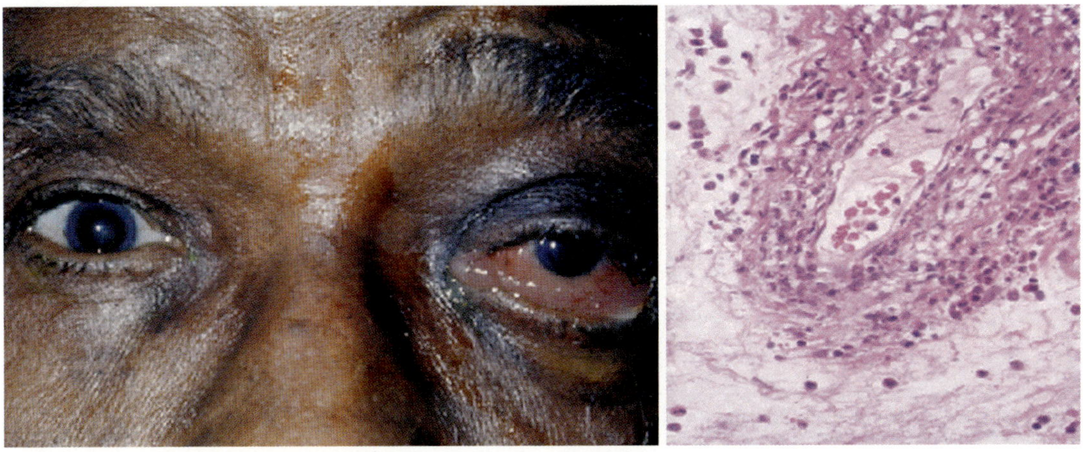

**Fig. 24.10** Wegener's granulomatosis in a 70-year-old woman with a left orbital apex syndrome. *Left*, external appearance of patient. *Right*, biopsy of abnormal tissue reveals a vasculitis. The patient had c-ANCA antibodies in her serum

Wegener's granulomatosis also is known as ANCA-associated vasculitis, as antineutrophil cytoplasmic antibodies are present in 80–90 % of cases [17, 18]. These antibodies are thought to be related to the pathogenesis of the disease. c-ANCA (which reacts with proteinase 3) is more commonly associated with Wegener's granulomatosis than p-ANCA (which reacts with myeloperoxidase), with the presence of c-ANCA antibodies having an overall sensitivity of 91 % and a specificity of 99 % for the disease [18].

Patients with Wegener's granulomatosis typically present with a several-month history of flu-like symptoms, including fever, myalgias, arthralgias, headache, malaise, anorexia, and weight loss. The condition most often affects the lower and upper respiratory tracts (85 %) and kidneys (80 %). Thus, affected patients often have pulmonary (dyspnea, cough, hemoptysis, obstructive symptoms) and/or renal (hematuria, proteinuria) manifestations; however, the peripheral nervous system may be affected, causing numbness, tingling, and weakness of the extremities. Cutaneous manifestations also are common, including rash, purpura, and nodules.

Ocular involvement, including conjunctivitis, episcleritis, retinal vasculitis, and uveitis, is common in patients with Wegener's granulomatosis, occurring in 50–60 % of patients [17, 19]. Orbital involvement is less frequent, being recognized in 15–20 % of patients [20–22]. Orbital disease can be primary or secondary to the extension of sinus disease. Orbital masses are a rare manifestation and are characterized by a refractory course and a high rate of local damage with significant visual morbidity, sometimes leading to a complete vision loss [23, 24]. Both of the systemic forms of Wegener's granulomatosis (pulmonary and renal) as well as its so-called "limited" form may involve the orbital apex or cavernous sinus [25].

The diagnosis of orbital apex syndrome associated with Wegener's granulomatosis usually is made by biopsy of a firm mass that demonstrates a vasculitis, granulomatous inflammation, and/or necrosis. Prior to biopsy, however, imaging may help distinguish the condition from other etiologies. CT scanning with contrast usually shows a hyperintense lesion relative to the nasal mucosa with obliteration of tissue planes and bony erosion [26]. MR imaging reveals lesions that are hypointense relative to orbital fat on both T1- and T2-weighted images and enhance after intravenous injection of gadolinium. Positron emission tomographic (PET) scanning may reveal high uptake [27, 28].

The current standard of management of patients with Wegener's granulomatosis is a combination of corticosteroids and immune modulators such as cyclophosphamide, methotrexate, or azathioprine to induce remission, followed by maintenance therapy to sustain the remission, prevent relapse, and allow repair of disease-related damage. Survival rates are up to 95% at 5-year follow-up and 80% at 10 years [29, 30]. More recently, rituximab combined with pulse corticosteroids has been found to be beneficial in patients who fail to respond to other immunomodulatory agents [31], including patients with orbital involvement [32].

### Churg-Strauss Syndrome

Churg-Strauss syndrome is a systemic allergic disease that initially manifests with asthma and allergic rhinitis. It is characterized by a necrotizing vasculitis of small- to medium-sized vessels and granulomatous inflammation that is rich in eosinophils (Fig. 24.11) [33].

Churg-Strauss syndrome primarily affects the lungs, sinuses, and peripheral nervous system. In 1990, the American College of Rheumatology determined that four of the following six criteria must be met to make the diagnosis: (1) asthma, (2) hyper-eosinophilia, (3) mononeuropathy or polyneuropathy, (4) pulmonary infiltrates, (5) paranasal sinus abnormality, and (6) extravascular eosinophil infiltration in biopsy specimens [34].

Ocular manifestations are rare in patients with Churg-Strauss syndrome but can be separated into two clinical presentations: ischemic vasculitis and orbital inflammation. Ischemic vasculitis may cause amaurosis fugax, ischemic optic neuropathy, and/or central or branch retinal artery occlusions. Orbital inflammation may be diffuse or may present as dacryoadenitis, myositis, periscleritis, and/or perineuritis. Both orbital apex syndrome and cavernous sinus syndrome have been reported in patients with Churg-Strauss syndrome [35].

The diagnosis of orbital involvement secondary to Churg-Strauss syndrome should be suspected when a patient with an orbital process has hematologic evidence of eosinophilia and a positive assay for p-ANCA. The findings on CT scanning and MR imaging are nonspecific and include lacrimal gland and extraocular muscle enlargements. Ultimately, the diagnosis can be confirmed by biopsy, with the key histologic feature being a necrotizing vasculitis associated with extravascular infiltration by eosinophils [36, 37].

The treatment of patients with orbital involvement by Churg-Strauss syndrome consists of corticosteroids, sometimes combined with methotrexate or cyclophosphamide; however, as orbital involvement is fairly infrequent in Churg-Strauss syndrome, therapy is almost always in context with treatment of the systemic disease. There have been some reports showing the benefit of other agents in

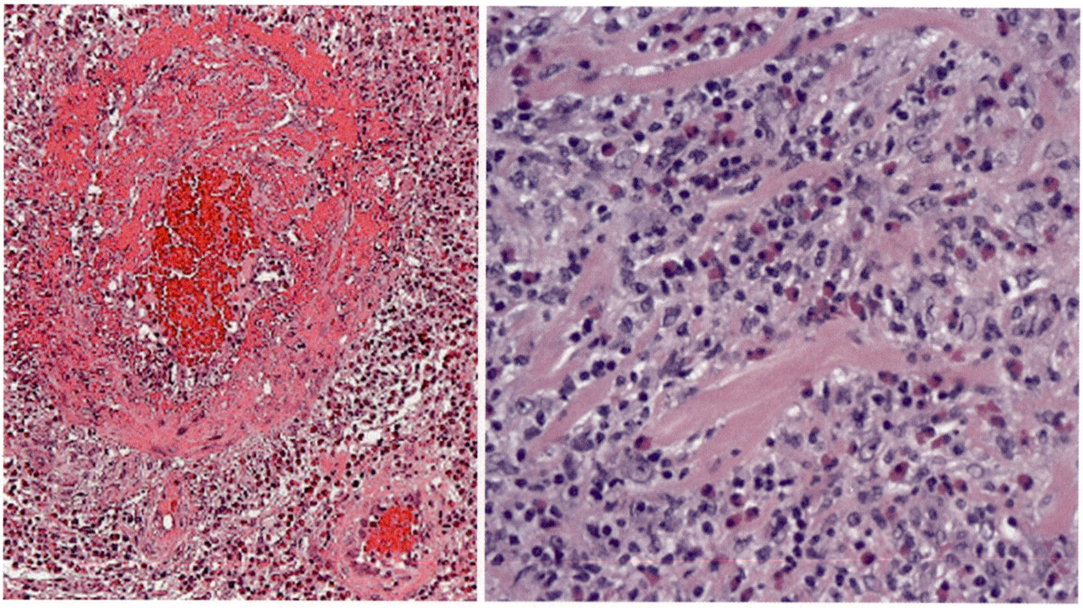

**Fig. 24.11** Histology of Churg-Strauss syndrome. Note intense necrotizing vasculitis rich in eosinophils

refractory or relapsing Churg-Strauss syndrome, although not specifically with respect to orbital involvement. Second-line drugs used in this setting include rituximab, infliximab, etanercept, mepolizumab, and omalizumab.

## Polyarteritis Nodosa

Polyarteritis nodosa is a systemic necrotizing vasculitis affecting small- and medium-sized arteries. Its cause is unknown, but an association with hepatitis B has been reported. The condition affects multiple organs, particularly the GI tract; the eyes and orbits are affected in approximately 10% of patients [19, 38]. Ocular manifestations usually are limited to retinal vasculitis, ischemic optic neuropathy, and scleritis, but patients with diffuse orbital inflammation characterized by proptosis, ophthalmoplegia, conjunctival injection and chemosis, and decreased vision have been described [39, 40].

The diagnosis of polyarteritis nodosa usually is based on the physical examination and laboratory studies. Laboratory findings generally are nonspecific but include an elevated ESR, eosinophilia, positive antinuclear antibody assay, and positive rheumatoid factor. CT scanning and MR imaging findings are nonspecific, but catheter angiography may show arterial dilation with aneurysm formation, arterial constriction by inflammation, or both. Orbital biopsies of affected tissue typically reveal a mixed arterial and venous vasculitis with variable fibrosis (Fig. 24.12).

Treatment of orbital vasculitis secondary to polyarteritis nodosa is identical with the treatment of the systemic disease. The mainstay of therapy is a combination of systemic corticosteroids and cyclophosphamide; however, other immunomodulatory agents such as azathioprine and methotrexate also have been used, and there are case reports of disease remission with the use of rituximab in polyarteritis nodosa, although not specifically in patients with orbital disease.

## Giant Cell Arteritis

Giant cell arteritis (GCA), also called temporal arteritis, is an idiopathic vasculitis of medium- to large-sized arteries. The condition is characterized histologically by segmental arterial inflammation consisting of giant cells, lymphocytes, plasma cells, and eosinophils in the media associated with thickening and disruption of its internal elastic lamina.

The systemic manifestations of GCA include headache, temple pain and/or tenderness, scalp tenderness, jaw claudication that may be mistaken for TMJ syndrome, migratory arthralgias, malaise, and fevers of unknown origin. Ocular manifestations include both anterior and retrobulbar ischemic optic neuropathy, central retinal

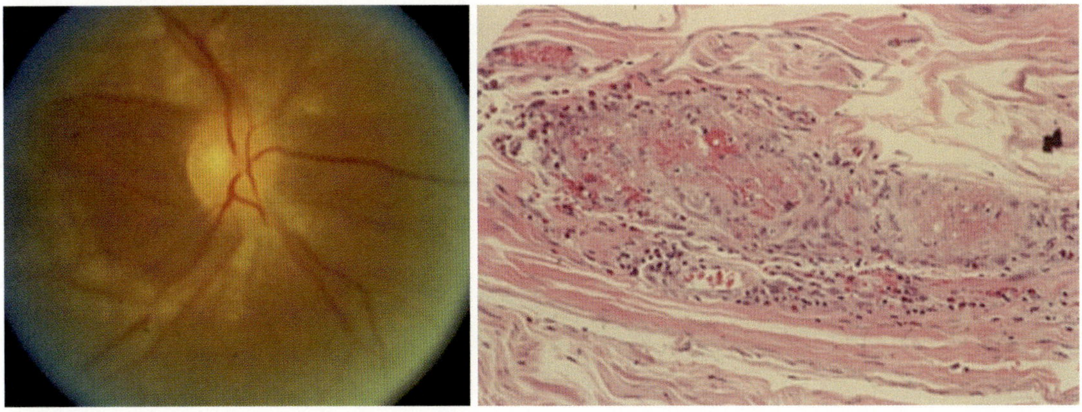

**Fig. 24.12** Polyarteritis nodosa (PAN) in a patient with a central retinal artery occlusion and a mass at the right orbital apex. *Left*, appearance of the right ocular fundus at the time of visual loss shows a partial central retinal artery occlusion. *Right*, biopsy of abnormal tissue at the orbital apex is consistent with PAN, showing a mixed arterial and venous vasculitis minimal variable fibrosis

artery occlusion, and diplopia from either ocular motor nerve paresis or extraocular muscle ischemia [41]. In addition, some patients develop an orbital ischemic syndrome characterized by corneal edema, cataract formation, hypotony, ophthalmoparesis, and visual loss from optic neuropathy [42]. A less common presentation of GCA is orbital inflammation; however, in this setting, patients can have signs and symptoms of an orbital apex syndrome (Fig. 24.13) [43–45].

The diagnosis of GCA-related orbital disease can be made from the combination of the clinical presentation, laboratory studies (elevated ESR, CRP, or both), imaging consisting of contrast enhancement of the orbit with an infiltrative appearance or a mass lesion on MR imaging, and, most importantly, a temporal artery biopsy showing giant cells, fragmentation or loss of the elastic lamina of arteries, and areas of fibrosis and necrosis [43, 45].

The treatment of a patient with an orbital apex syndrome caused by GCA is no different from the treatment of patients without orbital disease. All patients should be placed on high-dose corticosteroids, with a slow taper once there is an initial clinical and laboratory response. There is no consistently effective agent other than steroids for patients with GCA, although some authors advocate cyclophosphamide or methotrexate in cases that are refractory to steroids [45]. Other treatments suggested include external beam radiation, TNF-alpha inhibitors, and tocilizumab, an anti-interleukin-6 antibody.

## Systemic Lupus Erythematosus

Systemic lupus erythematosus (SLE) is a chronic, systemic autoimmune-mediated connective tissue disease causing a vasculitis that affects the eye and visual system in 20% of patients. In this condition, the deposition of pathogenic autoantibodies and immune complexes damages tissues and cells. Some common ocular manifestations of SLE include keratoconjunctivitis sicca, periocular skin lesions, retinal hemorrhages and vasculitis, retinal vaso-occlusive disease, iritis, scleritis, optic neuritis, ischemic optic neuropathy, and orbital inflammation. One rare clinical entity in the SLE spectrum is panniculitis, also known as lupus erythematosus profundus (LEP), which is a nodular inflammation of adipose tissue. Panniculitis involving orbital structures as the primary presenting symptom of SLE is quite unusual and only rarely has been reported in the literature [46]. Vascular inflammation consisting of a leukocytoclastic vasculitis affecting small vessels is a common finding in patients with SLE, with an incidence of 30–40%. It is related to immune complex deposition within the vessels walls.

The most common manifestations of SLE vasculitis are cutaneous lesions (e.g., nail-fold infarcts, palpable purpura, and digital gangrene) and polyneuropathy. The most common ocular findings are retinopathy, keratoconjunctivitis sicca, and uveitis [47]. Orbital involvement is infrequent, but there have been a number of case reports in the literature describing diffuse orbital

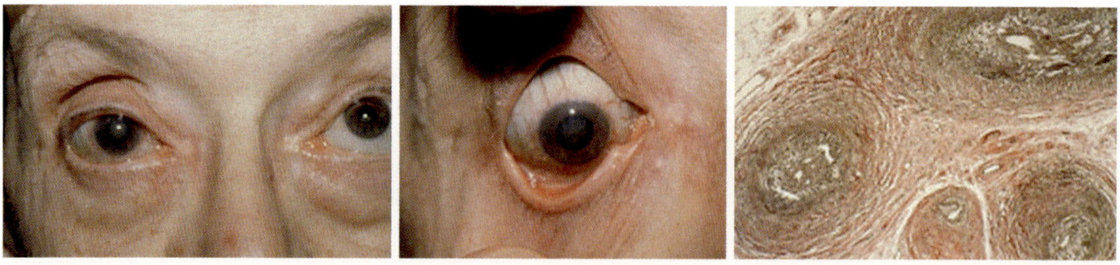

**Fig. 24.13** Giant cell (temporal) arteritis causing an orbital/ocular ischemic syndrome in a 76-year-old woman. *Left*, note right enophthalmos from fat atrophy due to ischemia. *Center*, the right eye is injected, and there is some corneal edema and a developing cataract. The intraocular pressure was low, and there was a general ophthalmoparesis. *Right*, the patient experienced a myocardial infarction and died. Pathology of the posterior orbital tissue revealed occlusion of the posterior ciliary arteries with fragmentation of the elastic lamina and a chronic inflammation characterized in part by giant cells

inflammation, orbital infarction, and myositis in association with SLE [48, 49].

The diagnosis of SLE can be made when 4 or more of 11 criteria (malar rash, discoid rash, photosensitivity, oral ulcers, nonerosive arthritis, pleuritis or pericarditis, renal disorder, neurologic disorder, hematologic disorder, immunologic disorder, positive ANA) are present (Table 24.2) [50]. In addition, the ANA assay is positive in 95 % of patients with SLE; thus, a negative ANA may be regarded as evidence against the condition, but a positive ANA is not diagnostic. If a patient meets the diagnostic criteria listed above and has a positive ANA, then no further test is required. On the other hand, if a patient has a positive ANA but does not meet the diagnostic criteria, he or she should undergo assays for antibodies to double-stranded DNA and smooth muscle nuclear antigen as positive results suggest the diagnosis.

**Table 24.2** 1997 update of the 1982 American College of Rheumatology revised criteria for classification of systemic lupus erythematosus [50]

| | |
|---|---|
| Malar rash | Fixed erythema, flat or raised, over the malar eminences |
| Discoid rash | Erythematous circular raised patches with adherent keratotic scaling and follicular plugging; atrophic scarring may occur |
| Photosensitivity | Exposure to ultraviolet light causes rash |
| Oral ulcers | Includes oral and nasopharyngeal ulcers, observed by physician |
| Arthritis | Nonerosive arthritis of two or more peripheral joints, with tenderness, swelling, or effusion |
| Serositis | Pleuritis or pericarditis documented by ECG or rub or evidence of effusion |
| Renal disorder | Proteinuria >0.5 g/d or 3+ or cellular casts |
| Neurologic disorder | Seizures or psychosis without other causes |
| Hematologic disorder | Hemolytic anemia or leukopenia (<4000/L) or lymphopenia (<1500/L) or thrombocytopenia (<100,000/L) in the absence of offending drugs |
| Immunologic disorder | Anti-dsDNA, anti-Sm, and/or antiphospholipid |
| Antinuclear antibodies | An abnormal titer of ANA by immunofluorescence or an equivalent assay at any point in time in the absence of drugs known to induce ANAs |

The classification is based on 11 criteria. For the purpose of identifying patients in clinical studies, a person is defined as having SLE if any 4 or more of the 11 criteria are present, serially or simultaneously, during any interval of observation

Similar to most of other orbital vasculitides, orbital inflammation related to lupus vasculitis usually is treated with systemic corticosteroids. Immunomodulatory agents, biologics and rituximab, infliximab, and belimumab also have shown to be beneficial [51].

## Tolosa-Hunt Syndrome

Tolosa-Hunt syndrome is the eponym used to describe idiopathic orbital inflammation causing painful ophthalmoplegia. It is characterized histologically by granulomatous inflammation consisting of epithelioid and occasional giant cells within the cavernous sinus, superior orbital fissure, orbital apex, or a combination of these structures [52–54]. It can affect people of any age with no sex predilection. The condition usually occurs spontaneously, although it has been reported to develop after ocular trauma [55].

The clinical manifestation of Tolosa-Hunt syndrome is an ophthalmoparesis associated with severe periorbital or hemicranial pain. In some cases, the ophthalmoparesis is associated with evidence of one or more ocular motor nerve paresis, whereas in other cases, it is related to inflammation of the extraocular muscles at the orbital apex. The periocular or hemicranial pain may precede the ophthalmoparesis by up to 2 weeks and typically is described as a severe, intense, boring, gnawing, or stabbing sensation. Pupillary reactions may be normal, or there may be either parasympathetic or sympathetic dysfunction. Tolosa-Hunt syndrome may have a relapsing and remitting course, and residual neurologic deficits may persist after remission [56].

The International Headache Society defined the diagnostic criteria of Tolosa-Hunt syndrome as follows: (1) one or more episodes of unilateral orbital pain persisting for weeks if untreated; (2) associated paralysis of one or more of the third, fourth, or sixth cranial nerves; and/or (3) demonstration of a granuloma by MR imaging or biopsy; (4) the paresis coincides with the onset of pain and follows it within 2 weeks; (5) pain and paresis resolve within 72 h when treated adequately with corticosteroids (see below), but in this setting, the condition should only be diagnosed after exclusion of other potentially causative lesions [57].

MR imaging should be the initial screening study in patients with suspected Tolosa-Hunt syndrome. Coronal fast spin-echo T2-weighted images and fat-saturated T1-weighted coronal and transverse images with and without contrast show high sensitivity for the detection and follow-up of the inflammatory lesion (Fig. 24.14) [58].

The findings are nonspecific, however, and cannot be differentiated from certain tumors, such as meningiomas or lymphomas, not to mention the granulomatous lesions caused by sarcoidosis [59]. Although high-resolution CT scanning also can demonstrate soft tissue changes in the orbital apex, superior orbital fissure, and/or cavernous sinus, it is not sensitive to soft tissue changes because of superimposed beam hardening and bone artifacts. Cerebral angiography may detect abnormalities of the cavernous portion of the internal carotid artery in patients with Tolosa-Hunt syndrome [60], but, again, the findings are nonspecific. Some reports have documented elevation of the ESR and a leukocytosis in the acute stage of Tolosa-Hunt syndrome [61], and some patients have antinuclear antibodies despite having no evidence of a connective tissue disorder. CSF examination tends to be unremarkable but may show an elevated protein concentration and a mild pleocytosis. Although biopsy of abnormal tissue in the orbital apex or cavernous sinus is rarely employed to establish the diagnosis of Tolosa-Hunt syndrome, it should be considered in patients with rapidly progressive neurological deficits, lack of steroid responsiveness, or persistent abnormalities on neuroimaging studies.

In the final analysis, the diagnosis of Tolosa-Hunt syndrome usually is one of exclusion, requiring a careful evaluation to eliminate out other etiologies of painful ophthalmoplegia and

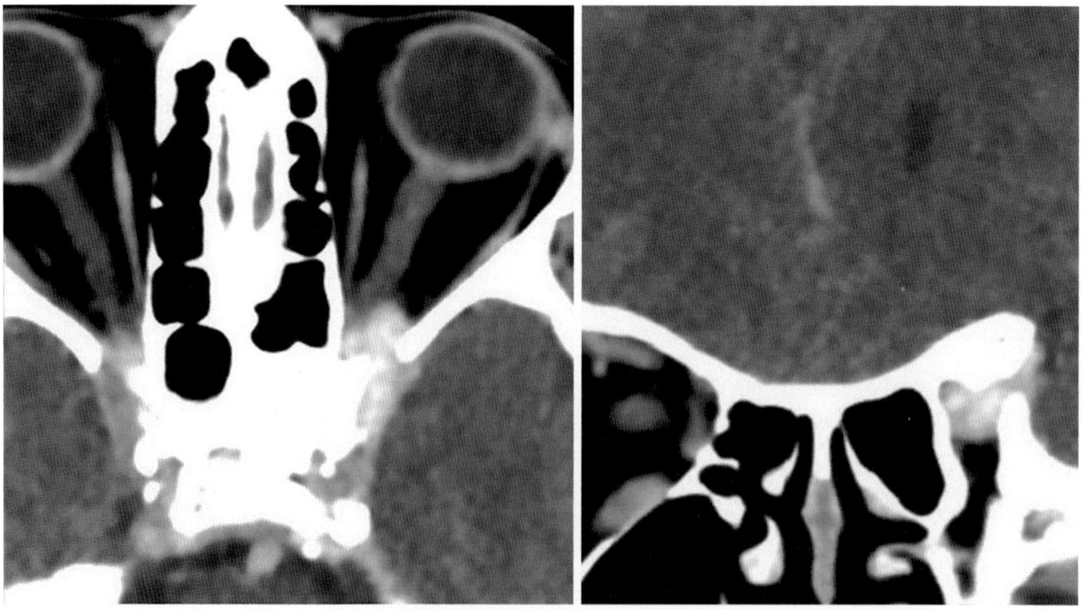

**Fig. 24.14** Tolosa-Hunt syndrome in a patient with left-sided ophthalmoparesis and a mild left optic neuropathy. CT scan, axial, and coronal views show an ill-defined mass in the left orbital apex and cavernous sinus

other forms of inflammation within the cavernous sinus and superior orbital fissure. Some authors have suggested excluding other causative conditions by using serologic and CSF studies and, occasionally, biopsy, followed by serial clinical and imaging examinations for at least 2 years after steroids have been ceased before the diagnosis can be made with some degree of assurance [62].

The treatment of Tolosa-Hunt syndrome consists of high-dose systemic steroids to which the condition is markedly sensitive. Indeed, as noted above, most patients have dramatic resolution of pain within 24–72 h after onset of treatment, although the ophthalmoparesis can take weeks to months to resolve. Methotrexate and azathioprine have provided clinical benefit in a limited number of patients with Tolosa-Hunt syndrome [63, 64]. Radiotherapy also reportedly alleviated symptoms of Tolosa-Hunt syndrome in a patient refractory to immunosuppressive therapy and in another patient who became steroid dependent [65].

## Idiopathic and Immunoglobulin G4 (IgG4)-Related Orbital Inflammation

Idiopathic orbital inflammatory syndrome is the third most common orbital disorder in adults after thyroid orbitopathy and lymphoproliferative disorders, with a peak incidence in middle age and a predilection for women [66, 67].

Based on the extent and location of involvement, it can be categorized as myositis, dacryoadenitis, anterior, apical, or diffuse. Histopathologic analysis of affected tissue shows a spectrum of granulomatous inflammation admixed with non-granulomatous inflammation and fibrosis (Fig. 24.15) [68].

In most cases, no cause can be found to account for the inflammatory process, hence the label "idiopathic" [69]; however, some cases are associated with autoimmune disease, trauma, or recent surgery [70], and an increasing number of cases once thought to be "idiopathic" have been found to have pathologic findings consisting of plasma cells containing IgG4 (Table 24.3) [71–73].

It remains unclear what percentage of case of "idiopathic" orbital inflammation is actually IgG4-related and, indeed, if elevated IgG4 is a cause of the condition or simply a marker of a form of the disorder. A recent article reported about a quarter of orbital lymphoproliferative disorders were related to IgG4 [74].

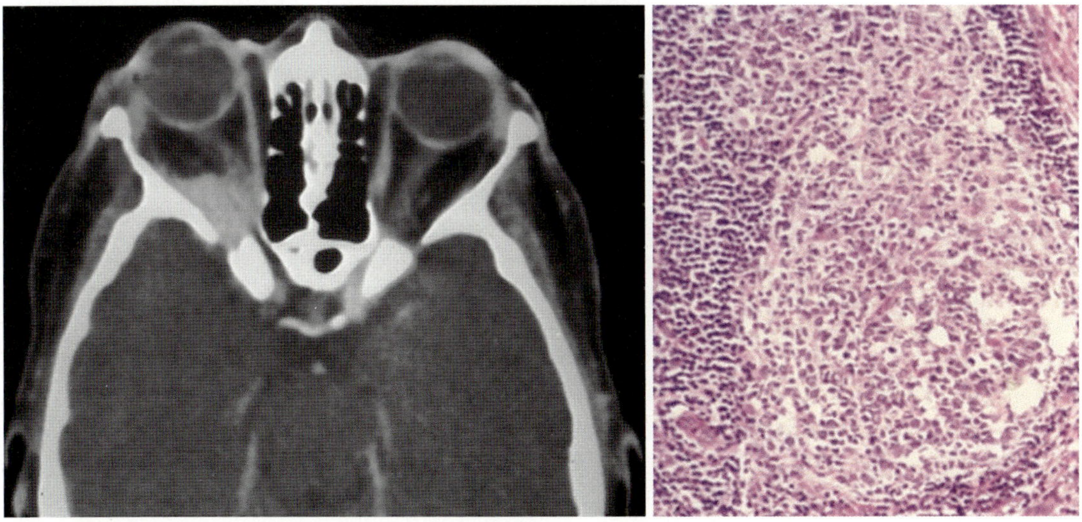

**Fig. 24.15** Patient with a right orbital apex syndrome characterized by the sudden development of right-sided orbital pain, injection, conjunctival chemosis, ophthalmoparesis, proptosis, and decreased vision associated with a right relative afferent pupillary defect. *Left*, axial CT scan shows a lesion at the orbital apex that is deviating the optic nerve medially. Because of concern for a lymphoma, the lesion was biopsied. *Right*, biopsy shows a nonspecific follicular inflammation. The lesion had both B- and T-lymphocytes. Staining for IgG4 was negative

**Table 24.3** Previously recognized conditions that comprise or may comprise parts of the IgG4-related disease spectrum

| Previous "idiopathic" conditions | Target organs |
|---|---|
| Orbital pseudotumor | Orbital adnexa |
| Mikulicz disease | Salivary and lacrimal glands |
| Kuttner's tumor | Submandibular glands |
| Eosinophilic angiocentric fibrosis | Sinuses and nasal cavities |
| Riedel's thyroiditis | Thyroid |
| Chronic sclerosing aortitis | Aorta |
| Fibrosing mediastinitis | Mediastinum |
| Retroperitoneal fibrosis | Retroperitoneum |
| Autoimmune pancreatitis/lymphoplasmacytic sclerosing pancreatitis | Pancreas |
| Sclerosing cholangitis | Biliary tree |
| Cutaneous pseudolymphoma | Skin |
| Multifocal fibrosclerosis | Various organs |

The clinical presentation of both idiopathic and IgG4-related orbital inflammations is typical, consisting of the sudden onset of pain that may increase or occur only with eye movement, redness, chemosis, proptosis, and periorbital edema. Decreased vision and diplopia also may be present depending on the extent of the inflammation and the structures affected.

Both idiopathic and IgG4-related orbital inflammations are diagnoses of exclusion, made either after other disorders have been eliminated from consideration or after a biopsy of affected tissue has been performed. The best imaging modality is contrast-enhanced, thin-section MR imaging with fat suppression. As with the clinical manifestations, the findings on MR imaging (and CT scanning) depend on the location of the inflammation and the structures involved. In patients with myositis, the affected extraocular muscle or muscles as well as their tendons tend to be enlarged, whereas patients with a dacryoadenitis show lacrimal gland enlargement. Diffuse orbital inflammation is characterized by poorly demarcated, enhancing soft tissue throughout the orbit, often associated with fat stranding [69]. Other imaging findings that may help to make a diagnosis of orbital inflammation include the absence of contiguous paranasal sinus process usually noted in patients with infectious orbital inflammation [70]. Biopsy is recommended for cases suspicious for an orbital malignancy or when a poor response to corticosteroids is seen.

As noted above, an increasing number of cases of orbital inflammation appear to be IgG4-related. Some patients in which this condition occurs have other IgG4-related inflammations involving the head and neck, including the salivary glands, thyroid gland, lymph nodes, sinonasal cavities, pituitary gland, and larynx. In other cases, periaortic inflammation may be present. The diagnostic criteria for IgG4-related disease are an increased serum concentration of IgG4 (>135 mg/dl) and/or a biopsy of affected tissue showing inflammation with infiltration by IgG4-positive cells (>40 % of IgG-positive plasma cells, absolute number of IgG4-positive plasma cells >10–40/HPF) (Fig. 24.16) [75].

For the investigation of the extent of systemic lesions, gallium scintigram and PET scanning may be helpful. CT scanning of affected organs may demonstrate enlargement or decreased attenuation, whereas at T2-weighted MR images may show relatively low signal intensity owing to increased cellularity and fibrosis [76]. Nevertheless, because the imaging features of IgG4-related disease are varied and difficult to distinguish from those of other inflammatory conditions such as Wegener's granulomatosis (see above), either serologic or histopathologic confirmation is required for definitive diagnosis [77].

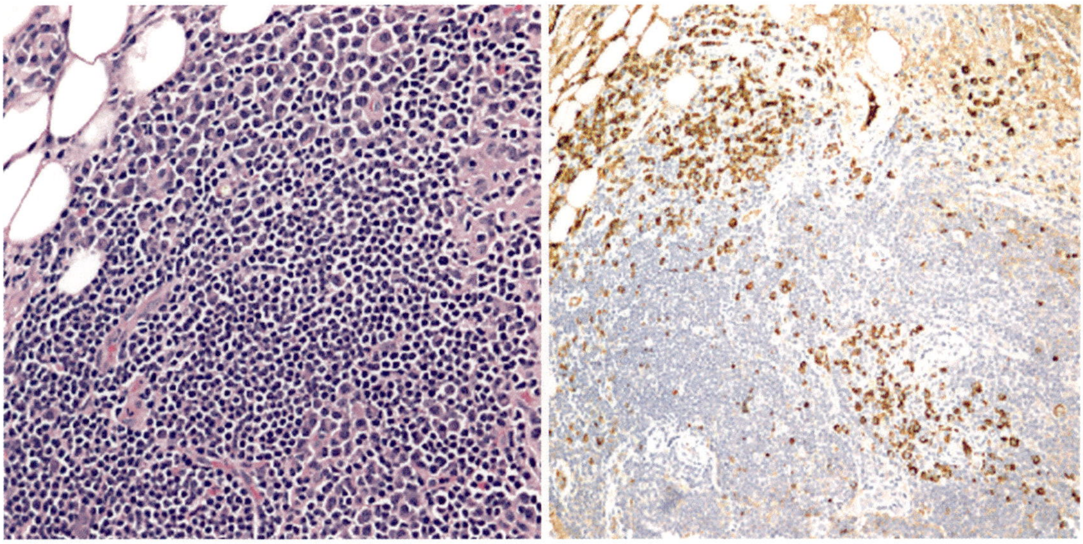

**Fig. 24.16** IgG4-positive inflammation in a patient with an orbital apex syndrome. *Left*, there is an inflammatory process consisting primarily of plasma cells and lymphocytes. *Right*, stain for IgG4 is markedly positive

Systemic corticosteroid therapy is the cornerstone of treatment for both idiopathic and IgG4-related orbital inflammations. Over 75 % of patients show dramatic improvement within 24–48 h of the start of treatment. Starting dosages of prednisone of 1.0–2.0 mg/kg/day usually are adequate. Once improvement occurs, treatment should be continued with a slow taper over weeks to months guided by clinical judgment. Intraorbital injections of corticosteroid have been reported as effective in selected patients; [78] however, we are reluctant to perform orbital injections in patients with inflammation because of the risk of hemorrhage. Low-lose radiation (20 Gy given in ten 2 Gy fractions) can be effective in patients with idiopathic inflammation but typically is reserved for elderly patients, for those unresponsive or intolerant to systemic corticosteroids, and for those in whom steroids are contraindicated [79, 80]. The role of radiotherapy for IgG4-related orbital inflammation has not established. For those patients who are refractory to both corticosteroids and radiotherapy, chemotherapeutic agents such as cyclophosphamide, methotrexate, and cyclosporine have been found to be helpful [81] and may be appropriate particularly for patients with known or suspected IgG4-related disease refractory to corticosteroids. Other therapies used in individual patients with severe or refractory orbital inflammation include cytotoxic agents such as chlorambucil and immunosuppressants such as azathioprine, intravenous immunoglobulin therapy, TNF-alpha inhibitors, monoclonal antibodies such as infliximab and adalimumab, and mycophenolate mofetil (Table 24.4) [82–84].

## Infectious

Inflammation caused by infections can cause an orbital apex syndrome. In most cases, the infection does not arise within the orbit but reaches it from adjacent structures such as the nasal cavity, paranasal sinuses, or CNS. In other cases, blood-borne organisms are responsible. Almost any organism can produce an infectious orbital apex syndrome. The most common are fungi, especially aspergillus species and mucormycosis; however, various bacteria such as *Mycobacterium tuberculosis*, *Streptococcus* species, *Staphylococcus* species, *Actinomyces* species, Gram-negative bacilli, and anaerobes as well as certain viruses, particularly herpes zoster, and spirochetes such as *Treponema pallidum* and *Borrelia burgdorferi* also can produce this clinical syndrome. There even are rare

**Table 24.4** Immunomodulators used for management of noninfectious orbital inflammation

| Categories | Mechanism of action | Adverse effects |
|---|---|---|
| Corticosteroids | | |
| Methylprednisolone | Inhibits multiple inflammatory cytokines | |
| Prednisone | Inhibits multiple inflammatory cytokines | Monitors bone density on long-term treatment. Mood swing, weight change, hyperglycemia, GI distress, loss of bone density |
| Immunosuppressants (steroid-sparing) | | |
| Azathioprine | Inhibits T-lymphocyte | Bone marrow suppression, GI distress, myalgias |
| Chlorambucil | Alkylates and cross-links DNA | |
| Cyclophosphamide | Alkylates and cross-links DNA | Cytotoxicity with hemorrhagic cystitis, bone marrow suppression, malignancy potential |
| Cyclosporine | Inhibits T-lymphocyte | Renal dysfunction, hypertension, liver toxicity |
| Methotrexate | Inhibits dihydrofolate reductase, inhibits lymphocyte proliferation | Useful steroid-sparing agent. Folate supplement may help to minimize adverse effects. Fatigue, GI distress, liver toxicity, hair loss, headaches, arthralgias |
| Mycophenolate mofetil | Inhibits B- and T-lymphocyte proliferation | Potential steroid-sparing. Hematuria, constitutional symptoms, cough, peripheral edema, arthralgias, GI distress, hematologic abnormalities |
| Monoclonal antibodies (biologics) | | |
| Belimumab | Inhibits B-lymphocytic stimulator | GI distress, pain |
| Adalimumab | Binds and inhibits tumor necrosis factor alpha | Demyelination disease, reactivation of infectious disease, bone marrow suppression, dermatitis, liver toxicity |
| Etanercept | Binds and inhibits tumor necrosis factor | |
| Infliximab | Binds and inhibits tumor necrosis factor alpha | |
| Omalizumab | Inhibits IgE binding to mast cells and basophils | Thrombocytopenia, cold symptoms |
| Rituximab | Binds to B-lymphocyte CD20 surface antigens | Worsening of infection (hepatitis, herpes, JC virus), bone marrow suppression, GI distress |
| Tocilizumab | Binds to and inhibits IL-6 receptors | Demyelinating disease, bone marrow suppression, infection |

reports of cases of orbital apex syndrome caused by parasitic infections. We consider some of these conditions in the sections below.

## Fungal Infections

Fungal infections are a not uncommon cause of an orbital apex syndrome, with mucormycosis and aspergillosis being the most frequent etiologies. Although a fungal orbital apex syndrome can occur in immunocompetent patients without apparent sinus disease [85–89], most cases occur in immunocompromised individuals and result from spread of the organisms from the paranasal sinuses directly or via the pterygopalatine fossa to the orbital apex and then to the cavernous sinus. Within the cavernous sinus, they invade the cavernous portion of the internal carotid artery, resulting in various complications, including cerebral infection, mycotic aneurysm formation, intracranial hemorrhage, subarachnoid hemorrhage, meningitis, cerebral abscess, and, ultimately, death [90–93]. The problem is that whereas invasive fungal sinusitis is easy to suspect and diagnose once a complete orbital apex syndrome has developed, by then it usually is too late to save the patient's vision or life. Invasive fungal sinusitis is difficult to diagnose early when the patient presents with only eye pain followed by diplopia or visual loss. Invasive fungal sinusitis is usually caused by Zygomycetes of the order Mucorales, *Aspergillus* species, or rarely, but increasingly, by *Scedosporium* [94, 95].

A fungal cause of an orbital apex syndrome should be suspected in patients with predisposing conditions including diabetes mellitus with and without ketoacidosis, chronic alcohol abuse, hematologic malignancies causing neutropenia, and immunosuppression as well as in any patient requiring immunomodulatory, antineoplastic, or long-term corticosteroid therapy [96–99]. Other risk factors for mucormycosis include iron overload states and the use of desferrioxamine and similar agents, whereas other risk factors for invasive aspergillosis include neutrophil defect and corticosteroid use.

Once the diagnosis of fungal orbital apex syndrome is suspected, one should obtain high-quality, contrast-enhanced, and fat-suppressed MR imaging of the orbits and paranasal sinuses looking for extra-sinus extension of disease or loss of contrast enhancement of the sinonasal mucosa. If the patient is deteriorating, immediate paranasal sinus or orbital apex biopsy is required to confirm the diagnosis and guide the treatment.

## Mucormycosis

Mucormycosis is a potentially life-threatening opportunistic fungal infection caused by the Mucorales order of Zygomycetes, most often *Rhizopus* and *Mucor* species (Fig. 24.17).

It generally affects patients with known predisposing conditions, such as poorly controlled diabetes mellitus; long-term treatment with steroids, antibiotics, cytotoxic agents, or desferrioxamine; lymphoproliferative disorders such as leukemia and lymphoma; organ transplantation; severe burns; hemochromatosis; previous treatment with antifungal drugs lacking activity against Zygomycetes; and possibly malnutrition. Although there are cases of orbital involvement by mucormycosis in healthy individuals, such cases are very rare [97, 100].

No serological method is available for the diagnosis of mucormycosis. Thus, the gold standard for the diagnosis, as it is with most other fungal infections, is tissue culture.

Early diagnosis of mucormycosis and rapid initiation of appropriate therapy within a few days of the onset of its clinical manifestations are crucial to control of the infection and ultimate survival. Early empiric systemic antifungal treatment is essential, as is treatment of the underlying medical condition or metabolic state, such as reversal of ketoacidosis or neutropenia and cessation of immunosuppression. Standard treatment for mucormycosis in immunocompromised patients requires discontinuation of immunosuppressive drugs like cyclosporine or mycophenolate mofetil, combined with systemic antifungal therapy and, in most cases, aggressive surgical debridement. The antifungal agent of choice is

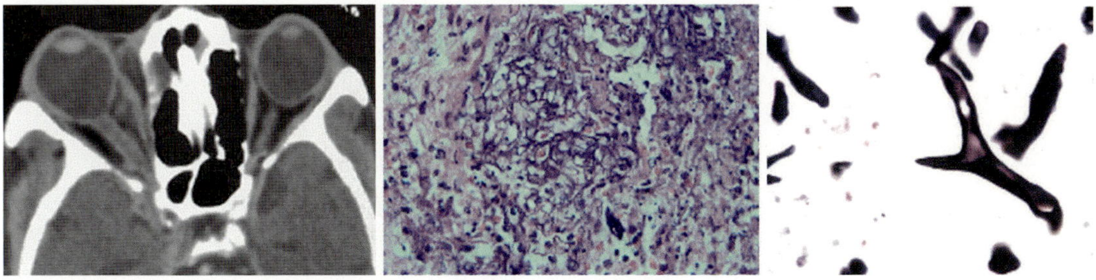

**Fig. 24.17** Mucormycosis causing an orbital apex syndrome in a diabetic patient with ketoacidosis who also abused alcohol. The patient presented with marked right ophthalmoparesis and loss of vision in the right eye. *Left*, axial CT scan shows thickening of the right optic nerve associated with abnormal tissue in the apex of the orbit and in the cavernous sinus. *Center*, biopsy of the abnormal tissue in the orbital apex shows an inflammatory reaction in which there are numerous fungi. *Right,* high-power fungal stain shows typical branching hyphal structure consistent with Mucorales species

amphotericin B alone or in combination with such drugs as flucytosine, fluconazole, itraconazole, or micafungin [101]. Lipid formulations of amphotericin B (LFABs) are less nephrotoxic than other preparations and can be used at higher doses and for a longer time.

## Aspergillosis

Aspergillosis is an infection caused by *Aspergillus* species. The most common subtype causing both paranasal sinus and orbital apex syndrome is *Aspergillus fumigatus*. As with other fungal infections, the diagnosis generally requires tissue for histopathologic examination and culture (Fig. 24.18) [102].

Aspergillosis can cause an orbital apex syndrome in three ways: as a solid mass called an aspergilloma, as an invasive infection, and, rarely, as an allergic process [103–108]. Aspergillomas may occur in patients with chronic, debilitating conditions [103, 104, 109, 110], but they more often are solitary lesions that arise in otherwise healthy persons without evidence of infection or other systemic diseases [111–113]. Aspergillomas in the orbit produce the nonspecific manifestations caused by all orbital masses, including proptosis, decreased vision, diplopia, and pain [114, 115]. Patients with orbital aspergillosis often have no evidence of systemic aspergillosis, with the organism having reached the orbit by direct extension from either the paranasal sinuses or the CNS.

In contrast to aspergillomas that tend to present in healthy individuals with subacute or even chronic manifestations, orbital apex or cavernous sinus syndromes caused by invasive aspergillosis tend to occur in immunocompromised patients and often have a more acute presentation with conjunctival injection, chemosis, and orbital or ocular pain associated with the general manifestations of orbital and/or cavernous sinus disease. As is the case with mucormycosis, early diagnosis by obtaining tissue for culture and histologic examination and aggressive treatment of invasive aspergillosis are crucial in preserving visual function, reversing visual deficits, and improving chances of survival, especially in immunocompromised individuals. Amphotericin B combined with aggressive debridement is the current standard of care for orbital aspergillosis. Intravenous amphotericin B was previously the agent of choice for invasive aspergillosis, but oral voriconazole is just as effective. Even with early diagnosis and treatment, patients with invasive aspergillosis causing an orbital apex or cavernous sinus syndrome have a poor prognosis [116]. Nevertheless, treatment of both aspergillomas and invasive aspergillosis can be successful with early recognition and aggressive therapy [107, 117–121]. Not surprisingly, the best results are in patients who

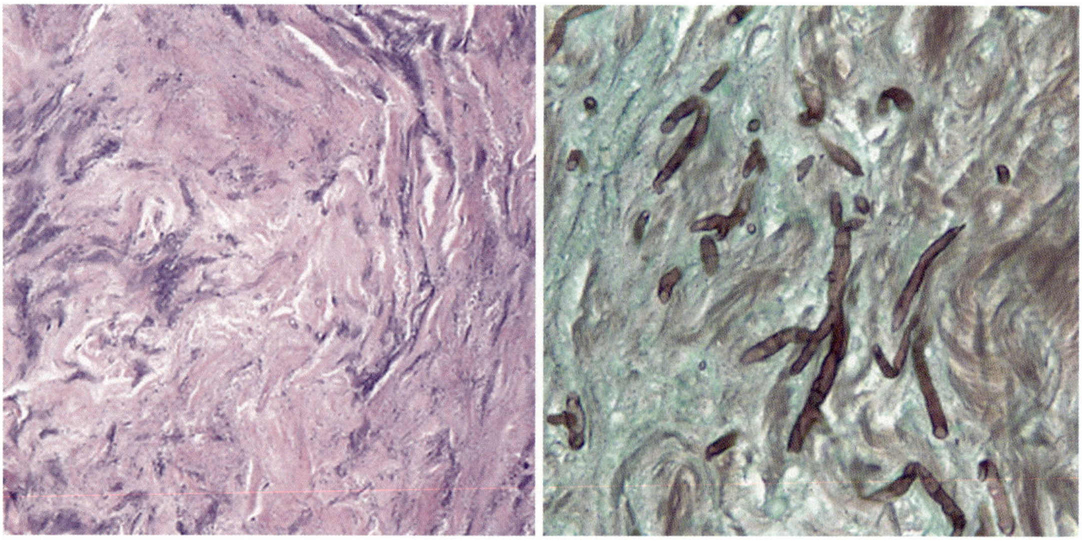

**Fig. 24.18** Aspergillus causing an orbital apex syndrome

are not immunocompromised. Unfortunately, most patients in whom invasive aspergillosis occurs are, in fact, immunocompromised, and in those individuals, the mortality is exceptionally high despite early diagnosis and treatment.

## Bacterial Infections

Bacterial infection can cause orbital apex as well as cavernous sinus syndromes. As is the case with fungal infections, the syndromes most commonly result from contiguous spread of organisms from the paranasal sinuses, although a case of orbital apex syndrome related to acute suppurative otitis media has been reported [122]. In many cases, there is associated septic cavernous sinus thrombosis (Fig. 24.19).

The bacteria most commonly implicated include *Staphylococcus aureus*, *Streptococcus pneumonia*, other streptococci, Gram-negative bacilli, and anaerobes [123–125]. Bilateral cavernous sinus involvement associated with CNS *Actinomyces israelii* has been reported [126, 127] as has a patient with orbital apex syndrome and cavernous sinus thrombosis caused by a mixed infection with *S. aureus* and *Pseudomonas aeruginosa* [128].

Bacterial infection as a cause of a cavernous sinus syndrome should be suspected in any patient who presents with acute cavernous sinus thrombosis. Appropriate culture and sensitivity studies of affected tissue usually are required to identify the causative organism, unless there is generalized sepsis, in which case cultures of blood, CSF, or both may be sufficient.

## Viral Infection

The most common viral cause of an orbital apex syndrome is the varicella-zoster virus. This virus can cause herpes zoster ophthalmicus, a localized disease usually characterized by a vesicular eruption in the periorbital region, conjunctival chemosis and injection, and severe lancinating periorbital pain (Fig. 24.20).

Herpes zoster ophthalmicus usually is triggered by reactivation of the virus that is dormant

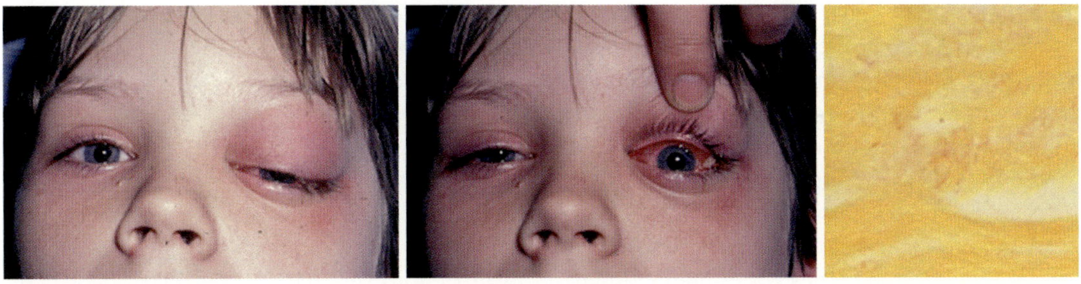

**Fig. 24.19** Left orbital cellulitis caused by *Pseudomonas aeruginosa*

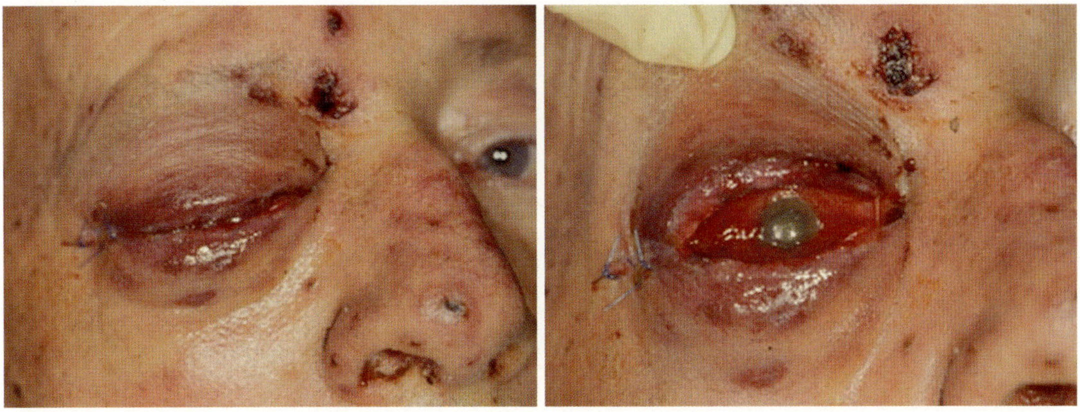

**Fig. 24.20** Herpes zoster ophthalmicus involving the right orbit

within the trigeminal nerve ganglia following a previous episode of chicken pox. Virus triggers include aging, immunosuppression, trauma, surgery, radiation therapy, and various infections such as tuberculosis and syphilis [129].

Ocular manifestations of herpes zoster ophthalmicus include blepharitis, keratoconjunctivitis, anterior uveitis, iritis, scleritis, acute retinal necrosis, and central retinal artery occlusion [130, 131]. Although patients with an orbital apex syndrome have been reported [132–138], more often, the virus causes an isolated abducens, oculomotor, or trochlear nerve paresis [136, 139–145]. The etiology of the orbital manifestations of herpes zoster ophthalmicus is unclear but may be due to a direct viral cytopathologic effect with infiltration and microinfarction in the long posterior ciliary vessels and nerves versus a reactive immunologic response to the virus that produces orbital edema.

The diagnosis of herpes zoster ophthalmicus is relatively straightforward and usually is based on the presence of the characteristic periorbital vesicular rash associated with pain. Therefore, often no tests are required for confirmation; however, when necessary, the virus can be identified and confirmed from vesicular fluid by performing either viral culture or the polymerase chain reaction (PCR). Testing for antibodies to the virus in the blood is rarely useful.

Although the effect of systemic steroids and antiviral therapy on herpes zoster ophthalmicus-related orbital apex syndrome has not been studied with a randomized controlled clinical trial, the combination treatment of systemic acyclovir and corticosteroids usually carries a good prognosis, especially in patients with intact immunity [146].

## Spirochetal Infections

Two spirochetes, *Treponema pallidum* and *Borrelia burgdorferi*, are responsible for virtually all of the very rare cases of orbital apex syndrome caused by spirochetes.

### Syphilis

The most common cause of ophthalmoplegia in patients with syphilis is basilar meningitis; however, some patients have been reported in whom a unilateral or bilateral ophthalmoparesis was associated with evidence of an optic neuropathy, suggesting involvement of the orbital apex [147]. We are unaware of any cases of a syphilitic gumma involving the orbital apex but see no reason that this could not occur.

The diagnosis of a syphilis is made by non-treponemal tests such as venereal disease research laboratory (VDRL) or rapid plasma reagin (RPR) tests and/or treponemal-specific tests such as the enzyme immunoassay (EIA) for anti-treponemal IgG, the *Treponema pallidum* hemagglutination (TPHA) test, the microhemagglutination test with *T. pallidum* antigen, the fluorescent treponemal antibody-absorption (FTA-ABS) test, and the enzyme-linked immunosorbent assay (ELISA). These tests can be performed on both serum and CSF. If a specimen is available, dark-field microscopy may help to identify the pathogen.

Syphilis usually is treated with penicillin. The dose and route of administration depend on the stage of the disease. In patients with ocular or orbital manifestations, visual acuity and clinical recovery occur early with early diagnosis and appropriate treatment.

### Lyme Disease

The ocular manifestations of Lyme borreliosis most often are conjunctivitis, episcleritis, and uveitis; however, the disease may involve the orbit and present as orbital myositis or as a sclerosing orbital inflammation [148–150].

Lyme borreliosis can be diagnosed clinically based on symptoms and physical findings such as erythema migrans, facial palsy, and/or arthritis, combined with a history of possible or definite exposure to infected ticks. The diagnosis is easily confirmed by serologic and/or CSF studies, such as Western blot and ELISA to detect IgM to *Borrelia* antigen and PCR to detect genetic material. It is known to be difficult to culture *Borrelia*.

Early-stage Lyme disease usually is treated with one of several antibiotics for 2–3 weeks. More advanced disease requires prolonged antibiotic therapy. With early detection and treatment, the prognosis usually is favorable.

## Mycobacterial Infection

Tuberculosis has been reported to cause both unilateral and bilateral orbital apex and cavernous sinus syndromes (Fig. 24.21) [151].

As is the case with aspergillosis (see above), the infection may result from a tuberculoma or from invasive disease [152]. Tuberculosis involving the orbit may result from hematogenous spread of the organisms from a distant site or from direct extension of infection from the adjacent bone, sinus, lacrimal gland, or lacrimal sac. Ocular involvement by tuberculosis occurs in 1.4–18 % of patients with established disease [153], with the majority of cases characterized by asymptomatic choroiditis. But involvement of ocular and adnexal tissue has been described, including the cranial nerves passing through the orbital apex. The incidence of tuberculous orbital apex syndromes is unknown but thought to be very low.

The diagnosis of tuberculosis is not straightforward due to the difficulty in obtaining tissue samples from the site of infection. This has led the clinicians to being reliant on the tuberculin skin test, although in patients with lymphadenopathy or pulmonary disease, it may be possible to culture the organism or demonstrate caseating granuloma on biopsy. MR imaging findings are variable but typically show enhancing meningeal lesions, including the dura of the optic nerve sheath and in one case along the maxillary division of the trigeminal nerve [154].

Tuberculosis can be treated with a variety of drugs, sometimes combined with systemic corticosteroids. The rationale behind the use of systemic corticosteroid in these cases is to treat the presumed inflammatory component to the disease and to prevent a Jarisch-Herxheimer-type reaction on commencing antibiotics. This regimen was rapidly effective and achieved a good outcome in a case of tuberculous orbital inflammation [154].

## Parasitic Infection

Preechawat et al. reported a single case of gnathostomiasis causing an orbital apex syndrome [155]. Gnathostomiasis, also called larval migrans profundus, is a food-borne parasitic infection caused by the nematode *Gnathostoma spinigerum* or *Gnathostoma hispidum*. Humans are accidental hosts, infected by eating third-stage larvae encapsulated in raw freshwater fish. The infection most commonly manifests with intermittent migratory swelling in the skin and subcutaneous tissues related to larval migration. The parasite may migrate to the CNS, resulting in encephalitis or meningitis and may also involve the eye and/or orbit, causing lid swelling, uveitis, secondary glaucoma, and hemorrhage in the vitreous, retina, or choroid [156]. Ophthalmoplegia, pupillary disorders, and optic neuropathy can be observed in patients with CNS involvement [157, 158]. The diagnosis of gnathostomiasis should be suspected when there is recurrent migratory swelling associated with peripheral and/or CSF eosinophilia in an individual with a history of eating raw fish. Detection of *Gnathostoma* antigens and antibodies con-

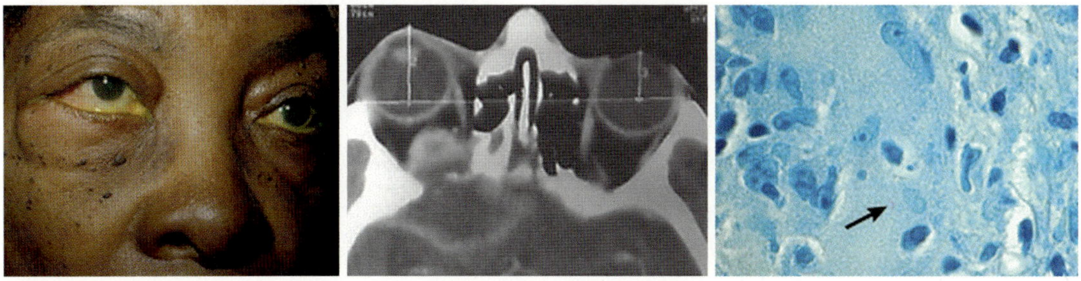

**Fig. 24.21** Right orbital apex syndrome from tuberculosis. *Left*, external appearance of the patient. *Center*, Axial CT scan shows a large mass in the orbital apex with erosion of the posterior orbital wall and abscess formation in the anterior right frontal lobe. *Right*, biopsy of the lesion shows a granulomatous reaction associated with the presence of rare mycobacteria (*arrow*)

firms the diagnosis. Albendazole and ivermectin may be effective for subcutaneous gnathostomiasis but not for intracranial or ocular involvement. In such cases, systemic corticosteroid therapy also may be required.

## References


1. Daniels DL, Mark LP, Mafee MF, et al. Osseous anatomy of the orbital apex. AJNR Am J Neuroradiol. 1995;16(9):1929–35.
2. Unger JM. Orbital apex fractures: the contribution of computed tomography. Radiology. 1984;150:713–7.
3. Wolfsberger S, Ba-Ssalamah A, Pinker K, et al. Application of three-tesla magnetic resonance imaging for diagnosis and surgery of sellar lesions. J Neurosurg. 2004;100:278–86.
4. Schick U, Hassler W. Neurosurgical management of orbital inflammations and infections. Acta Neurochir (Wien). 2004;146:571–80.
5. Islam N, Asaria R, Plant GT, et al. Giant cell arteritis mimicking idiopathic orbital inflammatory disease. Eur J Ophthalmol. 2003;13:221–4.
6. Newman LS, Rose CS, Maier LA. Sarcoidosis. N Engl J Med. 1997;336(17):1224–34.
7. Obenauf CD, Shaw HE, Sydnor CF, et al. Sarcoidosis and its ophthalmic manifestations. Am J Ophthalmol. 1978;86(5):648–55.
8. Collison JMT, Miller NR, Green WR. Involvement of orbital tissues by sarcoid. Am J Ophthalmol. 1986;102(3):302–7.
9. Jabs DA, Johns CJ. Ocular involvement in chronic sarcoidosis. Am J Ophthalmol. 1986;102(3):297–301.
10. Zarei M, Anderson JR, Higgins JN, et al. Cavernous sinus syndrome as the only manifestation of sarcoidosis. J Postgrad Med. 2002;48:119–21.
11. Segal EI, Tang RA, Lee AG, et al. Orbital apex lesion as the presenting manifestation of sarcoidosis. J Neuroophthalmol. 2000;20:156–8.
12. Prabhakaran VC, Saeed P, Esmaeli B, et al. Orbital and adnexal sarcoidosis. Arch Ophthalmol. 2007;125(12):1657–62.
13. Bezo C, Majzoub S, Nochez Y, et al. Ocular and neuro-ophthalmic manifestations of sarcoidosis: retrospective study of 30 cases. J Fr Ophthalmol. 2013;36(6):473–80.
14. American Thoracic Society. Statement on sarcoidosis. Am J Respir Crit Care Med. 1999;160(2):736–55.
15. Goldberg RA. Orbital steroid injections. Br J Ophthalmol. 2004;88(11):1359–60.
16. Perumal B, Black EH, Levin F, et al. Non-infectious orbital vasculitides. Eye. 2012;26(5):630–9.
17. Hoffman GS, Kerr GS, Leavitt RY, et al. Wegener granulomatosis. An analysis of 158 patients. Ann Intern Med. 1992;116:488–98.
18. Rao JK, Weinberger M, Oddone EZ, et al. The role of antineutrophil cytoplasmic antibody (c-ANCA) testing in the diagnosis of Wegener granulomatosis. A literature review and meta-analysis. Ann Intern Med. 1995;123:925–32.
19. Rothschild PR, Pagnoux C, Seror R, et al. Ophthalmologic manifestations of systemic necrotizing vasculitides at diagnosis: a retrospective study of 1286 patients and review of the literature. Semin Arthritis Rheum. 2013;42(5):507–14.
20. Anderson G, Coles ET, Crane M, et al. Wegener's granuloma. A series of 265 British cases seen between 1975 and 1985. A report by a sub-committee of the British Thoracic Society Research Committee. Q J Med. 1992;83:427–38.
21. Fauci AS, Haynes BF, Katz P, et al. Wegener's granulomatosis: prospective clinical and therapeutic experience with 85 patients for 21 years. Ann Intern Med. 1983;98:76–85.
22. Thorne JE, Jabs DA. Ocular manifestations of vasculitis. Rheum Dis Clin N Am. 2001;27:761–79.
23. Holle JU, Voigt C, Both M, et al. Orbital masses in granulomatosis with polyangiitis are associated with a refractory course and a high burden of local damage. Rheumatology. 2013;52(5):875–82.
24. Provenzale JM, Mukherji S, Allen NB, et al. Orbital involvement by Wegener's granulomatosis: imaging findings. AJR Am J Roentgenol. 1996;166:929–34.
25. Thajeb P, Tsai J-J. Cerebral and oculorhinal manifestations of a limited form of Wegener's granulomatosis with c-ANCA-associated vasculitis. J Neuroimaging. 2001;11:59–63.
26. Muhle C, Reinhold-Keller E, Richter C, et al. MRI of the nasal cavity, the paranasal sinuses and orbits in Wegener's granulomatosis. Eur Radiol. 1997;7:566–70.
27. Bertagna F, Treglia G, Rossioni P, et al. An unusual orbital localization of Wegener Granulomatosis detected by 18F-FDG PET/CT. Clin Nucl Med. 2013;39(8):711–2.
28. Beggs AD, Hain SF. F-18 FDG-position emission tomographic scanning and Wegener's granulomatosis. Clin Nucl Med. 2002;27(10):705–6.
29. Lagnford CA. Treatment of ANCA-associated vasculitis. N Engl J Med. 2003;349:3–4.
30. Pagnoux C, Mahr A, Hamidou MA, et al. Azathioprine or methotrexate maintenance for ANCA-associated vasculitis. N Engl J Med. 2008;359:2790–803.
31. Hughes J, Barkhoudarian G, Ciarlini P, et al. Refractory pituitary granulomatosis with polyangiitis (Wegener's) treated with rituximab. Endocr Pract. 2013;19(1):1–7.
32. Baslund B, Wiencke AK, Rasmussen N, et al. Treatment of orbital inflammation with rituximab in Wegener's granulomatosis. Clin Exp Rheumatol. 2012;30:7–10.
33. Cottin V, Cordier JF. Churg-Strauss syndrome. Allergy. 1999;54:535–51.

34. Masi AT, Hunder GG, Lie JT, et al. The American College of Rheumatology 1990 criteria for the classification of Churg-Strauss syndrome (allergic granulomatosis and angiitis). Arthritis Rheum. 1990;33:1094–100.
35. Tokumaru AM, Obata T, Kohyama S, et al. Intracranial meningeal involvement in Churg-Strauss syndrome. AJNR Am J Neuroradiol. 2002;23:221–4.
36. Pradeep TG, Prabhakaran VC, McNab A, et al. Diffuse bilateral orbital inflammation in Churg-Strauss syndrome. Ophthal Plast Reconstr Surg. 2010;26:57–9.
37. Takanashi T, Uchida S, Arita M, et al. Orbital inflammatory pseudotumor and ischemic vasculitis in Churg-Strauss syndrome: report of two cases and review of the literature. Ophthalmology. 2001;108:1129–33.
38. Abouzahir A, Bennouk Y, El Qatni M, et al. Ocular involvement in polyarteritis nodosa: two cases. J Fr Ophthalmol. 2012;35(9):724.
39. Ishida K, Yokota T, Wada Y, et al. Unilateral facial swelling and exophthalmos in a patient with polyarteritis nodosa. Intern Med. 1992;31:500–3.
40. Koike R, Yamada M, Matsunaga T, et al. Polyarteritis nodosa (PN) complicated with unilateral exophthalmos. Intern Med. 1993;32:232–6.
41. Hayreh SS, Podhajsky PA, Zimmerman B. Ocular manifestations of giant cell arteritis. Am J Ophthalmol. 1998;125:509–20.
42. Borruat FX, Bogousslavsky J, Uffer S, et al. Orbital infarction syndrome. Ophthalmology. 1993;100:562–8.
43. Cockerham KP, Cockerham GC, Brown HG, et al. Radiosensitive orbital inflammation associated with temporal arteritis. J Neuroophthalmol. 2003;23:117–21.
44. Fa'Amatuainu NA, Ng J, Kumar S, et al. Unusual presentations of giant cell arteritis (temporal arteritis). Int Med J. 2004;34:654–5.
45. Lee AG, Tang RA, Feldon SE, et al. Orbital presentations of giant cell arteritis. Graefes Arch Clin Exp Ophthalmol. 2001;239:509–13.
46. Ohsie LH, Murchison AP, Wojno TH. Lupus erythematosus profundus masquerading as idiopathic orbital inflammatory syndrome. Orbit. 2012;31(2):181–3.
47. Read RW. Clinical mini-review: systemic lupus erythematosus and the eye. Ocul Immunol Inflamm. 2004;12:87–99.
48. Jordan DR, McDonald H, Olberg B, et al. Orbital panniculitis as the initial manifestation of systemic lupus erythematosus. Ophthal Plast Reconstr Surg. 1993;9:71–5.
49. Stavrou P, Murray PI, Batta K, et al. Acute ocular ischaemia and orbital inflammation associated with systemic lupus erythematosus. Br J Ophthalmol. 2002;86:474–5.
50. Hochberg MC. Updating the American college of rheumatology revised criteria for the classification of systemic lupus erythematosus. Arthritis Rheum. 1997;40(9):1725.
51. Lateef A, Petri M. Biologics in the treatment of systemic lupus erythematosus. Curr Opin Rheumatol. 2010;22:504–9.
52. Hunt WE. Tolosa-Hunt syndrome: one cause of painful ophthalmoplegia. J Neurosurg. 1976;44:544–9.
53. Hunt WE, Meagher JN, LeFever HE, et al. Painful ophthalmoplegia. Its relation to indolent inflammation of the cavernous sinus. Neurology. 1961;11:56–62.
54. Aron-Rosa D, Doyon D, Sallamon G, et al. Tolosa-Hunt syndrome. Ann Ophthalmol. 1978;10:1161–8.
55. Granados-reyes GM, Soriano-Redondo E, Duran-Ferreras E. Tolosa-Hunt syndrome following traumatic eye injury. Rev Neurol. 2012;54(12):729–33.
56. Kline LB, Hoyt WF. The Tolosa-Hunt syndrome. J Neurol Neurosurg Psychiatry. 2001;71:577–82.
57. International Headache Society. The international classification of headache disorders. Cephalagia. 2004;24 Suppl 1:1–151.
58. Jain R, Sawhney S, Koul RL, et al. Tolosa-Hunt syndrome: MRI appearances. J Med Imaging Radiat Oncol. 2008;52(5):447–51.
59. Yousem DM, Atlas SW, Grossman RI, et al. MR imaging of Tolosa-Hunt syndrome. AJR Am J Roentgenol. 1990;154(1):167–70.
60. Julien J, Vallat JM, Vallat M, et al. Orbital phlebography in the diagnosis of painful ophthalmoplegia. Neuroradiology. 1975;9:163–6.
61. Zafrulla KM, Dhir SP, Jain IS. Tolosa-Hunt syndrome. Ind J Ophthalmol. 1977;25:21–6.
62. Forderreuther S, Straube A. The criteria of the International Headache Society for Tolosa-Hunt syndrome need to be revised. J Neurol. 1999;246:371–7.
63. Smith JR, Rosenbaum JT. A role for methotrexate in the management of non-infectious orbital inflammatory disease. Br J Ophthalmol. 2001;85:1220–4.
64. Hannerz J. Recurrent Tolosa-Hunt syndrome. Cephalalgia. 1992;12:45–51.
65. Mormont E, Lalous P, Vauthier J, et al. Radiotherapy in a case of Tolosa-Hunt syndrome. Cephalalgia. 2000;20:931–3.
66. Yuen SJ, Rubin PA. Idiopathic orbital inflammation: distribution, clinical features, and treatment outcome. Arch Ophthalmol. 2003;121(4):491–9.
67. Weber AL, Romo LV, Sabates NR. Pseudotumor of the orbit. Clinical, pathologic, and radiologic evaluation. Radiol Clin N Am. 1999;37(1):151–68.
68. Mombaerts I, Schlingemann RO, Goldschmeding R, et al. Idiopathic granulomatous orbital inflammation. Ophthalmology. 1996;103:2135–41.
69. LeBedis CA, Sakai O. Nontraumatic orbital conditions: diagnosis with CT and MR imaging in the emergent setting. RadioGraphics. 2008;28(6):1742–53.
70. Narla LD, Newman B, Spottswood SS, et al. Inflammatory pseudotumor. Radiographics. 2003;23:719–29.
71. Lindfield D, Attfield K, McElvanney A. Systemic immunoglobulin G4 (IgG4) disease and idiopathic

orbital inflammation; removing 'idiopathic' from the nomenclature? Eye. 2012;26(5):623–9.

72. Wallace ZS, Khosroshahi A, Jakobiec FA, et al. IgG4-related systemic disease as a cause of "idiopathic" orbital inflammation, including orbital myositis, and trigeminal nerve involvement. Surv Ophthalmol. 2012;57(1):26–33.
73. Schweier C, Kordic H, Chaloupka K. IgG4-related orbital inflammation. Klin Monbl Augenheilkd. 2013;230(4):370–3.
74. Japanese Study Group of IgG4-Related Ophthalmic Disease. A prevalence study of IgG4-related ophthalmic disease in Japan. Jpn J Ophthalmol. 2013;57(6):573–9.
75. Umehara H, Okazaki K, Masaki Y, et al. Comprehensive diagnostic criteria for IgG4-related disease (IgG4-RD). Mod Rheumatol. 2011;22:21–30.
76. Fujita A, Sakai O, Chapman MN, et al. IgG4-related disease of the head and neck: CT and MR imaging manifestation. Radiographics. 2012;32(7):1945–58.
77. Origuchi T, Yano H, Nakamura H, et al. Three cases of IgG4-related orbital inflammation presented as unilateral pseudotumor and review of the literature. Rheumatol Int. 2012;33(11):2931–6.
78. Leibovitch I, Prabhakaran VC, Davis G, et al. Intraorbital injection of triamcinolone acetonide in patients with idiopathic orbital inflammation. Arch Ophthalmol. 2007;125:1647–51.
79. Harris GJ. Idiopathic orbital inflammation: a pathogenetic construct and treatment strategy: the 2005 ASOPRS Foundation Lecture. Ophthal Plast Reconstr Surg. 2006;22:79–86.
80. Thorne JE, Volpe NJ, Wulc AE, Galetta SL. Caught by a masquerade: sclerosing orbital inflammation. Surv Ophthalmol. 2002;47:50–4.
81. Jacobs D, Galetta S. Diagnosis and management of orbital pseudotumor. Curr Opin Ophthalmol. 2002;13:347–51.
82. Patel AK, Hoch S, Shindler KS. Mycophenolate mofetil treatment of steroid-resistant idiopathic sclerosing orbital inflammation. Clin Exp Ophthalmol. 2011;39(9):912–3.
83. Hatton MP, Rubin PA, Foster CS. Successful treatment of idiopathic orbital inflammation with mycophenolate mofetil. Am J Ophthalmol. 2005;140(5):916–8.
84. Michalova K, Lim L. Biologic agents in the management of inflammatory eye disease. Curr Allergy Asthma Rep. 2008;8(4):339–47.
85. Badiee P, Jafarpour Z, Alborzi A, et al. Orbital mucormycosis in an immunocompetent individual. IJM. 2012;4:210–4.
86. Galetta SL, Wulc AE, Goldberg HI, et al. Rhinocerebral mucormycosis: management and survival after carotid occlusion. Ann Neurol. 1990;28:103–7.
87. Hurst RW, Judkins A, Bolger W, et al. Mycotic aneurysm and cerebral infarction resulting from fungal sinusitis: imaging and pathologic correlation. AJNR Am J Neuroradiol. 2001;22:858–63.
88. Breadmore R, Desmond P, Opeskin K. Intracranial aspergillosis producing cavernous sinus syndrome and rupture of internal carotid artery. Australas Radiol. 1994;38:72–5.
89. McLean FM, Ginsberg LE, Stanton CA. Perineural spread of rhinocerebral mucormycosis. AJNR Am J Neuroradiol. 1996;17:114–6.
90. Jones J, Katz SE, Lubow M. Scedosporium apiospermum of the orbit. Arch Ophthalmol. 1999;117:272–3.
91. Thiagalingam S, Fernando GT, Tan K, O'Donnell BA, et al. Orbital apex syndrome secondary to Pseudallescheria boydii fungal sinusitis in an immunocompetent patient. Clin Exp Ophthalmol. 2004;32:545–7.
92. Gamaletsou MN, Sipsas NV, Roilides E. Rhino-orbito-cerebral mucormycosis. Curr Infect Dis Rep. 2012;14(4):423–34.
93. Bray WH, Giangiacomo J, Ide CH. Orbital apex syndrome. Surv Ophthalmol. 1987;32:136–40.
94. Okada Y, Shima T, Nishida M, et al. Subarachnoid hemorrhage caused by Aspergillus aneurysm as a complication of transcranial biopsy of an orbital apex lesion. Neurol Med Chir (Tokyo). 1998; 38(7):432–7.
95. Balch K, Phillips PH, Newman NJ. Painless orbital apex syndrome from mucormycosis. J Neuroophthalmol. 1997;17(3):178–82.
96. Petrick M, Honegger J, Daschner F, et al. Fungal granuloma of the sphenoid sinus and clivus in a patient presenting with cranial nerve III paresis: case report and review of the literature. Neurosurgery. 2003;52:955–9.
97. Fairley C, Sullivan TJ, Bartley P, et al. Survival after rhino-orbital-cerebral mucormycosis in an immunocompetent patient. Ophthalmology. 2000; 107:555–8.
98. O'Toole L, Acheson JA, Kidd D. Orbital apex lesion due to Aspergillosis presenting in immunocompetent patients without apparent sinus disease. J Neurol. 2008;255(11):1798–801.
99. Thurtell MJ, Chiu AL, Goold LA, et al. Neuro-ophthalmology of invasive fungal sinusitis: 14 consecutive patients and a review of the literature. Clin Exp Ophthalmol. 2012;41(6):567–76.
100. Martin-Moro JG, Calleja JM, Garcia MB, et al. Rhino-orbito-cerebral mucormycosis: a case report and literature review. Med Oral Patol. 2008;13:792–5.
101. Chen SC, Playford EG, Sorrell TC. Antifungal therapy in invasive fungal infections. Curr Opin Pharmacol. 2010;10:522–30.
102. Weinstein JM, Sattler FA, Towfighi J, et al. Optic neuropathy and paratrigeminal syndrome due to Aspergillus fumigatus. Arch Neurol. 1982; 39:582–5.
103. Moling O, Lass-Floerl C, Verweji PE, et al. Case reports: chronic and acute Aspergillus meningitis. Mycoses. 2002;45:504–11.

104. Cunha BA. Central nervous system infections in the compromised host: a diagnostic approach. Infect Dis Clin N Am. 2001;15:567–90.
105. Kleinschmidt-DeMasters BK. Central nervous system aspergillosis: a 20-year retrospective series. JUM Pathol. 2002;33:116–24.
106. Golin V, Sprovieri SR, Cancado JE, et al. Aspergillosis of the central nervous system. Rev Paul Med. 1996;114:1274–7.
107. Walsh TJ, Hier DB, Caplan LR. Aspergillosis of the central nervous system: clinicopathological analysis of 17 patients. Ann Neurol. 1985;18:574–82.
108. Satoh H, Uozumi T, Kiya K, et al. Invasive aspergilloma of the frontal base causing internal carotid occlusion. Surg Neurol. 1995;44:483–8.
109. Pruitt AA. Nervous system infections in patients with cancer. Neurol Clin. 2003;21:193–219.
110. Wilms G, Lammens M, Dom R, et al. MR imaging of intracranial aspergilloma extending from the sphenoid sinus in an immunocompromised patient with multiple myeloma. J Belg Radiol. 1992;75:29–32.
111. Chang T, Teng MMH, Wang SF, et al. Aspergillosis of the paranasal sinuses. Neuroradiology. 1992;34:520–3.
112. Breen DJ, Clifton AG, Wilkins P, et al. Invasive aspergilloma of the skull base. Neuroradiology. 1993;35:216–7.
113. Haran RP, Chandy MJ. Intracranial Aspergillus granuloma. Br J Neurosurg. 1993;7:383–8.
114. Dortzbach RK, Segrest DR. Orbital aspergillosis. Ophthalmic Surg. 1983;14:240–4.
115. Swoboda H, Ullrich R. Aspergilloma in the frontal sinus expanding into the orbit. J Clin Pathol. 1992;45:629–30.
116. Qu Q, Wang X, Teng L. Five cases of invasive rhino-orbital-skull base aspergillosis with orbit apex syndrome initial presentation. Lin Chung Er Bi Yan Hou Tou Jing Wai Ke Za Zhi. 2010;24(9):396–9.
117. Muller FM, Trusen A, Weig M. Clinical manifestations and diagnosis of invasive aspergillosis in immunocompromised children. Eur J Pediatr. 2002;161:563–74.
118. Graham DA, Kinyoun JL, Georger DP. Endogenous Aspergillus endophthalmitis after lung transplantation. Am J Ophthalmol. 1995;119:107–9.
119. Polo JM, Fabrega E, Casafot F, et al. Treatment of cerebral aspergillosis after liver transplantation. Neurology. 1992;42:1817–9.
120. Scamoni C, Dario A, Pozzi M, et al. Drainage of Aspergillus "primitive" brain abscess with long-term survival. J Neurol Sci. 1990;34:155–8.
121. Camarata PJ, Dunn DL, Farney AC, et al. Continual intracavitary administration of amphotericin B as an adjunct in the treatment of Aspergillus brain abscess: case report and review of the literature. Neurosurgery. 1992;31:575–9.
122. Sethi A, Sareen D, Mrig S, et al. Acute suppurative otitis media: an unusual cause of orbital apex syndrome. Orbit. 2008;27:462–5.
123. Cannon ML, Antonio BL, McCloskey JJ, et al. Cavernous sinus thrombosis complicating sinusitis. Pediatr Crit Care Med. 2004;5:86–8.
124. Ebright JR, Pace MT, Niazi AF. Septic thrombosis of the cavernous sinuses. Arch Intern Med. 2001;161:2671–6.
125. Southwick RFS, Richardson Jr EP, Swartz MD. Septic thrombosis of the dural venous sinuses. Medicine. 1986;65:82–106.
126. Holland NR. CNS actinomyces presenting with bilateral cavernous sinus syndrome. J Neurol Neurosurg Psychiatry. 1998;64:4.
127. Ohta S, Nishizawa S, Namba H, et al. Bilateral cavernous sinus actinomycosis resulting in painful ophthalmoplegia. J Neurosurg. 2002;96:600–2.
128. Colson AE, Daily JP. Orbital apex syndrome and cavernous sinus thrombosis due to infection with Staphylococcus aureus and Pseudomonas aeruginosa. Clin Infect Dis. 1999;29:701–2.
129. Kurimoto T, Tonari M, Ishizaki N, et al. Orbital apex syndrome associated with herpes zoster ophthalmicus. Clin Ophthalmol. 2011;5:1603–8.
130. Schoenlaub P, Grange F, Nasica X, et al. Oculomotor nerve paralysis with complete ptosis in herpes zoster ophthalmicus: 2 cases. Ann Dermatol Venereol. 1997;124:401–3.
131. Pavan-Langston D. Herpes zoster ophthalmicus. Neurology. 1995;45(12):50–1.
132. Capoferri C, Martorina M, Menga M. Herpes zoster ophthalmoplegia in two hemodialysis patients. Neuro-Ophthalmology. 1997;17:49–51.
133. Lexa FJ, Galetta SL, Yousem DM, et al. Herpes zoster ophthalmicus with orbital pseudotumor syndrome complicated by optic nerve infarction and cerebral granulomatous angiitis: MR-pathologic correlation. AJNR Am J Neuroradiol. 1993;14:185–90.
134. Amanat LA, Cant JS, Green FD. Acute phthisis bulbi and external ophthalmoplegia in herpes zoster ophthalmicus. Ann Ophthalmol. 1985;17:46–51.
135. Chang-Godinich A, Lee AG, Brazis PW, et al. Complete ophthalmoplegia after zoster ophthalmicus. J Neuroophthalmol. 1997;17:262–5.
136. Marsh RJ, Dudley B, Kelly V. External ocular motor palsies in ophthalmic zoster: a review. Br J Ophthalmol. 1977;61:677–82.
137. Bourke RD, Pyle J. Herpes zoster ophthalmicus and the orbital apex syndrome. Aust N Z J Ophthalmol. 1994;22:77–80.
138. Vardy SJ, Rose GE. Orbital disease in herpes zoster ophthalmicus. Eye. 1994;8:577–9.
139. Goldsmith MO. Herpes zoster ophthalmicus with sixth nerve palsy. Can J Ophthalmol. 1968;3:279–83.
140. Deane JS, Bibby K. Bilateral optic neuritis following herpes zoster ophthalmicus. Arch Ophthalmol. 1995;113:972–3.
141. Archambault P, Wise JS, Rosen J, et al. Herpes zoster ophthalmoplegia: report of six cases. J Clin Neuroophthalmol. 1988;8:185–93.

142. Tatlipnar S, Sener E, Sarac OI, et al. Trochlear nerve palsy in herpes zoster ophthalmicus. Neuro-Ophthalmology. 2001;26:247–51.
143. Chang-Godinich A, Lee AG, Brazis PW, et al. Complete ophthalmoplegia after zoster ophthalmicus. J Neuroophthalmol. 1997;17(4):262–5.
144. Womack LW, Liesegang TJ. Complications of herpes zoster ophthalmicus. Arch Ophthalmol. 1983;101(1):42–5.
145. Marsh RJ, Cooper M. Ophthalmic herpes zoster. Eye. 1993;7:350–70.
146. Arda H, Mirza E, Gumus K, et al. Orbital apex syndrome in herpes zoster ophthalmicus. Case Rep Ophthalmol Med. 2012;2012:854503.
147. Keane JR. Melkersson's syndrome associated with syphilis. J Clin Neuroophthalmol. 1988;8: 249–51.
148. Zagorski Z, Biziorek B, Haszcz D. Ophthalmic manifestations of Lyme borreliosis. Przegl Epidemiol. 2002;56:85–90.
149. Mikkila HO, Seppala IJ, Viljanen MK, et al. The expanding clinical spectrum of ocular Lyme borreliosis. Ophthalmology. 2000;107(3): 581–7.
150. Nieto JC, Kim N, Lucarelli MJ. Dacryoadenitis and orbital myositis associated with Lyme disease. Arch Ophthalmol. 2008;126(8):1165–6.
151. Bafna S, Lee AG. Presumed tuberculosis presenting as a cavernous sinus syndrome. J Neuroophthalmol. 1997;17:207–8.
152. Rebai R, Boudawara MZ, Bahloul K, et al. Cavernous sinus syndrome secondary to tuberculous meningitis. Eur Neurol. 2002;47:125–6.
153. Bouza E, Merino P, Munoz P, et al. Ocular tuberculosis, a prospective study in a general hospital. Medicine. 1997;76:53–61.
154. Hughes EH, Petrushkin H, Sibtain NA, et al. Tuberculous orbital apex syndromes. Br J Ophthalmol. 2008;92:1511–7.
155. Preechawat P, Wongwatthana P, Poonyathalang A, et al. Orbital apex syndrome from gnathostomiasis. J Neuroophthalmol. 2006;26(3):184–6.
156. Biswas J, Gopal L, Sharma T, et al. Intraocular Gnathostoma spinigerum: clinicopathologic study of two cases with review of literature. Retina. 1994;14:438–44.
157. Boongird P, Phuapradit P, Siridej N, et al. Neurological manifestations of gnathostomiasis. J Neurol Sci. 1977;31:279–91.
158. Punyagupta S, Bunnag T, Juttijudata P. Eosinophilic meningitis in Thailand. Clinical and epidemiological characteristic of 162 patients with myeloencephalitis probably caused by Gnathostoma spinigerum. J Neurol Sci. 1990;96:241–56.

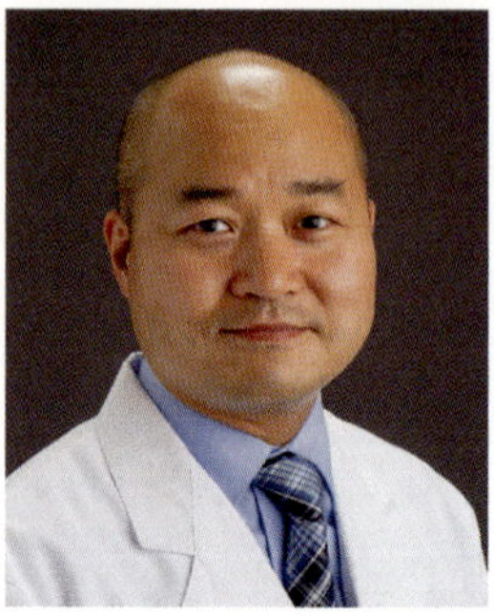

**Bokkwan Jun** Dr. Bokkwan Jun is a Neuro-Ophthalmologist and is currently assistant professor of Ophthalmology in University of Missouri, Columbia, MO, USA. He trained in Ophthalmology at Hanyang University, Neurology at Saint Louis University and Neuro-Ophthalmology at Johns-Hopkins University.

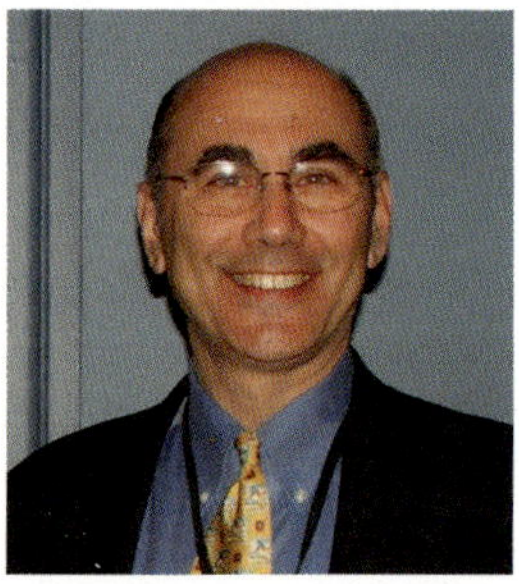

**Neil R. Miller** Dr. Neil Miller is currently Professor of Ophthalmology, Neurology, and Neurosurgery at the Johns Hopkins Medical Institutions and also the Frank B. Walsh Professor of Neuro-Ophthalmology. Dr. Miller was President of the North American Neuro-Ophthalmology Society from 2000 to 2002 and Chairman of its Executive Board from 2002 to 2004. He has been past President of the International Neuro-Ophthalmology Society on three occasions: in 1982, 1992, and 2008. He is also an emeritus member of the International Orbital Society. In 2009, he was given the Lifetime Achievement Award by the American Academy of Ophthalmology (AAO). He has authored or co-authored 500 articles, 90 chapters, and 13 books in the fields of neuro-ophthalmology and orbital disease. Many of Dr. Miller's previous fellows and residents hold faculty positions at major institutions throughout the United States and around the world.

# Pyoderma Gangrenosum

# 25

Elisabetta Miserocchi, Lorenzo Iuliano,
and Giulio Modorati

## Introduction

Pyoderma gangrenosum, first described by Brocq [1] and named by Brunsting [2] in 1930, is a rare, ulcerating, neutrophilic dermatosis primarily affecting patients aged 25–54 years, without a clear gender predilection. Epidemiologic data establishing disease incidence have yet to be published [3, 4].

## Clinical Presentation

A pyoderma gangrenosum lesion typically starts as a tender nodule, plaque, or sterile pustule that enlarges and erodes, over a course of days, into a sharply marginated ulcer with undermined, violaceous borders and a surrounding zone of erythema; pain is a characteristic feature. The skin and subcutis become necrotic, creating a friable wound bed often with a hemorrhagic or purulent exudate, sometimes extending as deep as the muscle. Cribriform or "sieve-like" atrophic scars often form as the lesions heal. Lesions typically are multiple and recurrent and tend to occur at areas of trauma, a process known as pathergy.

A hallmark of pyoderma gangrenosum is the purulent aspect of lesions, which seems to be infectious. No microorganism growth can be detected, but the caseating necrotic aspect of lesions is confounding about possible mycobacterial infection ("pseudotuberculous appearance") [5–10].

Pyoderma gangrenosum lesions in adults most frequently affect the lower extremities, but any anatomic site can be affected. In children (approximately 4 % of cases), it typically involves the lower extremities, buttocks, and perineal region, as well as the head and neck.

Pyoderma gangrenosum may also involve extracutaneous sites such as the eye, the lungs (aseptic pulmonary nodules), the spleen, and the musculoskeletal system in the form of sterile pyoarthrosis and neutrophilic myositis [4].

## Physiopathology

The pathophysiology of pyoderma gangrenosum remains poorly understood though is now believed to involve loss of innate immune regulation and altered neutrophil chemotaxis.

T-cells are involved in the regulation of both macrophage and neutrophil function, and helper T-cell abnormalities have been demonstrated in patients with pyoderma gangrenosum [11, 12].

E. Miserocchi, MD (✉) • L. Iuliano, MD
G. Modorati, MD
Ophthalmology, San Raffaele Scientific Institute,
Vita-Salute University, Milan 20132, Italy
e-mail: miserocchi.elisabetta@hsr.it;
iuliano.lorenzo@hsr.it; modorati.giulio@hsr.it


B. Mukherjee, H. Yuen (eds.), *Emergencies of the Orbit and Adnexa*,
DOI 10.1007/978-81-322-1807-4_25

It is not known whether the skin ulcers occur secondary to this immune dysfunction or if the lesions are the result of an inappropriate inflammatory response against some factor in the skin. Furthermore, emerging evidence of the clinical efficacy of tumor necrosis factor (TNF) alpha inhibitor therapy strongly suggests a key role for this cytokine in this disease [3, 13, 14].

## Association

Pyoderma gangrenosum is associated with underlying systemic diseases in at least half of patients; the remainder of cases are considered idiopathic. Inflammatory bowel disease (IBD), arthritis, and hematologic disorders are the most common disease associations [15, 16]. Although in most cases pyoderma gangrenosum was diagnosed after the associated disease, it may also precede or be the presenting sign of an underlying disease. The courses of the two diseases are sometimes, but not necessarily, parallel [17, 18].

Other association [3]:

- Less common: hematologic malignancy and other hematologic abnormality, monoclonal gammopathy, arthritis
- Rare: hidradenitis suppurativa, pyogenic arthritis, pyoderma gangrenosum and acne (PAPGA) syndrome, pulmonary disease, systemic lupus erythematosus, thyroid disease, solid organ malignancy, autoimmune hepatitis, sarcoidosis

## Diagnosis

Pyoderma gangrenosum remains a clinical diagnosis; it lacks specific serologic or histologic markers. Although no clinical criteria have been formally adopted, one proposed set requires the fulfillment of two major criteria [18–21]:

1. Rapid progression (margin expansion of 1–2 cm per day, or 50 % increase in ulcer size within 1 month) of a painful, necrolytic, cutaneous ulcer with an irregular, violaceous, and undermined border
2. Exclusion of other causes of cutaneous ulceration

and at least two minor criteria:

1. A history suggestive of pathergy or a clinical finding of cribriform scarring
2. Systemic diseases associated with PG
3. Histopathologic findings (sterile dermal neutrophilia, mixed inflammation, lymphocytic vasculitis)
4. Treatment response (rapid response to systemic corticosteroid treatment)

## Ocular Involvement

Ophthalmic involvement is rare. Isolated ocular localization of pyoderma gangrenosum is very rare, while an ophthalmic extension if other simultaneous cutaneous lesions are present makes the diagnosis easier. Pyoderma gangrenosum may involve the sclera, cornea, orbit, and ocular adnexa. Different ophthalmic segments may also be concurrently interested.

Scleral involvement clinically presents as a necrotizing scleritis (Fig. 25.1), where an abscess formation is the hallmark of the disease. Severe cases of sclerocorneal extension of the disease may result in cutaneous and scleral fistula, associated with hypopyon in the anterior chamber.

Regarding corneal involvement, cases of peripheral ulcerative keratitis (PUK) have been reported (Fig. 25.2). Pyoderma gangrenosum-associated PUK shares many similarities with collagen vascular disease-associated PUK. Residual corneal scarring with conjunctivalization and contiguous scleral thinning may be present after sclerokeratitis resolution [22–28].

Orbital involvement includes the eyelid, lacrimal sac, and the deep post-septal orbital tissues, including the lacrimal gland. Intraorbital (post-septal) extension is rare and tends to occur deep to the lateral canthus. Lacrimal sac involvement may be clinically confused with a chronic dacryocystitis. In the eyelid, necrosis appears characteristically to

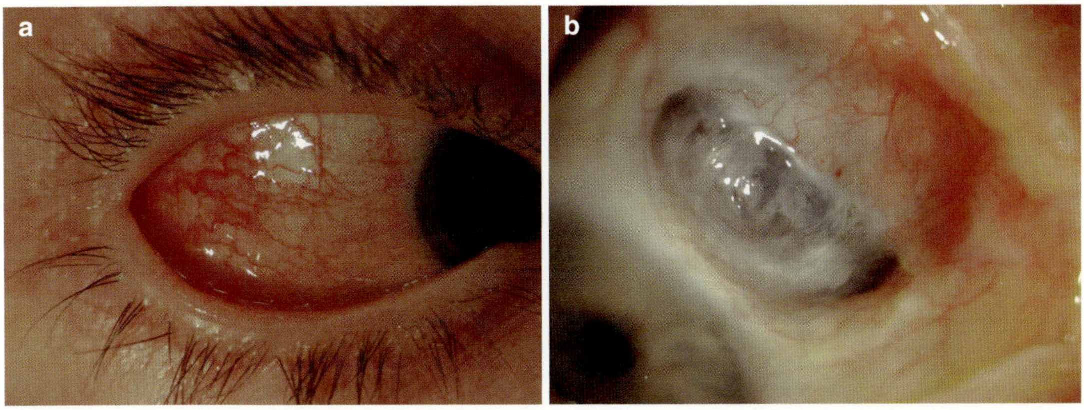


**Fig. 25.1** Two cases of necrotizing scleritis in patients with pyoderma gangrenosum associated with Crohn's disease. (**a**) Acute scleritis at presentation. Both episcleral and deep scleral vessels are markedly inflamed. Note the *white* circumscribed avascular area of necrosis. (**b**) Advanced phase. The uvea is visible under marked scleral thinning, next to an area of scleritis

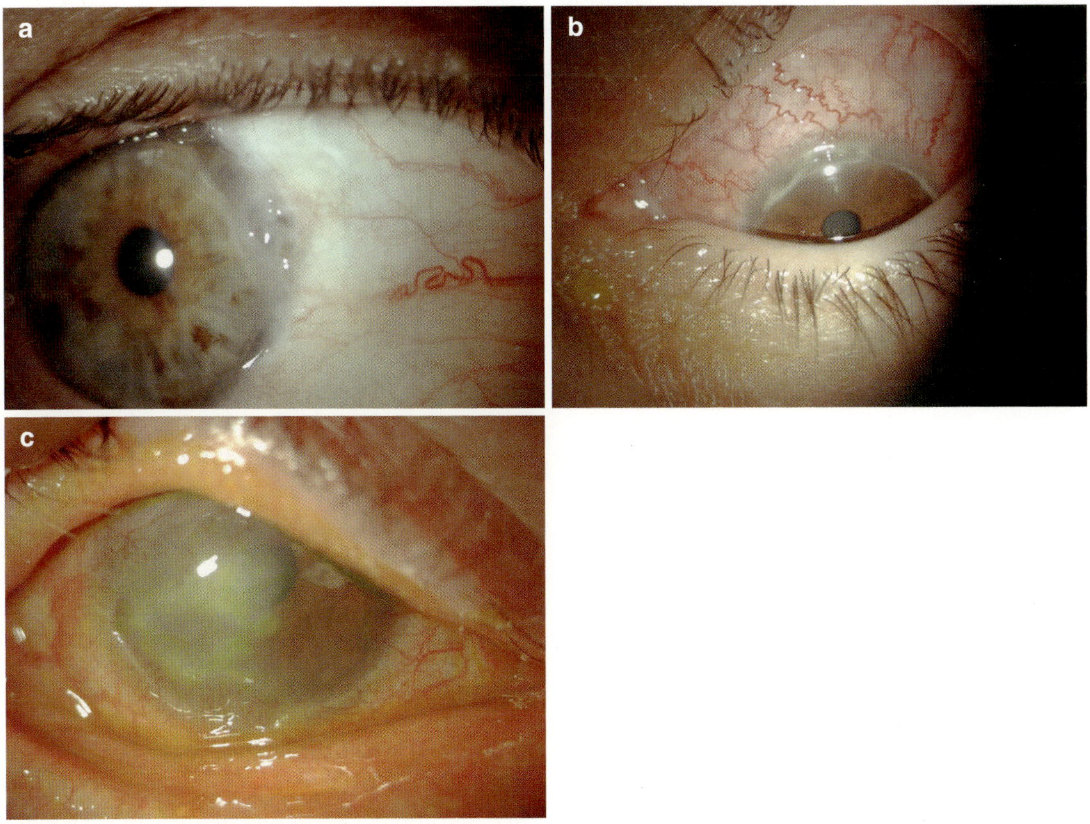


**Fig. 25.2** Typical clinical pictures of peripheral ulcerative keratitis. (**a**) A 52-year-old woman with rheumatoid arthritis. The lesion has a bullous-like aspect, invading the cornea and with adjacent dilated conjunctival vessels. (**b**) A 39-year-old woman with acute myeloid leukemia. The ulcerative keratitis is adjacent to an area of scleritis. (**c**) A 48-year-old man with Crohn's disease. Severe peripheral ulcerative keratitis in advanced phase, with stromal opacity, corneal neovascularization, and scleritis

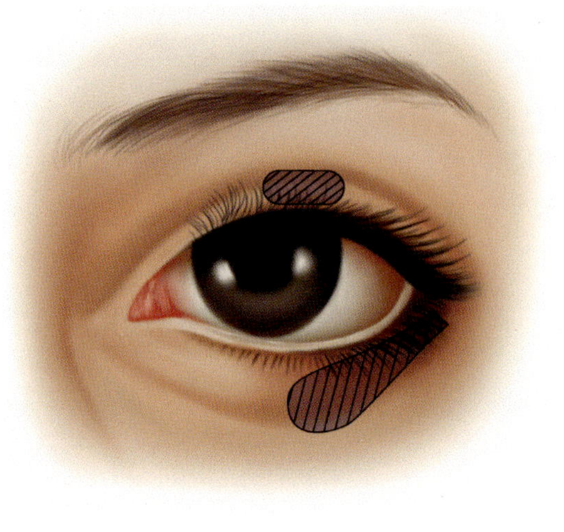

**Fig. 25.3** Diagram of eyelid involvement in pyoderma gangrenosum. The necrosis typically spares the marginal bar of upper lid tarsus (alongside the tarsomarginal artery) and favors the central one-third of the upper lid and lateral two-thirds of the lower lid

spare the marginal bar of upper lid tarsus (alongside the tarsomarginal artery) and to favor the central one-third of the upper lid and lateral two-thirds of the lower lid (Fig. 25.3). Healing process of periocular wounds may result also in a cicatricial ectropion [29–35].

## Workup

Once diagnosis has been done, it is imperative to exclude infection or malignancy as part of the initial workup, especially if the patient will undergo systemic immunosuppression.

Routine laboratory tests as an initial screen for hematologic disorders and liver or kidney dysfunction related to a variety of possible associated conditions.

- Systemic vasculitis: antinuclear antibody, coagulopathy panel including antiphospholipid antibody test, cryoglobulins, rheumatoid factor, circulating antineutrophil cytoplasmic antibodies
- IBD: fecal occult blood test and sigmoidoscopy/colonoscopy
- Hematologic disease: serum protein electrophoresis, urine spot protein, or urine protein electrophoresis, immunofixation electrophoresis, peripheral smear, bone marrow biopsy
- Infectious causes: HIV test, hepatitis serologies, and rapid plasma regain (if risk factors exist)

Radiologic examination (chest X-rays, computed tomography, magnetic resonance imaging) should be performed according to the clinical suspect. MRI is a powerful tool for evaluating the extent of extracutaneous pyoderma gangrenosum lesions in the periocular tissues. Acute inflammation shows marked homogeneous hyperintensity on fat-saturated T2-weighted image and hypointensity on T1-weighted image. Fibrosis reveals marked hypointensity on T2-weighted image and hyperintensity on T1-weighted image.

Wound care should be arranged by expert dermatologist. Pain specialist may be required for appropriate pain management.

## Treatment

No approved guidelines are available for the treatment of pyoderma gangrenosum ocular involvement. Current approach is aggressive, as an ocular extension of pyoderma gangrenosum makes the grade of disease severe. Usually combination of topical and systemic agents is required. Internal medicine expert consultation is mandatory in case of severe or refractory disease, requiring biological or immunosuppressive therapy. It should also be considered to raise the corticosteroid dose during any surgical procedure, to avoid healing problem or ulcer formation (both in the recipient and in the graft donor site) after surgery.

Ocular PG requires a different management according to the localization [3, 36]. Treatment may be topical and/or systemic. Topical treatment requires:

- High-penetrating corticosteroids (dexamethasone, difluprednate): drops or ophthalmic ointment are preferred, as dermatologic agents should be avoided in contact with the eye

- Fortified antimicrobic agents (vancomycin, gentamicin, and cefazolin)
- Artificial tear: drops or ophthalmic ointment of hyaluronate sodium 0.2–0.3 %

Topical tacrolimus should be avoided, since there is no experience about its ophthalmic use. Also intralesional agents (corticosteroid and cyclosporine A) should be avoided due to the lack of experience in ophthalmology. Furthermore, they should be used with caution as too frequent injections or an excessively high concentration can lead to pathergy and disrupt wound healing. Systemic agents are summarized in Table 25.1.

Granulocyte apheresis is a new therapeutic modality for IBD that exerts immunomodulatory

**Table 25.1** Systemic treatment for pyoderma gangrenosum

| Class | Agent | Dosage | Notes | Lab monitoring |
|---|---|---|---|---|
| Corticosteroid | Prednisone | 0.5–1 mg/kg/day oral | Response is usually rapid (2–3 days), halting lesion progression and preventing development of new lesions. Pulsed-dose steroids can also be used, but should be reserved for rapidly progressive disease. Consider tapering after intensive treatment | Blood pressure, blood glucose |
| | Methylprednisolone | Up to 0.8 mg/kg/day oral | | |
| T-cell inhibitor | Cyclosporine | 3–5 mg/kg/day (in divided doses), for up to 3 weeks | Should be used for acute control of pyoderma gangrenosum or in idiopathic disease, but is not appropriate as a long-term maintenance therapy for patients with chronic underlying conditions such as IBD | CBC, CMP |
| Anti TNF-α agents | Infliximab | 3–10 mg/kg infusion at 0, 2, 6, 8 weeks and then every 4–8 weeks | Frequently used to treat specific associated conditions including Crohn's disease. Adverse effects with all biologics include increased risk of infections (and reactivation of tuberculosis), hepatic necrosis indexes elevation, demyelinating disease, a lupus-like syndrome, and a possible increased risk of malignancy | CBC, CMP HBV, HCV, latent TBC |
| | Adalimumab | 40-mg subcutaneous injection every 1–2 weeks | | |
| | Etanercept | 25-mg subcutaneous injection 1–2 times weekly | | |
| Anti-neutrophilic agents | Colchicine | 1 mg bid or tid for 4–7 days oral | Demonstrated efficacy as an adjunct to corticosteroid therapy | |
| | Dapsone | 50–200 mg/day oral | | |
| Antimetabolite | Mycophenolate mofetil | 500–1,500 mg bid oral | Generally considered most effective as adjunctive treatments | CBC, CMP |
| | Methotrexate | 7.5–20 mg per week given with folic acid, oral | | |
| | Azathioprine | 2–2.5 mg/kg/day or 150 mg/day oral | | |

(continued)

**Table 25.1** (continued)

| Class | Agent | Dosage | Notes | Lab monitoring |
|---|---|---|---|---|
| Other | Intravenous immunoglobulin | From 0.5 mg to 1 g/kg/day for 2 days, or 0.4 g/kg/day for 5 days with the number of monthly treatments ranging from 2 to 6 | Very severe or refractory cases | |
| Alkylating agents | Cyclophosphamide | 2 mg/kg/day oral | The adverse effects associated with these medications including myelosuppression and hemorrhagic cystitis (with cyclophosphamide) generally limits their use to severe, refractory cases | CBC with differential |
| | Chlorambucil | 2–4 mg/day oral for 1 week followed by 2 mg/week | | |

*CBC* complete blood count, *CMP* complete metabolic panel

effects by selectively removing activated granulocytes and monocytes from peripheral blood, which efficacy in refractory lesions has been reported in several case reports.

The general management is reported in Fig. 25.4.

## PUK or Sclerokeratitis

PUK, necrotizing scleritis or sclerokeratitis management include:

- Hourly topical fortified antibiotic agents
- Hourly topical steroids
- Artificial tears

Conjunctival resection, removing collagenases localized in the conjunctiva adjacent to PUK and even temporarily interrupting the local immunologic events leading to corneal ulceration, is useful for many immune ulcerative conditions, but often makes matters worse in patients with pyoderma gangrenosum.

Cases of scleral or corneal perforation need expert consultation. Fibrin glue tissue adhesive or bandage contact lens may be used as initial management. Tectonic perforating keratoplasty must be promptly performed in case of corneal perforation. Small-incision surgery, when possible, might be advantageous to reduce the risk for a pathergic reaction [3, 27, 28].

## Lacrimal Sac

Isolated lacrimal sac involvement is almost impossible to diagnose. Dacryocystectomy with histological examination should be preferred to obtain a definitive diagnosis. A conjunctivodacryocystorhinostomy with Jones tube placement may be further performed to avoid epiphora. Systemic treatment is mandatory. Intralesional agents may be considered [33, 35].

## Eyelid

Systemic treatment is mandatory, while intralesional agents should be avoided.

In case of severe tissue loss, eyelid reconstruction should be performed with a different technique, according to lesion extension: direct synthesis, skin transposition, or full-thickness skin graft (usually supraclavicular or retroauricular) associated with a lateral tarsal strip procedure and scar tissue release [3, 29, 32].

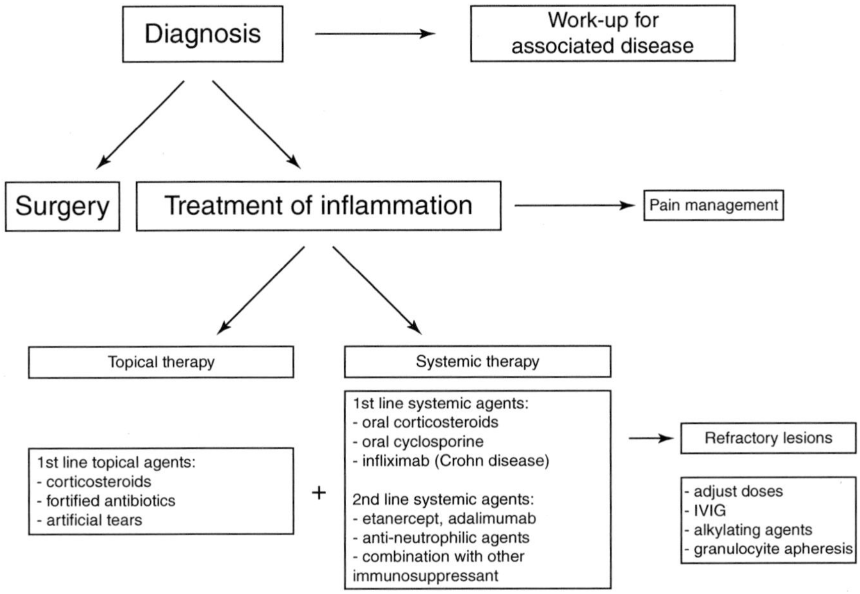


**Fig. 25.4** Diagram of pyoderma gangrenosum workup with ocular involvement

## Orbit and Lacrimal Gland

Orbital extension of pyoderma gangrenosum needs aggressive systemic therapy, as severe cases may be potentially life-threatening [3, 30, 35].

### Conclusion

Recognition of the clinical manifestation of pyoderma gangrenosum, in particular the most rare and atypical features of the disorder, including ocular symptoms, may be of crucial importance in making the diagnosis. Because the diagnosis is clinical, it is important for the ophthalmologist to consider pyoderma gangrenosum in the differential diagnosis of scleritis and orbital inflammation.

Further, physicians other than ophthalmologists and dermatologists should be aware of the possible existence of sterile neutrophilic collections in internal organs to avoid unnecessary invasive diagnostic investigations.

Although pyoderma gangrenosum is a rare disease, an early recognition of its manifestations can lead to the institution of adequate treatment, thereby improving the patient's prognosis.

## References

1. Brocq L. Nouvelle contribution a l'etude du phagedenisme geometrique. Ann Dermatol Syphiligr. 1916;6(1):1–39.
2. Brunsting LA, Goeckerman WH, O'Leary PA. Pyoderma (ecthyma) gangrenosum. Arch Dermatol. 1930;22:655–80.
3. Ahronowitz I, Harp J, Kanade S. Etiology and management of pyoderma gangrenosum. A comprehensive review. Am J Clin Dermatol. 2012;13(3):191–211.
4. Powell FC, Schroeter AL, Su WP, et al. Pyoderma gangrenosum: a review of 86 patients. Q J Med. 1985;55(217):173–86.
5. Vidal D, Puig L, Gilaberte M, et al. Review of 26 cases of classical pyoderma gangrenosum: clinical and therapeutic features. J Dermatol Treat. 2004;15(3):146–52.
6. Powell FC, Perry HO. Pyoderma gangrenosum in childhood. Arch Dermatol. 1984;120(6):757–61.
7. Kruger S, Piroth W, Amo Takyi B, et al. Multiple aseptic pulmonary nodules with central necrosis in association with pyoderma gangrenosum. Chest. 2001;119(3):977–8.
8. Vignon-Pennamen MD. The extracutaneous involvement in the neutrophilic dermatoses. Clin Dermatol. 2000;18(3):339–47.
9. Marie I, Levesque H, Joly P, et al. Neutrophilic myositis as an extracutaneous manifestation of neutrophilic dermatosis. J Am Acad Dermatol. 2001;44(1):137–9.
10. Wilson-Jones E, Winkelmann RK. Superficial granulomatous pyoderma: a localized vegetative form

of pyoderma gangrenosum. J Am Acad Dermatol. 1988;18(3):511–21.
11. Dean SM, Zirwas M. A second case of sunitinib-associated pyoderma gangrenosum. J Clin Aesthet Dermatol. 2010;3(8):34–5.
12. Freiman A, Brassard A. Pyoderma gangrenosum associated with isotretinoin therapy. J Am Acad Dermatol. 2006;55:S107–8.
13. Rostenberg Jr A. The Shwartzman phenomenon: a review with a consideration of some possible dermatological manifestations. Br J Dermatol. 1953;65(11):389–405.
14. Shwartzman G. Concerning the specificity and nature of the phenomenon of local skin reactivity to various bacterial filtrates. J Exp Med. 1930;51(4):571–83.
15. Prystowsky JH, Kahn SN, Lazarus GS. Present status of pyoderma gangrenosum. Review of 21 cases. Arch Dermatol. 1989;125:57–64.
16. Bennett ML, Jackson JM, Jorizzo JL, et al. Pyoderma gangrenosum: a comparison of typical and atypical forms with an emphasis on time to remission. Case review of 86 patients from 2 institutions. Medicine (Baltimore). 2000;79(1):37–46.
17. von den Driesch P. Pyoderma gangrenosum: a report of 44 cases with follow-up. Br J Dermatol. 1997;137(6):1000–5.
18. Ruocco E, Sangiuliano S, Gravina AG, et al. Pyoderma gangrenosum: an updated review. J Eur Acad Dermatol Venereol. 2009;23(9):1008–17.
19. Su WPD, Davis MDP, Weenig RH, et al. Pyoderma gangrenosum: clinicopathologic correlation and proposed diagnostic criteria. Int J Dermatol. 2004;43(11):790–800.
20. Su WP, Schroeter AL, Perry HO, et al. Histopathologic and immunopathologic study of pyoderma gangrenosum. J Cutan Pathol. 1986;13(5):323–30.
21. Powell FC, Schroeter AL, Perry HO, et al. Direct immunofluorescence in pyoderma gangrenosum. Br J Dermatol. 1983;108(3):287–93.
22. Ayyala RS, Armstrong S. Corneal melting and scleromalacia perforans in a patient with pyoderma gangrenosum and acute myeloid leukemia. Ophthalmic Surg Lasers. 1998;29:328–31.
23. Bishop P, Tullo A. Pyoderma gangrenosum and necrotising sclerokeratitis [letter]. Cornea. 1998;17:346–7.
24. Bouchard CS, Meyer MA, McDonnell JF. Bilateral peripheral ulcerative keratitis associated with pyoderma gangrenosum. Cornea. 1997;16:480–2.
25. Happle R, Schiffer HP, Kövary PM. Ocular involvement in pyoderma gangrenosum (letter). Arch Dermatol. 1977;113:1612.
26. Wilson DM, John GR, Callen JP. Peripheral ulcerative keratitis and extracutaneous neutrophilic disorder: report of a patient with rheumatoid arthritis, pustular vasculitis, pyoderma gangrenosum, and Sweet's syndrome with an excellent response to cyclosporine therapy. J Am Acad Dermatol. 1999;40:331–4.
27. Brown BA, Parker CT, Bower KS. Effective steroid-sparing treatment of peripheral ulcerative keratitis and pyoderma gangrenosum. Cornea. 2001;20:117–8.
28. Fournié P, Malecaze F, Coullet J, Arné J-L. Pyoderma gangrenosum with necrotizing sclerokeratitis after cataract surgery. J Cataract Refract Surg. 2007;33:1987–90.
29. Browning DJ, Proia AD, Sanfilippo FP. Pyoderma gangrenosum involving the eyelid. Arch Ophthalmol. 1985;103:551–2.
30. Newman WD, Frank HJ. Pyoderma gangrenosum of the orbit. Eye. 1993;7:89–94.
31. Miserocchi E, Modorati G, Foster CS, Brancato R. Ocular and extracutaneous involvement in pyoderma gangrenosum. Ophthalmology. 2002;109:1941–3.
32. Saito N, Yanagi T, Akiyama M, Lin HY, Kasai S, Fujita Y, Yamane N, Inokuma D, Kase A, Ono K, Minakawa H, Shimizu H. Pyoderma gangrenosum of the eyelid: report of two cases and review of the literature. Dermatology. 2010;221:211–5.
33. Cordero-Coma M, Pérez-Moreiras JV, Toribio A, Alonso-Orcajo N, Calleja S, Franco M, Ruiz de Morales JG. Refractory pyoderma gangrenosum of the orbit and the lacrimal sac. Orbit. 2012;31(4):249–51.
34. Teasley LA, Foster CS, Baltatzis S. Sclerokeratitis and facial skin lesions; a case report of pyoderma gangrenosum and its response to dapsone therapy. Cornea. 2007;26:215–9.
35. Rose GE, Barnes EA, Uddin JM. Pyoderma gangrenosum of the ocular adnexa. A rare condition with characteristic clinical appearances. Ophthalmology. 2003;110:801–5.
36. Agarwal A, Andrews JM. Systematic review: IBD-associated pyoderma gangrenosum in the biologic era, the response to therapy. Aliment Pharmacol Ther. 2013;38:563–72.

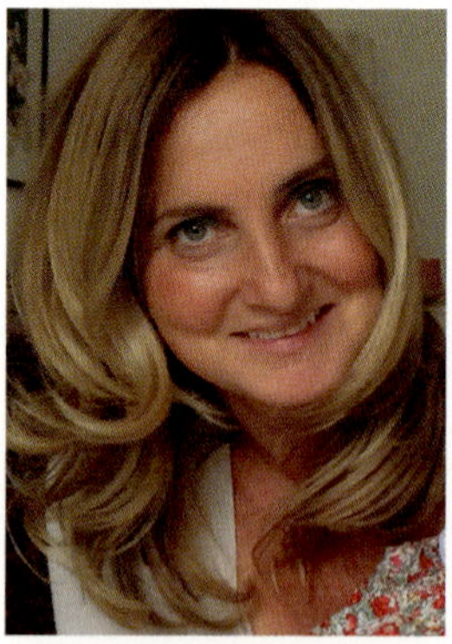

**Elisabetta Miserocchi** Dr. Elisabetta Miserocchi is a consultant ophthalmologist, based at University Hospital San Raffaele Milan, Italy. After graduating with a medical degree from the University of Milan in 1996, Dr. Miserocchi completed a four-year residency in the Department of Ophthalmology at the San Raffaele Hospital, including a research fellowship at the Massachusetts Eye and Ear Infirmary, part of Harvard Medical School, Massachusetts, USA, with Dr. Stephen Foster.

Her main areas of interest and activity are diagnosis and treatment of uveitis, pediatric uveitis associated with rheumatic diseases, ocular cicatricial pemphigoid, and herpetic ocular disease. Dr. Miserocchi is also currently participating in many international multicenter clinical trials on systemic immunosuppressive agents for non-infectious uveitis.

Dr. Miserocchi is a member of the International Uveitis Study Group in 2014 and the American Uveitis Society. She is widely published in peer-reviewed journals and has presented her work at a number of national and international congresses; she was awarded the SOI-SOE Lecture at the Società Oftalmologica Italiana 2012 annual meeting in Rome for new treatments in non-infectious uveitis. Dr. Miserocchi has conducted research and applied new therapies to further the diagnosis and treatment of non-infectious uveitis.

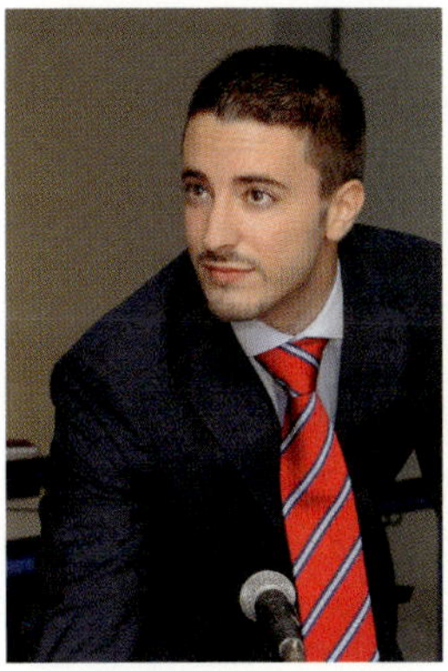

**Lorenzo Iuliano** Dr. Lorenzo Iuliano is a consultant ophthalmologist at the San Raffaele Scientific Institute of Milan, Italy. He graduated in 2010 at the Medical School of the Vita-Salute University of Milan and completed his five-year residency program in the Ophthalmology Department of the San Raffaele Scientific Institute of Milan, Italy. He is also a Fellow of the European Board of Ophthalmology.

Dr. Iuliano's main areas of interest are posterior segment diseases and uveitis, with a particular focus on vitreoretinal surgery. He is also currently participating as investigator in different international multicenter clinical trials on systemic immunosuppressive agents for non-infectious uveitis.

Dr. Iuliano is also widely active in spontaneous clinical research, which results are widely published in peer-reviewed journals. He also presented his work in different national and international congresses.

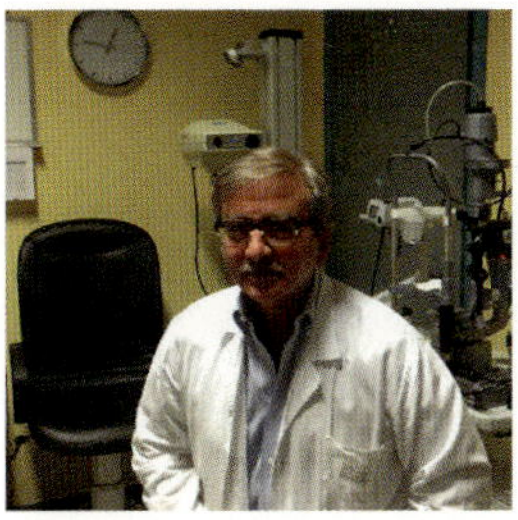

**Giulio Modorati** Dr. Giulio Modorati is a senior consultant ophthalmologist, based at University Hospital San Raffaele Milan, Italy. Graduated with a medical degree from the University of Milan, Dr Modorati completed a four-year residency in the Department of Ophthalmology at the San Raffaele Hospital.

Dr. Modorati's main areas of interest and activity are diagnosis and treatment of uveitis, AIDS, ocular oncology, and dry eye diseases. He is also currently involved as principal investigator in many international multicenter clinical trials on systemic immunosuppressive agents for noninfectious uveitis and ocular tumors.

Dr. Modorati is the Head of Ocular Oncology and Immunopathology Service at the San Raffaele Scientific Institute in Milan (Italy). He is widely published in peer-reviewed journals and has presented his work at a number of National and International Congresses.

# 26 Stevens-Johnson Syndrome, Toxic Epidermal Necrolysis and Other Mucocutaneous Syndromes

Bhaskar Srinivasan, Shweta Agarwal, and Geetha Iyer

## Introduction

Stevens-Johnson syndrome (SJS) and toxic epidermal necrolysis (TEN) are acute blistering diseases affecting the skin and mucous membrane including the ocular surface. The underlying aetiology of both are similar, and they differ only with respect to the amount of body surface area of desquamated epithelium with SJS being at the less severe end of the spectrum and TEN at the worse. Erythema multiforme major (EMM) which was a term interchangeably used for SJS is now known to be different and has infection as the etiology with predominantly an acral distribution of skin lesions, whereas both SJS and TEN are primarily due to adverse drug reaction and have more of a truncal and facial distribution of lesions. Ophthalmic manifestations are more common in both SJS and TEN and occur in 43–81 % patients in the acute phase [1, 2].

B. Srinivasan, MS(Ophthalmology) (✉)
S. Agarwal, MS(Ophthalmology) • G. Iyer, F.R.C.S.
Cornea, Refractive Surgery & Ocular Surface, Sankara Nethralaya, Chennai, Tamil Nadu 600006, India
e-mail: drbhaskar@hotmail.com; shwe20@yahoo.com; drgeethaiyer@gmail.com

## Aetiopathogenesis

Adverse idiosyncratic reaction to drugs is the commonest cause of SJS and TEN. Infections such as mycoplasma pneumonia and herpes are also known triggering factors. The most common medications causing these reactions are anticonvulsants, antimicrobials and nonsteroidal anti-inflammatory drugs (NSAID). The medications that cause SJS/TEN are listed in Table 26.1.

SJS occurs in individuals with lowered ability to detoxify reactive metabolites of drugs or due to an alteration of detoxifying enzymes due to a genetic basis or an acquired decrease in detoxifying enzymes as in acquired immune deficiency syndrome (AIDS). The incidence of SJS in AIDS is significantly more than the general population. The altered metabolite or drug act as haptens which bind to keratocytes and initiate a T cell immune reaction leading to keratocyte apoptosis. There is an increased incidence of HLA-B12, HLA-Aw33 and DRw5 in patients with the ocular lesions of Stevens-Johnson syndrome [1].

## Clinical Features

The typical interval between taking a drug and disease manifestation is between 1 and 3 weeks with a rapid recurrence when the patient is re-exposed to the same medication. The prodromal clinical features include fever, malaise, myalgia,


B. Mukherjee, H. Yuen (eds.), *Emergencies of the Orbit and Adnexa*,
DOI 10.1007/978-81-322-1807-4_26

**Table 26.1** Commonly implicated drugs causing SJS/TEN

| Drugs causing SJS | | |
|---|---|---|
| Antimicrobials | Anticonvulsants | Nonsteroidal anti-inflammatory drugs |
| Sulphonamides | Hydantoin derivatives (phenytoin) | Salicylates |
| Penicillins | Carbamazepine | Ibuprofen |
| Cephalosporins | Barbiturates | Pyrazolone derivatives |
| Ciprofloxacin | | |
| Rifampicin | | |
| Isoniazid | | |
| Chloroquine | | |

**Table 26.2** Differences between SJS/SJS-TEN overlap/TEN/EMM

| | SJS | SJS-TEN overlap | TEN | EMM |
|---|---|---|---|---|
| Type of lesion | Widespread macule or flat atypical target lesion | Widespread macule or flat atypical target lesion | Widespread macule or flat atypical target lesion | Localised typical target or raised atypical target lesion |
| Distribution of lesion | Trunk and head | Trunk and head | Trunk and head | Acral (extremities) |
| Extent of epithelial detachment (BSA) | <10 % | 10–30 % | >30 % | <10 % |
| Aetiology | Cutaneous adverse drug reaction | Cutaneous adverse drug reaction | Cutaneous adverse drug reaction | Infective aetiology? Viral |
| Histopathology | Necrotic reaction. Predominant dendritic cells and macrophages and TNF alpha | Necrotic reaction | Necrotic reaction | Significant inflammatory reaction with predominant T lymphocytes |
| Ophthalmic manifestation | Common | Common | Common | Rare |

upper respiratory tract infection, prostration and arthralgias that precede the skin and mucous membrane lesions.

*Skin Lesions* The cutaneous lesion consists of flat-topped erythematous macules which can form vesicles and bullae with epidermal necrosis having an atypical target lesion configuration. Skin lesion heals with residual hyperpigmentation and scarring. Nikolsky's sign (separation of apparently normal epithelium with minimal friction) is positive in patients with TEN.

The differences between SJS, TEN and EMM are mentioned in Table 26.2.

*Mucosal Lesions* These are in the form of bullous vesicles with clear or hemorrhagic fluid, and their rupture leads to mucosal ulceration and pseudomembrane and true membrane formation. The lesions heal in weeks with minimal subepithelial scarring.

## Ophthalmic Manifestations

### Acute Phase

The ophthalmic involvement in the acute stage can involve the lids, lid margin and the entire ocular surface involving the tarsal and bulbar conjunctiva, the limbal stem cells at the palisades of Vogt and the corneal epithelium. There could be varying grades of inflammation and denudation of these areas leading to loss of vision either in the acute phase secondary to corneal involvement with scaring or perforation or in the chronic phase as a sequelae of acute-phase insult. The sequence of events begin as injection, chemosis, pseudomembrane formation, true membrane formation, ulceration and symblepharon formation in conjunctiva. Conjunctival ulcers heal with subepithelial scarring causing destruction of goblet cell and meibomian gland orifice. Traditional grading of ocular involvement is given by Power et al. with a mild grade associated with minimal conjunctival changes and severe grade with extensive symblepharon and ankyloblepharon formation [3]. However, the grading does not guide us to a treatment algorithm and also does not correlate with chronic-stage ocular outcome. Corneal complications such as persistent epithelial defect, ulceration and melts are primarily due to lid pathology. Secondary bacterial infection can further complicate the condition. Rarely anterior uveitis can also occur. The initial eye findings resolve in 2–4 weeks. Figure 26.1 depicts the various ophthalmic and skin manifestations in the acute and subacute phase.

## Chronic Phase

Chronic sequelae include lid manifestation such as lid margin keratinisation, entropion/floppy lid and trichiasis and distichiasis formation. These changes cause blink-related microtrauma and exposure-related damage to ocular surface. Severe dry eye results from both lipid and aqueous tear deficiency. Repeated corneal epithelial breakdown due to microtrauma or inflammation causes limbal stem cell deficiency either in the

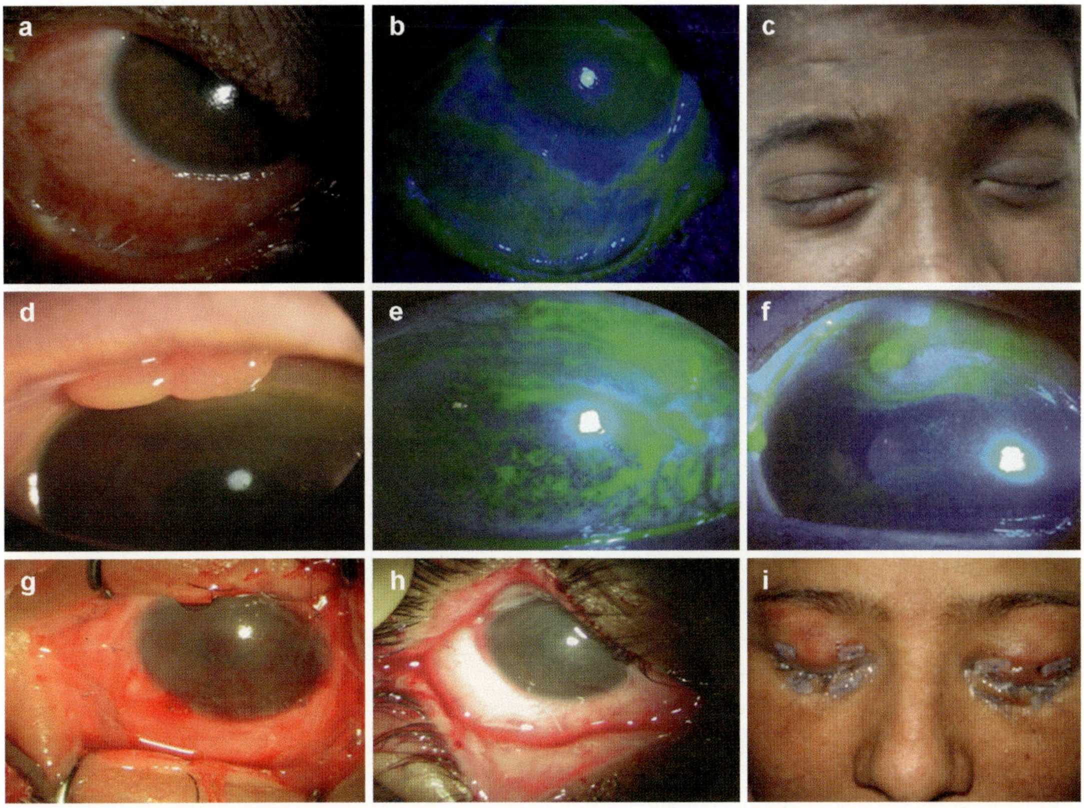


**Fig. 26.1** (**a**) Severe conjunctival inflammation. (**b**) Conjunctival ulceration staining with fluorescein. (**c**) Scarred skin lesion on face and forehead. (**d**) Conjunctival granuloma formations. (**e**) Corneal superficial punctate keratitis with conjunctival ulceration stating with fluorescein. (**f**) Conjunctival ulceration near the limbal area. (**g**) Amniotic membrane transplantation for the ocular surface in acute stage. (**h**) Amniotic membrane shown draping the entire ocular surface. (**i**) Amniotic membrane fixed using bolster so as to fix the membrane as deep in the fornix as possible to cover the tarsal and forniceal ulceration

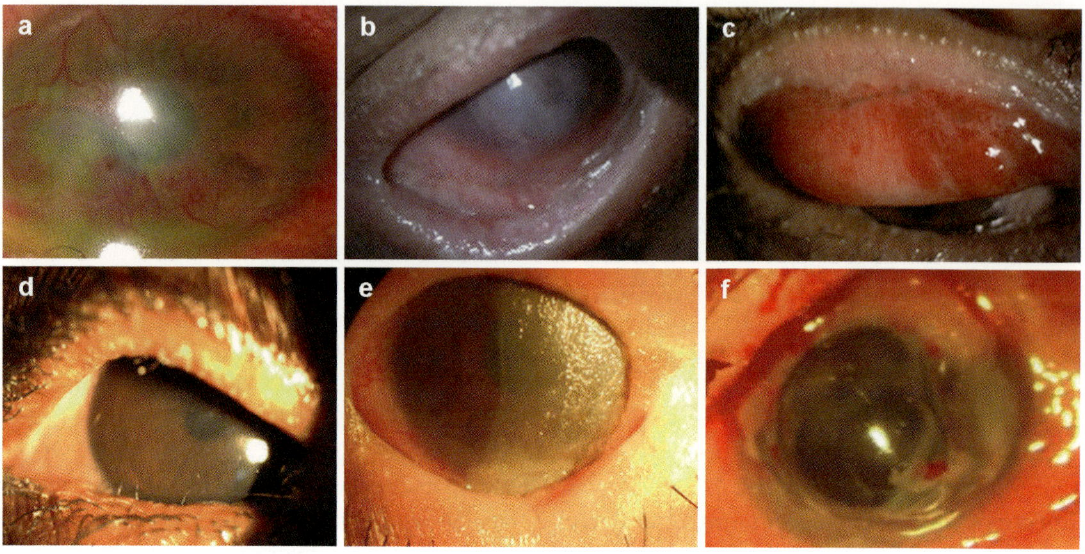


**Fig. 26.2** (**a**) Chronic surface inflammation resulting in limbal deficiency with vascularisation with thinning. (**b**) Anterior staphyloma formation corresponding to area of lid margin keratinisation. (**c**) Lid margin keratinisation responsible for repeated epithelial breakdown in these eyes. (**d**) Severe meibomian gland dysfunction with most of the glands being replaced by distichiatic lashes. (**e**) Symblepharon, ankyloblepharon, and ocular surface keratinisation. (**f**) Corneal infection and perforation

form of conjunctivalisation or squamous metaplasia of the ocular surface. Chronic sequelae can also include damage to the nasolacrimal system such as punctal stenosis, canalicular obstruction, nasolacrimal duct obstruction and dacryocystoceles. Figure 26.2 depicts the various chronic sequelae of the disease.

## Treatment

### Acute Phase

#### General Measures

Acute phase SJS patients are better managed in an intensive care or a burn unit setting and need to be co-managed by the dermatologist/internist and ophthalmologist. Extensive skin sloughing predisposes to fluid and electrolyte imbalance and sepsis, and most deaths due to SJS/TEN are attributed to sepsis. The goals of treatment are to maintain hydration, fluid electrolyte balance and prevent sepsis. Treatment for skin lesion includes antiseptic dressing for the wounds. Systemic antibiotics are not started as a routine and are reserved for culture-positive cases only. The role of systemic corticosteroids is controversial with their benefit in reducing inflammation vis-a-vis the risk of sepsis and delayed wound healing secondary to their use. There have been case reports of administering intravenous methylprednisolone 1,000 mg for 3–4 days in the acute stage that was associated with decreased incidence of chronic ophthalmic sequelae [4]. The other interventions in the acute phase that have been tried include systemic cyclosporine, intravenous cyclophosphamide, pentoxifylline (a TNF alpha inhibitor) and intravenous immunoglobulin (IVIG 1.5–2 g/kg) in order to suppress the inflammatory response.

### Ocular Measures

Ophthalmic measures aim to maintain the ocular hygiene and prevent development of superimposed infections, control inflammation, limit the cicatrisation process, prevent corneal melts and treat the dry eyes. Adequate hydration and cleansing of the ocular surface and lid margin with removal of crusts are important. A prophylactic antibiotic drop or ointment helps prevent infection. Preservative-free lubricants are used to moisten the ocular surface.

Topical steroids can reduce the acute inflammation but care should be taken due to the increased risk of secondary infection and corneal melts, especially in the presence of epithelial defects. A bandage contact lens can be placed in the presence of corneal epithelial defect. Symblepharon rings can be used to limit the symblepharon formation though it does not help in preventing the other chronic ocular sequelae.

### Surgical Intervention

The intervention that has shown reasonable promise in recent times is the use of amniotic membrane transplantation in the acute phase [5–7]. The entire ocular surface from lid margin to lid margin is draped with the membrane. This reduces inflammation, decreases scarring and promotes epithelial healing. The membrane is preferably sutured to the lid margin or secured with fibrin glue, and perilimbal sutures can be used to anchor the membrane to the ocular surface. These interventions usually need to be performed by the bedside. The use of PROKERA (Bio-Tissue, Miami) a polycarbonate ring with a sheet of amniotic membrane stretched across and fitted to the eye like a contact lens to cover the whole of the cornea and part of the bulbar conjunctiva has been also advocated; however, PROKERA does not cover the entire ocular surface up to the fornix. This procedure has shown to reduce chronic-stage sequelae of SJS. The indications for amniotic membrane grafting in acute SJS include eyes with severe inflammation, large tarsal or conjunctival ulcers or intense lid margin involvement with lash loss or those with early symblepharon formation. In case of corneal melts, tectonic procedures such as cyanoacrylate glue with bandage contact lens application, multilayered amniotic membrane grafts, lamellar patch grafts or full-thickness corneal grafts might be required to preserve the globe integrity. In case of infection, corneal scraping and detailed microbiological workup needs to be done and antibiotic chosen based on the sensitivity pattern.

## Chronic Phase

Following the acute phase (usually lasts 2 weeks–1 month), attention is directed to the severe dry eye which can be managed by punctal occlusion/cautery. Lid margin keratinisation (LMK) and tarsal pathologies cause corneal scarring and subsequent loss of vision and need to be addressed. Milder grades of LMK can be addressed by the use of a prosthetic replacement of the ocular surface ecosystem (PROSE) lens that acts as barrier between the lids and the ocular surface, thereby preventing the 'sandpaper effect' of the lids on the surface. Moderate to severe grades require excision of the keratinized strip of tarsal conjunctiva along the lid margin with replacement by mucus membrane graft harvested from the lip [8–10]. Punctal cautery for dryness and mucous membrane grafting for lid margin keratinisation serve as means to stabilise the ocular surface and have an important role in decreasing the ongoing damage to the ocular surface and the limbal stem cells. Nasolacrimal duct occlusion in patients with minimal dry eye might need a dacryocystorhinostomy with or without a Jones tube. Trichiasis or distichiasis can be treated by electroepilation or lid split and cryo application to destroy the hair follicles. Based on the severity, entropion needs to be treated by everting sutures, terminal eyelid margin rotation, grey-line splitting of anterior and posterior lamellae and anterior lamella recession or posterior lamella advancement, posterior lamella expansion and increasing posterior lamella height by various grafts. Figure 26.3 depicts the surgical intervention dose in SJS.

Ocular surface reconstruction can be done by releasing symblepharon, using mItomycin C judiciously intraoperatively and draping the ocular surface with amniotic membrane with or without mucous membrane grafts based on severity. Recently cultivated oral mucosal sheet of epithelium have been used to reconstruct the ocular surface and as a substitute for limbal stem cells in moist eyes.

Corneal scars, primary or progressive limbal deficiency and keratinisation are the sequelae that lead to decrease in vision in these eyes. Visual rehabilitative procedures, based on the cause for visual loss, include optical iridectomy, PROSE lenses and cataract extraction (challenging in the presence of multiple risk factors). Conventional penetrating keratoplasty carries a high risk of failure and end-stage disease

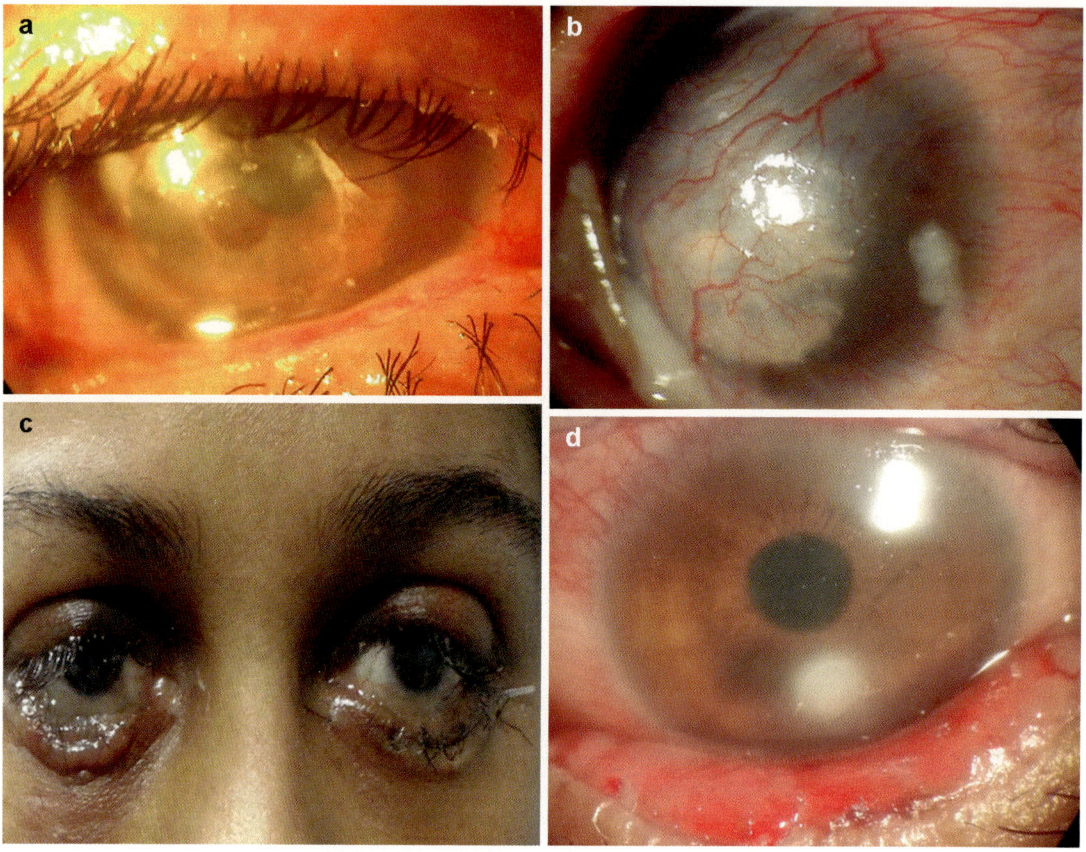

**Fig. 26.3** (**a**) Corneal thinning with impending perforation managed by a lamellar patch graft. (**b**) Persistent epithelial defect managed by a conjunctival hooding. (**c**) Surgery for lower lid entropion with everting sutures. (**d**) Surgery for the lid margin keratinisation which was excised and replaced by mucous membrane graft

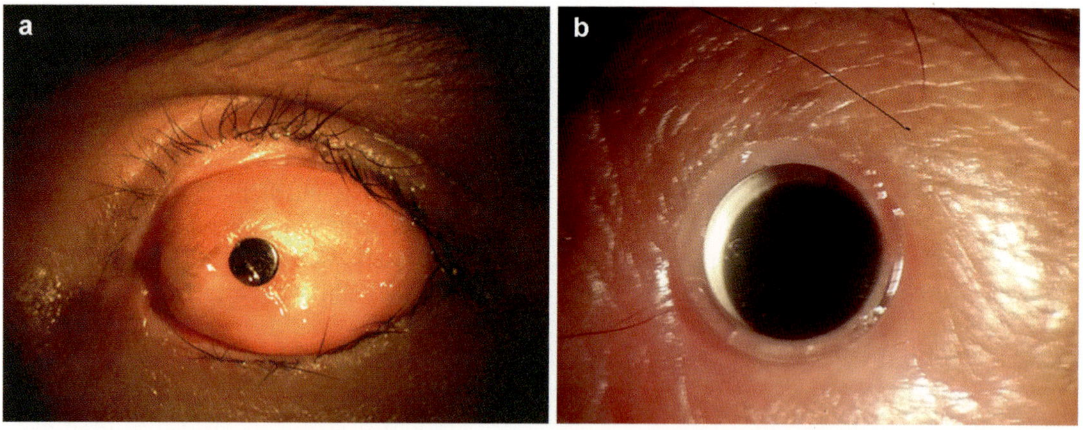

**Fig. 26.4** (**a**) Modified osteo-odonto-keratoprosthesis performed for an SJS patient. (**b**) Boston Type 2 keratoprosthesis performed for an SJS patient

warrants the placement of a keratoprosthesis (artificial corneal implant), namely, the modified osteo-odonto-keratoprosthesis (MOOKP) [11], tibial keratoprosthesis or the Boston type 2 Kpro [10]. Figure 26.4 depicts the role of keratoprosthesis in these patients.

**Table 26.3** Comprehensive approach to SJS/TEN

| Acute stage | Chronic stage | End stage | Concomitant issues |
|---|---|---|---|
| General measures | Trichiasis – electroepilation | Moist surface | Glaucoma |
| Ocular hygiene | Distichiasis – lid split and cryo application | Surface reconstruction with amniotic membrane and mucous membrane | Cataract |
| Lubricants? Topical steroids | Lid margin keratinization – excision with mucous membrane transplantation/ use of PROSE | Role of cultivated mucosal epithelial transplant (COMET) for fornix | Corneal melts/perforation tectonic procedures |
| Surgical measures AMT | Entropion – everting suture, eyelid margin rotation, grey-line splitting of anterior and posterior lamellae and anterior lamella recession or posterior lamella advancement, posterior lamella expansion and increasing posterior lamella height by various graft excisional procedures with excision of the anterior lamella and lash line | Minor salivary gland transplantation | Cyanoacrylate glue<br>Amniotic membrane<br>Lamellar keratoplasty<br>Penetrating keratoplasty |
| | Dry eye – Punctal cautery/PROSE | | |
| | | Keratinized surface | |
| | | MOOKP | |
| | | Boston type 2 keratoprosthesis | |
| | | Tibial keratoprosthesis | |

A comprehensive algorithmic approach to ophthalmic manifestations of SJS was earlier outlined by the authors (*Comprehensive approach to ocular consequences of Stevens-Johnson syndrome – the aftermath of a systemic condition. Graefes Arch Clin Exp Ophthalmol.*), based on the experience in 464 eyes of 232 SJS patients, and a gist of the same has been tabulated in Table 26.3.

## References


1. Yao FU, Gregory DG, et al. The ophthalmologist role in management of acute Stevens-Johnson syndrome and toxic epidermal necrolysis. Ocul Surf. 2010;8(4):31–41.
2. Palmon FE, Brilakis, HS, Webster GF, Holland EJ. Erythema multiforme, Stevens-Johnson syndrome, and toxic epidermal necrolysis. In: Krachmer, Cornea 3rd edition, Elseiver 2011:52;599–612.
3. Power WJ, Foster S, et al. Analysis of the acute ophthalmic manifestation of erythema multiforme/Stevens-Johnson syndrome/toxic epidermal necrolysis disease spectrum. Ophthalmology. 1994;102(11):1669–76.
4. Araki Y, Sotozono C, et al. Successful treatment of Stevens-Johnson syndrome with steroid pulse therapy at disease onset. Am J Ophthalmol. 2009;147(6):1004–11.
5. Gregory DG. Treatment of acute Stevens–Johnson syndrome and toxic epidermal necrolysis using amniotic membrane: a review of 10 consecutive cases. Ophthalmology. 2011;118(5):908–14.
6. Hsu M, Jayaram A, et al. Indications and outcome of amniotic membrane transplantation in management of acute Stevens-Johnson syndrome and toxic epidermal necrolysis: a case control study. Cornea. 2012;31(12):1394–140.
7. Ciralsy JB, Sippel KC, Gregory DG. Current ophthalmic treatment strategies for acute and chronic Stevens-Johnson syndrome and toxic epidermal necrolysis. Curr Opin Ophthalmol. 2013;24(00):1–8.
8. Di Pascuale MA, Espana E, et al. Correlation of corneal complications with eyelid cicatricial pathologies in patients with Stevens-Johnson syndrome and toxic

epidermal necrolysis syndrome. Ophthalmology. 2004;112(5):904–12.
9. Iyer G, Pillai VS, Srinivasan B, Guruswami S, Padmanabhan P. Mucous membrane grafting lid margin keratinization in Stevens-Johnson syndrome: results. Cornea. 2010;29:146–51.
10. Iyer G, Srinivasan B, Agarwal S, et al. Comprehensive approach to ocular consequences of Stevens-Johnson syndrome – the aftermath of a systemic condition. Graefes Arch Clin Exp Ophthalmol. 2014;252(3):457–67.
11. Iyer G, Pillai VS, Srinivasan B, et al. Modified osteo-odonto-keratoprosthesis – the Indian experience – results of the first 50 cases. Cornea. 2010;29(7): 771–6.

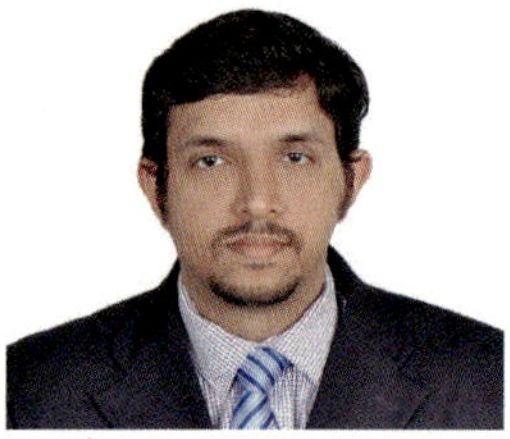

**Bhaskar Srinivasan** Dr. Bhaskar Srinivasan finished his graduation from Topiwala National Medical College, Mumbai, in 1997 and his masters in Ophthalmology (MS Ophthalmology) from Armed Forces Medical College, Pune, in 2002. He did his fellowship in cornea and external eye disease at Sankara Nethralaya, Chennai, following which he joined the same as faculty and is currently Senior Consultant Cornea and Refractive Services. His special interest is in managing various ocular surface diseases especially treating chemical injuries and Stevens–Johnson syndrome. He has experience with different kinds of keratoprosthesis and is a part of the ocular surface clinic at Sankara Nethralaya, a one of its kind in the world dealing with both ocular surface stem cell and various keratoprosthesis-based treatments. He is well versed in various kinds of corneal transplants (PK/DSEK/DALK), refractive surgery, and management of ocular surface tumors. He has 30 publications in peer-reviewed literature and has served as a faculty in various national and international conferences.

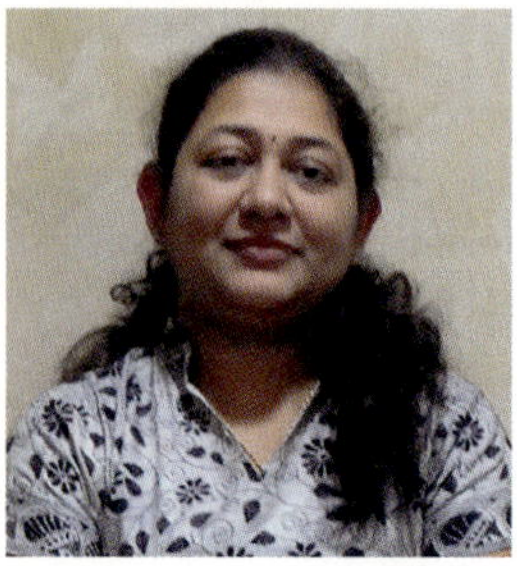

**Shweta Agarwal** Dr. Shweta Agarwal, D.O, a gold medalist from Pune university, completed her cornea fellowship from Sankara Nethralaya Chennai in 2009. She was awarded the Dr. D.S.Sardesai ophthalmology award from Pune university. She has quite a few publications in national and international journals and also a chapter on dry eyes in post graduate textbook of ophthalmology. She has been a primary investigator in two studies and a co-investigator in many studies related to cornea and ocular surface disorders funded by national agencies. She has been invited as a faculty in several national and international conferences. She was awarded the Best Cornea Free Paper in AIOC 2012. Her areas of interest are corneal diseases, ocular surface disorders, stem cells, and keratoprosthesis.

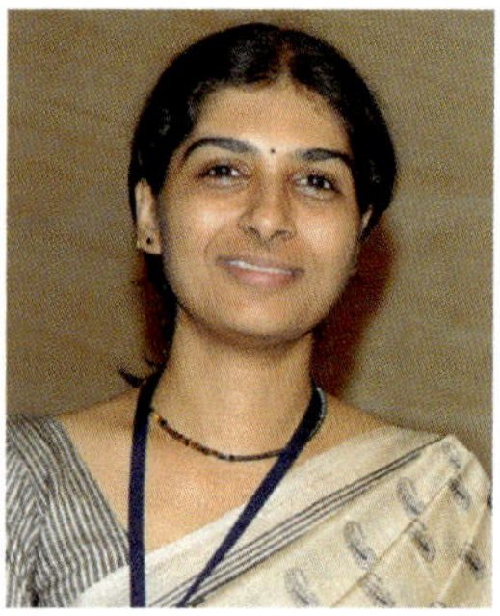

**Geetha Iyer** Dr. Geetha Iyer, FRCS (Glasgow), completed her basic medical training in 1999. She did her postgraduate training in Ophthalmology and fellowship in cornea and external disease from Sankara Nethralaya, Chennai, India. She was awarded the best postgraduate student following completion of her ophthalmology training at Sankara Nethralaya and has been adjudged twice as the Best Associate Consultant during the early years of her tenure. She has been the recipient of awards for the Best Cornea Paper at both regional and national conferences. She has done a short-term observership in Ocular Surface Disorders with Dr. Scheffer C G Tseng, Miami, USA, in October 2006 and in Boston Type 1 keratoprosthesis with Dr. Claes H Dohlman in November 2006. She was trained and is being guided by Prof. Giancarlo Falcinelli in performing the MOOKP procedure. She has so far done more than 100 keratoprosthesis surgeries (MOOKP, Boston Type 1 and 2 Kpro).

Dr. Geetha Iyer has to her credit publications in peer-reviewed journals and has conducted courses and presented papers in national and international meetings. She is actively involved in the management of ocular surface disorders and is currently working as Senior Consultant at the Ocular Surface Clinic and the Cornea Services, Sankara Nethralaya. Her areas of interest include pediatric penetrating keratoplasty, ocular surface tumors, ocular surface disorders including chemical injuries, stem cell transplants, keratoprosthesis, and in particular Stevens–Johnson Syndrome.

# 27 Idiopathic Orbital Inflammatory Disease

Dov Hersh and Geoffrey E. Rose

Idiopathic orbital inflammatory disease (IOID) is, realistically, an open-ended non-diagnosis in which a definite cause has not been found for the inflammation. The perceptive physician should, however, be aware that "inflammation is a tissue response and not a diagnosis", and that orbital inflammation can occur alongside almost any pathological process – such as ischemia, exposure to noxious substances (e.g. foreign bodies, or keratin from dermoid cysts), infections or malignancies. Irrespective of the underlying aetiology, inflammation will show a clinical improvement with systemic steroids, and it is therefore unwise to regard a "steroid response" as a diagnostic confirmation of IOID [1].

Inflammation accounts for about 5 % of orbital disease, affects all ages, and is a frequent reason for orbital biopsy [2]. Although "benign" on histopathological grounds, orbital inflammatory disease (OID) may have a clinically aggressive course that can endanger the globe, extraocular muscles and optic nerve. OIDs may be solely orbital, with no identified systemic abnormalities (termed "idiopathic OID", IOID), or associated with systemic inflammatory or sclerosing diseases, such as sarcoidosis or IgG4 sclerosing disease. IOID is an "umbrella" term commonly used to encompass dacryoadenitis, myositis and diffuse orbital soft-tissue inflammation for which no cause is found and, as our understanding of the mechanisms of inflammation improves, it is likely that the number of "idiopathic" presentations will decline.

The "classic" presentations of dacryoadenitis, myositis and diffuse OID are not mutually exclusive, and they can have significant overlap, as well as the inflammation spilling over to include scleritis or uveitis – particularly when associated with a systemic inflammatory disorder. OID can present in a hyperacute fashion (e.g. acute myositis) or as a subacute or chronic process. By taking a thorough history, particularly the temporal sequence of symptoms in relation to the patient's age, a tailored list of differential diagnosis for the OID can be formed; the differential diagnosis should further guide the clinical examination and relevant investigations, this often including biopsy (and sometimes re-biopsy) to assist the clinician in reaching a likely diagnosis and detecting threat to life or vision.

Several conditions may present with OID (Table 27.1), and it is imperative to exclude these before assigning a diagnosis of presumed IOID; "IOID" should always be considered as a temporary diagnosis. The astute physician will repeatedly

D. Hersh, BCom, MBBS, MMed, FRANZCO (✉)
Orbital Unit, Moorfields Eye Hospital,
162 City Road, London EC1V 2PD, UK
e-mail: dovhersh@gmail.com

G.E. Rose, MS, DSc, MRCP, FRCS, FRCOphth
Orbital, Lacrimal and Oculoplastic Service,
Moorfields Eye Hospital NHS Trust, London, UK


B. Mukherjee, H. Yuen (eds.), *Emergencies of the Orbit and Adnexa*,
DOI 10.1007/978-81-322-1807-4_27

**Table 27.1** Various orbital conditions that may present with orbital inflammation

| |
|---|
| Orbital inflammatory disease associated with systemic inflammatory conditions |
| Thyroid-associated eye disease |
| Neoplasms |
| Lymphoma and other lymphoproliferative disorders |
| Rhabdomyosarcoma |
| Choroidal malignant melanoma with extrascleral spread |
| Metastatic disease |
| Congenital malformations |
| Dermoid cyst |
| Lymphangioma |
| Carotico-cavernous fistula |
| Histiocytosis |
| Langerhans cell histiocytosis |
| Erdheim–Chester syndrome |
| Infectious diseases |
| Bacterial orbital cellulitis |
| Tuberculosis |
| Syphilis |
| Viral disease |
| Primary infection (e.g. mumps dacryoadenitis) |
| Secondary reactivation (e.g. herpes zoster) |
| Trauma and/or occult orbital foreign body |

Unknown cause (*IOID* idiopathic orbital inflammatory disease)

**Table 27.2** Systemic associations of orbital inflammatory disease

| |
|---|
| Sarcoidosis |
| ANCA-associated vasculitis |
| IgG4-related disease |
| Systemic lupus erythematosus |
| Crohn's disease |
| Churg–Strauss syndrome |
| Polyarteritis nodosa |
| Scleroderma |

reconsider the "non-diagnosis" (of IOID) and remain vigilant for later development of an orbital or systemic cause – particularly if the condition worsens during or after treatment.

## Systemic Inflammatory Conditions Associated with Orbital Inflammation

Several systemic inflammatory disorders have been associated with OID (Table 27.2), and the importance of detecting a systemic association is threefold. Firstly, if screening tests reveal an underlying systemic inflammatory disorder, it might be important to check for associated structural disease (e.g. retroperitoneal fibrosis in IgG4 disease). Secondly, OID associated with certain systemic inflammatory markers (ANCA-associated vasculitis being one such condition) can have a more protracted course and will often require more aggressive treatment for disease control [3]. Thirdly, development of novel biological agents (e.g. rituximab and anti-TNFα drugs) increases the prospect of targeted immunosuppression for specific diseases; clinical immunologists and rheumatologists have a leading role in exploring targeted treatments for systemic inflammation, and this work appears to be applicable to OID with underlying systemic aetiology – an example being the use of rituximab in the treatment of systemic ANCA-associated vasculitis [4].

Sarcoidosis is a chronic multisystem granulomatous inflammation that mainly affects the respiratory tract, skin and eyes, and the histopathology is characterised by non-caseating compact granulomas, asteroid bodies and Schaumann bodies. It is commoner in women and Afro-Caribbean people, with ocular involvement in up to a half of patients [5]. The commonest systemic manifestation is hilar lymphadenopathy and pulmonary fibrosis. Ophthalmic involvement includes conjunctival nodules, uveitis, chronic dacryoadenitis or more rarely optic neuropathy, myositis or fat infiltration. Skin disease may present as erythema nodosum, and much rarer manifestations include neurosarcoid and uveoparotid fever. Prior to treatment, serum angiotensin-converting enzyme (ACE) titres and calcium may be raised.

ANCA-associated vasculitis or granulomatous polyangiitis (previously known as Wegener's granulomatosis) is a necrotising granulomatous inflammation affecting predominantly small vessels. Typically the upper airway, lungs and kidneys are most affected, but periocular disease may affect a half of patients, and there can be a form of disease limited only to the eyes and/or orbit. Ophthalmic manifestations include conjunctivitis, scleritis, keratitis and retinal vasculitis, and the orbital disease can include aggressively fibrosing OID, dacryoadenitis, myositis or nasolacrimal duct obstruction. Tissues with significant disease activity usually display zonal granulomas, vasculitis and fibrinoid necrosis. Antibodies against proteinase 3 (PR3) or c-ANCA antibodies are highly (90 %) sensitive and specific for disseminated disease, but are positive in only about one-third of those with solely ophthalmic disease. With systemic involvement, ANCA-associated vasculitis has a significant morbidity and mortality and should be treated aggressively using a multidisciplinary approach [3].

Immunoglobulin G4-related disease (IgG4-RD) is a recently recognised systemic inflammatory disorder with diffuse tissue infiltration by IgG4-positive plasma cells on a background of fibrosis; elevated serum concentrations of IgG4 are also found in 60–70 % of patients. IgG4-RD has been linked to autoimmune pancreatitis, Mikulicz's disease, hepatic inflammatory pseudotumours, tubulo-interstitial nephritis, interstitial lung disease, retroperitoneal fibrosis and Hashimoto's thyroiditis [6]. Orbital IgG4-RD manifest mainly as sclerosing dacryoadenitis that may be bilateral, or as a more diffuse inflammation; the tissues show widespread IgG4-positive plasma cells, dense fibrosis and, for the lacrimal gland, loss of acini. Certain forms of IgG4-RD – for example, pancreatitis or sclerosing cholangitis – have been associated with a higher incidence of non-Hodgkin's lymphoma: to date there is no clear evidence linking orbital IgG4-RD and periocular lymphoma [7], but physicians should be aware of possible emergence of such a link.

Systemic lupus erythematosus (SLE) is a multisystem autoimmune collagen disease in which various autoantibodies (ENA, ANA) trigger a type 3 hypersensitivity reaction, resulting in occlusive vasculitis and fibrinoid necrosis. Ophthalmic complications include OID, Sjogren's syndrome, interstitial keratitis, scleritis and occlusive retinal vasculitis, and systemic manifestations include glomerulonephritis, pericarditis, malar rash and constitutional inflammatory symptoms (fevers, arthralgias, fatigue). Serological investigations include anti-nuclear antibodies (ANAs), double-stranded DNA (dsDNA) and extractable nuclear antigens (ENAs) that are all >90 % specific.

Crohn's disease, a progressive chronic granulomatous enteritis with frequent extra-intestinal complications, is most commonly associated with uveitis, episcleritis or, more rarely, myositis [8]. Patients with orbital myositis should be questioned about persistent gastrointestinal symptoms (diarrhoea, abdominal pain/cramping or faecal blood and mucus) and about any family history of Crohn's disease.

Churg–Strauss syndrome is a necrotising vasculitis with asthma, hypereosinophilia and multisystem vasculitis. Complications include myocarditis, coronary arteritis, granulomatous pneumonia, gastroenteritis, mononeuritis multiplex and atopy, and ophthalmic involvement include OID, ischemic optic neuropathy and retinal artery occlusion due to vasculitis. Classic histological findings are necrotizing arteritis, eosinophilic infiltration and extravascular granulomas, with laboratory evaluation showing raised serum IgE titre and p-ANCA antibodies. Early institution of therapy can reduce both systemic and ophthalmic complications [9].

## Orbital Biopsy

Open biopsy of affected orbital tissues is advisable in most cases of untreated clinical OID, to seek underlying causes for the process; it should, again, be remembered that "inflammation is a tissue response and not a diagnosis". Biopsy not only helps exclude serious underlying diseases – such as malignancy, infections or chemical inflammations – but also may show particular patterns of inflammation (such as granulomatous, necrotizing or sclerosing) that guide later medical therapy. To gain the most information before postinflammatory fibrosis, biopsy should, where possible, be taken from the epicentre of active inflammation: for example, biopsy of an extraocular muscle is best taken from the posterior third, and access to this area may be better through a transcutaneous (rather than transconjunctival) route. If the diagnosis remains in doubt, or the patient does not respond appropriately to therapy, the investigations and biopsy should be repeated. The pathologist should be given an adequate clinical history, the original location of specimens and a differential diagnosis so that the investigation can be tailored to the specific case – often guiding their choice of immunostaining, such as ER, GCDFP-15 or mammaglobin markers in suspected breast cancer metastases.

Orbital biopsy prior to systemic immunosuppression is advisable in all except three clinical scenarios: patients with a typical history and imaging for myositis or scleritis, patients with a rapid-onset painful orbital apex syndrome (where the morbidity of biopsy is far greater than the probability of missing malignancy) and patients with acute dacryoadenitis that improves within days of treatment and in which the lacrimal gland mass disappears within 3 months [1].

## Histopathological Variants of Orbital Inflammatory Disease

Although it should be remembered that incisional biopsy often takes only a few percent of the tissue and – as such – might not be representative of the entire lesion, several histopathological variants have been described. These variants include "classic", IgG4-RD, sclerosing, granulomatous, vasculitic and eosinophilic, and analysis of the cellular infiltrate, stromal changes, vascular changes and the changes in specific orbital structures can help to subclassify the inflammatory pattern and indicate the possibility of systemic associations [10].

Classic OID displays a polymorphic cellular infiltrate with variable degrees of inflammation and fibrosis, and the proportion of neutrophils, mast cells, lymphocytes, plasma cells, eosinophils, macrophages and fibroblasts is variable; B-lymphocytes have polyclonal immunophenotype and reactive lymphoid follicles (with germinal centres) are found. In IgG4-RD, tissue destruction is accompanied by IgG4-positive plasma cell infiltration and dense fibrosis; although there is some variation in the criteria for diagnosis of IgG4-RD, there are usually >30 IgG4-positive plasma cells per high-powered field [6]. The sclerosing variant of OID is paucicellular and dominated by hyalinised tissue with few fibroblasts. Granulomatous inflammation generally shows non-caseating granulomas, multinucleated giant cells and histiocytic infiltration; a diagnosis of sarcoidosis, ANCA-associated vasculitis, tuberculosis, ruptured dermoid cyst or retained foreign body should be considered with this pattern of inflammation. Vasculitic OID displays fibrinoid necrosis with destruction of arteriolar muscularis and elastic lamina, resulting in perivascular extravasations of erythrocytes and inflammatory cells, when clinical suspicion for associated systemic vasculitides (such as SLE and ANCA-associated vasculitis) should be high. With eosinophilic-dominant OID, eosinophils are scattered throughout the tissue, often found in cuffs around small blood vessels, or in the orbital fat. An association with systemic eosinophilia, such as Churg–Strauss syndrome, should be investigated.

## Clinical Presentations

Despite overlap in clinical features, there are three "classic" presentations of dacryoadenitis, myositis and diffuse orbital inflammation of the orbit.

### Dacryoadenitis

Acute dacryoadenitis, either solitary or with systemic association, presents as painful swelling and tenderness of the lacrimal gland – typically unilateral and associated with an S-shaped ptosis (Fig. 27.1a), palpebral lobe redness or inferonasal globe dystopia. Chronic disease – for example, that due to IgG4-RD or sarcoidosis – is more likely to be bilateral and painless (Fig. 27.1b) [11].

The differential diagnosis for childhood dacryoadenitis includes infection (particularly mumps and infectious mononucleosis), a leaking dermoid cyst or a possible foreign body, whereas that in adulthood should include malignant

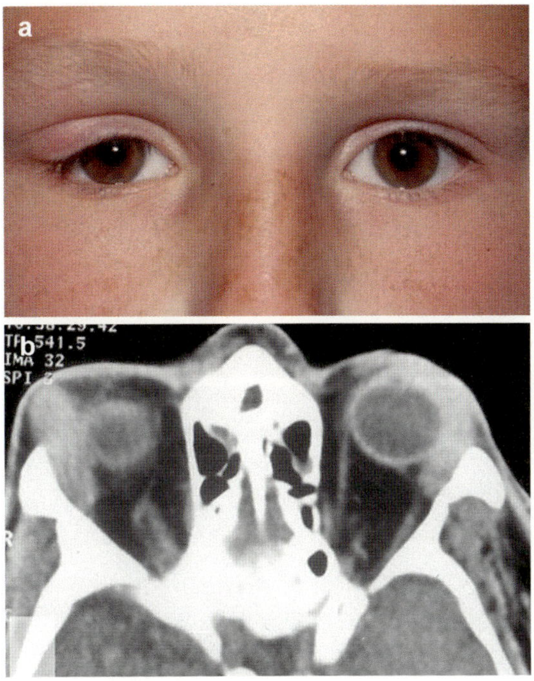


**Fig. 27.1** (**a**) S-shaped painful ptosis in a child with acute right dacryoadenitis. (**b**) Marked bilateral enlargement of the lacrimal glands with some "moulding" around the left globe, due to chronic dacryoadenitis

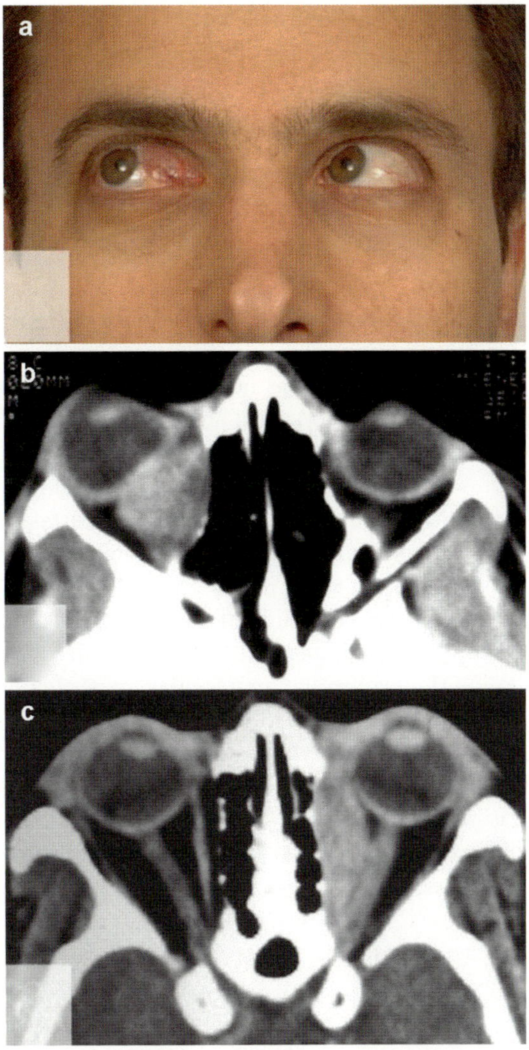


**Fig. 27.2** (**a**) Marked inflammation and swelling over the insertion of the right medial rectus in subacute orbital myositis. (**b**) Rhabdomyosarcoma presenting as a rapid onset of a well-defined mass inferonasally in the right orbit, the mass not being related to the extraocular muscles. (**c**) Acute idiopathic myositis of the left medial rectus, the muscle showing the typical involvement of tendon alongside the globe

infiltration. Systemic conditions associated with dacryoadenitis include IgG4-RD, sarcoidosis, SLE and ANCA-associated vasculitis.

Baseline serological investigation for dacryoadenitis includes full blood count, ACE, ANCA, thyroid function tests and C-reactive protein; where indicated, tuberculosis QuantiFERON, ANA, ENA, dsDNA and serum IgG4 should be ordered. Orbital imaging shows smooth enlargement of the lacrimal gland(s), without bone erosion, but with variable "spillage" of soft-tissue opacity into the adjacent orbital fat or over the orbital rim; slight enlargement or displacement of the neighbouring lateral and superior recti may be evident. Chest x-ray or high-resolution CT is recommended where sarcoidosis or tuberculosis is suspected.

## Myositis

Myositis is characterised by an acute or subacute inflammation of one or more of the extraocular muscles, is commoner in females and accounts for 8 % of all IOID [12]. Patients usually present, after a brief prodromal headache, with diplopia that is worse with eye movement. Depending on disease severity, presentation can range from mild chemosis and vascular injection over the involved muscle insertion to frank orbital inflammation, ptosis and proptosis (Fig. 27.2a).

Unilateral myositis occurs in 70–80 % and typically causes a restrictive strabismus, although children may present with bilateral disease. The horizontal recti are most commonly involved, but superior oblique inflammation and trochleitis are particularly associated with rheumatoid arthritis. The symptoms and signs of myositis may occur with thyroid eye disease (TED), orbital cellulitis, metastasis or paediatric rhabdomyosarcoma. TED is by far the commonest cause of restrictive strabismus in an inflamed orbit, and, as distinct from idiopathic myositis, this is usually bilateral, can be asymmetrical and is often associated with other signs of TED – as lid retraction or proptosis. A medial subperiosteal abscess due to infective ethmoiditis may cause a secondary medial rectus myositis, although such a patient may be systemically unwell. Intramuscular metastases, with poor prognosis, tend to cause single muscle enlargement, although this is generally painless. In children, the possibility of rhabdomyosarcoma should be kept in mind, although generally they do NOT involve the extraocular musculature (Fig. 27.2b).

Sarcoidosis, polymyositis, dermatomyositis, rheumatoid arthritis, SLE, ANCA-associated vasculitis and Crohn's disease are systemic conditions known to be associated with orbital myositis. Baseline investigations for myositis include full blood count, thyroid function tests and C-reactive protein; a neutrophilia should alert the physician to an infective cause such as orbital cellulitis. Serum ACE, c-ANCA, dsDNA, rheumatoid factor, ANA and anticardiolipin antibody titres should be ordered where clinically or pathologically indicated.

Myositis classically shows fusiform muscular enlargement, including its tendon (Fig. 27.2c), with some spillover of inflammation in the orbital fat; in contrast TED myopathy typically spares the muscle tendon. Bony involvement should raise the possibility of an underlying malignancy or infection. Active myositis tends to show a high signal on fat-suppressed T2 MRI sequences.

## Diffuse Orbital Inflammatory Disease

The presentation of diffuse OID – varying from an explosive onset of acute inflammation (Fig. 27.3a) to a chronic grumbling process (Fig. 27.3b) – varies according to the severity and anatomical extent of active inflammation, amount of induced fibrosis and degree of any mass effect. Diffuse OID is generally unilateral and can be associated with repeated recurrences, intracranial spread, or be linked to an underlying systemic disease. Whilst it often presents in the third and fourth decades, it has been reported at all ages and has no gender bias [3].

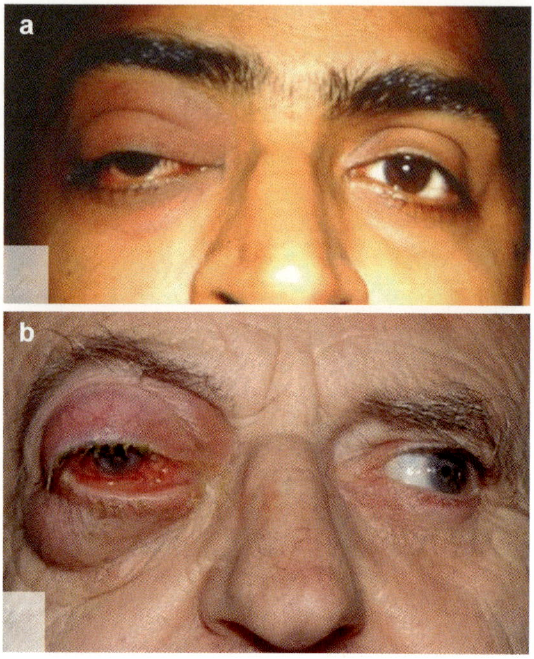

**Fig. 27.3** (**a**) Onset of major right orbital swelling, pain and proptosis over a few weeks, due to acute idiopathic orbital inflammatory disease. (**b**) Chronic sclerosing inflammation associated with chronic pain, a "frozen" and proptotic right globe and poor vision

The acute variant presents with a rapid onset of orbital swelling, pain and varying degrees of proptosis and ophthalmoplegia, and optic neuropathy may arise from optic nerve sheath inflammation or apical crowding. Signs of orbital congestion include raised intraocular pressure, chemosis or dilated episcleral veins. The differential diagnosis for acute OID primarily includes fulminant TED, trauma, infective orbital cellulitis, high-flow carotico-cavernous fistulae and inflammation due to tumour necrosis; in children, the additional differentials of rhabdomyosarcoma, neuroblastoma or histiocytic tumours should always be kept in mind. Infective orbital cellulitis is usually accompanied

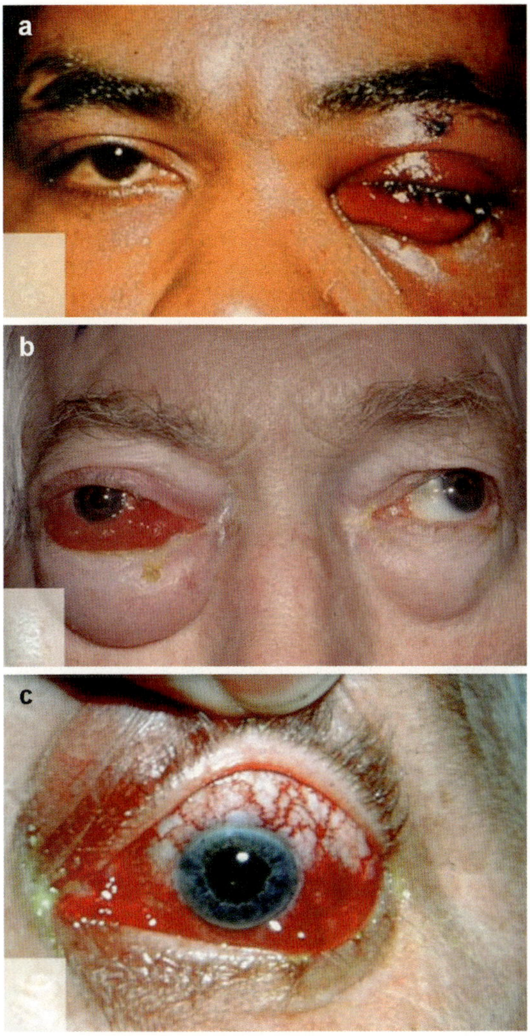


**Fig. 27.4** (**a**) Acute onset of left carotico-cavernous fistula in a young man after trauma. (**b**) A painful high-grade lymphoma of the right orbit, mimicking acute inflammation. (**c**) Patient with low-flow dural arteriovenous shunt, referred as subacute orbital inflammatory disease

by fever and a leukocytosis, and the symptoms and signs of sinus disease (particularly ethmoid sinusitis) may be evident clinically or radiologically. High-flow carotico-cavernous fistula is usually evident as pulsatile proptosis, audible orbital bruit and haemorrhagic chemosis, and suspicion should be high if these signs are present after trauma (particularly in younger patients, Fig. 27.4a), or in older patients with uncontrolled hypertension. Although angiography remains the most accurate investigation, Doppler ultrasonography may show retrograde blood and arterial wave-form within the

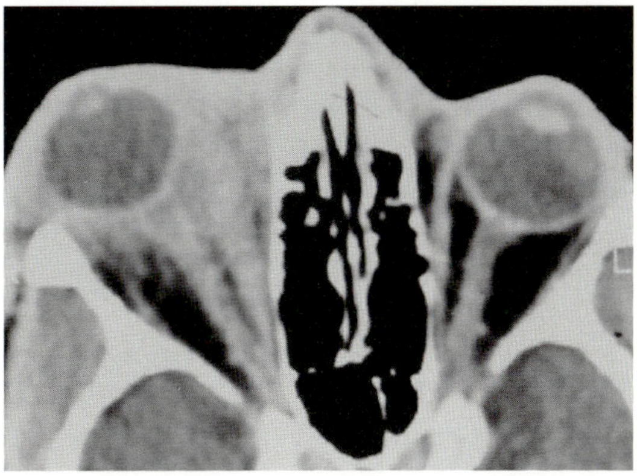

**Fig. 27.5** Axial CT of the orbits, showing subacute right orbital inflammation, manifests as ill-defined opacification of the peribulbar fat, some "cuffing" of the anterior part of the optic nerve and "streaked" opacities within the retrobulbar orbital fat

superior ophthalmic vein. Rhabdomyosarcoma is an embryological mesenchymal tumour of childhood that presents with rapid proptosis, ptosis and orbital inflammation, but unlike infective cellulitis, the periorbital swelling is not warm to touch. Langerhans cell histiocytosis arises from cells of the dendritic system and involves the orbit in 25% of cases [13] with osteolysis in the region of the zygomaticofrontal suture; children and teenagers typically present with acute or chronic periorbital swelling.

Lymphoproliferative disease should be considered in the differential diagnosis of chronic diffuse OID (Fig. 27.4b), together with subacute TED and low-flow carotico-cavernous fistula (Fig. 27.4c). The main differential for OID is TED; the latter also occurring in euthyroid and hypothyroid patients. The two conditions may be indistinguishable at presentation, although upper lid retraction, lateral flare and lid lag on downgaze are suggestive of TED, and imaging typically shows enlarged extraocular muscles with sparing of the anterior tendons.

Systemic associations for the diffuse form of OID are similar to those for dacryoadenitis and myositis (*v.s.*), and so the same investigations and imaging are appropriate. Imaging for diffuse OID usually shows ill-defined orbital opacification and "stranding" of fat (Fig. 27.5), with moderate contrast enhancement; involvement of bone should raise concerns about malignant infiltration or possibly infection. CT or CT-angiography can be useful where carotico-cavernous fistula is suspected. Orbital inflammation is best appreciated on fat-suppressed contrast-enhanced MRI, with hypointense signal on T1-weighted images (due to cellular infiltrate and fibrosis) and isointense, or slightly hyperintense, on fat-suppressed T2-weighting due to high water content [14]. In contrast, the sclerosing variant of OID is hypointense on fat-suppressed T2 and STIR imaging.

## Treatment

Treatment – the main indications being for pain, a threat to vision or loss of function – should be tailored to the patient's presentation, symptoms and any associated systemic disease.

For mild OID, a trial of a non-steroidal anti-inflammatory drug (NSAID) should be considered after biopsy, where indicated. If there is inadequate response to (or progression of disease despite) NSAID, then most OID – whether idiopathic or specific – will respond to high-dose oral corticosteroids, and these should be slowly tapered over several months to prevent early rebound [15]. Patients with frequent relapses or recurrent OID, or those who cannot get below 5 mg prednisolone, should be considered for an additional treatment; these include low-dose orbital radiotherapy or second-line immunosuppressive agents, such as azathioprine, mycophenolate mofetil or cyclophosphamide [15].

With greater understanding of the immune mechanisms underlying orbital inflammatory disease, various cytokine- and protein-specific biologic agents (e.g. rituximab, infliximab) are being investigated for use with OID and are likely to be used in recalcitrant cases [16, 17]. Intravenous immunoglobulins or plasmapheresis, probably by neutralising or removing auto-antibodies, have also been utilised in recalcitrant cases of OID [18]. Surgical debulking is useful where there is a persistent and significant orbital mass, or where there is steroid resistance – particularly with recurrent dacryoadenitis [11].

## References


1. Rose GE. A personal view: probability in medicine, levels of (un)certainty, and the diagnosis of orbital disease (with particular reference to orbital 'pseudotumor'). Arch Ophthalmol. 2007;125:1171–2.
2. Shields JA, Shields CL, Scartozzi R. Survey of 1264 patients with orbital tumors and simulating lesions: the 2002 Montgomery Lecture, part 1. Ophthalmology. 2004;111:997–1008.
3. Gordon LK. Orbital inflammatory disease: a diagnostic and therapeutic challenge. Eye. 2006;20:1196–206.
4. Stone JH, Merkel PA, Spiera R, et al. Rituximab versus cyclophosphamide for ANCA-associated vasculitis. N Engl J Med. 2010;363:221–32.
5. White ES, Lynch III JP. Sarcoidosis involving multiple systems: diagnostic and therapeutic challenges. Chest. 2001;119:1593–7.
6. Perez Alamino R, Espinoza LR, Zea AH. The great mimicker: IgG4-related disease. Clin Rheumatol. 2013;32:1267–73.
7. Lindfield D, Attfield K, McElvanney A. Systemic immunoglobulin G4 (IgG4) disease and idiopathic orbital inflammation; removing 'idiopathic' from the nomenclature? Eye. 2012;26:623–9.
8. Fraser C, Skalicky S, Gurbaxani A, McCluskey P. Ocular myositis. Curr Allergy Asthma Rep. 2013;13:315–21.
9. Pradeep TG, Prabhakaran VC, McNab A, Dodd T, Selva D. Diffuse bilateral orbital inflammation in Churg-Strauss syndrome. Ophthal Plast Reconstr Surg. 2010;26:57–9.
10. Mombaerts I, Goldschmeding R, Schlingemann RO, Koornneef L. What is orbital pseudotumour? Surv Ophthalmol. 1996;41:66–78.
11. Mombaerts I, Cameron D, Chanlalit W, Garrity J. Surgical debulking for idiopathic dacryoadenitis. A diagnosis and a cure. Ophthalmology. 2014;121:603–8.
12. Schoser BG. Ocular myositis: diagnostic assessment, differential diagnoses, and therapy of a rare muscle disease – five new cases and review. Clin Ophthalmol. 2007;1:37–42.
13. Margo CE, Goldman DR. Langerhans cell histiocytosis. Surv Ophthalmol. 2008;53:332–58.
14. Lutt JR, Lim LL, Phal PM, Rosenbaum JT. Orbital inflammatory disease. Sem Arthr Rheumtol. 2008;37: 207–22.
15. Ahn Yuen SJ, Rubin PAD. Idiopathic orbital inflammation – distribution, clinical features, and treatment outcome. Arch Ophthalmol. 2003;121:491–9.
16. Wilson MW, Shergy WJ, Haik BG. Infliximab in the treatment of recalcitrant idiopathic orbital inflammation. Ophthal Plast Reconstr Surg. 2004;20:381–9.
17. Ibrahim I, Barton A, Ibrahim A, Ho P. Idiopathic orbital inflammation successfully treated using Rituximab in a patient with rheumatoid arthritis. J Rheumatol. 2012;39:1485–6.
18. Symon Z, Schneebaum N, Eyal A, et al. Successful intravenous immunoglobulin therapy for resistant inflammatory pseudotumor of the orbit. Thyroid. 2005;14:398–9.

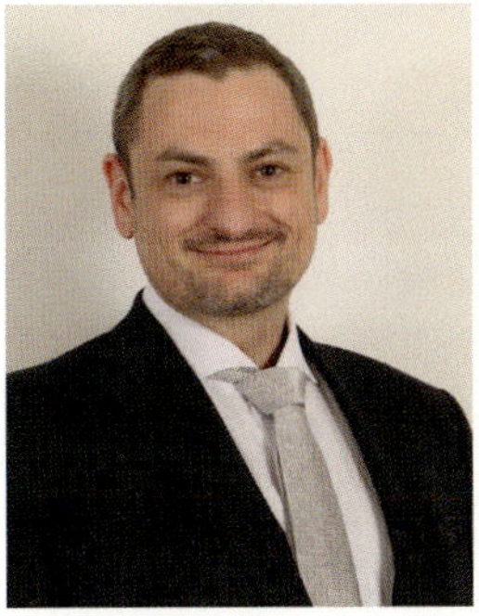

**Dov Hersh** Dr. Dov Hersh is an oculoplastic and ophthalmic surgeon based in Sydney, Australia. Dr Hersh undertook his comprehensive ophthalmic training at Sydney Eye Hospital and advanced oculoplastics subspecialty training at Bristol and Moorfields Eye Hospitals, UK. Dr Hersh is a clinical associate lecturer at Sydney University, Australia, and is an accredited investigator in a number of multinational oculoplastic clinical trials studying novel treatments for orbital inflammatory and thyroid eye disease. Prior to his medical career, Dr Hersh gained a B Com, specializing in IT. He has established telemedicine projects in developing countries.

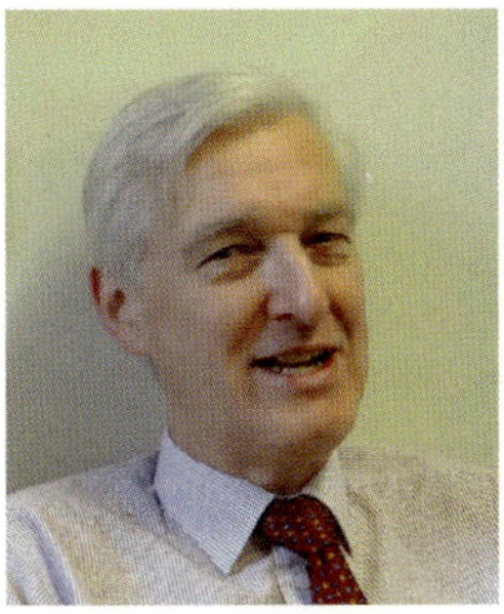

**Geoffrey E. Rose** Geoffrey Rose graduated BSc Pharmacology, MBBS, and MRCP. His postgraduate ophthalmic training culminated in award of FRCS in 1985 and FRCOphth at its foundation in 1988. In 1990, the University of London granted an MS doctorate for corneal research and, in 2004, a Doctor of Science in Ophthalmology and Ophthalmic Surgery.

Professor Rose was appointed consultant to Moorfields Eye Hospital, London, in 1990 and is also a Senior Research Fellow of the NIHR Biomedical Research Centre of the Institute of Ophthalmology. He served as the British Council member of the European Society of Ophthalmic Plastic and Reconstructive, is a Past-President of the British Oculoplastic Surgical Society, and is President of the European Society of Oculoplastic and Reconstructive Surgeons.

# 28 Management of Dysthyroid Optic Neuropathy

Shannon S. Joseph and Neil R. Miller

## Introduction

Dysthyroid optic neuropathy (DON) is one of the most serious complications of thyroid eye disease (TED). It occurs in 4–8.6 % of TED patients and can lead to permanent vision loss [1–3]. DON is defined as the impairment of optic nerve function in TED caused by the mechanical compression or distortion of the optic nerve [3]. This chapter will focus on the management options for DON, but we will first review its disease mechanism, clinical presentation, and diagnostic process.

## Mechanism of Disease

TED is an autoimmune phenomenon that involves both antigen-dependent and antigen-independent immune systems (Fig. 28.1).

The fundamental change that underlies most clinical manifestations of TED, including DON, is enlargement or expansion of orbital soft tissues [4–7]. The pathogenic processes leading to this soft tissue enlargement remain under investigation; however, current theories point to the orbital fibroblasts (OF) as the principal effector cells of this process [4, 5, 8]. The orbit contains two subpopulations of OFs: Thy1+ and Thy1- cells, each of which contributes to orbital soft tissue enlargement in TED in a unique manner. Thy1+ OFs overexpress the cell surface marker Thy1 (CD90) in TED. Upon stimulation by pro-inflammatory cytokines, such as interleukin-1β, these OFs proliferate and upregulate specific hyaluronan synthases, resulting in increased hyaluronan secretion [5, 9–12]. Hyaluronan is a hydrophilic glycosaminoglycan (GAG) that accumulates within the orbit and draws water into the extraocular muscles, orbital fat, and connective tissues, leading to swelling [9, 13–15]. Thy1- OFs, which do not express Thy1, are pre-adipocytes that can differentiate into mature adipocytes, leading to expansion of orbital fat [16]. In addition to the OFs, lymphocytes and macrophages contribute to orbital soft tissue swelling by infiltrating the tissue and generating inflammatory edema [17, 18]. Together, these mechanisms lead to the orbital soft tissue enlargement seen in TED.

As soft tissue volume increases within the rigid bony orbital walls, intraorbital pressure also increases, and mechanical compression occurs [18, 19]. When this compression affects the optic nerve, usually in the orbital apex, it can cause DON [20]. In some patients, the rise in orbital pressure leads to proptosis that, in turn, may

S.S. Joseph, MD, MSc
Ophthalmology, Johns Hopkins Hospital,
Baltimore, MD 21287, USA
e-mail: SJCShan@gmail.com

N.R. Miller, MD (✉)
Ophthalmology, Neurology and Neurosurgery,
Johns Hopkins Hospital, Baltimore, MD 21287, USA
e-mail: nrmiller@jhmi.edu


B. Mukherjee, H. Yuen (eds.), *Emergencies of the Orbit and Adnexa*,
DOI 10.1007/978-81-322-1807-4_28

serve as spontaneous orbital decompression, thus decreasing the risk for DON [21]. Proptosis typically occurs in patients with eyelid laxity and/or minimal orbital soft tissue fibrosis [21]. Conversely, patients with less eyelid laxity and more orbital fibrosis are less likely to have proptosis and more likely to have greater intraorbital pressure, resulting in an increased risk for DON [4]. Indeed, several studies have demonstrated that patients with DON typically do not have marked proptosis [1, 3, 20, 22].

As noted above, the location at which optic nerve mechanical compression occurs in the TED orbit is widely accepted to be the orbital apex. This theory is well supported by evidence from both radiographic imaging studies and histopathological studies [1, 6, 18, 20, 23–29]. Trokel et al. were the first to demonstrate using computed tomographic (CT) scanning crowding of the enlarged extraocular muscles at the orbital apex in patients with DON [30]. This significant correlation between apical crowding on CT and DON has since been confirmed in numerous studies [1, 23, 26–29] (Fig. 28.2a, b).

Nevertheless, what established the clinicopathological correlation between apical crowding and DON were the histopathological findings of exenterated orbital contents from a patient with

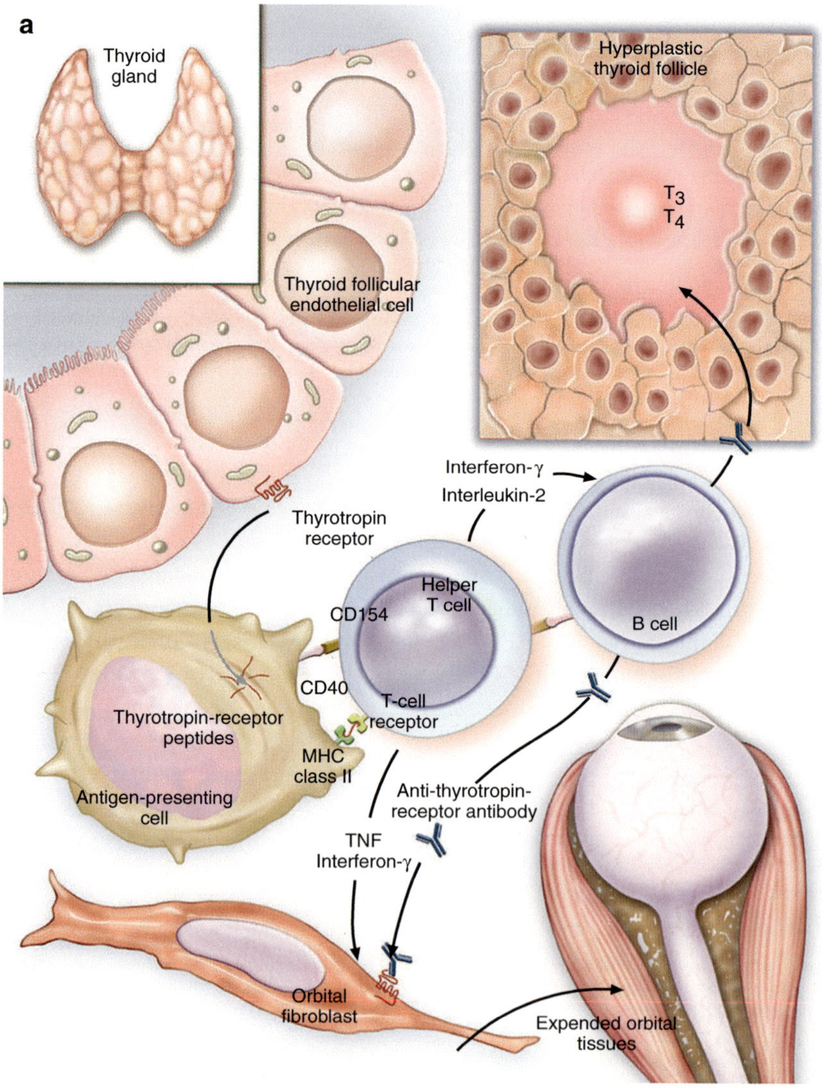


**Fig. 28.1** (a, b) Pathogenesis of thyroid eye disease

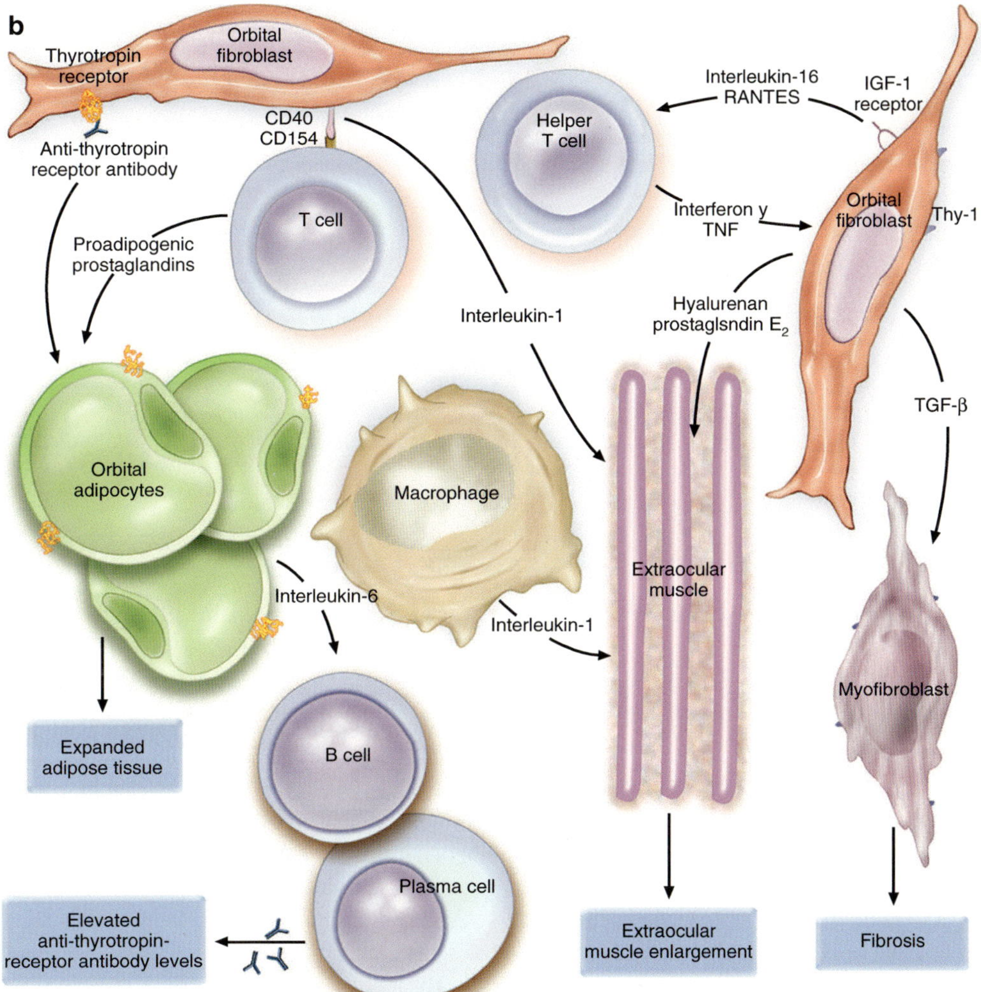


**Fig. 28.1** (continued)

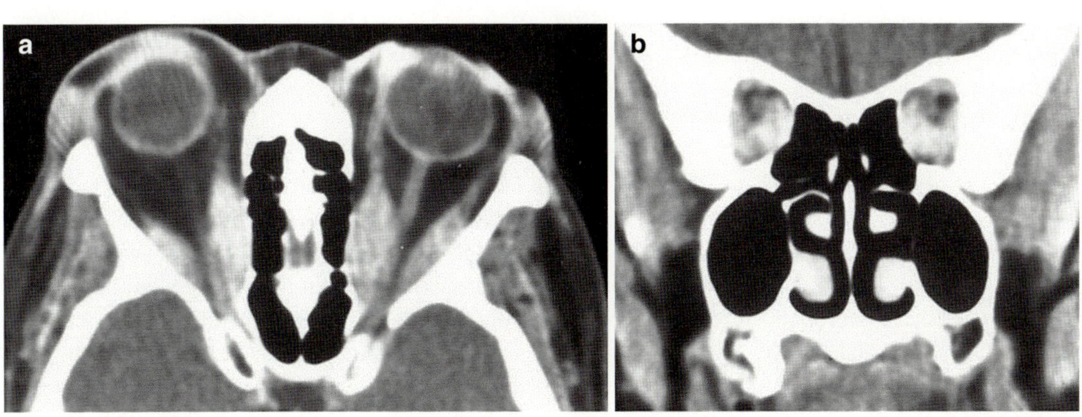


**Fig. 28.2** (**a**, **b**) Axial (**a**) and coronal (**b**) CT images show Apical crowding in a patient with thyroid eye disease and bilateral optic neuropathy

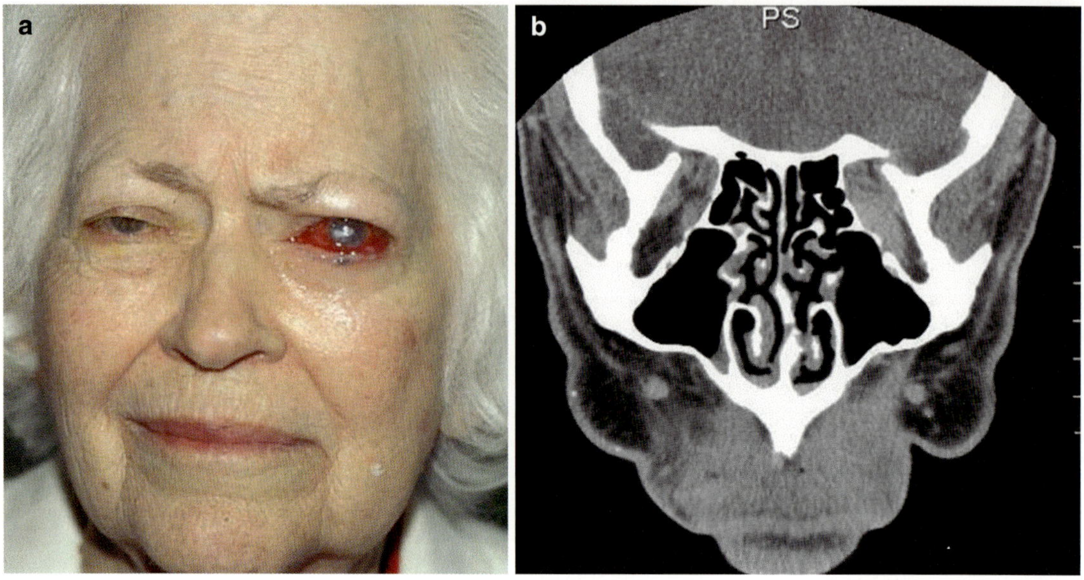


**Fig. 28.3** (**a**) Corneal ulceration causing decreased vision in the left eye of a patient who also had a left optic neuropathy. (**b**) Same patient from (**a**). Non-contrast CT scan, coronal view. Note crowding in the left orbital apex but not in the right

TED [18]. In this study, Hufnagel et al. used immunohistochemical stains to confirm the presence of partial optic nerve atrophy in their specimen. More importantly, they observed that the axon loss was most pronounced in the sections of the optic nerve from the orbital apex [18]. They noted no evidence of inflammatory infiltrate of the optic nerve [18]. Taken together, current evidence suggests that DON is caused by mechanical compression or distortion of the optic nerve at the orbital apex due to enlargement of orbital soft tissue. DON thus is a form of compressive optic neuropathy, and the goal of management for DON should be to decrease orbital soft tissue enlargement and/or increase the space in which the orbital soft tissue reside, thereby relieving the intraorbital pressure and compression, especially at the orbital apex.

## Clinical Presentation and Diagnosis

Compressive optic neuropathies typically present with decreased visual acuity, dyschromatopsia, visual field defects, a relative afferent pupillary defect (RAPD) (unless the condition is bilateral), and either normal-appearing optic disks or optic disk swelling [31]. The onset of DON is highly variable [1, 32–34]; it can be acute or insidious [35], progressing over days, weeks, or even months. Other ocular comorbidities, such as exposure keratopathy, glaucoma, and cataract, may be present as confounding factors [1, 32, 33], sometimes resulting in delayed diagnosis (Fig. 28.3a, b).

To identify the most diagnostically useful clinical features of DON, the European Group on Graves' Orbitopathy (EUGOGO) analyzed the clinical presentation of 94 eyes in 47 patients in a multicenter study [3]. Fifty-five of these eyes had definite DON. Of these 55 eyes, 80 % had reduced visual acuity compared with 32 % in those without DON, 77 % had dyschromatopsia compared with 7 % in those without DON, 45 % had an RAPD compared with none in those without DON, and 56 % had optic disk swelling compared with 5 % in those without DON [3]. Even though an RAPD and optic disk swelling were not very sensitive findings, they were highly specific, rendering them diagnostically valuable signs. Collectively, current evidence suggests that visual acuity, color vision, pupillary reaction to light, and optic disk appearance are arguably the four most important element of the clinical exam in diagnosing DON [3, 36, 37]. Other clinical features such as extraocular movement abnormalities, proptosis, and the clinical activity score (CAS, a score based on classic subjective features of inflammation such as swelling, redness, and pain) [38] have lower sensitivity and specificity in diagnosing DON. The EUGOGO survey found that extraocular movement restriction was slightly more common in eyes with DON than eyes without DON (71 % versus 52 % for upgaze, 18 % versus 0 % for downgaze, 33 % versus 5 % for abduction, 15 % versus 15 % for adduction) [3], but there was no significant difference in the amount of proptosis between eyes with DON and eyes without (62 % versus 63 %) [3]. As previously mentioned in this chapter, numerous studies have shown that proptosis does not correlate with the presence or severity of DON [3, 20, 22, 23, 36, 39]. The CAS for eyes with DON was slightly higher, but 39 % of patients with definite DON had a CAS less than 3 [3]. This finding is consistent with the previously reported observation that even though DON is, by definition, indicative of severe TED, patients with DON often lack or at least have relatively mild soft tissue stigmata of TED [1, 2, 20, 36, 40]. Resistance to retropulsion on clinical exam has been suggested to correlate with elevated intraorbital pressure and, therefore, DON [21, 41]; however, the sensitivity and specificity of this finding have not been assessed. In summary, although assessment of ocular motility and alignment, amount of proptosis, CAS, and degree of resistance to retropulsion are important elements of the clinical exam when assessing patients with known or suspected TED, they may not be the most sensitive or specific features for DON.

## Ancillary Testing

When DON is suspected based on clinical findings, or when the etiology is unclear, ancillary testing is necessary to ensure accurate diagnosis. Three ancillary testing modalities have been most commonly used in the diagnosis of DON: orbital imaging, perimetry, and visual evoked potentials (VEPs). We will discuss each of these tests in more detail, with a special focus on orbital CT scanning, one of the best diagnostic tests currently available for DON.

Magnetic resonance (MR) imaging, ultrasonography, and CT scanning are all commonly used to evaluate patients suspected of having TED. MR imaging provides the most detailed imaging of the orbital soft tissue anatomy and is useful in assessing if interstitial edema and evidence of active inflammation are present [42–44]. Ultrasonography is an economical and safe method of evaluating orbital soft tissue enlargement as well as changes in internal reflectivity of the extraocular muscles [42–44], but it requires an experienced ultrasonographer. In addition, a major disadvantage of both modalities is their inferiority to CT scanning in imaging bony structures [42–44]. DON occurs from mechanical compression or distortion of the optic nerve at the orbital apex. Therefore, orbital CT scanning, which provides precise imaging of the orbital bony structures, including the orbital apex, is the imaging modality of choice not only for the diagnosis of DON but also for determining its management [42–44].

Orbital CT scans to evaluate for DON are performed without intravenous contrast, using a spiral CT technique with 2-mm-thick slices in the axial plane. Coronal and sagittal images should be reconstructed [42]. Imaging features such as extraocular muscle enlargement, orbital fat compartment enlargement, orbital fat prolapse, proptosis, lacrimal gland displacement, superior ophthalmic vein dilation, medial bowing of the lamina papyracea, and apical crowding have all been described in patients with DON [1, 6, 23–29, 45–47]. Two of these features, extraocular muscle enlargement and apical crowding, have been shown to have the most reliable predictors of DON (Fig. 28.2a, b).

Numerous studies have documented a correlation between extraocular muscle enlargement on orbital CT scanning and DON [6, 23, 24, 27, 40, 45–47]. Feldon et al. performed the first quantitative volumetric assessment demonstrating that TED patients with DON have significantly higher extraocular muscle volume compared with those without DON [45]. To quantify extraocular muscle enlargement more reproducibly, Barrett et al. used a "muscle index" (MI): the percentage of orbital width occupied by the extraocular muscles measured in the plane at the midpoint between the orbital apex and the posterior globe [46]. Sensitivity and specificity varied depending on the level of MI used. The best combination was found to be for MI of 60 %, which was 79 % sensitive and 72 % specific for DON [48].

Another CT parameter that has been shown to be an excellent predictor of DON is optic nerve crowding at the orbital apex [1, 3, 23–29, 42]. Nugent et al. proposed a subjective grading scale for apical crowding based on coronal imaging at the apex: grade 0 represents no effacement of perineural fat planes by enlarged extraocular muscles; grade 1 represents 1–24 % of effacement; grade 2 represents 25–50 % of effacement; and grade 3 represents greater than 50 % effacement [28]. Studies have shown that grade 3 apical crowding on CT scanning has sensitivity ranging from 62 to 80 % and specificity ranging from 70 to 91 % [26, 28, 29]. With the advent of multidetector CT (MDCT) scanners, quantitative measures and precise image reformatting have become readily available. Goncalves et al. developed a more objective measure of apical crowding using MDCT: the orbital crowding index (CI) [49]. This is a ratio between the square area measurements of the extraocular muscles and the orbital bone area, measured at three well-defined coronal planes [49]. The best combination of sensitivity and specificity (92 % and 90 %, respectively) was found for a CI of 0.575 at 18 mm from the interzygomatic plane [49].

Collective evidence shows that orbital CT scanning is one of the best diagnostic tools currently available for DON. Every patient suspected of having DON based on the clinical examination, or for whom the diagnosis is unclear but DON is a possibility, should undergo this imaging technique. For patients with DON who require surgery, orbital CT scanning is also useful for preoperative planning, postoperative assessment, and, at some centers, intraoperative stereotactic navigation (see below) [43, 50].

Other ancillary tests that have been used to facilitate the diagnosis of DON include static perimetry and VEPs. It is well established that patients with DON can present with a variety of visual field defects on perimetry. Central and paracentral scotomata tend to be the most common, but arcuate and altitudinal scotomata have also been observed [34, 36, 37, 51, 52]. The EUGOGO multicenter survey reported that 71 % of eyes with definite DON had abnormal visual fields, compared with 13 % in eyes without DON, although the method of visual field testing was not standardized in this study [3]. Unfortunately, a myriad of ocular conditions can produce field defects, including exposure keratopathy, lenticular changes, glaucoma, other causes of optic neuropathy, retinal disorders, lid malposition, and refractive error. Many of these can be comorbidities of TED. Indeed, up to 70 % of TED patients without DON have also been reported to have reproducible visual field defects, many of which are also central or paracentral [53]. Moreover, static perimetry is also subject to nonophthalmologic factors such as technician errors, patient test-taking errors, and cognitive factors (usually on the part of the patient). In summary, static perimetry may be informative and should be obtained as part of the assessment of a patient suspected to have DON, but it is not very sensitive and is definitely not specific for DON.

Another test that has been used for both the diagnosis and monitoring of DON is VEPs. Patients with DON often have abnormal VEP latency and amplitude [1, 3, 54–59]. Several studies have reported on the remarkably high sensitivity of abnormal VEPs for DON [1, 3, 54–59]. For example, Neigel et al. observed that VEPs were abnormal in 94 % of 58 patients with DON versus 9.1 % in a control group [1]. Comparatively, the sensitivity of other tests were much lower in their study, including decreased visual acuity (52.6 %), RAPD (35 %), dyschromatopsia (64 %), and visual field defect (66 %) [1]. The most common changes in VEPs observed in DON are decreased amplitude and increased latency of both the P2 and the P100 peaks [54, 55, 57, 59]. Interestingly, after patients undergo treatment for DON with either steroids or surgical decompression, their VEPs tend to normalize, with the amplitudes improving more than the latencies [55, 57]. Nevertheless, although VEPs may be highly sensitive in facilitating the diagnosis of DON and monitoring patients after treatment, the test results are not very specific.

Factors such as opaque media, uncorrected refractive error, and other causes of optic neuropathy can affect results. Furthermore, the testing equipment is not readily available, so VEPs have not been widely adopted as a part of the routine diagnostic process for DON.

In summary, timely and accurate diagnosis is imperative to the successful management of DON [60]. Most cases of delayed diagnosis of compressive optic neuropathy are caused by failure to perform color vision or visual field testing, failure to check for an RAPD, and failure to obtain appropriate imaging studies [31]. There currently are no standardized diagnostic guidelines for DON. Based on the currently available evidence, however, all patients with DON should have periodic complete ophthalmologic assessments, with special attention to color vision testing, visual fields, pupillary responses to light stimulation, and the appearance of the optic disks. In cases concerning for DON, orbital CT scanning should be obtained to assess for the degree of enlargement of the extraocular muscles as well as apical crowding. If VEPs are available, they may yield additional information. If visual impairment is confirmed based on these tests and no other identifiable etiology can account for the impairment, then the diagnosis of DON is likely.

## Management of DON

Dysthyroid optic neuropathy, once diagnosed, mandates urgent and, sometimes, emergent, treatment. Once optic neuropathy develops, permanent visual loss may result, and by the time optic atrophy becomes apparent, visual recovery is unlikely. Hence, early and accurate diagnosis and treatment of DON may improve a patient's visual prognosis.

### Risk Factor Modification

The risk factors of DON include male gender, older age, smoking, and significant comorbidities such as diabetes mellitus (DM) [61]. One of the first steps in the management of DON is modification of risk factors. Smoking is a key modifiable behavioral risk factor for TED and DON [32]. Among patients with Graves' disease, smokers are more likely to develop TED (odds ratio 7.7, 95 % CI 4.3–13.7) [62] than nonsmokers, and smokers with TED also tend to have more severe disease and poorer response to treatment [62–64]. Bartalena et al. reported that in 150 patients with severe TED, 93.8 % of nonsmokers responded to treatment (high-dose oral prednisone followed by orbital radiotherapy), whereas only 68.2 % of smokers responded [63]. Similarly, Eckstein et al. observed that smoking influences the treatment response of TED in a dose-dependent manner, with delayed and decreased therapeutic response in smokers [64]. Therefore, to optimize response to therapy and prevent further progression of disease, smoking cessation should be discussed upon diagnosis and remain an integral part of management for all patients with TED and DON.

Diabetes mellitus also is an important risk factor for DON. Neigel et al. reported that 15.5 % of patients in their DON group were diabetics, compared with 1.7 % in their control group [1]. Similarly, Kalmann et al. noted that DON developed in 33.3 % of TED patients with DM compared with 2.9 % in the TED patients without DM [65]. TED patients with DM also seem to have a more recalcitrant course, developing more severe DON with a worse visual prognosis [1, 37, 65]. One proposed mechanism underlying this relationship is that diabetic microvascular changes in the optic nerve may sensitize it to compression [65]. No studies have evaluated whether or not there is a dose-response relationship between the severity of DM and the progression or therapeutic response of DON; however, upon diagnosing DON in a patient with DM, it would be prudent to alert the patient's primary care provider of this diagnosis and emphasize to the patient the importance of glycemic control.

### Systemic Thyroid Status

A major systemic factor that must be considered when managing patients with TED is their systemic thyroid status. Although patients may be hyperthyroid, hypothyroid, or euthyroid when they first develop symptoms and signs of TED, TED typically presents simultaneously or within 18 months of the onset of hyperthyroidism [66, 67]. No correlation between the level of thyroid dysfunction and DON has been reported in the literature, but evidence suggests that TED patients who are persistently dysthyroid have more severe eye disease than those who are euthyroid [68]. Therefore, the restoration and maintenance of normal thyroid function should be a key treatment goal in every patient with TED.

Three treatments are used to normalize thyroid function: radioablation using iodine-131, antithyroid medication, and total or partial thyroidectomy. Two large randomized controlled trials have shown that iodine-131 treatment is more likely than other forms of antithyroid therapy to be followed by the development or worsening of TED [68–73]. The mechanism underlying this phenomenon is likely related to the destruction of thyroid tissue by radioactive iodine therapy leading to the release of thyroid antigens that are shared between the thyroid and the orbital soft tissues, which subsequently exacerbates the autoimmune reaction within these tissues [5]. The risk factors for developing or worsening of TED triggered by radioablation include high pretreatment serum T3 levels (more than 5 nmol), high serum thyrotropin binding inhibiting immunoglobulins (TBII) levels, and an active smoking history [69, 70]. This adverse effect of radioactive iodine therapy may be prevented or at least reduced by concomitant administration of low-dose (0.5 mg/kg/day) systemic oral steroids beginning 1 week prior to radioablation and continuing for several months following radioablation [70]. In summary, euthyroidism should be the goal in all patients with TED. For patients who already have TED or who do not have TED but have the risk factors described above and in whom radioablation is to be performed, we recommend pre- and posttreatment with low-dose systemic corticosteroids.

## Treatments for DON

Three major treatment modalities may be used to treat DON: systemic glucocorticoids, orbital decompression, and orbital radiotherapy. Some patients may require a combination of these therapies. Because DON is rare, randomized controlled trials to assess the efficacy of the various treatment modalities are difficult to conduct. Most of the current literature consists of retrospective studies and will be reviewed below.

## Glucocorticoid Therapy

Glucocorticoids (GCs) have been used to treat TED for more than half a century [39, 74, 75]. GCs have anti-inflammatory properties and, at higher doses, are immunosuppressive. Specifically, GCs suppress lymphocytes, hinder recruitment of monocytes and macrophages, and inhibit the release of inflammatory mediators [76]. Not surprisingly, patients with more active orbital inflammation tend to be more responsive to GC therapy than those with long-standing or inactive disease associated with fibrotic orbital soft tissue [77]. In addition, GCs inhibit glycosaminoglycan synthesis in fibroblasts [78]. By reducing the inflammation and swelling of the orbital soft tissues, GCs decrease orbital soft tissue and extraocular muscle enlargement, reduce apical crowding, and relieve compression of the optic nerve.

Both local and systemic GC treatments for patients with TED with and without DON have been used. Local treatment consists of retrobulbar and subconjunctival injections of steroids [79]. The efficacy of this treatment for DON has not been extensively studied, but given the site of the compression, the risk of tissue injury from multiple intraorbital injections, and the large doses of systemic GCs usually required to control DON, we and others do not recommend this route of administration [80]. Instead, systemic GC administration is the route of choice for DON. The oral regimen routinely requires an initial large daily dose (1–2 mg/kg/day) with a prolonged taper over several months. As might be expected, this regimen is associated with significant systemic side effects [81]. Over the past two decades, five randomized controlled trials (RCTs) have shown that intravenous (IV) administration of glucocorticoids is superior to oral administration in treating both DON and severe TED without DON and is associated with fewer side effects [76]. Thus, the IV route is preferred over the oral route by most physicians [82].

For patients with DON, IV administration of GCs is typically given as daily doses of methylprednisolone (MP) for 3–5 days, following which a decision is made as to whether to continue daily or weekly IV administration or switch the patient to oral steroids. This regimen is similar to that used for other autoimmune or inflammatory conditions, such as systemic lupus erythematosus, rheumatoid arthritis, and giant cell arteritis [83–85], and it can lead to rapid visual recovery in patients with DON [86–89]. Guy et al. reported five patients with severe DON treated with IV MP, 1 g/day, for 3 days. All five patients experienced significant improvement in visual acuity, color vision, and visual field defects immediately after the completion of therapy [87]. A larger retrospective study by Mourits et al. examined the longer-term efficacy of IV pulse therapy for DON [88]. Sixty-two consecutive patients with DON were treated with four courses of IV MP, 500 mg every other day, followed by either an oral prednisone taper or orbital radiotherapy. Vision, proptosis, supraduction, and CAS all improved significantly by the first day after completion of therapy. Changes in other findings of DON such as visual field defects, dyschromatopsia, presence or absence of an RAPD, disk appearance, and results of VEPs were not documented in this study; however, by the time the disease had been stable for at least 6 months, 39 % of patients retained normal vision, whereas 61 % had to undergo surgical decompression for persistent or recurrent DON [88].

These retrospective studies support the short-term efficacy of IV pulse therapy with GCs for DON; however, if a majority of patients treated in this manner eventually have to undergo surgical decompression, should the first-line therapy be surgery instead of IV GCs? Wakelkamp et al. conducted a small randomized controlled trial to answer this question [89]. Nine patients were randomized to IV MP pulse therapy followed by an oral taper over 4 months. Six patients were randomized to immediate three-wall orbital decompression surgery. At 52 weeks, there was improvement in visual acuity, "total eye score," and CAS in 56 % of the steroid group compared with 17 % in the surgery group. Moreover, although 56 % of patients in the steroid group eventually required surgical decompression or orbital radiotherapy, 83 % of the surgery group required subsequent steroid treatment, orbital radiotherapy, or both. Therefore, immediate surgery has no advantage over initial pulse therapy, at least in this study. This result is not surprising as, in contrast to GC treatment, surgery does not have a targeted effect on either the underlying immune response or the ongoing orbital inflammation in TED [89]. In fact, surgery may generate additional stress and inflammation in the orbital soft tissue. Thus, we believe that IV GC pulse therapy should be the first line of therapy for DON unless the patient has a contraindication to steroid use.

There is currently no standardized dosing regimen for IV GC pulse therapy or for the subsequent oral prednisone taper in patients with DON. No RCTs have been conducted to determine the most efficacious regimen. There also is no clear evidence regarding the benefit of adjuvant radiotherapy for DON after GC therapy. Based on the available evidence, most would agree with a regimen of IV MP, 1 g/day, for three consecutive days, repeated in the second week if necessary. If the response is sufficient, an oral prednisone taper can be initiated at the completion of the pulse therapy. If the response is insufficient or if the patient cannot tolerate or has contraindications to steroid treatment, either orbital decompression surgery or radiation therapy should be considered [90–92].

Systemic GC therapy is well known to have a multitude of adverse effects, many of which have serious health consequences and some of which can be lethal. Four studies that specifically investigated the use of IV GC pulse therapy for DON observed the following side effects: peptic ulcer, osteoporosis, abscess formation, increased insulin requirement, weight gain, cushingoid appearance, hypertension, central retinal vein occlusion, and irritability [86–89]. Other known serious GC side effects such as gastrointestinal (GI) bleed, liver dysfunction, and adrenal insufficiency were not reported by the authors of these studies, but this may be due to the small sample size in each. Indeed, much larger studies have been conducted on IV GC treatment for moderate-to-severe TED, which typically involves weekly infusions of IV GCs with a cumulative dose ranging from 4.2 to 12 g [92]. A meta-analysis of a total of 1,461 patients with moderate-to-severe TED treated with IV GCs reported a morbidity and mortality rate of 6.5 % and 0.6 %, respectively [76]. The mortalities were due to acute liver failure and cerebrovascular or cardiovascular events [92–97]. All but one of these patients had received a cumulative dose of at least 8 g when the fatal adverse event occurred [92]. Therefore, it would appear that the higher the cumulative dose of GCs, the greater the risk for a serious and potentially fatal adverse effect.

The most common serious adverse effect reported in TED patients treated with IV GCs is acute liver damage (ALD) [97, 98]. The estimated total frequency of GC-associated ALD is 1 %, with 30 % of these cases being lethal [61]. The mechanism underlying this serious complication is unclear, but studies suggest three major risk factors: fatty liver (steatosis), autoimmune hepatitis, and subclinical viral hepatitis [92, 98]. To minimize risk of ALD, the following tests should be obtained prior to initiating GC therapy for DON: liver function tests, liver ultrasound, non-organ-specific autoantibodies that may be associated with autoimmune hepatitis (microsomal antibodies, anticentromeric antibodies, antimitochondrial antibodies, and smooth muscle antibodies) [98], and viral markers for hepatitis B and C [92].

Cardiovascular and GI risk factors also should be assessed prior to initiating systemic GC therapy for DON. These include hypokalemia, cardiac arrhythmia, uncontrolled hypertension, uncontrolled diabetes, and history of a GI bleed [92]. Therefore, in addition to the aforementioned hepatic workup, the following tests should also be performed: complete blood count, basic metabolic panel, fasting glucose test, lipid panel, urinalysis (urine culture), and fecal occult test. If testing suggests that a patient is at high risk for developing an adverse effect from GC therapy, alternate treatment modalities should be considered. In addition, once GC therapy is initiated, all patients should be monitored closely for side effects.

## Surgical Orbital Decompression

For patients with DON who do not respond to IV GC pulse therapy or for those who have contraindications to or cannot tolerate the side effects of GCs, surgical decompression should be considered [99]. The goal of surgical decompression is to remove parts of the rigid bony orbital walls and/or orbital fat, thereby effectively expanding the available orbital space. This allows the enlarged and congested orbital soft tissue to expand into newly available space, relieving the orbital pressure and reducing the compression on the optic nerve [99, 100]. Numerous techniques to decompress the TED orbit have been developed since the early 1900s. We will discuss the major techniques that are in use today.

The orbit has several bony regions that could be subject to decompression: the anterior lateral wall, the deep lateral wall, the orbital floor, and the medial wall [101] (Fig. 28.4).

The anterior lateral wall consists of the zygoma and is covered by the temporalis muscle and buccal fat. The deep lateral wall consists of the greater wing of the sphenoid and the lesser wing of the sphenoid anterior to the tip of the superior orbital fissure. The orbital floor overlies the maxillary sinus. The medial wall overlies the ethmoid sinuses. Although decompression of each of these areas has been shown to be effective to varying degrees in treating severe TED, it is the decompression of the posterior medial wall that is especially important in the treatment of DON [101] as the posterior medial wall is in close proximity to the orbital apex, the location at which the optic nerve compression occurs.

The medial wall can be approached either endoscopically or non-endoscopically (Fig. 28.5). Kennedy et al. first described using the intranasal endoscope to perform medial and inferior orbital wall decompression to treat DON [102]. In this approach, a total ethmoidectomy is first performed. The middle turbinate is retained to

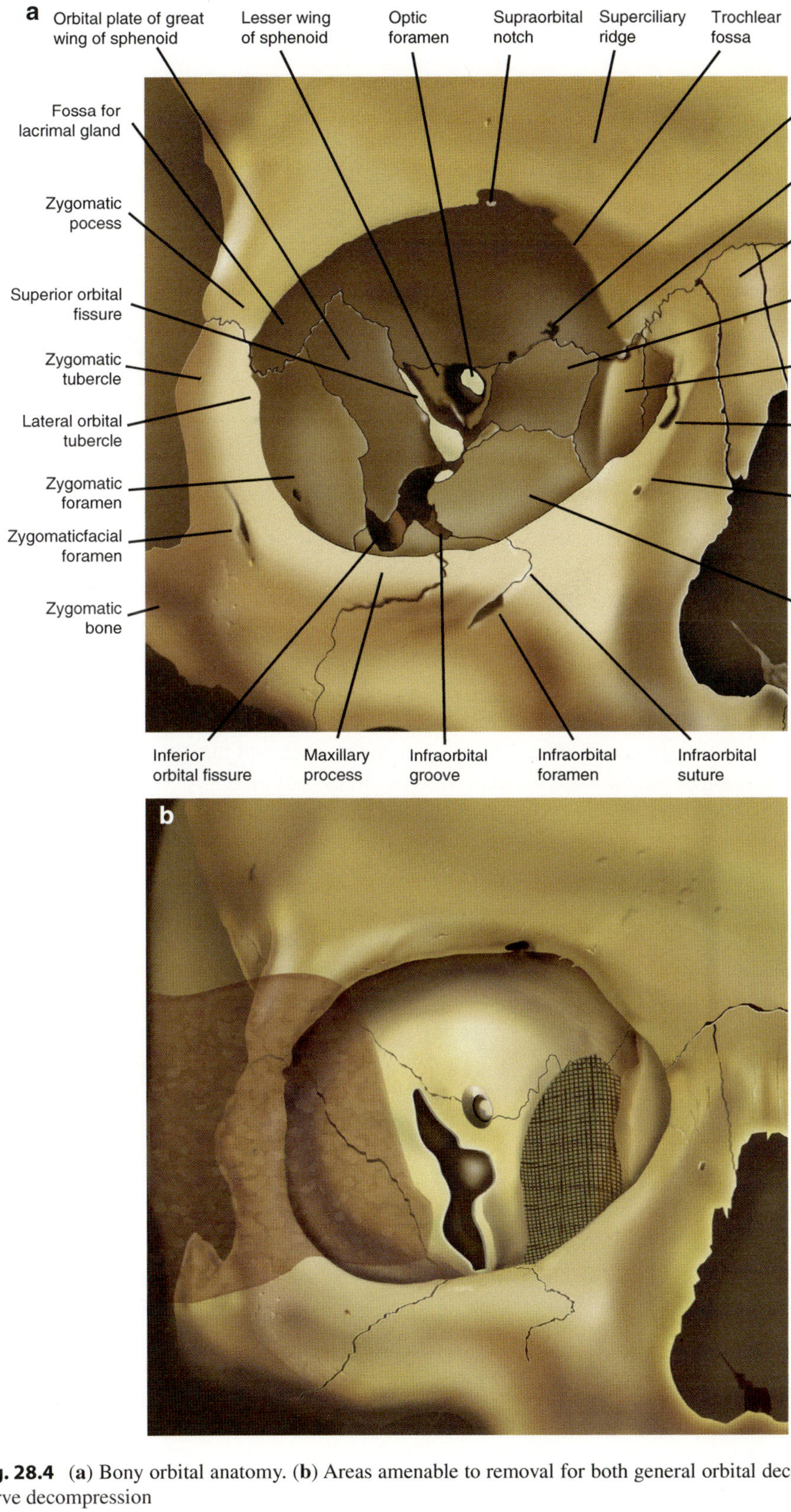


**Fig. 28.4** (**a**) Bony orbital anatomy. (**b**) Areas amenable to removal for both general orbital decompression and optic nerve decompression

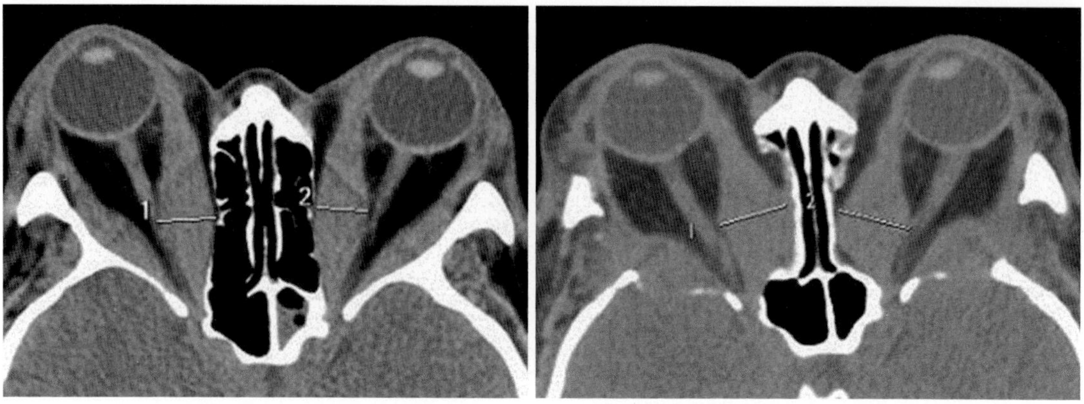


**Fig. 28.5** Preoperative and postoperative CT scans showing results of bilateral posterior orbital decompressions for thyroid eye disease characterized in part by bilateral optic neuropathy. Note expansion of the medial rectus muscles into the space previously occupied by the anterior and ethmoid sinuses. The patient has also had bilateral lateral and intracranial decompressions because of his severe proptosis

prevent the prolapse of orbital fat over the sphenoid osteum and decreases the risk of a postoperative cerebrospinal fluid (CSF) leak. The lamina papyracea is then removed in piecemeal fashion, leaving a small piece intact in the frontal recess to prevent prolapsing fat from obstructing the frontal sinus. The exposed periorbita is incised from the face of the sphenoid anteriorly to facilitate decompression of the orbital contents into the ethmoid sinus. This approach has comparable efficacy as but fewer side effects than the previously used transantral approach involving a Caldwell-Luc antrostomy and external ethmoidectomy [102–106].

Non-endoscopic techniques can also effectively decompress the posterior medial wall and orbital floor. The medial wall can be approached by a transcaruncular or transcutaneous route. The orbital floor can be accessed through the inferior fornix transconjunctivally, with or without an additional lateral canthotomy (the "swinging eyelid approach) or through a subciliary incision [107–116]. Although the more minimally invasive approaches are typically preferred, in patients with significant periorbital swelling or conjunctival chemosis, these smaller incisions may not provide sufficient posterior access. In such settings, larger incisions such as a coronal incision may be more reasonable. A combined approach using both endoscopic and transconjunctival or transcutaneous incisions has also been reported to be beneficial for the treatment of DON [117, 118].

The transcaruncular approach is a technique that is particularly well studied and is now commonly performed by most oculoplastic surgeons to decompress the medial wall in the treatment of DON [109, 110] (Fig. 28.6). The incision is made between the plica and the caruncle. Blunt dissection is carried out medially to the posterior lacrimal crest. The periorbita is incised posterior to the posterior lacrimal crest and elevated to expose the medial orbital wall. The entire medial orbital wall and parts of the inferior orbital wall are then removed. The osteotomy extends superiorly to the level of the anterior and posterior ethmoidal arteries (that are identified and cauterized), anteriorly to the posterior lacrimal crest, inferiorly to the bony maxilloethmoidal strut, and laterally to the infraorbital canal [119]. Posteriorly, the bone inferior and posterior to the posterior ethmoidal artery is removed to decompress the orbital apex. The advantages of the transcaruncular approach over the transcutaneous approaches include more rapid entry into the orbit, less manipulation of ocular adnexal structures, and better cosmetic outcome [110]. Retrospective studies have found the transcaruncular approach to be efficacious in the treatment of DON patients who are refractory to IV GC therapy, with significant improvement in visual acuity, color vision, and visual fields [110, 120].

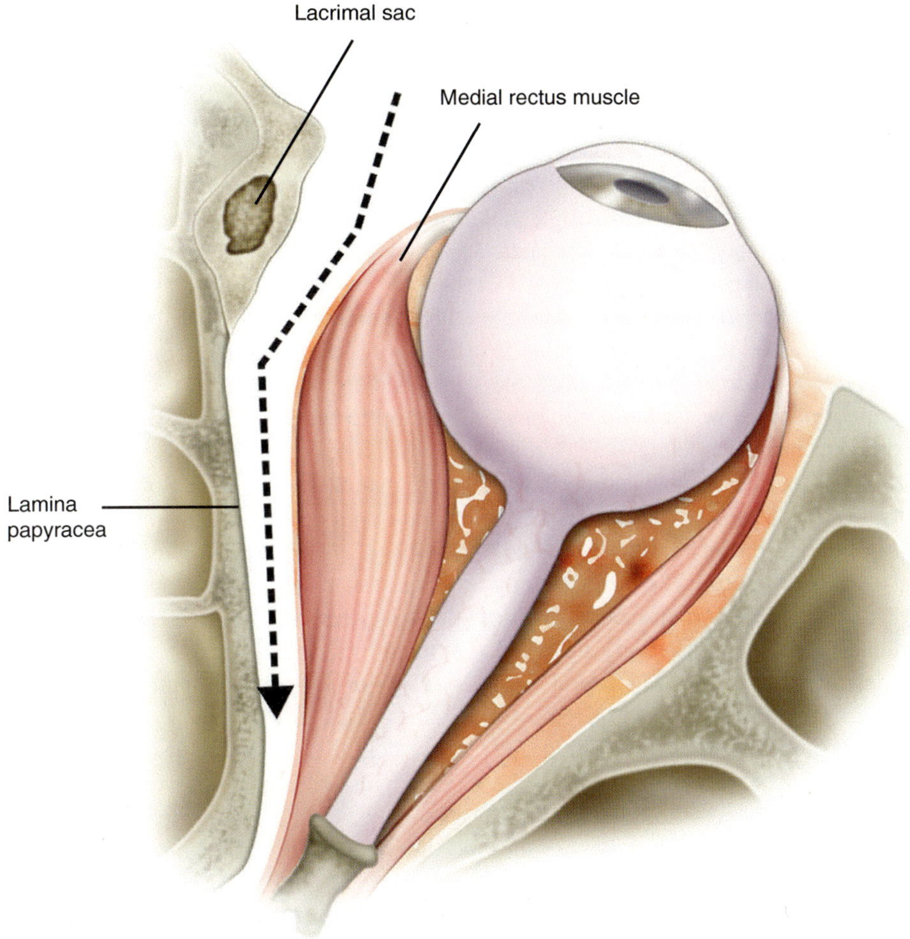


**Fig. 28.6** Schematic drawing of the transcaruncular approach to the optic nerve. For DON, a total ethmoidectomy would be performed

In addition to removal of the medial wall and orbital floor, some surgeons also decompress the lateral wall at the same time. This approach is called the "three-wall decompression" [121, 122]. Others perform a "balanced decompression," removing parts of the medial and lateral walls but leaving the orbital floor intact [119]. Retrospective case series have shown each of these approaches to be efficacious in treating TED, but none has been studied with respect to treatment of DON [82, 119, 121, 122]. We believe that all surgical procedures are of equal benefit as long as they result in sufficient posterior decompression. Removal of the lateral wall alone or removal of bone from the anterior medial wall or floor only usually is not beneficial. Nevertheless, a study by Choe et al.. evaluated the outcome of medial wall (transcaruncular approach) versus lateral wall decompression in patients with DON and found no significant difference in the clinical outcome measures (visual acuity, color vision, pupillary reaction, visual field) between these two approaches [123] although the lateral wall group achieved more proptosis reduction than the medial wall group. Although this study suggests that lateral wall decompression is as effective as medial wall decompression in treating DON, we have not found this to be the case.

Lateral orbital wall decompression was the earliest orbital decompression technique described for the treatment of TED and remains one of the most popular techniques used today. For the treatment of TED without DON, lateral wall decompression is frequently the first line of surgical approach for many surgeons. The traditional technique, used in the aforementioned Choe et al. study, involves a lateral canthal incision and removal of part of the zygoma from approximately the frontozygomatic suture to just above the zygomatic arch [119, 124, 125]. This allows the orbital contents to decompress into the region of the temporalis muscle [125]. The medullary space of the sphenoid bone can also be removed to allow further decompression. A modified technique of lateral wall decompression, called the deep lateral wall approach, was described by Goldberg et al. in the early 1990s [101]. In this technique, the lateral wall is removed medially up to the inferior orbital fissure, anteriorly to posterior to the orbital rim, superomedially to the superior orbital fissure, and posteriorly up to the dura of the middle cranial fossa. The lateral wall, including the marrow of the sphenoid, is removed with a high-speed surgical drill using a cutting and/or diamond burr tip [121]. The advantages of the deep lateral wall decompression technique include posterior axial displacement of the globe rather than sideways or inferior displacement and significantly lower risk of consecutive strabismus, sinusitis, and CSF leak [101, 126]. The efficacy of the deep lateral approach in treating DON has not yet been assessed.

In addition to bony decompression, another technique that can reduce orbital pressure in patients with TED is orbital fat resection [21, 101, 104, 120, 127–130]. The normal orbit has approximately 8 mL of orbital fat. This volume is increased in TED. Both the superior and inferior orbital fat compartments can be decompressed. The superior compartment can be accessed through an upper lid crease incision and the lower compartment through a subciliary incision [21]. After the orbital septum is opened, prolapsing orbital fat can be removed with blunt dissection and electrocautery. Traction on the anterior orbital fat facilitates access to the intraconal fat. Electrocautery is used to excise the fat and to coagulate any directly visualized vessels and obtain hemostasis. Typically 2 ml of fat can be removed from the superior fat compartment and 3–6 ml from the inferior fat compartment. Orbital fat resection alone can lead to an average reduction of 1.8 mm in proptosis [127, 129]. Kazim et al. reported a case series of eight orbits in five patients with DON that was refractory to both systemic GC therapy and radiotherapy. Orbital imaging in these patients suggested that enlargement of orbital fat was more significant than that of the extraocular muscles as determined by direct volumetric measurement or by estimation based on the appearance of normal or only modestly enlarged extraocular muscles or straightened optic nerves [21]. Fat decompression alone was performed, and DON was reversed in all eight patients. Therefore, orbital fat resection alone may be sufficient in reversing DON for a subset of patients with an enlarged orbital fat compartment but without major compression of the optic nerve by enlarged extraocular muscles at the orbital apex [21].

Each of the surgical approaches above carries various risks and potential adverse effects. The most common adverse effect of surgical orbital decompression is new-onset or worsened diplopia, also called "consecutive diplopia" [111, 131]. It occurs in 10–30 % of patients [132]. Preoperative restriction in extraocular movement is a risk factor for consecutive diplopia [133]. Indeed, in this setting, we do not consider postoperative diplopia a complication of surgery. Instead, we explain to the patient prior to surgery that they have no diplopia because the generalized pressure in the orbit is affecting all of their extraocular muscles equally but that once this pressure is relieved by the decompression procedure, some of their enlarged extraocular muscles may be selectively affected (e.g., the medial and inferior recti), whereas others may not (e.g., the lateral rectus). The risk of postoperative diplopia also is significantly higher with the medial wall and orbital floor approach than with the lateral wall approach [126, 134, 135]. Consecutive diplopia is mostly caused by the displacement of the rectus muscles away from the orbital axis: the medial rectus is displaced toward the ethmoid sinus, and the inferior rectus muscle is displaced toward the orbital floor [136–138]. The amount of displacement is directly correlated with the degree of consecutive diplopia [137]. The risk of consecutive diplopia may be lowered if the maxilloethmoidal strut is left intact [139]. Medial wall decompression may also lead to CSF and sinusitis. Orbital floor decompression carries a risk of hypoesthesia of the lower eyelid and cheek due to damage to the infraorbital nerve. This may resolve postoperatively within weeks to months but occasionally persists. Other potential complications of orbital decompression may be caused by intraoperative damage to the rectus muscles, optic nerve, and, in rare cases, even the ocular motor nerves.

Intraoperatively, there are areas of the orbit that cannot be visualized easily or directly, increasing the risk for iatrogenic injury. Stereotactic-guided intraoperative navigation has become more popular in recent years and is most commonly used in neurosurgery to assist with localization in patients with marked distortion of normal anatomy due to infiltrative and destructive tumors. During orbital decompression, stereotactic guidance can allow precise localization and extent of bone removal in real time. In addition, distances to important anatomical structures such as the optic nerve, the orbital roof, and the skull base can be assessed [140], thus potentially reducing the risk of iatrogenic injury and serious complications such as breach of the cranial dura mater or damage to the optic nerve [50]. A case-controlled series of seven patients who underwent stereotactic-guided balanced orbital decompression with maximum debulking of the lateral wall showed this technique to be particularly helpful with minimally invasive techniques and with deep lateral wall decompression [50].

In summary, orbital decompression using a variety of techniques is efficacious in treating DON, particularly when posterior structures are decompressed, but randomized controlled studies are needed to assess the relative effectiveness of each of these approaches [82, 104]. The cost-effectiveness of stereotactic intraoperative guidance also needs to be determined.

## Orbital Radiotherapy

Low-dose orbital radiation has been used to treat DON for several decades. Its mechanism of action is via nonspecific anti-inflammatory effects by interfering with the nitric oxide pathway [77, 141]. Moreover, lymphocytes are exquisitely radiosensitive; thus, even low doses of radiation are sufficient to induce apoptosis or disrupt the function of the lymphocytes that infiltrate the orbit in TED [142]. Radiation also may reduce the capability of orbital fibroblasts to synthesize and secrete glycosaminoglycans [143]. It is not surprising, then, that orbital radiation is most effective in the actively inflammatory phase of TED, and its effects are mostly on soft tissue inflammatory changes and extraocular movements and diplopia [143]. Unfortunately, the effects of orbital radiation tend to be delayed. Thus, radiation usually is not used as a first-line treatment for DON, which requires much more urgent approach. Rather, it usually is used in combination with systemic GC therapy and/or surgical decompression to maintain remission [143] or in patients who have failed, cannot tolerate, or decline such therapy.

The exact role that orbital radiation should play in the management of DON remains controversial. Some studies have suggested that it is at least as effective as *oral* GC in treating moderately severe TED and DON [36, 91, 144–148]. There may also be a synergistic effect between the two treatments [91]. However, as IV GC pulse therapy has been established as the first-line medical treatment for most patients with DON, no studies have compared the efficacy of orbital radiation against IV GC pulse therapy. Although a non-randomized study of 39 patients with moderate-to-severe TED showed that orbital radiation provided no additional benefit to IV GC pulse therapy [149], there have been no randomized controlled studies to show that or it is consistently efficacious even as adjuvant therapy in DON. A small case series by Guy et al. reported the benefit of treating DON with IV GC pulse therapy followed by oral GCs and orbital radiation to prevent recurrence [87].

The conventional protocol for orbital radiation for DON using linear accelerators is to deliver a total of 20 Gy divided over 10 days with 4–6 mV photon beams aimed through lateral ports at the retrobulbar tissue of each orbit [141]. Care is taken to avoid the radiosensitive lens and the pituitary gland [141]. However, Kahaly et al.

found that a lower-dose regimen (1 Gy per week for 20 weeks) had similar response rates and was better tolerated compared with the conventional regimen [150]. Other studies have shown that cumulative dose of as low as 2.4 Gy can have similar effects as 16 Gy [151, 152]. Further randomized studies need to assess not only the efficacy of orbital radiation as either primary or adjuvant therapy for DON but also the optimum regimen.

Orbital radiotherapy, with modern standardized protocols, is well tolerated and relatively safe [77, 82, 152–154]. Mild acute side effects include skin erythema, temporary hair loss at the entry ports, and conjunctival injection [145, 150]. In some patients, orbital radiation results in transient worsening of orbital inflammation, for which oral steroid may be helpful [155]. The lens receives 4 % of the total radiation dose using current protocols with linear accelerators. With these protocols, the incidence of cataract is equivalent to that of the general population [152, 153]. A more significant risk of orbital radiation is radiation-induced retinopathy, but this occurs rarely and almost exclusively in patients with diabetes mellitus or severe hypertension [82, 152, 153]. Therefore, severe hypertension and/or diabetes mellitus may be contraindications to orbital radiation for DON. As such patients also may not be good candidates for GC therapy, most will require orbital decompression. Finally, although there is a theoretical cumulative lifetime risk of up to 1.2 % of developing secondary malignancy in the radiated field after low-dose orbital radiation [156], we and others are unaware of such a phenomenon being described in the literature [152, 153]. Nevertheless, given this theoretical risk, we tend to restrict the use of orbital radiation in TED both with and without DON to adult patients.

## Other Therapeutic Agents

Lacking in our current treatment repertoire for TED and DON are therapeutic agents that specifically target their underlying pathogenetic mechanisms. Nevertheless, several novel biologic agents are under investigation for moderate-to-severe TED. Evidence is currently limited to small, uncontrolled studies, but several RCTs are underway, and some of the agents being assessed may prove to be efficacious for DON. Small case series and case reports have suggested possible beneficial effects of rapamycin, cyclosporine, etanercept, and rituximab in treating TED. Systemic rapamycin, a fibroblast and T-cell inhibitor, has been shown to be effective in one case of DON that was refractory to both oral GC treatment and orbital decompression [157]. The combination of oral prednisone and cyclosporine, the latter also a T-cell inhibitor, was more effective than either treatment alone in treating TED [158, 159]. Etanercept, an antibody against tumor necrosis factor-alpha, was partially effective in a small uncontrolled study [160]. Lastly, several small retrospective reports and two open-label studies have shown that rituximab, an anti-CD20 monoclonal antibody, may be effective in treating TED [161–170]. Salvi et al. reported that visual acuity in one patient with DON improved from count fingers to 10/10 within 1–3 h after rituximab treatment [162]. Therefore, rituximab may act rapidly enough to be a treatment option for DON. Two randomized controlled trials are currently being conducted to evaluate the efficacy of rituximab in treating TED.

## Future Directions

The management of TED and DON remains a challenge because there are currently no disease-modifying treatment options available. This is due in part to the incomplete understanding of the pathogenesis of this disease. The ultimate goal should be to use targeted therapy to treat early TED and prevent its progression to more severe TED and DON. Until this goal becomes a reality, efforts should be focused on developing a standardized diagnostic algorithm for DON, conducting multicentered RCTs to evaluate the relative efficacies of the currently available therapies, and developing more standardized treatment protocols for DON.

## Summary of Management Protocol for DON

- Treatment should be initiated as soon as possible once the diagnosis has been made.
- Intravenous glucocorticoid pulse therapy should be the first line of treatment for most patients.
  - Patients should be evaluated for risk factors of developing IV GC-associated adverse effects prior to the initiation of therapy.
  - Conventional regimen is 1 g of IV methylprednisolone per day for three consecutive days given as 30–60 min infusions.
  - Improvement should be noted within 1–2 weeks, at which point the patient should be transitioned to either an oral prednisone taper starting at 1 mg/kg/day and decreasing by 10 mg at various intervals or a weekly IV dose of methylprednisolone.
  - Recurrence may occur during the tapering process or after completion of taper, in which case a decision needs to be made regarding retreatment with steroids versus orbital decompression or radiation.
  - Patients should be monitored for serious adverse effects during GC treatment.
- For patients with contraindications to, who cannot tolerate, or who decline IV GC therapy and for those in whom no improvement is noted after 2 weeks of GC therapy, either surgical decompression or orbital radiation should be considered.
  - Various combinations of medial wall, lateral wall, orbital floor, and orbital fat decompression can be performed as long as the approach involves decompression of the posterior orbit.
  - Endoscopic, external, or combination approaches can be used.
  - Minimally invasive techniques are preferred when possible.
  - Stereotactic intraoperative guidance may be beneficial.
  - Surgical decompression may lead to rapid resolution of DON within days.
- Orbital radiation may be beneficial in selected patients with DON.
  - May be first-line treatment in patients who are not candidates for, cannot tolerate, or decline treatment with GCs and who also are not candidates for or decline orbital decompression.
  - May be used as adjuvant therapy to IV GC and/or surgical decompression to maintain remission.
  - Conventional protocol is 10–20 Gy given over 10–20 days, but lower doses may be effective.
  - Severe hypertension and diabetes mellitus with retinopathy should be considered absolute contraindications to orbital radiation.
  - Diabetes without retinopathy is a relative contraindication to orbital radiation.
  - Should probably not be used in children and adolescents due to a theoretical risk of secondary malignancy.
- Patients with TED and DON should be followed in multidisciplinary centers.
- Smoking cessation should be attempted in all patients.
- A euthyroid state should be restored and maintained in all patients, but should not delay the treatment for DON.
- Quality of life may be seriously limited in patients with TED despite treatments.

## References

1. Neigel JM, Rootman J, Belkin RI, et al. Dysthyroid optic neuropathy. The crowded orbital apex syndrome. Ophthalmology. 1988;95:1515–21.
2. Bartley GB. The epidemiologic characteristics and clinical course of ophthalmopathy associated with autoimmune thyroid disease in Olmsted County, Minnesota. Trans Am Ophthalmol Soc. 1994;92: 477–588.
3. McKeag D, Lane C, Lazarus JH, et al. Clinical features of dysthyroid optic neuropathy: a European Group on Graves' Orbitopathy (EUGOGO) survey. Br J Ophthalmol. 2007;91:455–8.
4. Bahn RS. Graves' ophthalmopathy. N Engl J Med. 2010;362:726–38.
5. Wiersinga WM. Autoimmunity in Graves' ophthalmopathy: the result of an unfortunate marriage

between TSH receptors and IGF-1 receptors? J Clin Endocrinol Metab. 2011;96:2386–94.
6. Hallin ES, Feldon SE. Graves' ophthalmopathy: I. Simple CT estimates of extraocular muscle volume. Br J Ophthalmol. 1988;72:674–7.
7. Monteiro ML, Portes AL, Moura FC, Regensteiner DB. Using frequency-doubling perimetry to detect optic neuropathy in patients with Graves' orbitopathy. Jpn J Ophthalmol. 2008;52:475–82.
8. Douglas RS, Gupta S. The pathophysiology of thyroid eye disease: implications for immunotherapy. Curr Opin Ophthalmol. 2011;22:385–90.
9. Kaback LA, Smith TJ. Expression of hyaluronan synthase messenger ribonucleic acids and their induction by interleukin-1beta in human orbital fibroblasts: potential insight into the molecular pathogenesis of thyroid-associated ophthalmopathy. J Clin Endocrinol Metab. 1999;84:4079–84.
10. Han R, Smith TJ. T helper type 1 and type 2 cytokines exert divergent influence on the induction of prostaglandin E2 and hyaluronan synthesis by interleukin-1beta in orbital fibroblasts: implications for the pathogenesis of thyroid-associated ophthalmopathy. Endocrinology. 2006;147:13–9.
11. Koumas L, Smith TJ, Feldon S, et al. Thy-1 expression in human fibroblast subsets defines myofibroblastic or lipofibroblastic phenotypes. Am J Pathol. 2003;163:1291–300.
12. Khoo TK, Coenen MJ, Schiefer AR, et al. Evidence for enhanced Thy-1 (CD90) expression in orbital fibroblasts of patients with Graves' ophthalmopathy. Thyroid. 2008;18:1291–6.
13. Hansen C, Rouhi R, Forster G, Kahaly GJ. Increased sulfatation of orbital glycosaminoglycans in Graves' ophthalmopathy. J Clin Endocrinol Metab. 1999;84:1409–13.
14. Kahaly G, Forster G, Hansen C. Glycosaminoglycans in thyroid eye disease. Thyroid. 1998;8:429–32.
15. Tallstedt L, Norberg R. Immunohistochemical staining of normal and Graves' extraocular muscle. Invest Ophthalmol Vis Sci. 1988;29:175–84.
16. Sorisky A, Pardasani D, Gagnon A, Smith TJ. Evidence of adipocyte differentiation in human orbital fibroblasts in primary culture. J Clin Endocrinol Metab. 1996;81:3428–31.
17. Weetman AP, Cohen SB, Oleesky DA, Morgan BP. Terminal complement complexes and C1/C1 inhibitor complexes in autoimmune thyroid disease. Clin Exp Immunol. 1989;77:25–30.
18. Hufnagel TJ, Hickey WF, Cobbs WH, et al. Immunohistochemical and ultrastructural studies on the exenterated orbital tissues of a patient with Graves' disease. Ophthalmology. 1984;91:1411–9.
19. Riemann CD, Foster JA, Kosmorsky GS. Direct orbital manometry in patients with thyroid-associated orbitopathy. Ophthalmology. 1999;106:1296–302.
20. Trobe JD. Optic nerve involvement in dysthyroidism. Ophthalmology. 1981;88:488–92.
21. Kazim M, Trokel SL, Acaroglu G, Elliott A. Reversal of dysthyroid optic neuropathy following orbital fat decompression. Br J Ophthalmol. 2000;84:600–5.
22. Mourits MP, Lombardo SH, van der Sluijs FA, Fenton S. Reliability of exophthalmos measurement and the exophthalmometry value distribution in a healthy Dutch population and in Graves' patients. An exploratory study. Orbit. 2004;23:161–8.
23. Kennerdell JS, Rosenbaum AE, El-Hoshy MH. Apical optic nerve compression of dysthyroid optic neuropathy on computed tomography. Arch Ophthalmol. 1981;99:807–9.
24. Trokel SL, Jakobiec FA. Correlation of CT scanning and pathologic features of ophthalmic Graves' disease. Ophthalmology. 1981;88:553–64.
25. Feldon SE, Weiner JM. Clinical significance of extraocular muscle volumes in Graves' ophthalmopathy: a quantitative computed tomography study. Arch Ophthalmol. 1982;100:1266–9.
26. Giaconi JA, Kazim M, Rho T, Pfaff C. CT scan evidence of dysthyroid optic neuropathy. Ophthalmic Plast Reconstr Surg. 2002;18:177–82.
27. Enzmann D, Marshal Jr WH, Rosenthal AR, Kriss JP. Computed tomography in Graves' ophthalmopathy. Radiology. 1976;118:615–20.
28. Nugent RA, Belkin RI, Neigel JM, et al. Graves orbitopathy: correlation of CT and clinical findings. Radiology. 1990;177:675–82.
29. Birchall D, Goodall KL, Noble JL, Jackson A. Graves ophthalmopathy: intracranial fat prolapse on CT images as an indicator of optic nerve compression. Radiology. 1996;200:123–7.
30. Trokel SL, Hilal SK. Submillimeter resolution CT scanning of orbital diseases. Ophthalmology. 1980;87:412–7.
31. Miller NR, Newman NJ, Biousse V, Kerrison JB, editors. Walsh and Hoyt's clinical neuro-ophthalmology. 6th ed. Philadelphia: Lippincott Williams & Wilkins; 2005.
32. Wiersinga WM. Management of Graves' ophthalmopathy. Nat Clin Pract Endocrinol Metab. 2007;3:396–404.
33. Dayan CM, Dayan MR. Dysthyroid optic neuropathy: a clinical diagnosis or a definable entity? Br J Ophthalmol. 2007;91:409–10.
34. Henderson JW. Optic neuropathy of exophthalmic goiter (Graves' disease). Arch Ophthalmol. 1958;59:471–80.
35. Klingele TG, Hart WM, Burde RM. Management of dysthyroid optic neuropathy. Ophthalmologica. 1977;174:327–35.
36. Trobe JD, Glaser JS, Laflamme P. Dysthyroid optic neuropathy. Clinical profile and rationale for management. Arch Ophthalmol. 1978;96:1199–209.
37. Day RM, Carroll FD. Optic nerve involvement associated with thyroid dysfunction. Trans Am Ophthalmol Soc. 1961;59:220–38.
38. Douglas RS, Tsirbas A, Gordon M, et al. Development of criteria for evaluating clinical response in thyroid eye disease using a modified Delphi technique. Arch Ophthalmol. 2009;127:1155–60.
39. Day RM, Carroll FD. Corticosteroids in the treatment of optic nerve involvement associated with thyroid dysfunction. Trans Am Ophthalmol Soc. 1967;65:41–51.

40. Feldon SE, Muramatsu S, Weiner JM. Clinical classification of Graves' ophthalmopathy. Identification of risk factors for optic neuropathy. Arch Ophthalmol. 1984;102:1469–72.
41. Anderson RL, Tweeten JP, Patrinely JR, et al. Dysthyroid optic neuropathy without extraocular muscle involvement. Ophthalmic Surg. 1989;20:568–74.
42. Muller-Forell W, Kahaly GJ. Neuroimaging of Graves' orbitopathy. Clin Endocrinol Metab. 2012;26:259–71.
43. Kirsch E, von Arx G, Hammer B. Imaging in Graves' orbitopathy. Orbit. 2009;28:219–25.
44. Kahaly GJ. Imaging in thyroid-associated orbitopathy. Eur J Endocrinol. 2001;145:107–18.
45. Feldon SE, Lee CP, Muramatsu SK, Weiner JM. Quantitative computed tomography of Graves' ophthalmopathy. Extraocular muscle and orbital fat in development of optic neuropathy. Arch Ophthalmol. 1985;103:213–5.
46. Barrett L, Glatt HJ, Burde RM, Gado MH. Optic nerve dysfunction in thyroid eye disease: CT. Radiology. 1988;167:503–7.
47. Lima Bda R, Perry JD. Superior ophthalmic vein enlargement and increased muscle index in dysthyroid optic neuropathy. Ophthalmic Plast Reconstr Surg. 2013;29:147–9.
48. Monteiro ML, Gonçalves AC, Silva CT, et al. Diagnostic ability of Barrett's index to detect dysthyroid optic neuropathy using multidetector computed tomography. Clinics (Sao Paulo). 2008;63:301–6.
49. Goncalves AC, Silva LN, Gebrim EM, et al. Quantification of orbital apex crowding for screening of dysthyroid optic neuropathy using multidetector CT. AJNR Am J Neuroradiol. 2012;33:1602–7.
50. Millar MJ, Maloof AJ. The application of stereotactic navigation surgery to orbital decompression for thyroid-associated orbitopathy. Eye. 2009;23:1565–71.
51. Hedges Jr TR, Scheie HG. Visual field defects in exophthalmos associated with thyroid disease. Arch Ophthalmol. 1955;54:885–92.
52. Igersheimer J. Visual changes in progressive exophthalmos. Arch Ophthalmol. 1955;53:94–104.
53. Labonia AF, Carnovale-Scalzo G, Paola A, et al. Subclinical visual field alterations are commonly present in patients with Graves' Orbitopathy and are mainly related to the clinical activity of the disease. Exp Clin Endocrinol Diabetes. 2008;116:347–51.
54. Salvi M, Spaggiari E, Neri F, et al. The study of visual evoked potentials in patients with thyroid-associated ophthalmopathy identifies asymptomatic optic nerve involvement. J Endocrinol Metab. 1997;82:1027–30.
55. Lipski A, Eckstein A, Esser J, et al. Course of pattern-reversed visual evoked cortical potentials in 30 eyes after bony orbital decompression in dysthyroid optic neuropathy. Br J Ophthalmol. 2011;95:222–6.
56. Setala K, Raitta C, Valimaki M, et al. The value of visual evoked potentials in optic neuropathy of Graves' disease. J Endocrinol Invest. 1992;15:821–6.
57. Tsaloumas MD, Good PA, Burdon MA, Misson GP. Flash and pattern visual evoked potentials in the diagnosis and monitoring of dysthyroid optic neuropathy. Eye. 1994;8:638–45.
58. Perez-Rico C, Rodriguez-Gonzalez N, Arevalo-Serrano J, Blanco R. Evaluation of multifocal visual evoked potentials in patients with Graves' orbitopathy and subclinical optic nerve involvement. Doc Ophthalmol. 2012;125:11–9.
59. Ambrosio G, Ferrara G, Vitale R, De Marco R. Visual evoked potentials in patients with Graves' ophthalmopathy complicated by ocular hypertension and suspect glaucoma or dysthyroid optic neuropathy. Doc Ophthalmol. 2003;106:99–104.
60. Ebner R. Dysthyroid optic neuropathy (DON). Semin Ophthalmol. 2002;17:18–21.
61. Marcocci C, Pinchera A, Marino M. A treatment strategy for Graves' orbitopathy. Nat Clin Pract Endocrinol Metab. 2007;3:430–6.
62. Prummel MF, Wiersinga WM. Smoking and risk of Graves' disease. JAMA. 1993;269:479–82.
63. Bartalena L, Marcocci C, Tanda ML, et al. Cigarette smoking and treatment outcomes in Graves ophthalmopathy. Ann Intern Med. 1998;129:632–5.
64. Eckstein A, Quadbeck B, Mueller G, et al. Impact of smoking on the response to treatment of thyroid associated ophthalmopathy. Br J Ophthalmol. 2003;87:773–6.
65. Kalmann R, Mourits MP. Diabetes mellitus: a risk factor in patients with Graves' orbitopathy. Br J Ophthalmol. 1999;83:463–5.
66. Marcocci C, Bartalena L, Bogazzi F, et al. Studies on the occurrence of ophthalmopathy in Graves' disease. Acta Endocrinol. 1989;120:473–8.
67. Wiersinga WM, Smit T, van der Gaag R, Koornneef L. Temporal relationship between onset of Graves' ophthalmopathy and onset of thyroidal Graves' disease. J Endocrinol Invest. 1988;11:615–9.
68. Prummel MF, Wiersinga WM, Mourits MP, et al. Effect of abnormal thyroid function on the severity of Graves' ophthalmopathy. Arch Intern Med. 1990;150:1098–101.
69. Tallstedt L, Lundell G, Torring O, et al. Occurrence of ophthalmopathy after treatment for Graves' hyperthyroidism. N Engl J Med. 1992;326:1733–8.
70. Bartalena L, Marcocci C, Bogazzi F, et al. Relation between therapy for hyperthyroidism and the course of Graves' ophthalmopathy. N Engl J Med. 1998;338:73–8.
71. Sridama V, DeGroot LJ. Treatment of Graves' disease and the course of ophthalmopathy. Am J Med. 1989;87:70–3.
72. Marcocci C, Bartalena L, Bogazzi F, et al. Relationship between Graves' ophthalmopathy and type of treatment of Graves' hyperthyroidism. Thyroid. 1992;2:171–8.
73. Winsa B, Rastad J, Akerstrom G, et al. Retrospective evaluation of subtotal and total thyroidectomy in Graves' disease with and without endocrine ophthalmopathy. Eur J Endocrinol. 1995;132:406–12.
74. Day RM, Carroll FD. Corticosteroids in the treatment of optic nerve involvement associated with

thyroid dysfunction. Arch Ophthalmol. 1968;79: 279–82.
75. Brown J, Coburn JW, Wigod RA, et al. Adrenal steroid therapy of severe infiltrative ophthalmopathy of Graves' disease. Am J Med. 1963;34:786–95.
76. Zang S, Ponto KA, Kahaly GJ. Clinical review: intravenous glucocorticoids for Graves' orbitopathy: efficacy and morbidity. J Clin Endocrinol Metab. 2011;96:320–32.
77. Bartalena L, Pinchera A, Marcocci C. Management of Graves' ophthalmopathy: reality and perspectives. Endocr Rev. 2000;21:168–99.
78. Smith TJ. Dexamethasone regulation of glycosaminoglycan synthesis in cultured human skin fibroblasts. Similar effects of glucocorticoid and thyroid hormones. J Clin Invest. 1984;74:2157–63.
79. Garber MI. Methylprednisolone in the treatment of exophthalmos. Lancet. 1966;1:958–60.
80. Marcocci C, Bartalena L, Panicucci M, et al. Orbital cobalt irradiation combined with retrobulbar or systemic corticosteroids for Graves' ophthalmopathy: a comparative study. Clin Endocrinol. 1987;27:33–42.
81. Bartalena L, Marcocci C, Pinchera A. Treating severe Graves' ophthalmopathy. Baillieres Clin Endocrinol Metab. 1997;11:521–36.
82. Bartalena L, Baldeschi L, Dickinson A, et al. Consensus statement of the European Group on Graves' orbitopathy (EUGOGO) on management of GO. Eur J Endocrinol. 2008;158:273–85.
83. Isenberg DA, Morrow WJ, Snaith ML. Methyl prednisolone pulse therapy in the treatment of systemic lupus erythematosus. Ann Rheum Dis. 1982;41: 347–51.
84. Weusten BL, Jacobs JW, Bijlsma JW. Corticosteroid pulse therapy in active rheumatoid arthritis. Semin Arthritis Rheum. 1993;23:183–92.
85. Mazlumzadeh M, Hunder GG, Easley KA, et al. Treatment of giant cell arteritis using induction therapy with high-dose glucocorticoids: a double-blind, placebo-controlled, randomized prospective clinical trial. Arthritis Rheum. 2006;54:3310–8.
86. Kendall-Taylor P, Crombie AL, Stephenson AM, et al. Intravenous methylprednisolone in the treatment of Graves' ophthalmopathy. BMJ. 1988;297:1574–8.
87. Guy JR, Fagien S, Donovan JP, Rubin ML. Methylprednisolone pulse therapy in severe dysthyroid optic neuropathy. Ophthalmology. 1989;96: 1048–52. discussion 1052–1043.
88. Ph Mourits M, Kalmann R, Sasim IV. Methylprednisolone pulse therapy for patients with dysthyroid optic neuropathy. Orbit. 2001;20:275–80.
89. Wakelkamp IM, Baldeschi L, Saeed P, Mourits MP, et al. Surgical or medical decompression as a first-line treatment of optic neuropathy in Graves' ophthalmopathy? A randomized controlled trial. Clin Endocrinol. 2005;63:323–8.
90. Bartalena L, Marcocci C, Chiovato L, et al. Orbital cobalt irradiation combined with systemic corticosteroids for Graves' ophthalmopathy: comparison with systemic corticosteroids alone. J Clin Endocrinol Metab. 1983;56:1139–44.
91. Marcocci C, Bartalena L, Bogazzi F, et al. Orbital radiotherapy combined with high dose systemic glucocorticoids for Graves' ophthalmopathy is more effective than radiotherapy alone: results of a prospective randomized study. J Endocrinol Invest. 1991;14:853–60.
92. Marcocci C, Marino M. Treatment of mild, moderate-to-severe and very severe Graves' orbitopathy. Clin Endocrinol Metab. 2012;26:325–37.
93. Weissel M, Hauff W. Fatal liver failure after high-dose glucocorticoid pulse therapy in a patient with severe thyroid eye disease. Thyroid. 2000;10:521.
94. Marino M, Morabito E, Brunetto MR, et al. Acute and severe liver damage associated with intravenous glucocorticoid pulse therapy in patients with Graves' ophthalmopathy. Thyroid. 2004;14:403–6.
95. Lendorf ME, Rasmussen AK, Fledelius HC, Feldt-Rasmussen U. Cardiovascular and cerebrovascular events in temporal relationship to intravenous glucocorticoid pulse therapy in patients with severe endocrine ophthalmopathy. Thyroid. 2009;19:1431–2.
96. Gursoy A, Cesur M, Erdogan MF, et al. New-onset acute heart failure after intravenous glucocorticoid pulse therapy in a patient with Graves' ophthalmopathy. Endocrine. 2006;29:513–6.
97. Salvi M, Vannucchi G, Sbrozzi F, et al. Onset of autoimmune hepatitis during intravenous steroid therapy for thyroid-associated ophthalmopathy in a patient with Hashimoto's thyroiditis: case report. Thyroid. 2004;14:631–4.
98. Marino M, Morabito E, Altea MA, et al. Autoimmune hepatitis during intravenous glucocorticoid pulse therapy for Graves' ophthalmopathy treated successfully with glucocorticoids themselves. J Endocrinol Invest. 2005;28:280–4.
99. Eckstein A, Schittkowski M, Esser J. Surgical treatment of Graves' ophthalmopathy. Clin Endocrinol Metab. 2012;26:339–58.
100. Otto AJ, Koornneef L, Mourits MP, Deen-van Leeuwen L. Retrobulbar pressures measured during surgical decompression of the orbit. Br J Ophthalmol. 1996;80:1042–5.
101. Goldberg RA. The evolving paradigm of orbital decompression surgery. Arch Ophthalmol. 1998;116: 95–6.
102. Kennedy DW, Goodstein ML, Miller NR, Zinreich SJ. Endoscopic transnasal orbital decompression. Arch Otolaryngol Head Neck Surg. 1990;116: 275–82.
103. Graham SM, Carter KD. Combined-approach orbital decompression for thyroid-related orbitopathy. Clin Otolaryngol Allied Sci. 1999;24:109–13.
104. Boboridis KG, Bunce C. Surgical orbital decompression for thyroid eye disease. Cochrane Database Syst Rev. 2011;12:CD007630.
105. Asaria RH, Koay B, Elston JS, Bates GE. Endoscopic orbital decompression for thyroid eye disease. Eye. 1998;12:990–5.
106. McCord Jr CD, Moses JL. Exposure of the inferior orbit with fornix incision and lateral canthotomy. Ophthalmic Surg. 1979;10:53–63.

107. McCord Jr CD. Current trends in orbital decompression. Ophthalmology. 1985;92:21–33.
108. Anderson RL, Linberg JV. Transorbital approach to decompression in Graves' disease. Arch Ophthalmol. 1981;99:120–4.
109. Shorr N, Baylis HI, Goldberg RA, Perry JD. Transcaruncular approach to the medial orbit and orbital apex. Ophthalmology. 2000;107:1459–63.
110. Liao SL, Chang TC, Lin LL. Transcaruncular orbital decompression: an alternate procedure for Graves ophthalmopathy with compressive optic neuropathy. Am J Ophthalmol. 2006;141:810–8.
111. Paridaens DA, Verhoeff K, Bouwens D, van Den Bosch WA. Transconjunctival orbital decompression in Graves' ophthalmopathy: lateral wall approach ab interno. Br J Ophthalmol. 2000;84:775–81.
112. Chang EL, Bernardino CR, Rubin PA. Transcaruncular orbital decompression for management of compressive optic neuropathy in thyroid-related orbitopathy. Plast Reconstr Surg. 2003;112:739–47.
113. Leone Jr CR, Bajandas FJ. Inferior orbital decompression for dysthyroid optic neuropathy. Ophthalmology. 1981;88:525–32.
114. Sasim IV, de Graaf ME, Berendschot TT, et al. Coronal or swinging eyelid decompression for patients with disfiguring proptosis in Graves' orbitopathy? Comparison of results in one center. Ophthalmology. 2005;112:1310–5.
115. Baldeschi L. Correction of lid retraction and exophthalmos. Dev Ophthalmol. 2008;41:103–26.
116. Rosen N, Ben Simon GJ. Orbital decompression in thyroid related orbitopathy. Pediatr Endocrinol Rev. 2010;7 Suppl 2:217–21.
117. Graham SM, Carter KD. Combined endoscopic and subciliary orbital decompression for thyroid-related compressive optic neuropathy. Rhinology. 1997;35: 103–7.
118. Schaefer SD, Soliemanzadeh P, Della Rocca DA, et al. Endoscopic and transconjunctival orbital decompression for thyroid-related orbital apex compression. Laryngoscope. 2003;113:508–13.
119. Graham SM, Brown CL, Carter KD, et al. Medial and lateral orbital wall surgery for balanced decompression in thyroid eye disease. Laryngoscope. 2003; 113:1206–9.
120. McCann JD, Goldberg RA, Anderson RL, et al. Medial wall decompression for optic neuropathy but lateral wall decompression with fat removal for non vision-threatening indications. Am J Ophthalmol. 2006;141:916–7.
121. Goldberg RA, Weinberg DA, Shorr N, Wirta D. Maximal, three-wall, orbital decompression through a coronal approach. Ophthalmic Surg Lasers. 1997; 28:832–43.
122. Cansiz H, Yilmaz S, Karaman E, et al. Three-wall orbital decompression superiority to 2-wall orbital decompression in thyroid-associated ophthalmopathy. J Oral Maxillofac Surg. 2006;64:763–9.
123. Choe CH, Cho RI, Elner VM. Comparison of lateral and medial orbital decompression for the treatment of compressive optic neuropathy in thyroid eye disease. Ophthalmic Plast Reconstr Surg. 2011;27: 4–11.
124. Dollinger J. Die Druckentlastung der Augenhöhle durch Entfernung der äusseren Orbitawand bei hochgradigenvExophthalmos und konsekutiver Hornhauterkrankungen. Dtsch Med Wochenschr. 1911;37: 1988–90.
125. Kroll AJ, Casten VG. Dysthyroid exophthalmos. Palliation by lateral orbital decompression. Arch Ophthalmol. 1966;76:205–10.
126. Goldberg RA, Perry JD, Hortaleza V, Tong JT. Strabismus after balanced medial plus lateral wall versus lateral wall only orbital decompression for dysthyroid orbitopathy. Ophthalmic Plast Reconstr Surg. 2000;16:271–7.
127. Olivari N. Transpalpebral decompression of endocrine ophthalmopathy (Graves' disease) by removal of intraorbital fat: experience with 147 operations over 5 years. Plast Reconstr Surg. 1991;87:627–41. discussion 642–623.
128. O'Malley MR, Meyer DR. Transconjunctival fat removal combined with conservative medial wall/ floor orbital decompression for Graves orbitopathy. Ophthalmic Plast Reconstr Surg. 2009;25:206–10.
129. Trokel S, Kazim M, Moore S. Orbital fat removal. Decompression for Graves orbitopathy. Ophthalmology. 1993;100:674–82.
130. Unal M, Leri F, Konuk O, Hasanreisoglu B. Balanced orbital decompression combined with fat removal in Graves ophthalmopathy: do we really need to remove the third wall? Ophthalmic Plast Reconstr Surg. 2003;19:112–8.
131. Douglas RS, Goldberg RA, Smith TJ. A symposium on thyroid-associated ophthalmopathy, also known as Graves' orbitopathy at the Jules Stein Eye Institute at the University of California, Los Angeles. Thyroid. 2008;18:931.
132. Boulos PR, Hardy I. Thyroid-associated orbitopathy: a clinicopathologic and therapeutic review. Curr Opin Ophthalmol. 2004;15:389–400.
133. Nunery WR, Nunery CW, Martin RT, et al. The risk of diplopia following orbital floor and medial wall decompression in subtypes of ophthalmic Graves' disease. Ophthalmic Plast Reconstr Surg. 1997;13: 153–60.
134. Garrity JA, Fatourechi V, Bergstralh EJ, et al. Results of transantral orbital decompression in 428 patients with severe Graves' ophthalmopathy. Am J Ophthalmol. 1993;116:533–47.
135. Ben Simon GJ, Wang L, McCann JD, Goldberg RA. Primary-gaze diplopia in patients with thyroid-related orbitopathy undergoing deep lateral orbital decompression with intraconal fat debulking: a retrospective analysis of treatment outcome. Thyroid. 2004;14:379–83.
136. Trokel SL, Cooper WC. Symposium: extraocular muscle problems associated with graves' disease. Orbital decompression: effect on motility and globe position. Ophthalmology. 1979;86:2064–70.
137. Abramoff MD, Kalmann R, de Graaf ME, et al. Rectus extraocular muscle paths and decompression surgery

for Graves orbitopathy: mechanism of motility disturbances. Invest Ophthalmol Vis Sci. 2002;43:300–7.
138. Inoue Y, Tsuboi T, Kouzaki A, et al. Ophthalmic surgery in dysthyroid ophthalmopathy. Thyroid. 2002; 12:257–63.
139. Seiff SR, Tovilla JL, Carter SR, Choo PH. Modified orbital decompression for dysthyroid orbitopathy. Ophthalmic Plast Reconstr Surg. 2000;16:62–6.
140. Tavassol F, Kokemuller H, Muller-Tavassol C, et al. A quantitative approach to orbital decompression in Graves' disease using computer-assisted surgery: a compilation of different techniques and introduction of the "temporal cage". J Oral Maxillofac Surg. 2002;70:1152–60.
141. Dolman PJ, Rath S. Orbital radiotherapy for thyroid eye disease. Curr Opin Ophthalmol. 2002;23:427–32.
142. Bartalena L, Marcocci C, Tanda ML, et al. Orbital radiotherapy for Graves' ophthalmopathy. Thyroid. 2002;12:245–50.
143. Tanda ML, Bartalena L. Efficacy and safety of orbital radiotherapy for graves' orbitopathy. J Clin Endocrinol Metab. 2012;97:3857–65.
144. Kazim M, Trokel S, Moore S. Treatment of acute Graves orbitopathy. Ophthalmology. 1991;98:1443–8.
145. Prummel MF, Mourits MP, Blank L, et al. Randomized double-blind trial of prednisone versus radiotherapy in Graves' ophthalmopathy. Lancet. 1993;342:949–54.
146. Donaldson SS, Bagshaw MA, Kriss JP. Supervoltage orbital radiotherapy for Graves' ophthalmopathy. J Clin Endocrinol Metab. 1973;37:276–85.
147. Kazim M, Goldberg RA, Smith TJ. Insights into the pathogenesis of thyroid-associated orbitopathy: evolving rationale for therapy. Arch Ophthalmol. 2002;120:380–6.
148. Hurbli T, Char DH, Harris J, et al. Radiation therapy for thyroid eye diseases. Am J Ophthalmol. 1985;99: 633–7.
149. Ohtsuka K, Sato A, Kawaguchi S, et al. Effect of steroid pulse therapy with and without orbital radiotherapy on Graves' ophthalmopathy. Am J Ophthalmol. 2003;135:285–90.
150. Kahaly GJ, Rosler HP, Pitz S, Hommel G. Low- versus high-dose radiotherapy for Graves' ophthalmopathy: a randomized, single blind trial. J Clin Endocrinol Metabol. 2000;85:102–8.
151. Gerling J, Kommerell G, Henne K, et al. Retrobulbar irradiation for thyroid-associated orbitopathy: double-blind comparison between 2.4 and 16 Gy. Int J Radiat Oncol Biol Phys. 2003;55:182–9.
152. Marcocci C, Bartalena L, Rocchi R, et al. Long-term safety of orbital radiotherapy for Graves' ophthalmopathy. J Clin Endocrinol Metab. 2003;88:3561–6.
153. Wakelkamp IM, Tan H, Saeed P, et al. Orbital irradiation for Graves' ophthalmopathy: is it safe? A long-term follow-up study. Ophthalmology. 2004;111:1557–62.
154. Burch HB, Wartofsky L. Graves' ophthalmopathy: current concepts regarding pathogenesis and management. Endocrine Rev. 1993;14:747–93.
155. Cockerham KP, Kennerdell JS. Does radiotherapy have a role in the management of thyroid orbitopathy? Br J Ophthalmol. 2002;86:102–4.
156. Snijders-Keilholz A, De Keizer RJ, Goslings BM, et al. Probable risk of tumour induction after retro-orbital irradiation for Graves' ophthalmopathy. Radiother Oncol. 1996;38:69–71.
157. Chang S, Perry JD, Kosmorsky GS, Braun WE. Rapamycin for treatment of refractory dysthyroid compressive optic neuropathy. Ophthalmic Plast Reconstr Surg. 2007;23:225–6.
158. Kahaly G, Schrezenmeir J, Krause U, et al. Ciclosporin and prednisone v. prednisone in treatment of Graves' ophthalmopathy: a controlled, randomized and prospective study. Eur J Clin Invest. 1986;16:415–22.
159. Prummel MF, Mourits MP, Berghout A, et al. Prednisone and cyclosporine in the treatment of severe Graves' ophthalmopathy. N Engl J Med. 1989;321:1353–9.
160. Paridaens D, van den Bosch WA, van der Loos TL, et al. The effect of etanercept on Graves' ophthalmopathy: a pilot study. Eye. 2005;19:1286–9.
161. Salvi M, Vannucchi G, Campi I, et al. Treatment of Graves' disease and associated ophthalmopathy with the anti-CD20 monoclonal antibody rituximab: an open study. Eur J Endocrinol. 2007;156: 33–40.
162. Salvi M, Vannucchi G, Curro N, et al. Small dose of rituximab for graves orbitopathy: new insights into the mechanism of action. Arch Ophthalmol. 2012;130:122–4.
163. Salvi M, Vannucchi G, Campi I, et al. Rituximab treatment in a patient with severe thyroid-associated ophthalmopathy: effects on orbital lymphocytic infiltrates. Clin Immunol. 2009;131:360–5.
164. Salvi M, Vannucchi G, Campi I, et al. Efficacy of rituximab treatment for thyroid-associated ophthalmopathy as a result of intraorbital B-cell depletion in one patient unresponsive to steroid immunosuppression. Eur J Endocrinol. 2006;154:511–7.
165. El Fassi D, Nielsen CH, Hasselbalch HC, Hegedus L. Treatment-resistant severe, active Graves' ophthalmopathy successfully treated with B lymphocyte depletion. Thyroid. 2006;16:709–10.
166. Katoh N, Matsuda M, Ishii W, et al. Successful treatment with rituximab in a patient with stiff-person syndrome complicated by dysthyroid ophthalmopathy. Intern Med. 2010;49:237–41.
167. Khanna D, Chong KK, Afifiyan NF, et al. Rituximab treatment of patients with severe, corticosteroid-resistant thyroid-associated ophthalmopathy. Ophthalmology. 2010;117:133–9. e132.
168. Krassas GE, Stafilidou A, Boboridis KG. Failure of rituximab treatment in a case of severe thyroid ophthalmopathy unresponsive to steroids. Clin Endocrinol. 2010;72:853–5.
169. Silkiss RZ, Reier A, Coleman M, Lauer SA. Rituximab for thyroid eye disease. Ophthalmic Plast Reconstr Surg. 2010;26:310–4.
170. Madaschi S, Rossini A, Formenti I, et al. Treatment of thyroid-associated orbitopathy with rituximab – a novel therapy for an old disease: case report and literature review. Endocrine Pract. 2010;16:677–85.

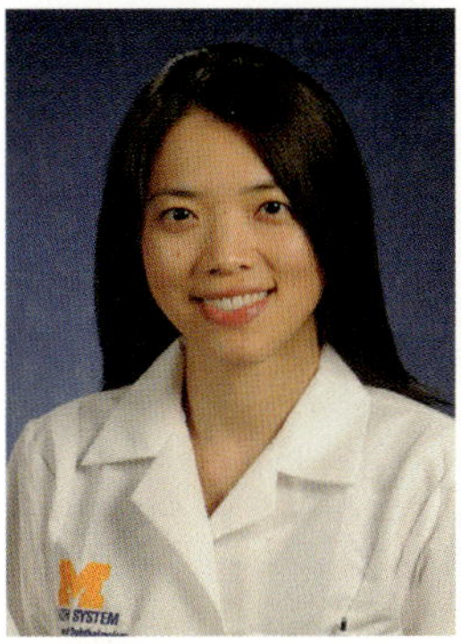

**Shannon S. Joseph** Shannon S. Joseph, M.D., M.Sc. is an oculoplastic and orbital surgeon. She completed her medical school and residency training at the Johns Hopkins University School of Medicine, followed by an oculoplastic and orbital surgery fellowship accredited by the American Society of Ophthalmic Plastic and Reconstructive Surgery at the University of Michigan.

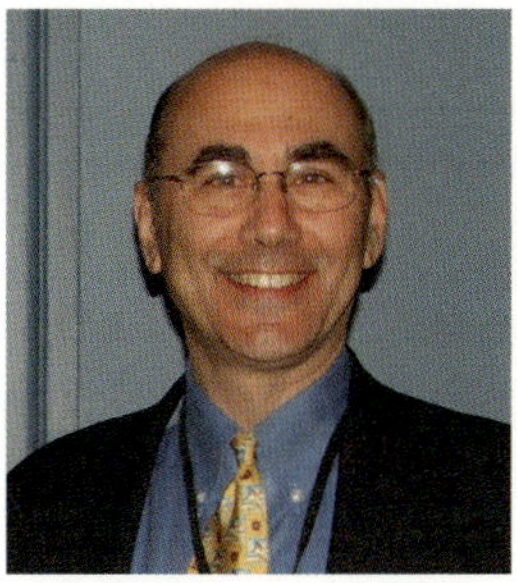

**Neil R. Miller** Dr. Neil Miller is currently Professor of Ophthalmology, Neurology, and Neurosurgery at the Johns Hopkins Medical Institutions and also the Frank B. Walsh Professor of Neuro-Ophthalmology. Dr. Miller was President of the North American Neuro-Ophthalmology Society from 2000 to 2002 and Chairman of its Executive Board from 2002 to 2004. He has been past President of the International Neuro-Ophthalmology Society on three occasions: in 1982, 1992, and 2008. He is also an emeritus member of the International Orbital Society. In 2009, he was given the Lifetime Achievement Award by the American Academy of Ophthalmology (AAO). He has authored or co-authored 500 articles, 90 chapters, and 13 books in the fields of neuro-ophthalmology and orbital disease. Many of Dr. Miller's previous fellows and residents hold faculty positions at major institutions throughout the United States and around the world.

# Management of Severe Exposure Keratopathy

29

Darmayanti Siswoyo
and Tjahjono D. Gondhowiardjo

## Introduction

Exposure keratopathy is seen in severe thyroid orbitopathy with proptosis caused by the drying of the ocular surface. Typically, this is caused by lagophthalmos. Progressive proptosis with eyelid retraction and meibomian gland inflammation may worsen corneal exposure and progress to corneal ulceration and perforation and can end with blindness if not managed properly [1].

## The Interplay Within the Tear Film, the Ocular Surface, and the Eyelid in Tear Flow Dynamic

A proper focus of any visual object in the macula cannot be obtained without an optically smooth ocular surface, which can only be produced through the interplay within the tear film, the ocular surface (cornea and conjunctiva), and the dynamic tear flow pumping mechanism by blinking of eyelids. The eyelids play a crucial role in the secretion, distribution, and drainage processes of the tear fluid. Moreover, since the delicate mixture of the tear fluid is not secreted from a single source, the blinking serves to combine the various components of the tear film.

During blinking, the normal healthy eyelids push the tear film evenly across the ocular surface. Blinking also assists pumping of the tear lake into the proximal part of lacrimal drainage system. However, the time between each blinking is the critical period to have a stable and optimal tear film in order to obtain a smooth optical ocular surface. An optimal tear film quality and quantity could maintain its stability for a certain period before discontinuity (dry spots) of the tear film form. The tear film also has a buffering capacity to overcome any corneal or conjunctival surface irregularities.

In reverse, any abnormalities of either the lid function or ocular surface may in turn jeopardize the tear film quality, changing the volume of the tear lake, and its buffering capabilities. These conditions may subsequently decrease the "tear breakup time," which clinically contributes to the so-called dry eye syndrome [3, 5, 8].

If the blinking mechanism is affected severely and reduced by lagophthalmos either due to

D. Siswoyo (✉)
Oculoplastic & Eye Reconstructive Surgery, Jakarta-Eye-Center, Jakarta, Indonesia 10310, Indonesia
e-mail: darmayanti_spm@yahoo.com; yanti@jec.co.id

T.D. Gondhowiardjo, PhD
Corneal & Refractive Surgery, Jakarta-Eye-Center, Jakarta, Indonesia 10310, Indonesia

Eye Department, Cipto Mangunkusumo – Kirana Hospital, Jakarta, Indonesia 10310, Indonesia
e-mail: tdg@jec.co.id; tgondh@yahoo.com


B. Mukherjee, H. Yuen (eds.), *Emergencies of the Orbit and Adnexa*,
DOI 10.1007/978-81-322-1807-4_29

proptosis as well as lid retraction as in thyroid eye disease, severe exposure keratopathy may occur (Fig. 29.1).

## Clinical Manifestations

Although Graves' orbitopathy can present with a number of clinical signs, it is very unusual for patient to present with all of them.

The most frequent sign is upper eyelid retraction (Fig. 29.2a, b), which affects 90–98 % of patients at some stage [2].

The contour of the retracted upper eyelid often shows lateral flare, an appearance that is almost pathognomonic for Graves' ophthalmopathy (GO) [2]. Proptosis is a very frequent sign, and if associated with significant upper or lower lid retraction, then these patients are more likely to demonstrate incomplete eyelid closure or lagophthalmos.

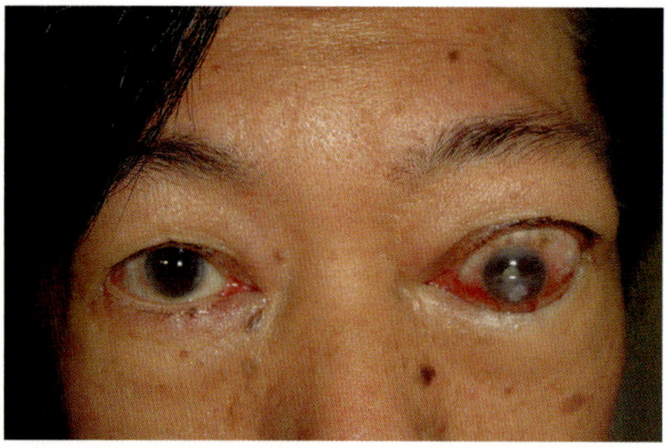

**Fig. 29.1** Left eye severe keratopathy

Many such patients, especially those with eyelid retraction, will show punctate inferior corneal staining with fluorescein, sometimes with thinning and very occationally corneal perforation. Corneal ulceration can develop when normal corneal protection is lost. This occurs in those patients who not only cannot close their eyes but also whose cornea remains visible when the eyelids are closed due to poor Bell's phenomenon, the normal protective upward movement of the eyeball (Fig. 29.3a). Although this reflex is absent in 10 % of individuals, it is more likely to be affected in GO due to a very tight and thickened inferior rectus limiting the upward excursion of the eyeball (Fig. 29.3b).

## Corneal Examination

Corneal sensitivity is tested by applying soft cotton fibers to the unanesthetized cornea and comparing the blink reaction with that of the fellow eye. Conduct a slit-lamp exam that focuses on the presence of punctate epithelial erosions or abrasions highlighted with fluorescein staining, and pay particular attention to the inferior cornea where lid excursion ends. Also, record the tear breakup time. Any epithelial defects or corneal ulcers should be carefully documented [7].

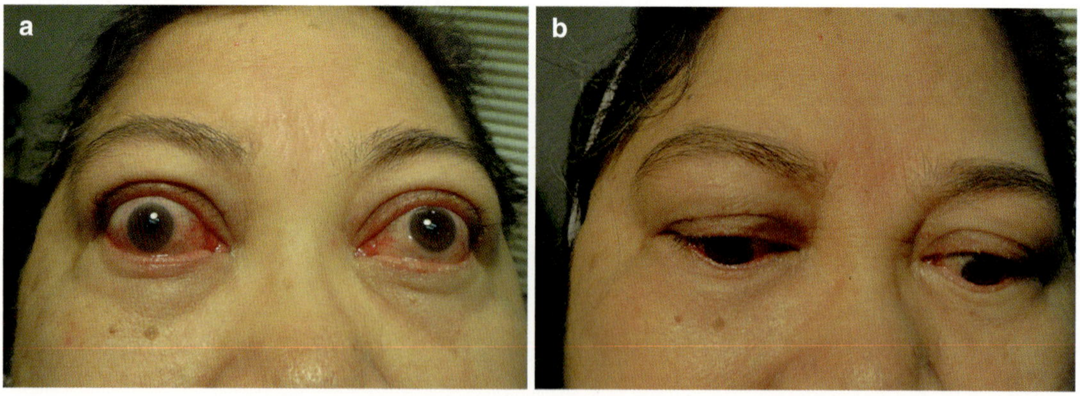


**Fig. 29.2** (**a**) Upper lid retraction on both eyelids. (**b**) Upper lid retraction on both eyelids

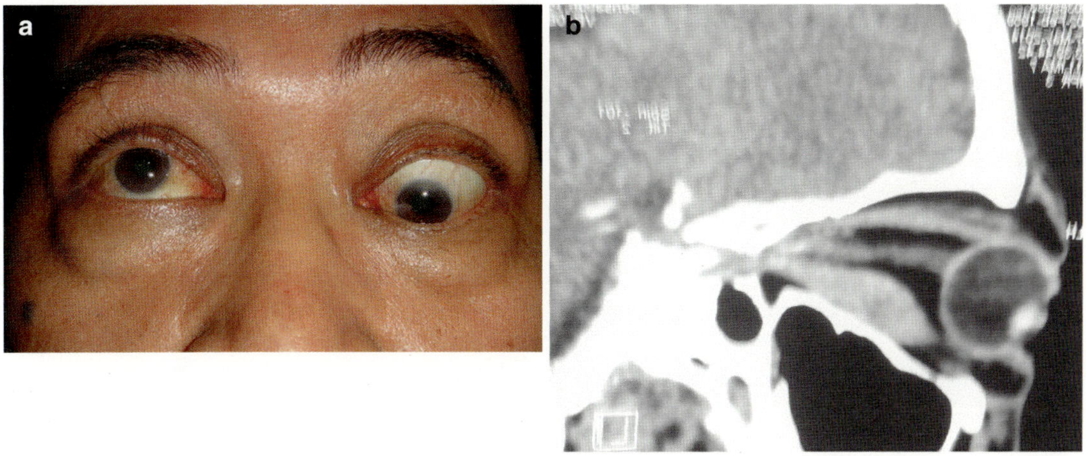


**Fig. 29.3** (**a**) Poor Bell's phenomenon, limiting upward movement of the left eyeball. (**b**) Thick left inferior rectus muscle

## Management

### Severe Exposure Keratopathy in Active State of Disease

Medical management of thyroid orbitopathy: see 4.3.1.1 (covered extensively by Dr. Miller).

### Medical Management of Keratopathy

Medical therapy includes intensive topical lubricants and antibiotics and serum eye drops [9, 11]. In case of delayed repair of the epithelial surface and marked corneal inflammatory reaction, the corneal surface can be shielded with amniotic membrane transplantation. Amniotic membrane can be used as an adjunctive approach to reduce inflammation and promote epithelial wound healing [9].

Medical therapy is a temporary measure, awaiting clinical improvement after intravenous glucocorticoid for 3 days or while preparing for surgery, usually orbital decompression.

### Surgical Intervention

Severe keratopathy is an emergency which should be managed properly to prevent blindness.

There are three components that usually cause exposure keratopathy secondary to lagophthalmos: severe proptosis, lid retraction (both upper and lower), and involvement of the inferior recti leading to a loss of normal Bell's phenomenon [10].

The surgical approach as an emergency surgical intervention in order to cover the cornea effectively with a very simple technique is blepharotomy (full-thickness eyelid transection) for upper eyelid lengthening [4]. A transverse anterior blepharotomy as described by Korneff and reported by Elner holds promise to both simplify the procedure and improve the outcome of the upper eyelid restriction repair [6].

### Blepharotomy Surgical Technique

1. Mark the skin incision on the lid crease level (Fig. 29.4).
2. Local anesthesia with pehacain and bupivacaine 0.5 % 1: 1, subcutaneously (Fig. 29.5).
3. Stitch control to make a good skin incision, then skin incision (Fig. 29.6a, b)
4. Dissect orbicularis muscle in a horizontal plane (Fig. 29.7).
5. Local anesthetic subconjunctival injection (Fig. 29.8).
6. Incise the orbital septum (Fig. 29.9).

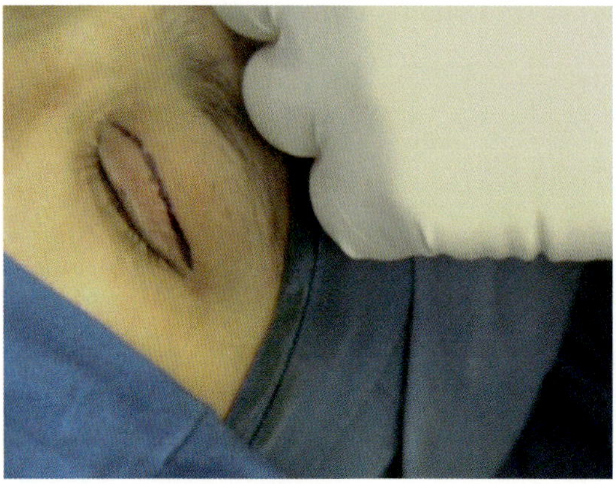

**Fig. 29.4** Skin incision marked

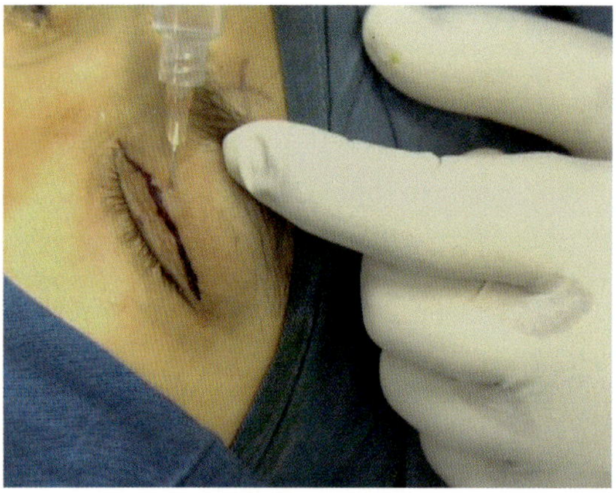

**Fig. 29.5** Local anesthetic injected

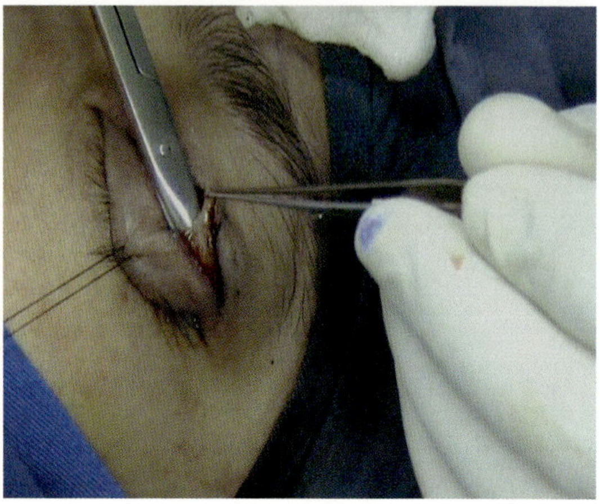

**Fig. 29.7** Orbicularis muscle dissection

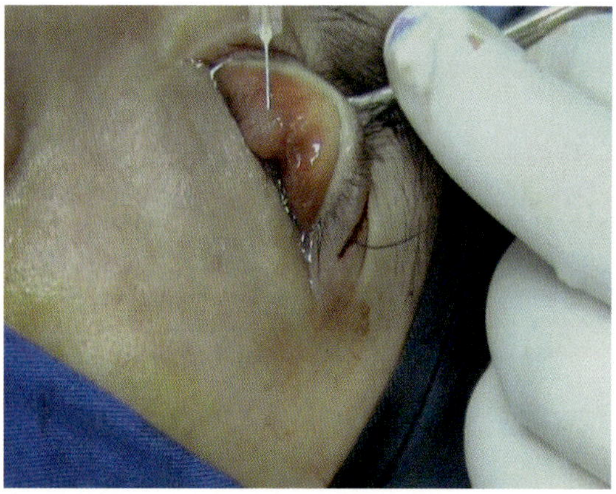

**Fig. 29.8** Subconjunctival injection with local anesthetic

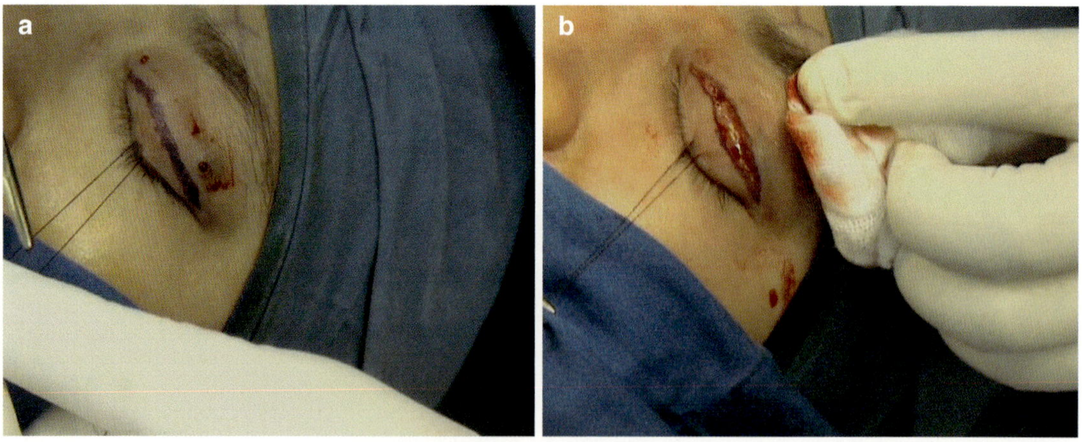


**Fig. 29.6** (**a**) Stitch controlled to make a good skin incision. (**b**) Skin incision

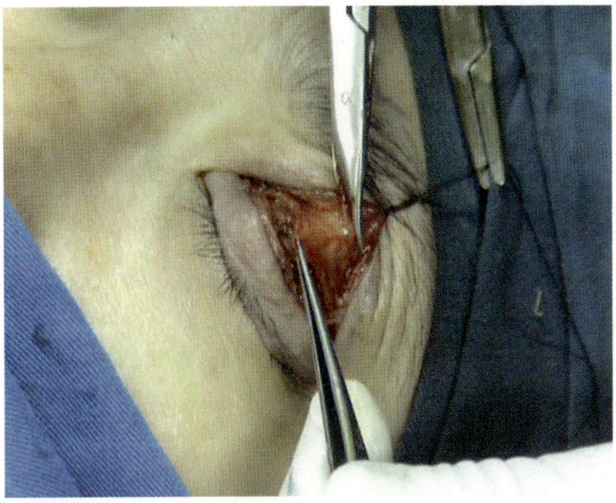

**Fig. 29.9** Orbital septum incision

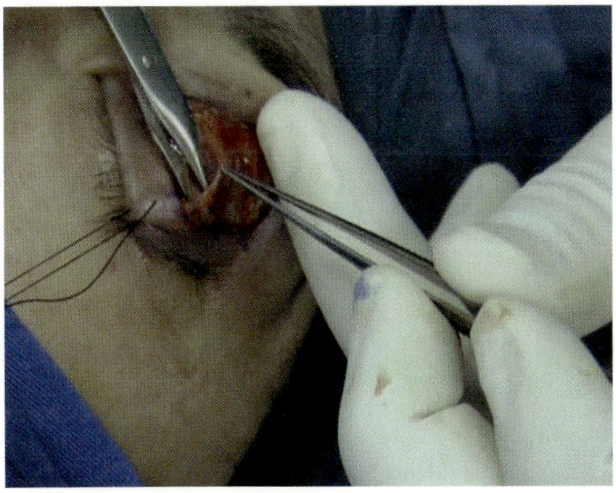

**Fig. 29.10** Levator complex cut from the tarsal plate

7. Cut the levator complex from the tarsal plate (Fig. 29.10).
8. Incise the conjunctiva in the lateral third (Fig. 29.11a) and then the medial third (Fig. 29.11b) and then cut the medial third of the conjunctiva (Fig. 29.11c). Once the medial and lateral third of the conjunctiva have been cut (Fig. 29.11d), ask the patient to open the eyes, gradually step by step transect the conjunctiva medially and laterally, controlling the desired height and contour of the lid, and leave the remaining bridge of conjunctiva intact at the center over the pupil.
9. In case of more severe upper lid retraction, free up the levator muscle from the conjunctiva underneath (Fig. 29.12 a, b) while controlling the position of the upper lid by asking the patient to look up and straight, and leave the central bridge of intact conjunctiva as small as a rope (Fig. 29.12c) to maintain a good contour of the lid. If the retraction is very severe, the conjunctiva could be transected as well.
10. Create skin fold with suturing the lower skin incision, upper border of the tarsal plate, upper skin incision at the center (Fig. 29.13a), and medial (Fig. 29.13b) and lateral lid (Fig. 29.13c), and then suture the rest of the lower and upper skin incision, the end result of the upper lid position (Fig. 29.13d)

Management for severe keratopathy in inactive state: medical therapy with lubricant/artificial tears and/or blepharotomy with local anesthesia. Always consult an endocrinologist before doing the surgery.

There are other procedures to manage upper lid retraction (Fig. 29.14a) such as levator recession with or without spacers and marginal myotomy, but in my experience, the result is much more predictable with blepharotomy procedure, and it is a very simple procedure (Fig. 29.14b).

If, however, the orbit appears extremely tense and very chemotic, it might be appropriate to proceed to decompression in order to relieve both the proptosis and the congestive element associated with crowded orbit [9].

There are some circumstances when it is appropriate to release the inferior rectus at the time of eyelid blepharotomy, for example, when the eye is not only displaced downward by mass effect but severely hypotropic due to significant inferior rectus involvement causing an absence of Bell's phenomenon associated with exposure keratopathy.

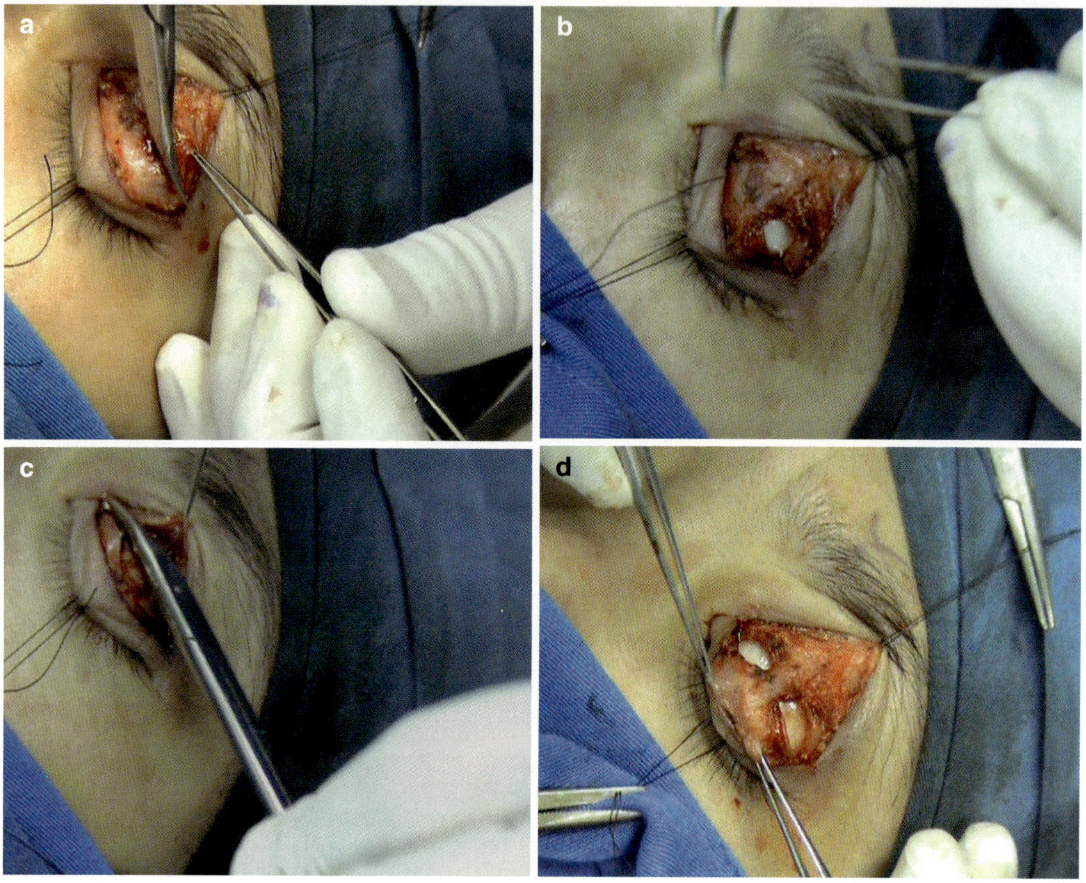


**Fig. 29.11** (**a**) Cut the lateral third of the conjunctiva. (**b**) The lateral third of the conjunctiva has been cut. (**c**) Cut the medial third of the conjunctiva. (**d**) The medial and lateral third of the conjunctiva have been cut

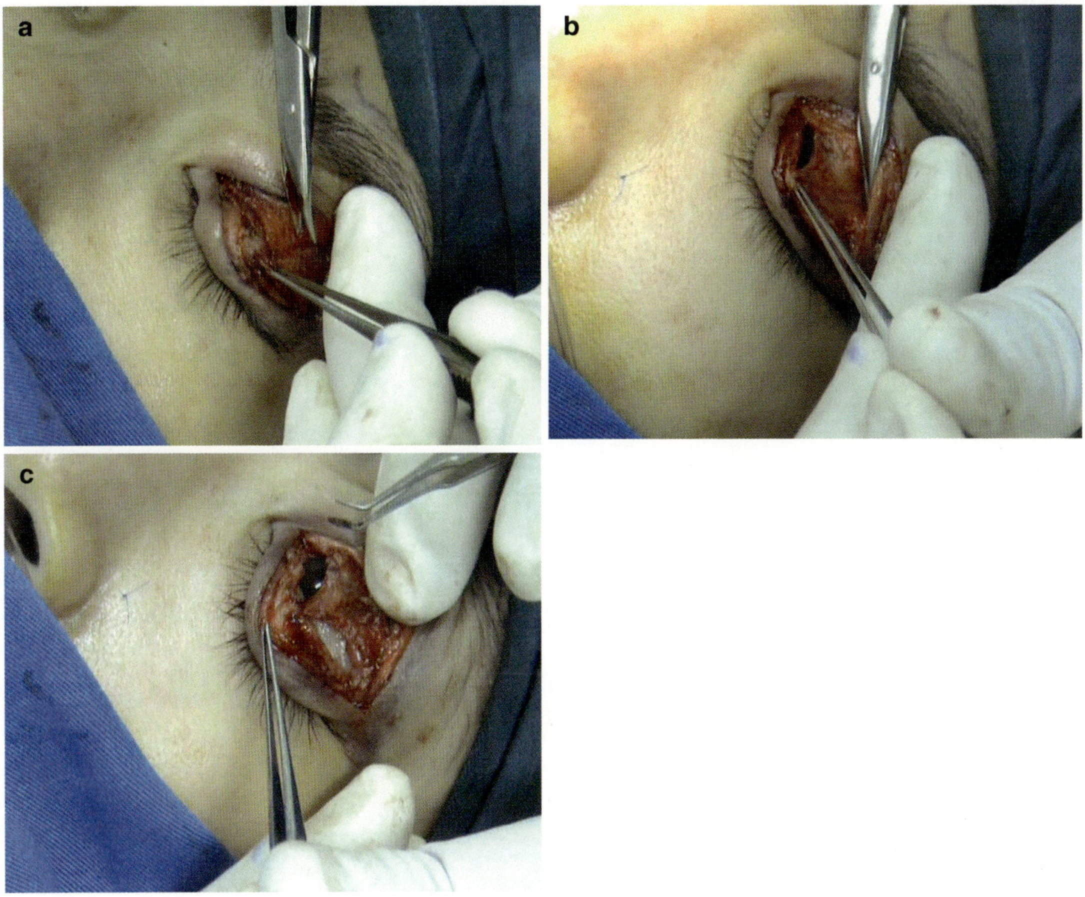


**Fig. 29.12** (**a**) Levator muscle dissected from the conjunctiva underneath. (**b**) Levator muscle dissected from the conjunctiva underneath. (**c**) Central bridge of intact conjunctiva left as small as a rope

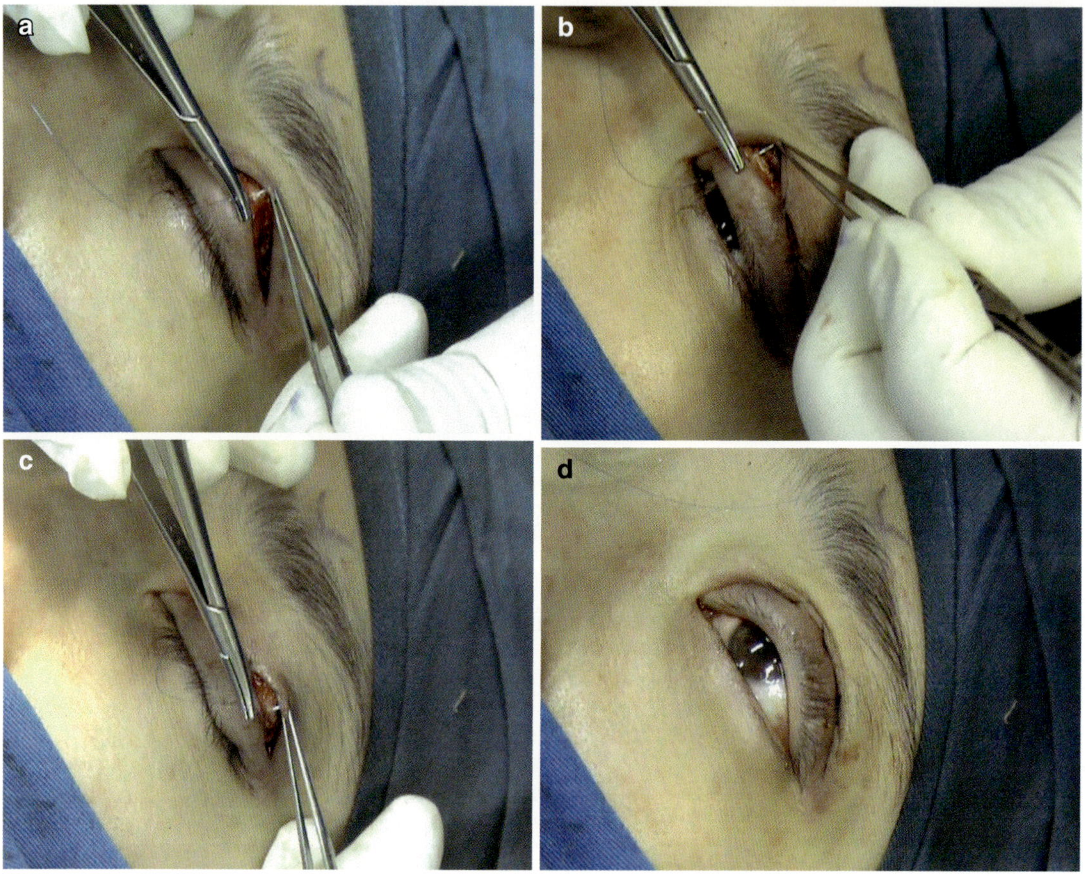


**Fig. 29.13** (**a**) Skin fold created by suturing the lower skin incision, upper border of the tarsal plate, and upper skin incision at the center lid. (**b**) Upper skin incision at the medial lid. (**c**) Upper skin incision at the lateral lid. (**d**) The rest of the lower and upper skin incision sutured for end result

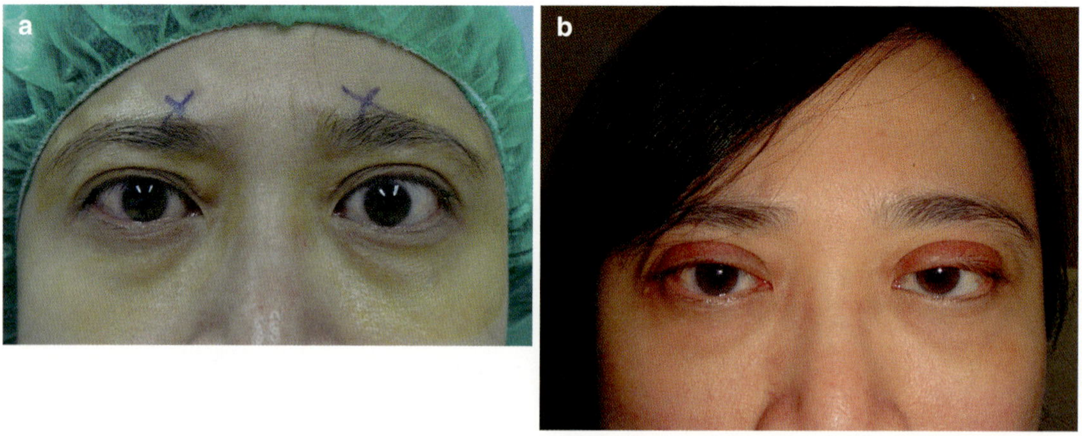


**Fig. 29.14** (**a**) Retraction of both upper lids. (**b**) 2 weeks after blepharotomy of both upper lids

## References


1. Bothun ED, Scheurer RA, Harrison AR, Lee MS. Update on thyroid eye disease and management. Clin Ophthalmol. 2009;3:543–51.
2. Dickinson AJ. Clinical manifestation in Graves' Orbitopathy. In: Wiersinga WM, Kahaly GJ, editors. A multidisciplinary approach. Karger. 2007. p. 1–26. ISBN 978-3-8055-8342-8.
3. Doane MG. Tear spreading, turnover, and drainage. In: Holly F, editor. The preocular tear film in health, disease, and contact lens wearer. p. 652–62 @ 1986 Dry Eye Institute. Library of Congress Catalog Card No: 86-71801, ISBN 0-9616938-0-0.
4. Hintschich C, Haritoglou C. Full thickness eyelid transection (blepharotomy) for upper eyelid lengthening in lid retraction associated with Graves' disease. Br J Ophthalmol. 2003;89:413–6.
5. Holly FJ. Tear film formation and rupture: an update. In Holly FJ, editor. The preocular tear film in health, disease, and contact lens wearer. p. 634–45 @ 1986 Dry Eye Institute. Library of Congress Catalog Card No: 86-71801, ISBN 0-9616938-0-0.
6. Kazim M. Graves' orbitopathy: new and future treatment. In: Rootman J, editor. Orbita disease, present status and future challenges. Taylor & Francis; 2005. p. 285–300.
7. Lawrence SD, Orris CL. In: Scott IU, Fekrat S, Nelson CC, editors. Lagophthalmos evaluation and treatment, ophthalmic pearls: oculoplastic. Eye Net Magazine; April 2008.
8. Lin SP, Brenner H. Stability of the tear film. In: Holly FJ, editor, The preocular tear film in health, disease, and con- tact lens wearer. p. 670–76 @ 1986. Dry Eye Institute. Library of Congress Catalog Card No: 86-71801, ISBN 0-9616938-0-0.
9. Neoh C, Ecstein A. Eyelid surgery in Graves' orbitopathy. In: Wiersnga WM, Kahaly GJ, editors. A multidisciplinary approach. Karger; 2007. p. 188–200.
10. Rootman J. In: Rootman J, editor. Surgical paradigms in the management of thyroid orbitopathy in orbital disease, present status and future challenges. T & F Informa; 2005. p. 273–83.
11. Verity DH, Rose GE. Acute thyroid eye disease (TED): principles of medical and surgical management. Eye. 2013;27:308–19.


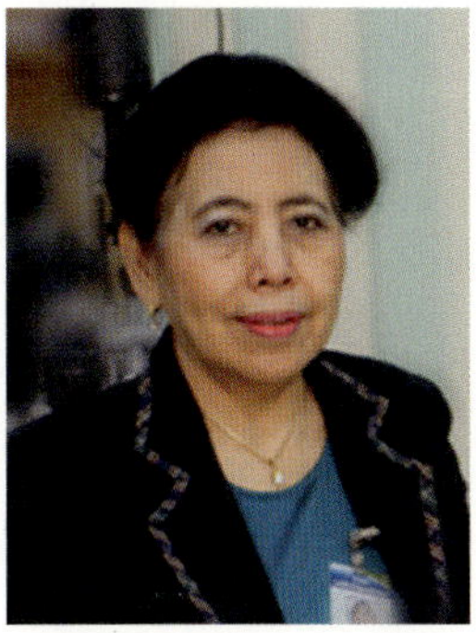

**Darmayanti Siswoyo**
Dr. Darmayanti Siswoyo is currently consultant of Ophthalmic Plastic & Reconstructive Surgery, Jakarta Eye Center Hospital, Indonesia.

She is the past Head of Ophthalmic Plastic & Reconstructive Surgery, Sub Department, Department of Ophthalmology, Faculty of Medicine, University of Indonesia.

She is also the past Head of Indonesian Ophthalmic Plastic & Reconstructive & Eye Tumor Surgery Association. She graduated from Department of Ophthalmology University of Indonesia in 1987.

She underwent orbital reconstruction training at Cranio Facial Center, Department of Plastic surgery, Royal Adelaide Hospital, South Australia in 1987.

She also underwent Oculoplastic & Reconstructive Surgery training at Department of Plastic Surgery, Kansai Medical Faculty and Department of Ophthalmology, Hamamatsu Hospital, Japan in 1992.

She is also National Speaker, Didactic Course Instructor, Wet Lab Instructor in Oculoplastic and Reconstructive Surgery in Indonesia since 1988 and International Speaker in Oculoplastic & Reconstructive Surgery since 1996.

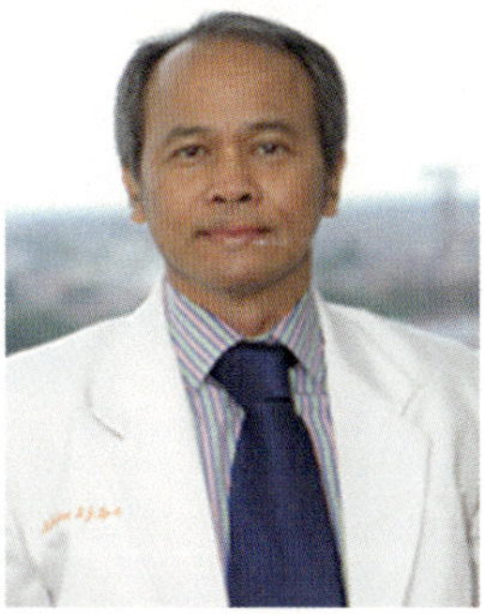

**Tjahjono D. Gondhowiardjo**
Dr. Tjahjono D. Gondhowiardjo is currently consultant of Refractive and Corneal surgery, Jakarta Eye Center Hospital, Indonesia.

His clinical expertise in corneal problems were derived from Prof. Gabriel van Rij and Prof. Hennie Volker-Dieben, the two best corneal surgeons in the Netherlands in that era.

He is the past Head of the Department of Ophthalmology Medical faculty University of Indonesia-Cipto Mangunkusumo National Hospital (1997–2004).

He is the past Vice Chairman of Indonesian Eye Bank (2005–2010).

He is also past APAO Asian Coordinator for Education (2009–2011) & then Vice President of APAO Asian Coordinator for Education (2010–2012).

His role was recognized by APAO Distinguish Service Award (2004) & the Arthur Liem's Award for Leadership in 2010.

He is currently Chaiman of the Indonesian College of Ophthalmology (2010–now), and a life member of the Indonesian Academy of Sciences.

He plays the main role in the development and progress of the Indonesian Ophthalmology within the last decade.

# Acute Medical Management of Non-thyroid Orbital and Eyelid Inflammation

30

David H. Verity and Geoffrey E. Rose

## Introduction

The acute medical management of non-thyroid orbital and lid inflammation depends on the likely aetiology, this either being deduced from the history and clinical findings or – where there is an intention to treat with immunosuppressants or immunomodulators – from the clinical features and histology of representative tissue(s). Since many diseases can manifest with orbital inflammation (Table 30.1) – including both benign and neoplastic disorders[1] – the clinician should almost always obtain a tissue biopsy before starting treatment with glucocorticoids or other immunomodulatory agents.[2] The hackneyed term 'pseudotumour' is misleading and should no longer be used, chiefly because suppression of orbital inflammatory signs *without a tissue diagnosis* can mask more sinister pathology and delay appropriate treatment: for example, empirical steroid suppression of the inflammation of an aggressive B-cell lymphoma delays staging and appropriate chemotherapy and/or radiotherapy. Thus, treatment with glucocorticoids without a histological diagnosis is rarely indicated, and, with few exceptions, a tissue biopsy should precede treatment.

[1] Neoplastic disease can manifest with orbital inflammation, including rhabdomyosarcoma, lymphoma (this carrying a worse prognosis than lymphoma presenting *without* inflammation), haematological malignancy and necrosis of a primary or secondary orbital neoplasm.

[2] The exceptions being (i) thyroid eye disease, (ii) myositis/scleritis spectrum and (iii) orbital apical lesions in which biopsy poses an unacceptable risk of irreversible sight loss.

D.H. Verity, MD, MA, FRCOphth (✉)
Adnexal Service, Moorfields Eye Hospital,
London EC1V 2PD, UK
e-mail: david.verity@moorfields.nhs.uk

G.E. Rose, MS, DSc, MRCP, FRCS, FRCOphth
Orbital, Lacrimal and Oculoplastic Service,
Moorfields Eye Hospital NHS Trust, London, UK
e-mail: geoff.rose@moorfields.nhs.uk


B. Mukherjee, H. Yuen (eds.), *Emergencies of the Orbit and Adnexa*,
DOI 10.1007/978-81-322-1807-4_30

**Table 30.1** Causes of orbital inflammation

| |
|---|
| (A) *Infectious disease* |
| Bacterial, viral, fungal and parasitic disease |
| (B) *Idiopathic inflammations* |
| Thyroid eye disease |
| Myositis |
| Scleritis |
| Sarcoidosis |
| Granulomatous polyangiitis (GPA; previously termed Wegener's granulomatosis). |
| IgG4-related disease |
| Reactive lymphoid hyperplasia |
| Inflammatory bowel disease |
| Histiocytic disease [1] |
| Rarer vasculitic causes of orbital inflammation: |
| *Churg–Strauss syndrome* |
| *Polyarteritis nodosa* |
| *Systemic lupus erythematosus and rheumatoid arthritis* |
| *Temporal arteritis* |
| *Dermatomyositis* |
| (C) *Neoplastic disease* |
| Rhabdomyosarcoma |
| Necrosis of primary or secondary orbital neoplasia |
| Haematological malignancy |
| Lymphoma |
| (D) *Miscellaneous* |
| Cystic lesions: |
| Congenital dermoid cyst |
| Congenital conjunctival cyst |
| Encysted foreign body (including parasitic disease) |
| Lymphangioma |
| Retained foreign body |

In this chapter, the acute medical management of common eyelid, periorbital and orbital inflammations is summarised. Emphasis is given throughout to the importance of avoiding empirical treatment, and management should be based on representative histopathology to avoid dangerous delays in diagnosis.

## Preseptal Inflammation and Infection

### Idiopathic Eyelid Inflammation

Severe lipogranulomatous (non-infective) lid inflammations can be particularly difficult to manage, and where the underlying pathology is in doubt with a prolonged 'cellulitis', a full-thickness tissue biopsy should be performed to exclude dermatomyositis, discoid lupus erythematosus and neoplasia – with sebaceous cell carcinoma being a recognised cause of recalcitrant lid inflammation (or 'unilateral blepharitis'). The inflammatory changes seen in severe lipogranulomatous disease are due to retained sebaceous secretions from the glands of Zeiss or Meibom, with acne rosacea and/or seborrhoeic dermatitis frequently being present in such severe cases. Histology shows focal or diffuse inflammation which can involve the entire lid and lead to formation of localised abscesses. Treatment with topical steroid drops and oral doxycycline or lymecycline is generally effective, with topical and oral antibiosis being added where there is evidence for secondary infection; biopsy should be reserved for resistant cases.

## Preseptal Infections

Acute staphylococcal meibomitis and bacterial infections of the lash follicles or associated glands of Zeiss or Moll present as tender localised swellings that usually resolve spontaneously or discharge; medical management in the form of topical antibiosis usually suffices, with drainage reserved for refractory cases. Acutely infected lacrimal dacryocoeles are best managed by marsupialising the dilated ductule into the conjunctival sac and evacuation of pus, this leading to rapid resolution. Actinomyces is a common cause of canaliculitis and is reliably cured with canaliculotomy and evacuation of debris and stones, antibiotic drops being largely ineffective. Meibomian ducts per se rarely become infected, causing chronic discharge of oil onto the ocular surface, and may require evacuation of debris and any associated calcific concretions. In the presence of major underlying meibomian gland dysfunction or rosacea, a prolonged (3–6 month) course of oral doxycycline or lymecycline should be considered.

Infections of brow hair follicles and epidermoid cysts can also lead to local abscess formation (Fig. 30.1), with local antibiotic preparations

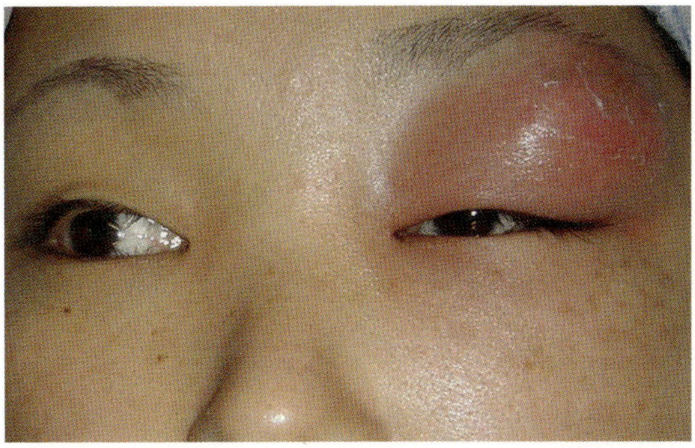

**Fig. 30.1** Acute brow abscess rapidly resolving with surgical drainage

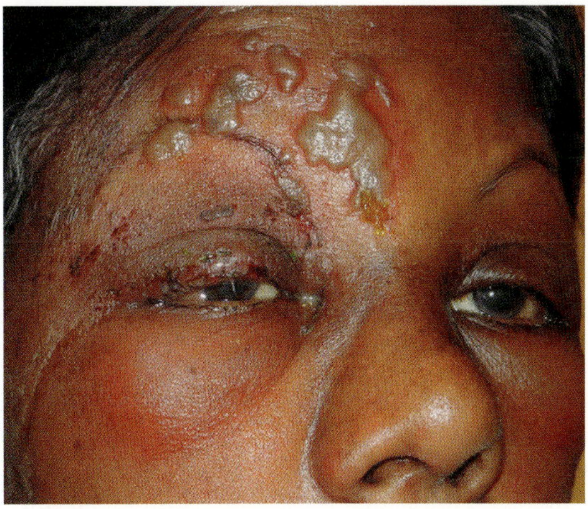

**Fig. 30.2** Acute herpes zoster ophthalmicus with vesicle formation above the brow. Note dependent oedema in the lower lid

being insufficient to prevent a wider cellulitis developing. In such cases, prompt drainage of localised loculations of pus usually leads to rapid resolution.

The presentation of herpes zoster ophthalmicus (HZO; Fig. 30.2) is well known: treatment with an oral antiviral such as acyclovir (800 mg five times a day), famciclovir (500 mg tid) or valaciclovir (1 g tid) is initiated immediately and continued for 7–10 days. Rarely, herpes zoster can also cause orbital inflammation, this including apical involvement with visual loss. Oral corticosteroids reduce the duration of acute pain and accelerate cutaneous healing, but do not decrease the incidence of postherpetic neuralgia, and should be reserved for patients who are relatively healthy and who have no contraindication to their use.

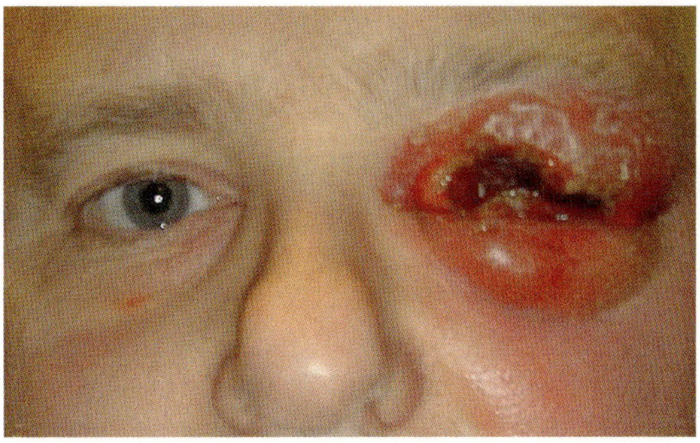

**Fig. 30.3** Acute necrotising fasciitis of the left upper lid

## Necrotising Fasciitis (NF)

Rapidly progressive periorbital inflammation with tissue necrosis strongly suggests a diagnosis of necrotising fasciitis (NF) and is a medical emergency (Fig. 30.3) [2]. A proportion of patients are diabetic or have a history of local injury, but many have no identifiable risk factors. NF carries a high risk of septicaemia, organ failure, disseminated intravascular coagulation (DIC) and death. The immediate management involves demarcation of the area to determine the extent of disease and its progression, very high-dose antibiosis to treat streptococcal species[3] and surgical debridement down to healthy tissues (with repeat tissue excision where there is progression at any stage) unless there is prompt response to initial medical treatment. The management of this emergency is shared between the ophthalmologist, internist and microbiologist, and the importance of early and aggressive therapy cannot be overstated, with these authors having treated a number of patients whose late presentation resulted in dire systemic complications and even death.

[3]The most common causative bacteria in NF have been grouped into two types: Type 1 includes polymicrobial infections, consisting of anaerobes, gram-negative bacilli and enterococci. Type 2 includes group A beta-haemolytic *Streptococcus* with or without associated staphylococcal infection.

## Systemic Inflammatory Disease with Eyelid Involvement

Idiopathic inflammations which can affect the eyelids include eczema (Fig. 30.4a), discoid lupus erythematosus (Fig. 30.4b), sarcoidosis (typically presenting with cutaneous plaques; Fig. 30.4c), xanthogranuloma and dermatofibrosis. Where the underlying aetiology is uncertain, tissue biopsy and discussion with the histopathologist or dermopathologist are essential. The advice of a dermatologist should be sought in refractory cases or where there is dermatopathy elsewhere, with treatment being directed at the underlying aetiology – this typically being in the form of topical glucocorticoid or tacrolimus for severe eczema and similar *systemic* treatment for sarcoidosis and xanthogranuloma where there is evidence either for deeper orbital disease or peripheral involvement.

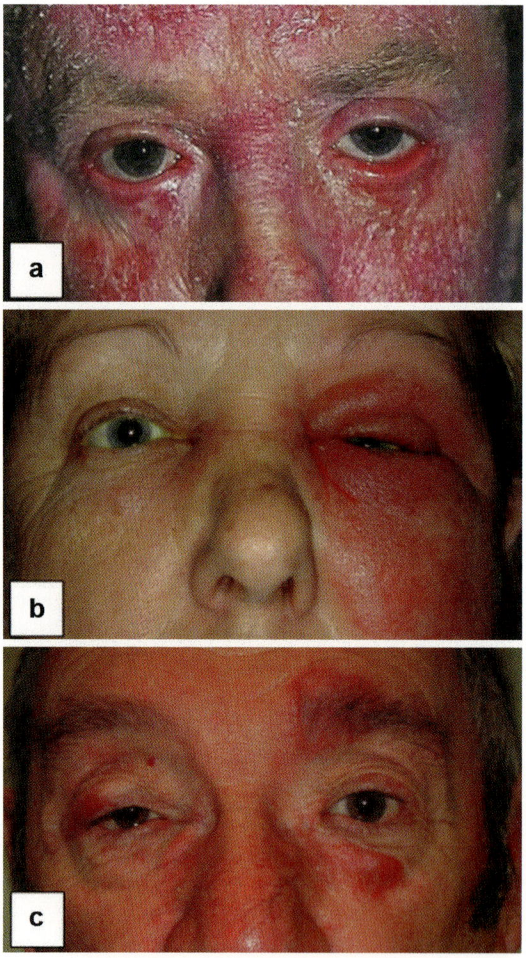


**Fig. 30.4** Idiopathic inflammatory diseases presenting with eyelid inflammation: (**a**) Severe eczema affecting the face and eyelids. (**b**) Atypical presentation of discoid lupus erythematosis with facial swelling and dacryoadenitis. (**c**) Acute sarcoid plaques

## Acute Inflammation of the Lacrimal Sac (Dacryocystitis)

Acute dacryocystitis typically presents with medial canthal and lower lid inflammation, and rupture of a distended and inflamed sac can lead to an acquired lacrimo-cutaneous fistula. Such infected mucocoeles are best managed with oral or parenteral antibiosis and lacrimal drainage surgery – via an external or endoscopic route – once the inflammation has subsided, this typically occurring within a week or 2. Lid swellings *above* the medial canthal tendon – whether inflamed or otherwise – should be viewed with suspicion, and CT imaging, with a view to tissue biopsy, is indicated since these lesions are likely to represent neoplasia in or around the lacrimal sac; in contrast, swellings *beneath* the medial canthal tendon are generally 'benign' lacrimal sac mucocoeles.

## Orbital Cellulitis: Inflammation Due to Orbital Infection

'Orbital cellulitis', whilst strictly referring to all forms of orbital inflammation, generally implies an *infective* process, this typically microbial and sinus in origin, with rarer cases of viral or fungal infection in immune-compromised patients. In all patients with a suspected infective aetiology, the immediate priority is high-dose antibiosis, with these authors favouring parenteral treatment in all but the most mild of cases [3]. Any delay to effective treatment carries a small but significant risk of both sight loss (due to orbital congestion or ischaemia) and systemic morbidity (including cerebral abscesses, septicaemia, organ failure and death). For this reason, all patients suspected of an orbital infection should immediately be started on broad-spectrum antibiotic before any investigation(s) is performed, these potentially delaying treatment. Typically, and particularly in children, the delay incurred in arranging orbital imaging (CT being the modality of choice for orbital pathology and *not* MRI) can have devastating consequences and should always be preceded by immediate administration of broad-spectrum antibiotic. Once performed, investigations such as blood tests and cultures (although infrequently contributory) and dedicated orbital CT imaging can then be performed. A subperiosteal or orbital collection (Fig. 30.5) should be drained unless there is a clear documented improvement in the physical signs. In children, such collections tend to resolve on medical treatment, but drainage should be undertaken without delay where there is evidence for visual compromise or where it cannot be excluded due to an incomplete or unreliable examination.

Orbital infections typically derive from microbial sinus disease, and an accurate history is essential both in determining the likely aetiology and to guide management. Where a retained foreign body is suspected based on the history,

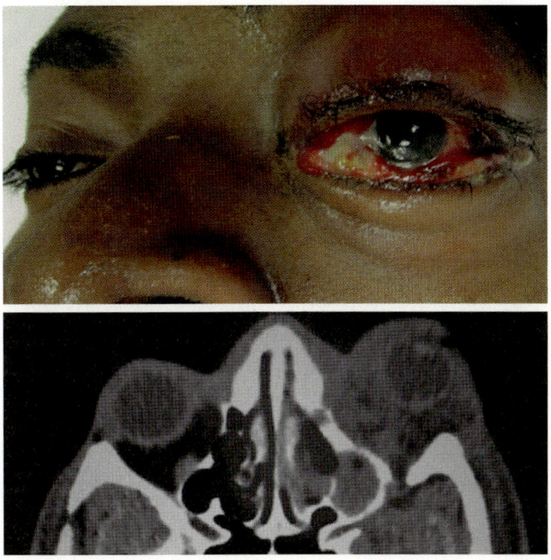

**Fig. 30.5** Orbital cellulitis complicated by orbital abscess spontaneously discharging through the inferomedial conjunctival fornix

careful attention to the soft tissue windows on orbital imaging can identify retained organic material – this often having similar radiodensity to the adjacent inflamed tissues. In such cases, consideration should be given to orbital exploration where the signs do not rapidly abate on parenteral antibiosis; in such cases, exploration of the original soft tissue entry track will typically yield release of further inflammatory debris and retained material. In rare cases, foreign bodies can become encysted and present years later with recurrent bouts of orbital inflammation; CT imaging in such cases reveals a cystic lesion, and careful examination of the overlying skin will often reveal a scar from the previous entry site.

## Non-infective Orbital Inflammations

### Orbital 'Pseudotumour'

The term 'pseudotumour' should no longer be used as it is misleading and blunts clinical acumen. Irrespective of the underlying aetiology, most cases of orbital inflammation will 'respond' to oral glucocorticoids – these causes including primary and secondary neoplasms (such as lymphoma) and inflammatory diseases at risk of serious systemic involvement (such as GPA and IgG4 disease) [4]. With prolonged empirical steroid treatment of 'pseudotumour', the patient is exposed both to the risks of such treatment and the inevitable delay in true diagnosis, this potentially having profound implications for the patient. For this reason, tissue biopsy is indicated in orbital inflammation that fails to respond to a short course of high-dose non-steroidal anti-inflammatories. The exceptions to this guiding principle include thyroid eye disease (being considered a distinct form of orbital inflammation), orbital myositis and scleritis (having a typical presenting history) and orbital apex lesions, where the risks of immunosuppression *without a diagnosis* must be weighed up against the relatively high risk of sight loss following a deep orbital biopsy.

## Idiopathic Orbital Inflammatory Disease (IOID)

Also referred to as non-specific orbital inflammation (NSOI), idiopathic orbital inflammatory disease can involve isolated orbital structures (e.g. trochleitis, scleritis, myositis and dacryoadenitis), spill over into neighbouring structures or diffusely involve all orbital soft tissues [5]. Occasionally such chronic inflammations can lead to severe fibrosis, also known as sclerosing orbital inflammation, although all forms of IOID can lead to loss of function with a prolonged inflammatory phase. Orbital biopsy, to exclude malignancy and other infiltrative diseases, is essential, and the histology should comment on the presence or absence of vasculitis (this requiring full systemic review), granuloma formation (suggestive of sarcoidosis or GPA) and cellular atypia or neoplasia, since the latter can show an impressive response to glucocorticoid treatment, at least in the early stages. Aggressive lymphocytic and haematological neoplasms, in addition to primary and secondary orbital neoplasms, can likewise present with acute orbital inflammatory signs, once again emphasising the importance of obtaining an accurate past medical history in all such patients.

### Dacryoadenitis

Lacrimal gland inflammation can either be due to an acute neutrophilic inflammation, usually presumed to be viral in origin, or present as a more indolent, predominantly lymphocytic, inflammation, occasionally associated with an idiopathic inflammatory disorder such as sarcoidosis or granulomatous polyangiitis (GPA).

The natural history of *acute* dacryoadenitis is one of a prodromal ache followed by unilateral or bilateral painful lacrimal gland enlargement with tearing, mild ocular injection and upper lid swelling with an 'S'-shaped configuration (Fig. 30.6). CT imaging identifies an enlarged gland – this often being severalfold larger than normal. Untreated, dacryoadenitis can persist for several months, and where the symptoms are not promptly alleviated with non-steroidal anti-inflammatories (with oral antibiosis for more severe cases) or

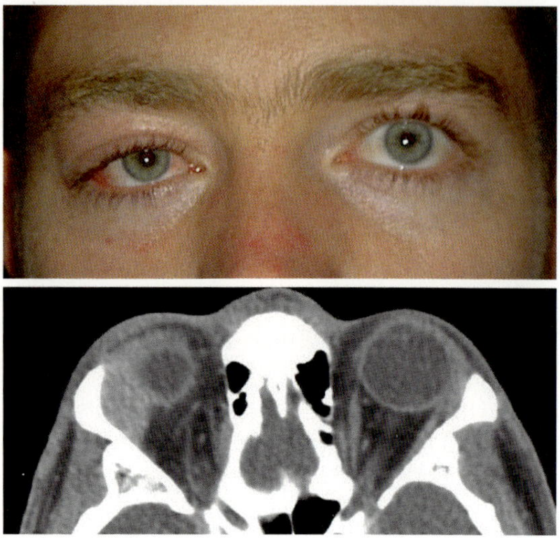

**Fig. 30.6** Acute dacryoadenitis with CT identifying enlarged orbital lobe of lacrimal gland

where there is *persistent* glandular enlargement after 3–4 months – irrespective of treatment – consideration should be given to performing a biopsy to exclude a vasculitic or neoplastic process.

In contrast, *chronic* inflammation of the lacrimal gland usually presents as a relatively painless, non-tender swelling which may be bilateral. CT imaging identifies diffusely enlarged glands which mould around the globe; biopsy and systemic investigations are essential before immunosuppression is initiated.

Representative biopsies are best obtained from the orbital lobe of the gland via an upper lid skin-crease incision, following which the patient can be treated with a rapidly tapering course of oral steroid, this typically beginning at 60–80 mg daily for 3 days – with appropriate gastric protection – and reducing to 20 mg daily within 7–10 days, with a slower taper thereafter, the rate of taper being guided by the clinical response and tissue diagnosis. In most cases, histology identifies chronic inflammation with a B-cell predominance (i.e. without other characteristic features), and the patient shows a rapid clinical improvement. Where the clinical history and histology suggest a systemic disorder such as sarcoidosis or IgG4 disease, the patient should be referred to the appropriate physician for further investigation.

## Scleritis and Myositis

Forming a disease continuum, both scleritis and myositis can be isolated and idiopathic in origin or be associated with other systemic inflammatory disorders, these including sarcoidosis, GPA and systemic lupus erythematosus. Scleritis typically presents acutely with localised or diffused 'brick red' scleral inflammation (Fig. 30.7), although occasionally marked inflammatory signs are absent if the posterior sclera alone is involved. Ultrasonography typically reveals thickening of the sclera, and accumulation of inflammatory oedema within the optic nerve sheath accounts for the so called 'T-sign'. In its most severe form, patients can present with profound visual loss, this typically responding promptly to high-dose glucocorticoids and often leading to a rapid reduction in pain and improvement in vision. Where patients fail to respond to such treatment, other vasculitic disorders such as GPA, sarcoidosis and lupus should be considered and investigations directed accordingly.

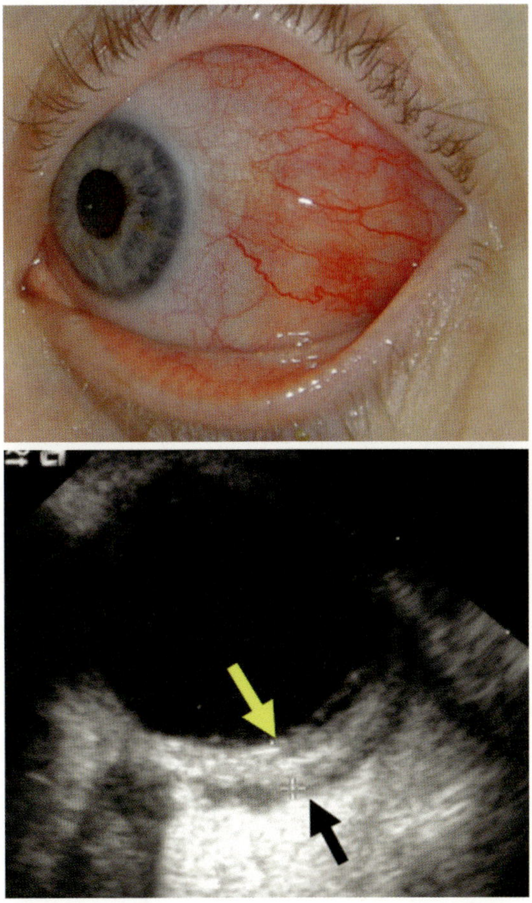

**Fig. 30.7** Scleritis, with ultrasound identifying gross thickening of sclera (delineated by the two *arrows*) and oedema within the optic nerve sheath

Orbital myositis has a characteristically rapid onset, presenting after a short prodromal period with acute orbital ache (often on waking), ocular redness and diplopia. Occurring most often in young women, the pain and diplopia are worse on attempted ductions *away* from the field of action of the affected muscle. CT imaging reveals enlarged muscle(s), the inflammatory process including the tendon sheath (in contrast to thyroid eye disease in which the tendon is spared), with the medial rectus being most commonly affected muscle (Fig. 30.8), followed by involvement of the superior rectus, lateral rectus, levator complex, superior oblique and inferior rectus in decreasing frequency. Where the clinical presentation is typical for myositis, initial management with a rapidly tapering high-dose course of oral glucocorticoids is acceptable, with patients often reporting almost instantaneous improvement in symptoms. Where there is doubt, or the disease relatively mild, oral non-steroidal anti-inflammatory drugs are often used, with a low threshold for performing a muscle biopsy for atypical or resistant cases before considering radiotherapy or second-line immunosuppression (these including methotrexate, cyclosporine and cyclophosphamide) [6].

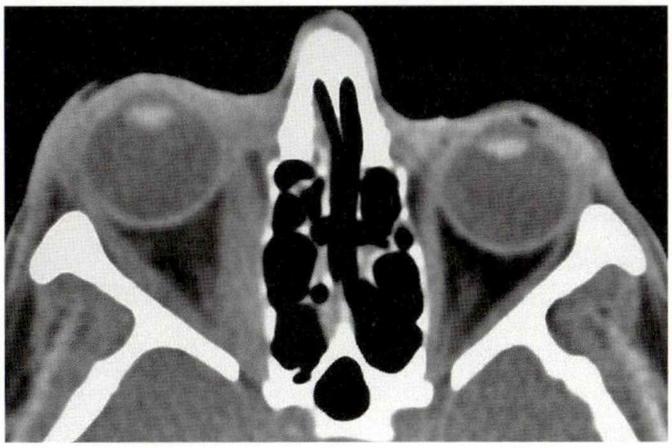

**Fig. 30.8** Orbital myositis: CT image identifying enlargement of the medial rectus muscle belly *and* tendinous insertion

## Sarcoidosis

A relatively common vasculitic disease of unknown aetiology, sarcoidosis can involve the eye and ocular adnexa and occasionally be the presenting feature of systemic disease. Typically, the patient reports a painless fullness of the upper lids, with more severe cases presenting with an 'S'-shaped ptosis. On further questioning, the patient frequently admits to systemic symptoms including a peripheral rash, arthralgia and respiratory symptoms.

Although lacrimal gland swelling per se is not an indication for treatment, and is not sight threatening, a debulking biopsy of the gland(s) – where there is evidence for bilateral involvement or unilateral disease not responding to NSAIDs – frequently gives the diagnosis as well as reducing the size of the gland, this often being the patient's chief concern. Note that in all cases, biopsy of the *orbital* portion of the lacrimal gland should be performed via an upper lid skin-crease approach; tissue from the subconjunctival *palpebral* lobe rarely yields representative histology, jeopardises the integrity of the lacrimal ductules and does not reduce the bulk of the gland.

Other acute adnexal presentations of sarcoid include periocular inflammatory plaques (Fig. 30.4c), acute unilateral lacrimal gland inflammation, sight-threatening orbital apical inflammation with associated 'apical' signs (Fig. 30.9a) and inflammatory deposits within the optic nerve itself (Fig. 30.9b), the latter causing a rapid and profound (but reversible) visual decline. In most cases high-dose glucocorticoid treatment is highly effective, although second-line immunosuppression should be considered where the patient cannot be weaned off treatment without recurrent inflammatory relapses.

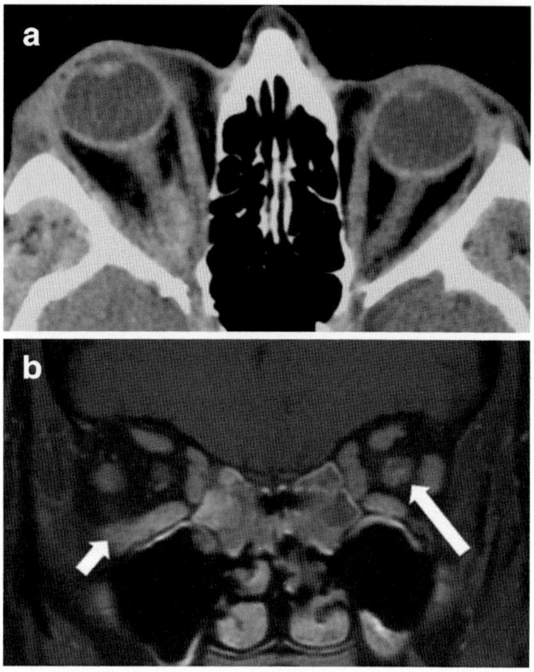


**Fig. 30.9** Sarcoidosis with imaging identifying acute orbital apical inflammation. (**a**) A second patient, whose imaging is shown in (**b**), presented with orbital inflammation and an inferolateral sarcoid mass (*short arrow*). Three weeks later, she presented with marked *contralateral* visual loss due to optic nerve inflammation (*long arrow*), which responded promptly to high-dose oral steroid

## Granulomatous Polyangiitis (GPA; Previously Termed Wegener's Granulomatosis)

GPA is a multisystem ANCA-associated vasculitis of uncertain aetiology, with a peak age of onset in the fourth and fifth decades of life. Approximately 60 % of all patients suffer acute intraocular inflammation, with acute orbital inflammation occurring in about 20 % of patients. Adnexal disease, which can lead to visual loss in up to half of all patients, includes scleritis, dacryoadenitis, dacryocystitis, optic neuritis, an inflammatory mass effect, tissue ischaemia and a more diffuse form of disease leading to deposition of collagenous plaque *en face* with the orbital wall or at the orbital apex (Fig. 30.10). GPA is associated with c-ANCA,[4] and histology identifies various degrees of granulomatous inflammation involving small and medium-sized arterioles, necrosis and, in chronic cases, collagen deposition. Management includes urgent systemic review, chiefly to exclude granulomatous glomerulonephritis and respiratory tract disease, and initiation of high-dose tapering corticosteroids, with a low threshold for second-line immunosupression – such as pulsed cyclophosphamide,

[4] c-ANCA has an overall sensitivity of 91 % and specificity of 99 % for GPA.

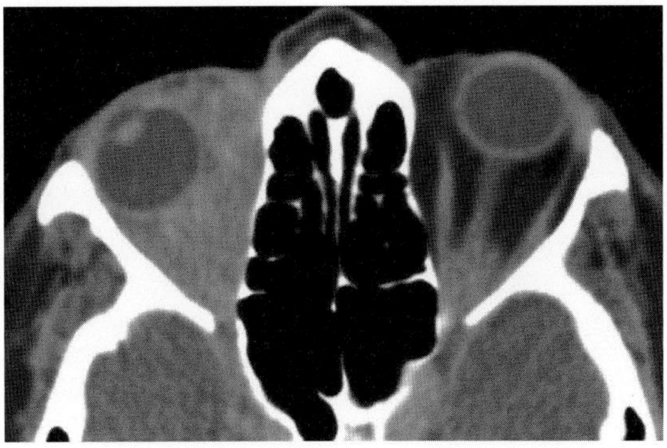

**Fig. 30.10** CT imaging of a patient with chronic orbital granulomatous polyangiitis. Note the diffuse right intraorbital intraconal and extraconal soft tissue mass obliterating the normal structures. The eye is now enophthalmic due to intraorbital fibrosis. The inflammatory mass extends into the orbital apex and the superior and inferior orbital fissures

methotrexate or azathioprine. Progressive orbital inflammation requires adequate systemic immunosupression *even in the absence of systemic disease*, and effective management requires a clear dialogue between the orbital surgeon and rheumatologist given the toxicity profiles of such second-line agents.

## Reactive Lymphoid Hyperplasia (RLH)

Frequently presenting with symmetrical inflammatory changes of the orbital soft tissues, RLH is a *relatively* innocuous polyclonal lymphoid expansion, with histology revealing germinal centres surrounded by a mantle zone of layers of small lymphocytes. Management with high-dose tapering oral steroid is generally successful; low-dose orbital radiotherapy also plays a role, and, for refractive cases, rituximab can be used with appropriate screening and monitoring [7]. Where disease is progressive, the original pathology should be reviewed and immunohistochemistry performed to exclude other forms of IOID, such as IgG4 disease and GPA. Consideration should also be given to undertaking a further biopsy of core representative tissue to exclude lymphoma.

## IgG4 Disease

In the past decade, IgG4-related disease has emerged as a distinct inflammatory disorder characterised by tissue infiltration with IgG4-rich plasma cells, elevation of serum IgG4 levels and sclerosis of the involved organ(s). Predominantly affecting middle-aged and elderly men, it can cause inflammatory lesions within most organs – in particular the pancreas, thyroid, aorta, lungs and retroperitoneum. Adnexal structures commonly involved include the lacrimal gland, extraocular muscles, lacrimal sac and infraorbital nerve [8,9]. Following a confirmatory biopsy of the involved adnexal structure(s), review by a general physician or rheumatologist should be sought to exclude disease elsewhere. Acute adnexal inflammation is managed with oral non-steroidal medication for mild cases and oral corticosteroid for more severe inflammations; resistant cases require disease control and maintenance therapy with long-term immunosuppressive therapies such as methotrexate, azathioprine or cyclophosphamide. Recent reports indicate that mycophenolate mofetil (MMF) or rituximab can also be effective as second-line steroid-sparing alternatives in managing IgG4-related inflammation [10,11].

## References


1. Verity DH, Meligonis G, Rose GE. Benign histiocytic disorders of the orbit (chapter 241). In: Albert DM, Miller JW, editors. Albert and Jakobiec's "Principles and Practice of Ophthalmology". 3rd ed. Philadelphia: Saunders; 2008.
2. Amrith S, Hosdurga Pai V, Ling WW. Periorbital necrotizing fasciitis – a review. Acta Ophthalmol. 2013;91:596–603.
3. Verity DH, Rose GE. Infectious processes of the orbit (chapter 232). In: Albert DM, Miller JW, editors. Albert and Jakobiec's "Principles and Practice of Ophthalmology". 3rd ed. Philadelphia: Saunders; 2008.
4. Espinoza GM. Orbital inflammatory pseudotumors: etiology, differential diagnosis, and management. Curr Rheumatol Rep. 2010;12:443–7.
5. Perumal B, Black EH, Levin F, Servat JJ. Non-infectious orbital vasculitides. Eye. 2012;26:630–9.
6. Smith JR, Rosenbaum JT. A role for methotrexate in the management of non-infectious orbital inflammatory disease. Br J Ophthalmol. 2001;85:1220–4.
7. Talaulikar D, Tridgell D, Leong D, Dahlstrom JE, Cherian M, Prosser I, et al. Novel therapeutic option for orbital atypical lymphoid hyperplasia. Clin Exper Ophthalmol. 2010;38:892–4.

8. Takahashi Y, Kitamura A, Kakizaki H. Bilateral optic nerve involvement in immunoglobulin G4-related ophthalmic disease. J Neuroophthalmol. 2014;34:16–9.
9. Hardy TG, McNab AA, Rose GE. Enlargement of the infraorbital nerve: an important sign associated with orbital reactive lymphoid hyperplasia or immunoglobulin G4-related disease. Ophthalmology. 2014;121:1297–303.
10. Moss HE, Mejico LJ, de la Roza G. IgG4-related inflammatory pseudotumor of the central nervous system responsive to mycophenolate mofetil. J Neurol Sci. 2012;318:31–5.
11. Khosroshahi A, Carruthers MN, Deshpande V, Unizony S, Bloch DB, Stone JH. Rituximab for the treatment of IgG4-related disease: lessons from 10 consecutive patients. Medicine. 2012;91:57–66.

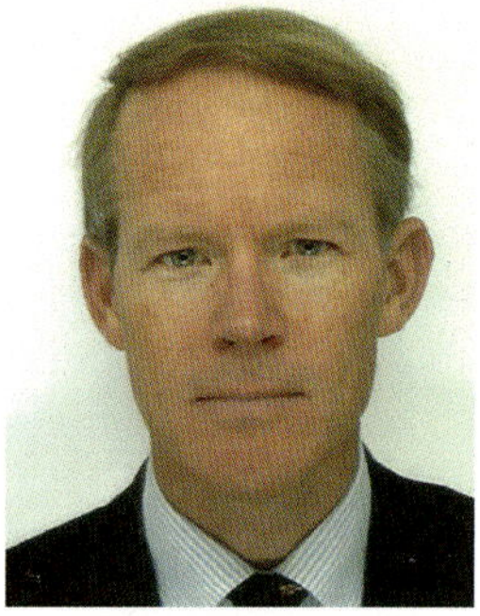

**David H. Verity** Dr. Verity is a Consultant Ophthalmic Surgeon, and Adnexal Service Director, Moorfields Eye Hospital, London.

He is a Honorary Senior Clinical Lecturer, University College London.

Trained in ophthalmology in the UK, Dr. Verity undertook two Fellowships in ophthalmic adnexal disease before joining the Consultant staff at Moorfields Eye Hospital in 2004.

He is a Full Member of the British Oculoplastic Surgery Society (current Treasurer), Treasurer Elect for the European Society of Ophthalmic Plastic and Reconstructive Surgery, and Full Member of the International Society of Ocular Oncology.

In 2009, he was elected to the Orbital Society, in 2010 became Editor-in Chief of the journal ORBIT, and in 2016 became Oculoplastic Section Editor for the Journal of Ophthalmic and Vision Research.

His medical publications in peer-reviewed journals and books include 90(+) publications, and with a wide range of research interests, he is an active national and international teacher and surgical trainer.

Dr. Verity also has a life-long interest in the charitable work of the St John Eye Hospital Group. In 2014, he was invested in the Order of St John, and in 2016 he joined the Board as Trustee of the Hospital Group.

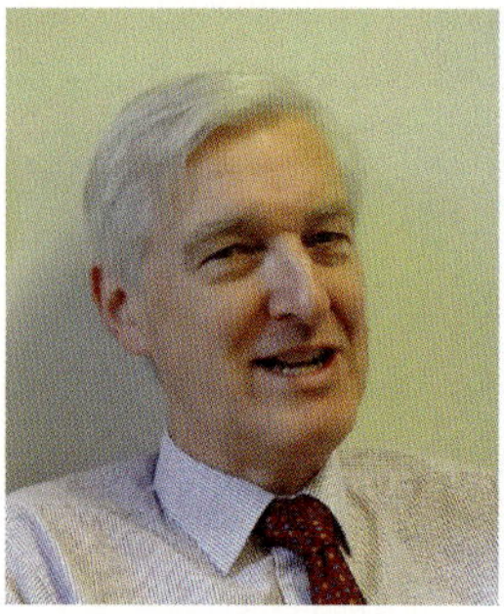

**Geoffrey E. Rose** Geoffrey Rose graduated BSc Pharmacology, MBBS, and MRCP. His postgraduate ophthalmic training culminated in award of FRCS in 1985 and FRCOphth at its foundation in 1988. In 1990, the University of London granted an MS doctorate for corneal research and, in 2004, a Doctor of Science in Ophthalmology and Ophthalmic Surgery.

Professor Rose was appointed consultant to Moorfields Eye Hospital, London, in 1990 and is also a Senior Research Fellow of the NIHR Biomedical Research Centre of the Institute of Ophthalmology. He served as the British Council member of the European Society of Ophthalmic Plastic and Reconstructive, is a Past-President of the British Oculoplastic Surgical Society, and is President of the European Society of Oculoplastic and Reconstructive Surgeons.

# Acute Surgical Management of Non-thyroid related, Non-infectious Orbital and Lid Inflammation

31

Kelvin Kam-lung Chong

## Introduction

Non-thyroid related, non-infectious orbital and eyelid inflammation involves a broad spectrum of conditions ranging from idiopathic, systemic, and specific causes of orbital and periocular inflammation to rarer conditions, e.g., Tolosa-Hunt syndrome and acute mucocutaneous syndromes including pyoderma gangrenosum, Stevens-Johnson syndrome, and toxic epidermal necrosis.

Idiopathic orbital inflammation (IOI) or idiopathic orbital inflammatory disease (IOID), previously known as orbital pseudotumor, is the commonest cause of non-thyroid related, non-infectious orbital and lid inflammation. Diagnosis of IOI is by exclusion of infectious, systemic, or specific etiologies, e.g., autoimmune thyroid disease, IgG4-related disease, sarcoidosis, histiocytosis, granulomatosis with polyangiitis (Wegener's granulomatosis), Crohn's disease, systemic lupus erythematosus, giant cell arteritis, Churg-Strauss syndrome, and other connective tissue diseases systemic evaluation, blood tests (serum thyroid function, ANA, ANCA, ACE, IgG4) and other ancillary investigations, e.g., chest radiographs [1, 2]. Histopathological examination of involved tissues is recommended to establish the diagnosis of IOI and to classify specific subtypes, e.g., sclerosing IOI, IOI with tissue eosinophilia [3]. Congenital lesions, e.g., ruptured dermoid cysts and lymphangiomas, are differential diagnoses of pediatric IOID. On the other hand, neoplastic conditions e.g. extrascleral extension of retinoblastoma, choroidal melanoma, lymphoproliferative disease in adult, and primary or metastatic orbital tumors, e.g., rhabdomyosarcoma in children, and vascular lesions e.g. carotid-cavernous fistula, acute hemorrhage or thrombosis of pre-existing venolymphatic malformation may have inflammatory presentations mimicking IOI [1].

K.K.-l. Chong, MB, ChB (Hon), FHKAM, FCOphth
Ophthalmology and Visual Science,
Prince of Wales Hospital, Alice Ho Miu Ling
Nethersole Hospital, The Chinese University
of Hong Kong, Hong Kong, Hong Kong SAR, China
e-mail: chongkamlung@cuhk.edu.hk

## Surgical Biopsy

Orbital biopsy is often performed after orbital imaging [4] (computerized tomography or magnetic resonance imaging) rule out primary vascular lesion, to identify the extent (localized versus generalized) of involvement, tissue(s) affected (eyelids/preseptal tissues, extraocular muscle, lacrimal gland, sclera/Tenon, optic nerve sheath, orbital apex), nature (vascularity, cystic, abscess, calcification, bony), and any extraorbital extent (sinus, intracranial, infratemporal fossa) of the lesion(s). Surgical approach is chosen using the most direct route to the most accessible (usually


B. Mukherjee, H. Yuen (eds.), *Emergencies of the Orbit and Adnexa*,
DOI 10.1007/978-81-322-1807-4_31

the anterior-most portion) and least risky part of the lesion(s), taken into account of the surgeons' experience. For more anterior-located or palpable lesions, upper lid crease, subbrow, subciliary skin incision, or caruncular, tarsal or forniceal conjunctival incision is usually enough for exposure [5]. For deeper lesions, subperiosteal approach using transcaruncular incision in medial-based lesions [6], upper lid crease incision for superiorly and laterally located lesion [7], and inferior forniceal conjunctival or swinging-eye incisions [8] are preferred. Endonasal transethmoidal approach, with or without retraction of the medial rectus, is an evolving alternative for medial lesions [9]. Small, apical lesions may require combined lateral orbitotomy with marginotomy [10], transcaruncular medial orbitotomy with retraction of the nearby rectus muscle, and occasionally even craniotomy approach to achieve adequate exposure.

Tissues obtained should be sent for histological and preferably microbiological examination while subsequent immunohistochemical, electron microscopic examination and other special stainings will be performed based on the initial hematoxylin and eosin staining results. Intraoperative frozen section examination allows rapid confirmation of adequate and representative sampling and is useful in more complicated or previously treated cases or biopsied.

## Debulking

In selected cases with suspected or confirmed orbital inflammation, surgical debulking of the lesion, preserving essential structures may improve proptosis and associated mass effects, e.g. mechanical ptosis, periocular swelling, compressive optic neuropathy, congestive orbitopathy (pain, redness and swelling), and exposure keratopathy. Mombaerts et al. reported 80 % (37 of 46) of patients with idiopathic dacryoadenitis fully recovered clinically after deliberately large debulking of the orbital lobe and injection of 40–80 mg triamcinolone to the remaining lacrimal gland [11]. All patients were off systemic steroid shortly postoperatively. The authors suggested, with mechanism not well understood, the affected lacrimal gland(s) patients with idiopathic dacryoadenitis was both diagnostic, and often therapeutic appeared superior to systemic steroid with higher response, lower recurrence and treatment-related complication rates [11].

## Curettage

In cases of unifocal orbital Langerhans cell histiocytosis (LCH) or eosinophilic granuloma, curettage of the lesions with intralesional steroid often leads to very favorable outcome [12].

## Intra-/perilesional Steroid

Mohammad et al. used betamethasone suspension of 2–4 ml (1 ml contains 2 mg betamethasone sodium phosphate and 5 mg betamethasone dipropionate) injecting inside the inflamed lacrimal gland, around the inflamed extraocular muscle, or periocularly in the diffuse, along with oral nonsteroidal anti-inflammatory drugs for 2, achieved quick and sustained response in his series of 47 IOI patients [13].

## Canthotomy, Cantholysis, and Surgical Decompression

While lateral canthotomy and cantholysis are performed in tight orbits with compartment syndrome, surgical decompression may occasionally be for compressive optic neuropathies not responding to medical treatment. Detailed management of compressive optic neuropathy and compartment syndrome have been covered elsewhere in the book and will not be repeated here [14].

## Tarsorrhaphy and Skin Graft

In cases of acute mucocutaneous syndromes, e.g., pyoderma gangrenosum, Stevens-Johnson syndrome, and toxic epidermal necrosis, lateral, paramedian, or total temporary tarsorrhaphy and sometimes skin graft may be required for cicatricial lid retraction and lagophthalmos to improve exposure keratopathy and avoid corneal breakdown.

## References


1. Gordon LK. Orbital inflammatory disease: a diagnostic and therapeutic challenge. Eye (Lond). 2006; 20(10):1196–206. Review.
2. Wallace ZS, Khosroshahi A, Jakobiec FA, Deshpande V, Hatton MP, Ritter J, Ferry JA, Stone JH. IgG4-related systemic disease as a cause of "idiopathic" orbital inflammation, including orbital myositis, and trigeminal nerve involvement. Surv Ophthalmol. 2012;57(1): 26–33.
3. Pemberton JD, Fay A. Idiopathic sclerosing orbital inflammation: a review of demographics, clinical presentation, imaging, pathology, treatment, and outcome. Ophthal Plast Reconstr Surg. 2012;28(1):79–83.
4. Pakdaman MN, Sepahdari AR, Elkhamary SM. Orbital inflammatory disease: pictorial review and differential diagnosis. World J Radiol. 2014;6(4):106–15.
5. Cho KJ, Paik JS, Yang SW. Surgical outcomes of transconjunctival anterior orbitotomy for intraconal orbital cavernous hemangioma. Korean J Ophthalmol. 2010;24(5):274–8.
6. Shorr N, Baylis HI, Goldberg RA, Perry JD. Transcaruncular approach to the medial orbit and orbital apex. Ophthalmology. 2000;107(8):1459–63.
7. Harris GJ, Logani SC. Eyelid crease incision for lateral orbitotomy. Ophthal Plast Reconstr Surg. 1999;15(1):9–16.
8. Kakizaki H. Tip for preventing chemosis after swinging eyelid procedure. Orbit. 2011;30(2):82.
9. Wu W, Selva D, Jiang F, Jing W, Tu Y, Chen B, Shi J, Sun MT, Qu J. Endoscopic transethmoidal approach with or without medial rectus detachment for orbital apical cavernous hemangiomas. Am J Ophthalmol. 2013;156(3):593–9.
10. Goldberg RA, Shorr N, Arnold AC, Garcia GH. Deep transorbital approach to the apex and cavernous sinus. Ophthal Plast Reconstr Surg. 1998;14(5):336–41.
11. Mombaerts I, Cameron JD, Chanlalit W, Garrity JA. Surgical debulking for idiopathic dacryoadenitis: a diagnosis and a cure. Ophthalmology. 2014;121(2): 603–9.
12. Margo CE, Goldman DR. Langerhans cell histiocytosis. Surv Ophthalmol. 2008;53(4):332–58.
13. El Nasser A Mohammad A. Local steroid injection for management of different types of acute idiopathic orbital inflammation: an 8-year study. Ophthal Plast Reconstr Surg. 2013;29(4):286–9.
14. Lima V, Burt B, Leibovitch I, Prabhakaran V, Goldberg RA, Selva D. Orbital compartment syndrome: the ophthalmic surgical emergency. Surv Ophthalmol. 2009;54(4):441–9.


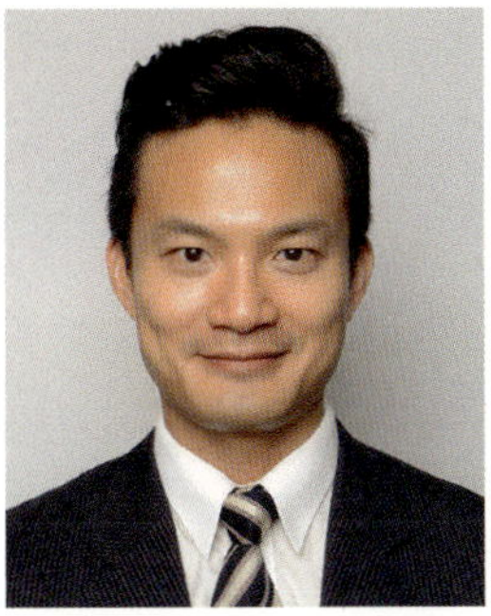

**Kelvin Kam-lung Chong** Dr. Kelvin Chong is a surgeonscientist in orbital and oculoplastic surgery and related cell biology. He graduated at the top of his class in the Bachelor of Medicine and Surgery (CUHK) program. He was awarded the Li Po Chun Charitable Trust Fund Overseas Postgraduate Scholarship where he continued later as an international clinical and research fellow at the University of California at Los Angeles (UCLA) (preceptor: Prof. Robert Goldberg) and LA Biomedical Institute (Preceptor: Prof. Terry Smith and Dr Raymond Douglas). His awards included the City Lion Club Gold Medal, Action for Vision Eye Foundation Young Researcher of the Year, Exemplary Eye Resident Award, Achievement Awards from American Academy of Ophthalmology and Asia Pacific Academy of Ophthalmology. Dr. Chong serves as the Coordinator of Orbital and Oculoplastic Surgery at the teaching hospital of the CUHK, the Prince of Wales Hospital and the CUHK Eye Center. He is the current vice President of Hong Kong Society of Ophthalmic Plastic and Reconstructive Surgery (HKSOPRS), Secretary of the Asia-Pacific Society of Ophthalmic Plastic and Reconstructive Surgery (APSOPRS).

# General Approach and Algorithm for Managing Acute Infections of the Orbit and Eyelid

32

Hunter Kwok-Lai Yuen

## Introduction

Acute eyelid infection and orbital infection are characterized by various cardinal signs of inflammation including pain, redness, swelling, and warmth. Eyelid infection is more easily identified clinically with redness and swelling over the eyelid, whereas distinguishing orbital infection and orbital inflammation can sometimes be difficult as orbital infection and other orbital inflammatory processes can have similar presentation. Since the orbit is a confined space, swelling or edema secondary to any inflammatory process can lead to proptosis as well as compression of the structures within the orbit [1]. Typical presentations for orbital infection include red eye, proptosis, ophthalmoplegia, and pain. In severe cases, the eyeball and optic nerve can be compressed leading to choroidal folds or compressive optic neuropathy [2]. Performing a complete medical history, along with complete physical examination with visual acuity testing, and laboratory and radiologic testing will narrow down the differential diagnosis. Blood tests should be guided by clinical suspicion; these include complete blood count, erythrocyte sedimentation rate (ESR), C-reactive protein, antinuclear antibody (ANA), cytoplasmic antineutrophil cytoplasmic antibodies (C-ANCAs), rheumatoid factor (RF), serum protein electrophoresis, angiotensin-converting enzyme (ACE), and thyroid function studies. Radiologic orbital evaluation commonly involves computerized tomography (CT) scan or magnetic resonance imaging (MRI) with intravenous contrast and is very helpful to narrow down the differential diagnoses and assess the location and extent of the disease process. Patients with atypical presentation or those who are unresponsive to medical treatment may even require an orbital biopsy for pathological diagnosis [3]. Microbiological tests including Gram stain, culture, and sensitivity tests are helpful to identify the causative microorganisms and to guide the antimicrobial treatments. In cases of atypical infections, HIV infection or other causes of immunodeficiency status should be excluded [4].

## Eyelid Infection

Eyelid infection should be considered as the first differential diagnosis if a patient presented with redness, swelling, and pain over the eyelid. Allergic eyelid disorders including acute allergic edema can also have similar presentation, but patients with allergic eyelid disorder may have a

H.K.-L. Yuen, FRCOphth, FRCSEd
Department of Ophthalmology and Visual Sciences, The Chinese University of Hong Kong, Hong Kong Eye Hospital, Hong Kong, Hong Kong SAR, China
e-mail: hunterklyuen@gmail.com


B. Mukherjee, H. Yuen (eds.), *Emergencies of the Orbit and Adnexa*,
DOI 10.1007/978-81-322-1807-4_32

history of insect bites, angioedema, urticaria, and occasionally drug usage. Patient may have itchiness in allergic eyelid disorder, especially in contact dermatitis. Moreover, allergic eyelid tends to be painless with the presence of pitting periorbital and lid edema. The differentiation is important as eyelid infection requires the use of antimicrobial medication, whereas antihistamine is required in case of acute allergic edema [5].

Acute eyelid and orbital infections are usually caused by viral or bacterial infection; fungal infection and atypical infection such as *Mycobacteria* infection tend to have different clinical presentation. The two most common forms of acute viral eyelid infections are herpes simplex and herpes zoster infection. Primary herpes simplex infection is caused by herpes simplex virus (HSV). This is typically affects children as unilateral condition. HSV eyelid infection may be more severe in those patients with atopic dermatitis and immunodeficiency status. The clinical features include crops of small vesicles which rupture, crust, and heal within a few days. Uncommon complications include follicular conjunctivitis and keratitis. The condition tends to be self-limiting and can be treated with acyclovir ointment [6].

Herpes zoster is a more common viral eyelid infection which is caused by varicella zoster virus (VZV). It typically affects elderly but may occur at earlier age and be more severe in immunocompromised patients. When this affects the first branch of the fifth nerve or trigeminal nerve, this is also known as herpes zoster ophthalmicus. The clinical features include pain in the distribution of first branch of the fifth nerve, a maculopapular rash over the forehead and eyelid which later became vesicles, pustules to crusting ulceration, and periorbital eyelid edema. In severe cases, this may cause scarring of the eyelid. Patients can have other ocular complications including conjunctivitis, keratitis, uveitis, scleritis, or even optic neuritis and cranial nerve palsy. The treatment includes the systemic antiviral agents such as acyclovir, valacyclovir, or famciclovir. Topical acyclovir or penciclovir cream and steroid-antibiotic combination ointment can be applied to the affected skin as well [6].

There are also various forms of bacterial eyelid infections; these include blepharitis, stye or infected chalazion, impetigo, erysipelas, and necrotizing fasciitis. Blepharitis is the commonest form of mild chronic eyelid infection and is related to poor lid hygiene, excessive meibomian gland secretion, and *Staphylococci* infection. In some cases, there may be eyelid hyperemia, telangiectasia, crusting, and redness suggestive of acute infective element. The treatment includes lid hygiene, antibiotic ointment, weak topical steroids, and artificial tear substitutes [7].

Stye is an acute infection of lash follicle unit caused by *Staphylococci* infection; sometimes this is associated with pustule formation. Chalazion is a chronic lipogranulomatous inflammation of the meibomian gland which produces a nodular lesion around the lid margin. Chalazion can be infected leading to a tender erythematous nodule. Both stye and infected chalazion can be treated with hot compress and topical antibiotics with or without steroid. Incision and drainage should be considered if there is abscess collection. Systemic antibiotics are required in case of secondary cellulitis [8].

Impetigo is the superficial skin infection caused by *Staph. aureus* or *Strep. pyogenes*. Children are more often affected, and patient may have erythematous macules which rapidly developed into vesicles and bullae. These vesicles and bullae will rupture and produce golden-yellow crust. The infection may spread into other parts of the face. Treatment includes the use of topical antibiotic and systemic antibiotic such as flucloxacillin or erythromycin [9].

Erysipelas, also known as St. Anthony's Fire, is an acute subcutaneous cellulitis caused by *Strep. pyogenes* through a site of skin injury. This is characterized by a well-defined indurated erythematous subcutaneous plaque. The treatment is with oral antibiotics such as phenoxymethylpenicillin, amoxicillin with clavulanate, or ampicillin-sulbactam [5].

More severe form of eyelid infection can also be called preseptal cellulitis, and possible etiological factors include endogenous infection foci, trauma, postoperative wound infection, chalazion, or idiopathic in nature. Even though eyelid infections are often localized in nature, in severe cases, patient can potentially have systemic symptoms such as fever and elevated WBC count. If left untreated, these can cause postseptal orbital cellulitis or even systemic bacteremia [5, 10].

Necrotizing fasciitis is an extremely rare rapidly progressive infection with necrosis of tissue caused by *Strep. pyogenes* or occasionally *Staph. aureus* infection. This is characterized by blackish discoloration of skin due to tissue thrombosis with gangrene. Necrotizing fasciitis is a potentially vision threatening or even life-threatening condition and has to be treated aggressively with tissue debridement and systemic antibiotics [11].

## Orbital Cellulitis

There are various causes of orbital inflammatory diseases and can be broadly divided into infective and noninfective causes. Orbital cellulitis should be the first differential diagnosis whenever one is faced with orbital inflammatory process. Orbital cellulitis can be classified as preseptal or postseptal cellulitis. In case of orbital cellulitis, bacterial infection is more common than viral, fungal, or parasitic infection. *Mycobacteria* infection may occasionally be encountered and tends to have a more indolent course [12]. Orbital fungal infections such as mucormycosis and aspergillosis can have aggressive clinical behavior, and a high of suspicious is required for prompt diagnosis [13].

Preseptal cellulitis refers to those infections localized to the eyelids and periocular structures anterior to the orbital septum. Common causes include skin trauma such as laceration or insect bites and spread of local infection from acute hordeolum or dacryocystitis or from remote infection of the upper respiratory tract or middle ear by hematogenous spread. Clinically, preseptal cellulitis is identified by unilateral, tender, erythematous periorbital and eyelid edema. Proptosis is absent; vision, optic nerve function, and ocular motility are unimpaired. Treatment is systemic antibiotic such as phenoxymethylpenicillin, amoxicillin with clavulanate, or ampicillin-sulbactam [5, 10].

Postseptal cellulitis refers to the infection that has extended behind the orbital septum. This is more severe than preseptal cellulitis and can lead to visual loss. The causes include sinus-related infection especially ethmoidal sinusitis, extension of preseptal cellulitis, local spread from adjacent dacryocystitis or dental infection, hematogenous spread of infection, trauma, or postsurgical infection. Other than the clinical features of preseptal cellulitis, patients will have proptosis, painful ophthalmoplegia, and optic nerve dysfunction. Possible complications secondary to orbital cellulitis include subperiosteal abscess (SPA), orbital abscess, cavernous sinus thrombosis, and cranial nerve palsy. Subperiosteal abscesses can expand rapidly causing more extensive complications such as orbital and cerebral abscesses. Vision loss can result due to central retinal artery occlusion, optic atrophy, septic optic neuritis, or thromboembolic lesions to the retina, choroid, or optic nerve [14–16].

If a patient is having postseptal cellulitis, hospital admission with imaging is essential. Contrast CT scan, including axial and coronal views, is required. Axial views should include low narrow cuts of the frontal lobes to rule out peridural and parenchymal brain abscess formation. Coronal views are helpful in determining the presence and extent of any SPA. MRI may be helpful in defining orbital abscesses and in evaluating the possibility of cavernous sinus disease. Patients may also have fever and elevated WBC count in their complete blood count. ENT surgeons or maxillofacial surgeons should be consulted if there is evidence of paranasal sinus infection or dental infection, respectively [16].

Antibiotic therapy is needed, and sometimes anaerobic coverage is required especially in case of sinus infection. Surgical indications to drain an orbital abscess include patients $\geq 9$ years of age, large SPA, frontal sinusitis, non-medial SPA, suspicion of anaerobic infection, recurrent SPA after drainage, chronic sinusitis, acute optic nerve or retinal compromise, or dental infection [14, 15, 17]. If drainage of the orbital abscess is required, a Gram stain of the pus can be performed, and this can be a useful guide in terms of selecting appropriate antibiotics for treatment. The exact pathogen can be identified by microbiological culture tests. Fungal infection including aspergillosis and mucormycosis should be considered in refractory cases [18, 19].

## Lacrimal Infections

Infection of the lacrimal system includes infective dacryoadenitis, dacryocystitis, and canaliculitis. Infective dacryoadenitis is infection of the lacrimal gland, usually caused by viral or bacterial infection. Patient will have inflammatory changes over the superolateral aspect of the orbit, where the lacrimal gland is situated [20]. Acute dacryocystitis is characterized by a painful erythematous swelling over the lacrimal sac region, often associated with nasolacrimal duct obstruction. Other than systemic antibiotic treatment, patient may require surgical intervention such as drainage of abscess and external or endoscopic dacryocystorhinostomy [21]. Patient with canaliculitis will have inflammatory changes with sprouting and discharge around the punctum and concretions within the lacrimal canaliculus. There are various causes for canaliculitis, and *Actinomyces* infection is a common cause [22]. There will be a more detail discussion for various lacrimal infections in Chaps. 39 and 40 of this book.

## Summary

There is a wide variety of acute eyelid, orbital, and lacrimal infections; some of these infections can threaten vision or even life. It is important to consider, and work up for, a wide range of differential diagnoses with appropriate imaging and laboratory tests. Prompt treatment with appropriate antimicrobial agent is essential. Surgical intervention such as incision or drainage of abscess, orbitotomy with exploration, or dacryocystorhinostomy may be required. The flowchart in Fig. 32.1 summarizes the diagnostic pathway

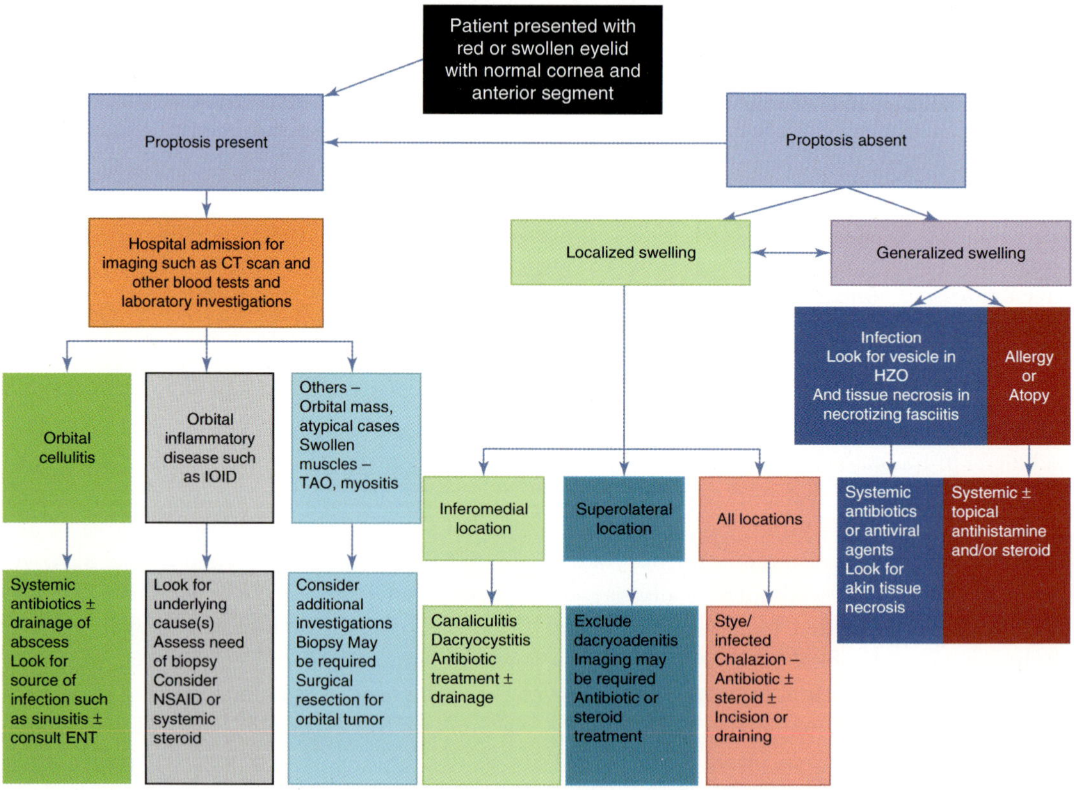


**Fig. 32.1** The diagnostic pathway for patients with red or swollen eyelid with normal cornea and anterior segment

for patients with red or swollen eyelid with normal cornea and anterior segment.

## References


1. Chandler JR, Langenbrunner DJ, Steven ER. The pathogenesis of orbital complications in acute sinusitis. Laryngoscope. 1970;80:1414–28.
2. Chaudhry IA, Shamsi FA, Elzaridi E, et al. Outcome of treated orbital cellulitis in a tertiary eye care center in the Middle East. Ophthalmology. 2007;114(2):345–54.
3. Yuen SJ, Rubin PA. Idiopathic orbital inflammation: distribution, clinical features, and treatment outcome. Arch Ophthalmol. 2003;121:491–9.
4. Lam Choi VB, Yuen HK, Biswas J, Yanoff M. Update in pathological diagnosis of orbital infections and inflammations. Middle East Afr J Ophthalmol. 2011; 18(4):268–76.
5. Kanski JJ. Clinicalophthalmology. A synopsis. London: Butterworths; 2009.
6. Newman H, Gooding C. Viral ocular manifestations: a broad overview. Rev Med Virol. 2013;23(5):281–94.
7. Suzuki T. Meibomitis-related keratoconjunctivitis: implications and clinical significance of meibomian gland inflammation. Cornea. 2012;31 Suppl 1:S41–4.
8. Lindsley K, Nichols JJ, Dickersin K. Interventions for acute internal hordeolum. Cochrane Database Syst Rev. 2010;9:CD007742.
9. Barza M, Baum J. Ocular infections. Med Clin North Am. 1983;67(1):131–52. Review.
10. Holds JB. San Francisco: American Academy of Ophthalmology; 2007–2008. Infectious and inflammatory disorders. Basic and Clinical Science Course. Section 7. Orbit, Eyelids, and Lacrimal system.
11. Tambe K, Tripathi A, Burns J, Sampath R. Multidisciplinary management of periocular necrotising fasciitis: a series of 11 patients. Eye (Lond). 2012; 26(3):463–7.
12. Madge SN, Prabhakaran VC, Shome D, Kim U, Honavar S, Selva D. Orbital tuberculosis: a review of the literature. Orbit. 2008;27:267–77.
13. Klotz SA, Penn CC, Negvesky GJ, Butrus SI. Fungal and parasitic infections of the eye. Clin Microbiol Rev. 2000;13:662–85.
14. Garcia GH, Harris GJ. Criteria for nonsurgical management of subperiosteal abscess of the orbit: analysis of outcomes 1998–1998. Ophthalmology. 2000;107: 1454–8.
15. Todman MS, Enzer YR. Management versus surgical intervention of orbital cellulitis: the importance of subperiosteal abscess volume as a new criterion. Ophthal Plast Reconstr Surg. 2011;27:255–9.
16. Tovilla-Canales JL, Nava A, Tovilla Y, Pomar JL. Orbital and periorbital infections. Curr Opin Ophthalmol. 2001;12:335–41.
17. Harris GJ. Subperiosteal abscess of the orbit: age as a factor in the bacteriology and response to treatment. Ophthalmology. 1994;101:585–95.
18. Levin LA, Avery R, Shore JW, Woog JJ, Baker AS. The spectrum of orbital aspergillosis: a clinicopathological review. Surv Ophthalmol. 1996;41:142–54.
19. Shatriah I, Mohd-Amin N, Tuan-Jaafar TN, Khanna RK, Yunus R, Madhavan M. Rhino-orbito-cerebral mucormycosis in an immunocompetent patient: case report and review of literature. Middle East Afr J Ophthalmol. 2012;19(2):258–61.
20. Goold LA, Madge SN, Au A, Leibovitch I, McNab A, Tumuluri K, Selva D. Acute suppurative bacterial dacryoadenitis: a case series. Br J Ophthalmol. 2013;97(6):735–8.
21. Lee TS, Woog JJ. Endonasal dacryocystorhinostomy in the primary treatment of acute dacryocystitis with abscess formation. Ophthal Plast Reconstr Surg. 2001;17(3):180–3.
22. Freedman JR, Markert MS, Cohen AJ. Primary and secondary lacrimal canaliculitis: a review of literature. Surv Ophthal mol. 2011;56(4):336–47.


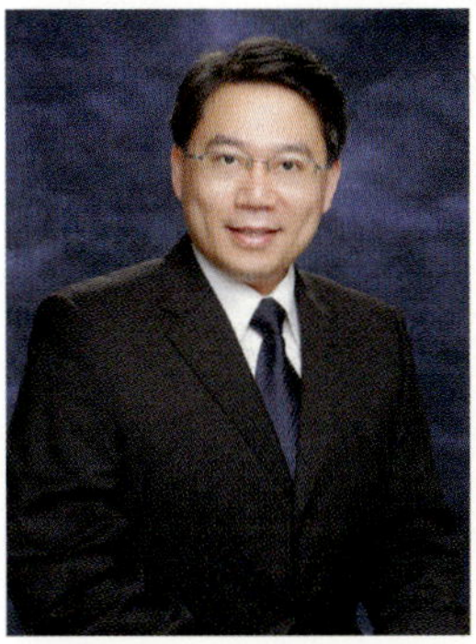


**Hunter Kwok-Lai Yuen** Dr. Hunter Kwok-Lai Yuen is the consultant ophthalmologist and head of the Oculoplastic & Orbital Surgery Service at Hong Kong Eye Hospital. Dr. Yuen was awarded as one of Ten Outstanding Youth Persons in 2007. Subsequently, he received The Fourth Hong Kong Volunteer Award in year 2011. He received Achievement Award and Distinguished Service Award from the Asian Pacific Academy of Ophthalmology in 2012. Moreover, he is the present first Vice President of Asia Pacific Society of Ophthalmic Plastic and Reconstructive Surgery (APSORPS), President of the Hong Kong Society of Ophthalmic Plastic and Reconstructive Surgery, Honorary Secretary of Asia-Pacific Society of Ocular Oncology and Pathology (APSOOP), and editorial member and reviewer of several journals.

# 33 Diagnosis and Treatment of Bacterial Infections of the Orbit

Emmy Yuen-mei Li and Hunter Kwok-Lai Yuen

## Non-necrotizing

### Introduction

Acute bacterial infection of the orbit is associated with diffuse edema of the orbital tissues with infiltration of inflammatory cells. There are usually cardinal signs of inflammation including pain, redness, swelling, and warmth. Since the orbit is a confined space, tissue edema secondary to the inflammatory process may lead to proptosis, as well as compression of the structures within the orbit causing conjunctival injection, ophthalmoplegia, and, in severe case, compressive optic neuropathy resulting in visual loss.

Conventionally, in the Chandler classification, orbital cellulitis was grouped into five different stages [1]:

Stage 1 – *Preseptal cellulitis*, with inflammation localized anterior to the orbital septum. There are eyelid swelling, erythema, and tenderness yet no orbital signs.

Stage 2 – *Orbital cellulitis*, where infection extends posterior to the orbital septum leading to diffuse orbital edema yet without discrete abscess. There are eyelid edema and erythema, proptosis, and chemosis with limited or normal extraocular movement and normal visual acuity.

Stage 3 – *Subperiosteal abscess*. There is pus collection between periorbital and orbital bones, which can displace the orbital contents, causing proptosis and ophthalmoplegia.

Stage 4 – *Intraorbital abscess*, with pus collection within orbital tissues. There are severe exophthalmos, chemosis, complete ophthalmoplegia, and visual impairment.

Stage 5 – *Cavernous sinus thrombosis*, caused by extension of infection posterior to the orbit. There are bilateral orbital pain, chemosis, proptosis, and ophthalmoplegia. It can be associated with meningitis, intracranial abscess formation, and sepsis.

A more practical and commonly used approach is to divide orbital infections into preseptal or postseptal cellulitis. Preseptal cellulitis refers to those infections localized to the eyelids and periocular structures anterior to the orbital septum where postseptal cellulitis describes an infection involving the soft tissues posterior to the orbital septum. In general, postseptal cellulitis

E.Y. Li, MBBS,MPH, FRCS, FCOphthHK, FHKAM (✉)
Ophthalmology, Hong Kong Eye Hospital, Hong Kong, Hong Kong SAR, China
e-mail: dr.emmyli@gmail.com

H.K.-L. Yuen, FRCOphth, FRCSEd
Department of Ophthalmology and Visual Sciences, Hong Kong Eye Hospital, The Chinese University of Hong Kong, Hong Kong, Hong Kong SAR, China
e-mail: hunterklyuen@hotmail.com


B. Mukherjee, H. Yuen (eds.), *Emergencies of the Orbit and Adnexa*,
DOI 10.1007/978-81-322-1807-4_33

is more severe and may be associated with sight and life-threatening complications [2, 3].

## Preseptal Cellulitis

Preseptal cellulitis occurs more commonly than orbital cellulitis and is generally associated with a more favorable prognosis. Preseptal cellulitis can occur alone or as a spread of infection from adjacent soft tissues of the face, ocular adnexa, and paranasal sinuses. There may be a history of trauma, insect bites, foreign bodies, chalazion or hordeola, dacryocystitis, skin infection like impetigo, sinusitis, upper respiratory tract infection, or recent periocular/oral procedures [3].

The typical presentations of preseptal cellulitis are eyelid edema and erythema. As the infection is superficial, patients have no orbital signs. Evaluation should start with relevant history to identify predisposing factors like trauma, surgery, or adjacent infection. A comprehensive ophthalmic examination, including assessment of visual acuity, pupillary response, extraocular movement, intraocular pressure, anterior segment biomicroscopy, and dilated fundal examination, is recommended. The distinctive features to differentiate preseptal cellulitis from orbital cellulitis are normal vision, absence of proptosis, absence of afferent pupillary defect, and absence of pain and limitation on extraocular movement. Care should be taken to identify any wound suggestive of trauma, especially perforating injuries that may affect the globe integrity or suggestive of a possible foreign body [4, 5].

The primary strategy in the treatment of preseptal cellulitis is the prompt initiation of appropriate antibiotic therapy. Given the predisposing factors of preseptal cellulitis, the choice of antibiotics should target towards causative agents of sinusitis and upper respiratory tract infection, in particular *Staphylococcus* and *Streptococcus* species. In cases with history of local trauma, coverage for *Staphylococcus aureus* is mandatory. Mild preseptal cellulitis in adults and children over 1 year old can be treated with empiric broad-spectrum oral antibiotics in outpatient setting. Those who require hospital admission for intravenous antibiotics are children less than 1 year of age, immunocompromised individuals, and patients who fail to respond to oral treatment and with development of more severe infection or systemic toxicity [4, 6–10]. A negative immunization history against *Haemophilus influenzae* and *Streptococcus pneumoniae* is considered a relative indication for early admission. Surgical interventions are usually not required in preseptal cellulitis, unless associated with the development of eyelid abscess or in the presence of foreign body [9]. Percutaneous drainage and debridement of an eyelid abscess can be performed through a direct incision over the area of fluctuance under local anesthesia. Loculation in the cavity should be broken with a curette and the wound packed with ribbon gauze to promote further drainage. Expressed material should be sent for microbiological evaluation, especially culture and sensitivity to guide subsequent antibiotic therapy. Any concurrent sinusitis should be treated and appropriate referral arranged [6].

## Orbital Cellulitis

Orbital cellulitis refers to infections that involve the tissues posterior to the orbital septum, including the extraocular muscles and orbital fat within the bony orbit. In contrast to preseptal cellulitis, it may result in more significant complications. Permanent visual loss has been reported in the range of 11–26 % of cases, as results of compressive optic neuropathy, toxic optic neuritis, panophthalmitis, or exposure keratopathy due to proptosis. Intracranial complications, though rare, include cavernous thrombosis, meningitis, brain abscess, and subdural empyema. Therefore accurate diagnosis, close observation, and expeditious treatment are of paramount importance [11–13].

Orbital cellulitis can affect all age groups yet it occurs more commonly in the pediatric population (Fig. 33.1). The most common cause is a direct extension of infection from the adjacent paranasal sinuses, in particular the ethmoid sinus through the thin lamina papyracea. The inflamed mucosa in sinusitis leads to closure of ostia and

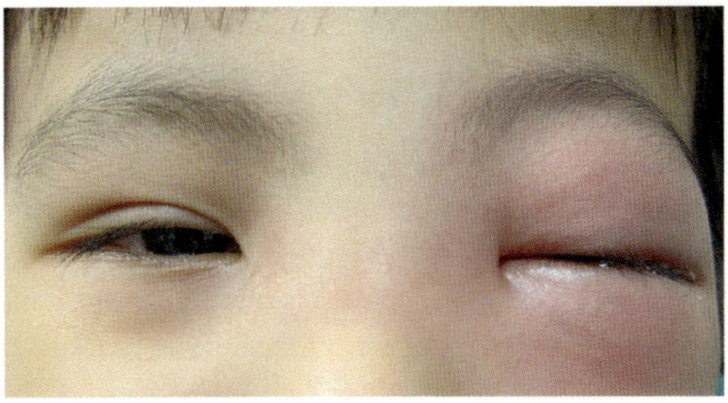

**Fig. 33.1** Orbital cellulitis in the left eye with periorbital swelling and erythema

blocks the sinus drainage, which promotes proliferation and accumulation of bacteria, resulting in suppuration and extension to the orbit through the thin bones of orbital walls, foramina, and venous and lymphatic channels. Other predisposing factors include trauma, especially those associated with orbital fracture or foreign bodies, dacryocystitis, untreated preseptal cellulitis, endophthalmitis, and dental infections or procedures [14–16]. Orbital cellulitis following ophthalmic surgery is uncommon, but has been reported after strabismus surgery, eyelid surgery, lacrimal surgery, cataract extraction, scleral buckling, and peribulbar injection [17–20]. Though uncommon, it can be the presenting feature of retinoblastoma in children [21]. Hematogenous spread in the setting of bacteremia is also possible.

Patients with orbital cellulitis typically present with more severe edema and erythema of periorbital tissues and may be associated with decreased vision, proptosis, pain with eye movement, and ophthalmoplegia with or without diplopia. The presence of fever is variable. Apart from identifying predisposing factors, like history of sinusitis, trauma, or surgery, a thorough ophthalmic examination is required, especially to identify any complications from the disease, e.g., the presence of relative afferent pupillary defect signifying compressive optic neuropathy, exposure keratopathy secondary to proptosis, elevated intraocular pressure, venous stasis, or even central retinal artery occlusion due to raised intraorbital pressure [22]. Systemic examination including assessment of vital signs should be performed. Blood cultures should be taken, and a lumbar puncture may be necessary if signs of meningitis are present. Urgent imaging is indicated to assess the anatomic extent of disease, to identify subperiosteal or orbital abscess that requires exploration and drainage, to look for sources of contiguous spread like sinusitis, and to rule out intracranial extension.

Before the introduction of the *Haemophilus influenzae* type B (HiB) vaccine, *H. influenzae* was one of the most commonly reported organisms associated with orbital infections [9]. In a more recent study on microbiology of pediatric orbital cellulitis, *Staphylococcus aureus* was the most common species isolated (one-third being methicillin-resistant *S. aureus* (MRSA)), followed by *Streptococcus* species. Anaerobic bacteria, including *Peptococcus*, *Peptostreptococcus*, and *Bacteroides*, are less common causes and are associated with infections following animal bites [10]. Blood cultures are usually negative. Cultures from ocular secretions and nasal swab can be performed, but there may be normal flora contaminants; thus organisms recovered from abscess or nasal drainage are the most reliable source of causative agents.

## Medical Management

Early diagnosis and aggressive proper management of orbital cellulitis are essential to avoid vision- or life-threatening complications. Intravenous antibiotics should be started promptly based on empiric coverage for the common causative microorganisms, typically the gram-positive *Staphylococcus* and *Streptococcus* species. Vancomycin should be considered early if the local resistance profile suggests high prevalence of methicillin-resistant staphylococcal infection. Second- or third-generation cephalosporin, clindamycin, or metronidazole is often added to provide coverage of gram-negative and anaerobic organisms [23, 24]. Treatment should be modified based on clinical response as well as culture and sensitivity results. Consultation with the infectious disease/microbiology team may be helpful. For patients with concurrent sinusitis, nasal decongestant and nasal irrigation can promote drainage of the sinus [25]. Intranasal corticosteroid can also be considered to facilitate drainage by reducing mucosal edema [26]. The use of systemic corticosteroids is still debatable. Although suppression of the immune system may lead to worsening of the infection, there are multiple theoretical advantages. Firstly, the reduction of tissue edema and cell migration may decrease compression on orbital structures to avoid irreversible visual loss and may facilitate drainage to accelerate recovery from sinusitis. Secondly, by inhibiting fibroblast proliferation, corticosteroids can reduce scarring of orbital tissues and potential long-term sequelae. In a retrospective study by Yen, it was concluded that the use of intravenous corticosteroids in the acute management of pediatric orbital cellulitis with subperiosteal abscess did not adversely affect clinical outcome [27]. In a prospective trial by Pushker, oral corticosteroids were offered after initial response to intravenous antibiotics, and it was observed that such adjunct hastened resolution of inflammation with a low risk of exacerbating infection [28].

### Surgical Management

Surgical intervention should be considered for those who fail to respond or deteriorate on medical therapy, demonstrate worsening of visual function, and develop pupillary changes or in the presence of subperiosteal/orbital abscess. The need for immediate surgical drainage of subperiosteal abscess (SPA) depends on the clinical picture, as medical therapy alone may suffice. Garcia outlined nine indications for surgical drainage in pediatric SPA based on a prospective case: patients age 9 years old or above, large size of SPA, non-medially located SPA, recurrent SPA after prior drainage, frontal sinusitis, chronic sinusitis, presence of ocular complications, suspected anaerobic infection, or infection of dental origin. In this study, more than 90 % of patients who met the criteria resolved without surgical intervention [29].

There are several situations that require surgical intervention without delay; these include the presence of orbital abscess; cases associated with retained orbital foreign body especially those of organic nature; fulminant infection of an ocular/adnexal structure, e.g., endophthalmitis, dacryocystitis, and concurrent sinusitis with completely opacified sinuses; and those with cavernous sinus or intracranial involvement. The surgical approach depends on the location of the abscess. The common options include transnasal, transcaruncular, or transcutaneous (Lynch incision) approach for medially located abscess, subbrow or lid crease incision for superiorly located abscess, and transconjunctival/transforniceal or subciliary incision for inferiorly located abscess.

## Necrotizing

Necrotizing fasciitis is a rapidly progressing necrotizing infection of the subcutaneous tissue and superficial fascia with secondary necrosis of overlying skin (Fig. 33.2) [30]. Periorbital necrotizing fasciitis, although rare, is a sight- and life-threatening ophthalmic emergency, with a reported rate of vision loss of 13.8 % and mortality of 8.5 % [31]. In a review of case reports on periorbital necrotizing fasciitis over the past 20 years, one-third has bilateral involvement. The reported predisposing factors include trauma, surgery (including dental procedure, sinus surgery, blepharoplasty, laser resurfacing, conjunctivo-dacryocystorhinostomy, and tumor excision), immunosuppression, and coexisting infections [31]. The diagnosis of necrotizing fasciitis is largely clinical. Patients commonly present with acute periorbital swelling and severe pain. There is initially violaceous discoloration of skin and fluid-filled bullae, which helps to distinguish it from preseptal cellulitis. The lesion usually turns gangrenous within 24 h. In the later

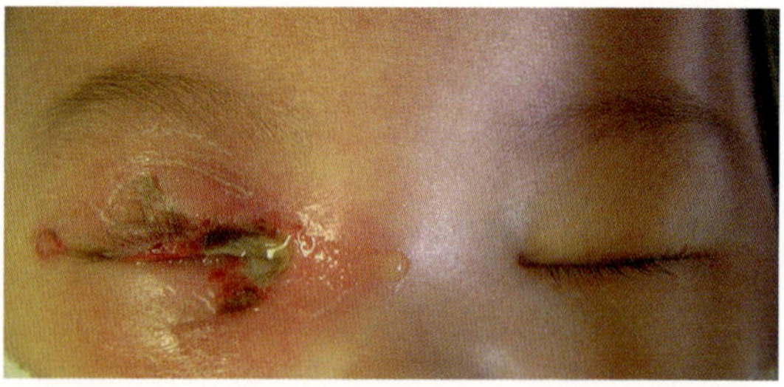

**Fig. 33.2** Necrotizing fasciitis in the right eye with blanched appearance and eyelid necrosis

stage, there may be tense edema with crepitus and local anesthesia due to destruction of the cutaneous nerves. Patient may have high fever, signs of systemic toxicity, or even multi-organ failure or disseminated intravascular coagulation [30]. CT and MRI may help in making an early diagnosis by identifying soft tissue edema infiltrating the fascial planes and the presence of subcutaneous emphysema.

Necrotizing fasciitis can be divided into two types on the basis of microbiological culture: Type 1 necrotizing fasciitis is polymicrobial caused by both aerobic and anaerobic organisms, which is more commonly seen in immunocompromised patients, and Type 2 necrotizing fasciitis is by single organisms like *Streptococci* or *Staphylococci* or a combination of the two. The most common causative agent for periorbital necrotizing fasciitis from previous reports is *Streptococcus pyogenes*, followed by *Pseudomonas*. Other microorganisms reported include *Staphylococcus albus*, *Streptococcus viridans*, *Streptococcus epidermis*, *Propionibacterium acnes*, *Citrobacter*, *Enterococci*, and *Serratia* and *Burkholderia pseudomallei* [30–32].

Prompt initiation of high-dose antibiotics combined with timely surgical debridement helps to reduce both morbidity and mortality, though there were a few reports describing successful management of periorbital necrotizing fasciitis with intravenous antibiotic therapy alone. Antimicrobial therapy should consist of a combination of beta-lactam antibiotics, such as penicillin or cephalosporin, which is effective against *Streptococcal* infection and clindamycin which inhibits protein synthesis and decreases the production of streptococcal toxin. If polymicrobial infection is suspected, aminoglycosides and/or metronidazole should be added to extend coverage for gram-negative and anaerobic microorganisms. Surgical debridement decreases the bacterial load and the level of hyaluronic acid, which facilitates the bacterial dissection through the connective tissue. Repeated debridement may be necessary (Fig. 33.3). Once the acute infection has settled, reconstructive surgery can be planned at a later stage. The use of hyperbaric oxygen to limit extension of ischemic tissue, as well as intravenous immunoglobulin and heparinization to neutralize superantigen activity have been proposed, yet their exact role remains controversial in view of isolated reports [30, 32].

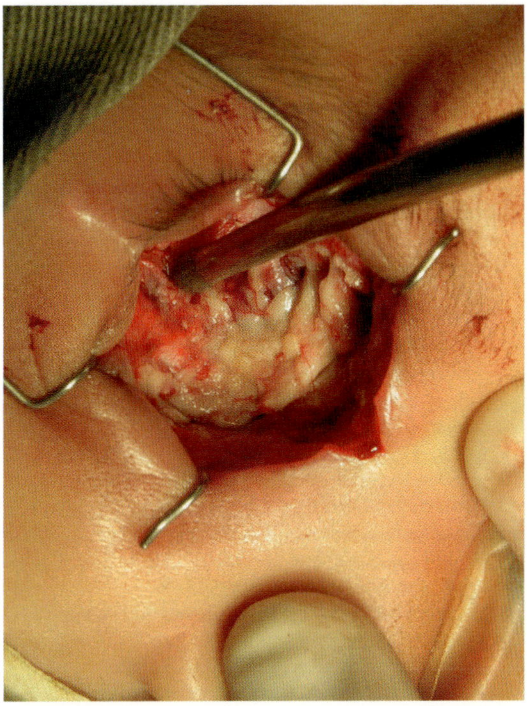

**Fig. 33.3** Surgical debridement of necrotic retrobulbar orbital content

The causes of visual loss from periorbital necrotizing fasciitis include central retinal artery occlusion, corneal perforation, or orbital spread of the infection necessitating removal of orbital contents including the eyeball. Other major morbidities are the loss of skin and soft tissue leading to cosmetic disfigurement and functional limitation. Mortality is the result of systemic complications like septicemia, shock, and multi-organ failure. Advanced age over 50 is considered a significant risk factor. Other factors associated with mortality are toxic shock syndrome, Type 1 necrotizing fasciitis with facial involvement, and blindness caused by necrotizing fasciitis [30, 31]. Therefore, vigilance, close monitoring, and prompt action are critical to save lives and vision in periorbital necrotizing fasciitis.

## References


1. Chandler JR, Langenbrunner DJ, Steven ER. The pathogenesis of orbital complications in acute sinusitis. Laryngoscope. 1970;80:1414–28.
2. Chaudhry IA, Shamsi FA, Elzaridi E, et al. Outcome of treated orbital cellulitis in a tertiary eye care center in the Middle East. Ophthalmology. 2007;114(2):345–54.
3. Lessner A, Stern GA. Preseptal and orbital cellulitis. Infect Dis Clin North Am. 1992;6:933–52.
4. Howe L, Jones NS. Guidelines for the management of periorbital cellulitis/abscess. Clin Otolaryngol. 2004;29:725–8.
5. Israele V, Nelson JD. Periorbital and orbital cellulitis. Pediatr Infect Dis J. 1987;6:404–10.
6. Smith TF, O'Day D, et al. Clinical implications of preseptal (periorbital) cellulitis in childhood. Pediatrics. 1978;62(6):1006–9.
7. Uzcategui N, Warman R. Clinical practice guidelines for the management of orbital cellulitis. J Pediatr Ophthalmol Strab. 1998;35(2):73–9.
8. Donahue SP, Schwartz G. Preseptal and orbital cellulitis in childhood. A changing microbiologic spectrum. Ophthalmology. 1998;105(10):1902–5.
9. Ambati BK, Ambati J. Periorbital and orbital cellulitis before and after the advent of Haemophilus influenzae type B vaccination. Ophthalmology. 2000;107(8):1450–3.
10. McKinley SH, Yen MT, Miller AM, Yen KG. Microbiology of pediatric orbital cellulitis. Am J Ophthalmol. 2007;144(4):497–501.
11. Mortimore S, Wormald PJ. The Groote Schuur hospital classification of the orbital complications of sinusitis. J LaryngolOtol. 1997;111(8):719–23.
12. Schmitt NJ, Beatty RL, et al. Superior ophthalmic vein thrombosis in a patient with dacryocystitis-induced orbital cellulitis. Ophthal Plast Reconstr Surg. 2005;21:387–9.
13. Yeh CH, Chen WC, et al. Intracranial brain abscess preceded by orbital cellulitis and sinusitis. J Craniofac Surg. 2010;21(3):934–6.
14. Cox NH, Knowles MA, et al. Pre-septal cellulitis and facial erysipelas due to Moraxella species. Clin Exp Dermatol. 1994;19:321–3.
15. Kikkawa DO, Heinz GW, et al. Orbital cellulitis and abscess secondary to dacryocystitis. Arch Ophthalmol. 2002;120(8):1096–9.
16. Molarte AB, Isenberg SJ. Periorbital cellulitis in infancy. J Pediatr Ophthalmol Strab. 1989;26:232–4.
17. Allen MV, Cohen KL, et al. Orbital cellulitis secondary to dacryocystitis following blepharoplasty. Ann Ophthalmol. 1985;17(8):498–9.
18. Weakley DR. Orbital cellulitis complicating strabismus surgery: a case report and review of the literature. Ann Ophthalmol. 1991;23(12):454–7.
19. Lopez PF, Marx J, et al. Endophthalmitis and orbital cellulitis after radial keratotomy. Ophthalmology. 1995;102(12):1902–7.
20. Hofbauer JD, Gordon LK, et al. Acute orbital cellulitis after peribulbar injection. Am J Ophthalmol. 1994;118:391.
21. Walinjkar J, Krishnakumar S, Gopal L, Ramesh A, Khetan V. Retinoblastoma presenting with orbital cellulitis. J AAPOS. 2013;17(3):282–6.
22. Proctor CM, Magrath GN, de Castro LE, Johnson JH, Teed RG. Orbital cellulitis complicated by central retinal artery occlusion. OphthalPlastReconstr Surg. 2013;29(2):e59–61.
23. Harris GJ. Subperiosteal abscess of the orbit. Arch Ophthalmol. 1983;101:751–7.
24. Jones DB, Steinkuller PG. Strategies for the initial management of acute preseptal and orbital cellulitis. Trans Am Ophthalmol Soc. 1988;86:94–108.
25. Brown CL, Graham SM. Nasal irrigations: good or bad? Curr Opin Otolaryngol Head Neck Surg. 2004;12:9–13.
26. Mygind N. Effects of corticosteroid therapy in non-allergic rhinosinusitis. Acta Otolaryngol. 1996;116:164–6.
27. Yen MT, Yen KG. Effect of corticosteroids in the acute management of pediatric orbital cellulitis with subperiosteal abscess. OphthalPlastReconstr Surg. 2005;21(5):363–6.
28. Pushker N, Tejwani LK, Bajaj MS, Khurana S, Velpandian T, Chandra M. Role of oral corticosteroids in orbital cellulitis. Am J Ophthalmol. 2013;156(1):178–83.
29. Garcia GH, Harris GJ. Criteria for nonsurgical management of subperiosteal abscess of the orbit: analysis of outcomes 1988–1998. Ophthalmology. 2000;107(8):1454–6.
30. Lazzeri D, Lazzeri S, Figus M, Tascini C, Bocci G, Colizzi L, Giannotti G, Lorenzetti F, Gandini D, Danesi R, Menichetti F, Del Tacca M, Nardi M, Pantaloni M. Periorbital necrotising fasciitis. Br J Ophthalmol. 2010;94(12):1577–85.
31. Amrith S, HosdurgaPai V, Wong W. Periorbital necrotizing fasciitis; a review. Acta Ophthalmol. 2013;91(7):596–603.
32. Seal DV. Necrotizing fasciitis. Curr Opin Infect Dis. 2001;14(2):127–32.

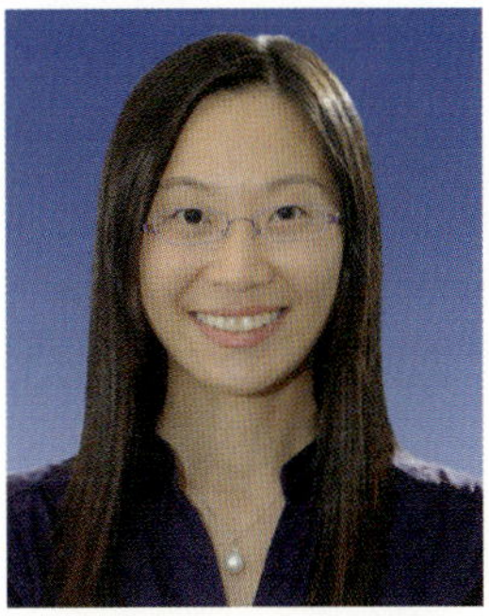

**Emmy Yuen-mei Li** Dr. Emmy Li graduated from the University of Hong Kong in 2004 with First Class Honor. She was admitted as fellow of the Royal College of Surgeons of Edinburgh in 2010 and fellow of the College of Ophthalmologists of Hong Kong in 2011. She is currently an Honorary Clinical Assistant Professor at the Department of Ophthalmology and Visual Sciences of the Chinese University of Hong Kong and an Associate Consultant of the Hong Kong Eye Hospital.

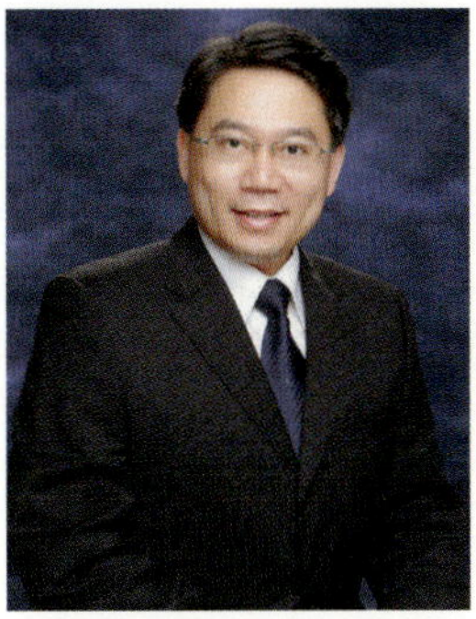

**Hunter Kwok-Lai Yuen** Dr. Hunter Kwok-Lai Yuen is the consultant ophthalmologist and head of the Oculoplastic & Orbital Surgery Service at Hong Kong Eye Hospital. Dr. Yuen was awarded as one of Ten Outstanding Youth Persons in 2007. Subsequently, he received The Fourth Hong Kong Volunteer Award in year 2011. He received Achievement Award and Distinguished Service Award from the Asian Pacific Academy of Ophthalmology in 2012. Moreover, he is the present first Vice President of Asia Pacific Society of Ophthalmic Plastic and Reconstructive Surgery (APSORPS), President of the Hong Kong Society of Ophthalmic Plastic and Reconstructive Surgery, Honorary Secretary of Asia-Pacific Society of Ocular Oncology and Pathology (APSOOP), and editorial member and reviewer of several journals.

# 34 Viral and Fungal Infections of the Orbit

Mohammad Javed Ali

## Introduction

Viral and fungal infections of the orbit, although not as common as bacterial etiologies, still remain important causes of orbital inflammations and proptosis. The past decade has seen a resurgence of a variety of fungal and viral agents involving orbits due to rising trends of HIV infections and other immunosuppressive comorbidities like diabetes; however the incidence may vary based on regional epidemiology. The modalities of orbital invasion can be contiguous from sinuses or oropharynx or through direct deposition from foreign bodies or from septicemia. The present chapter would discuss the various microbial factors, specific symptomatology, clinical signs, investigative modalities, management, complications, and outcomes of viral and fungal infections of the orbit.

## Viral Orbital Infections

### Herpes Infections

Viral infections of the orbit are uncommon and may mimic a bacterial cellulitis in early phases and hence need a high degree of suspicion, directed investigations, and appropriate management to prevent widespread damage and long-term sequelae. The most well-defined viral orbital infection is caused by herpes simplex virus (HSV) and herpes zoster virus (HZV) [1]. The varicella zoster virus can cause both chicken pox and shingles. In most of the cases, the primary infection usually occurs during childhood, following which the virus travels in a retrograde fashion to the dorsal root ganglia or sensory ganglia, where it may remain dormant for long periods. When the patient is immunosuppressed or when the virus-specific cell-mediated immunity decreases, it gets reactivated and travels along the trigeminal nerve or its branches to the orbit. Apart from the classical dermatomal pattern of skin lesions, orbital involvement may be in the form of retrobulbar neuritis, third, fourth, and sixth cranial nerve palsies manifesting with diplopia and ophthalmoplegia [1]. Most of these clinical features recover to a certain extent in 6–8 months, but may have a long-term sequelae [1].

Paraskevas et al. [2] described a case of a painful ophthalmoplegia with simultaneous orbital myositis with the involvement of the trigeminal nucleus and oculomotor nerve. Magnetic resonance imaging demonstrated abnormal signal intensity in recti muscles along with the trigeminal nucleus in brain stem. Serum and CSF were positive for HZV DNA, and the patient was effectively treated with acyclovir and methylprednisolone successfully. Rozenbaum O et al. [3]

M.J. Ali, FRCS, FRCGP
Ophthalmic Plastic Surgery, L.V. Prasad Eye Institute, Hyderabad 50034, Telangana, India
e-mail: drjaved007@gmail.com


B. Mukherjee, H. Yuen (eds.), *Emergencies of the Orbit and Adnexa*,
DOI 10.1007/978-81-322-1807-4_34

described a case of HSV-2-induced diffuse orbital cellulitis as a first presenting symptom of acute retinal necrosis. Although orbital inflammation resolved rapidly following initiation of antiviral, the intraocular inflammation worsened and the patient's vision could not be salvaged. Tornerup et al. [4] similarly presented a case of acute retinal necrosis presenting with signs of orbital inflammation, proptosis, and optic neuritis. CT scan was suggestive of thickened optic nerves, and polymerase chain reaction isolated HSV-1 DNA from the vitreous samples. The patient was successfully treated with intravenous acyclovir and oral prednisolone. Lee MS et al. [5] based on their case suggested that retrobulbar neuritis can precede acute retinal necrosis in HIV+ patients.

## HIV Infections and Acquired Immunodeficiency Syndrome (AIDS)

With increasing incidence of HIV infections, newer features of orbital infections and presentations are being unraveled. In a large epidemiological study on ocular manifestations in AIDS, among the 553 patient studies, 3 patients each presented with retrobulbar neuritis, lateral rectus palsy, and ptosis secondary to involvement of oculomotor nerve [6]. Opportunistic infections like varicella zoster and orbital tuberculosis with their sequelae may occur when the CD4 counts drop below 500 cells per microliter [6]. HIV infection-related orbital involvement with malignancies like Kaposi sarcomas and lymphomas are well known. Scheschonka et al. [7] reported AIDS-related Kaposi sarcoma of the lacrimal gland and discussed the role of a high suspicion and imaging modalities in managing these cases. Rarely orbital complications with the use of antiretroviral drugs have been reported to cause enophthalmos due to atrophy of the orbital fat secondary to lipodystrophic effect of the drugs [8].

## Other Viral Infections of the Orbit

Numerous other viral infections rarely cause orbital infections notably Epstein-Barr virus, hepatitis B virus, hepatitis C virus, and dengue virus. Epstein-Barr virus (EBV) may involve the orbit through its role in promoting orbital and adnexal lymphomas. Chronic infections with EBV have been reported to present as orbital myositis in conjunction with a generalized myositis with ineffective immunotherapy and poor prognosis [9]. EBV has also been reported and quantified in certain idiopathic orbital inflammatory pseudotumors and may present with the entire spectrum of proptosis, diplopia, chemosis, and periocular edema [10].Chronic EBV infections have also been reported to cause orbital Langerhans cell histiocytosis in pediatric age group, presenting as bilateral proptosis with extensive orbital bony wall involvement [11].

Urticaria and periorbital edema can rarely be a prodromal presenting sign of an acute hepatitis B infection [12]. Numerous viral agents have been implicated in orbital neoplasia with their typical orbital symptomatology. Notable among these are hepatitis C virus, herpes simplex virus 8 (HHV-8), and human papillomavirus (HPV) [13, 14].

## Fungal Orbital Infections

Fungal infections are the second common etiological cause of orbital infections after bacterial infections. There is an increasing trend in the diagnosis of sino-orbital fungal infections with the rise of HIV infection and other immunosuppressed states like diabetes and post-organ transplants. Although aspergillosis is more common, mucormycosis is the most virulent infection [15].

### Mucormycosis

Mucormycosis, also known as phycomycosis or zygomycosis, is the most aggressive fungal orbital infection, most commonly seen in patients with diabetic ketoacidosis and occasionally in post-renal transplant patients [16, 17]. It is caused by fungi in the order *Mucorales* and species implicated include *Mucor*, *Rhizopus*, and *Absidia* [18]. The infection usually starts when the respiratory tract and sinuses are inoculated by the ubiquitous spores. In the event of immunosuppression, the hyphae of the organism tend to invade tissues and are characteristically known to invade blood vessels causing infarction and the typical black eschar [19]. Orbit and intracranial invasion is usually secondary to sinus infections, can be rapid, and lead to quick mortality if untreated. The earliest feature can be painful ophthalmoplegia with rapidly developing proptosis and orbital cellulitis and sudden loss of vision [16]. Imaging with a CT scan and MRI would demonstrate hazy sinuses with destruction of sino-orbital walls and soft tissue density alterations in the orbit.

Upon suspicion, a prompt multidisciplinary approach is needed. Tissues should be obtained for microbiology workup and histopathological examination. Diagnosis is clinched by demonstrating large nonseptate-branching hyphae. The underlying cause like diabetic ketoacidosis should be aggressively treated, and wide surgical excision with frozen section control is usually performed followed by thorough irrigation with antifungal agents along with their systemic use [20, 21]. On occasions exenteration and extended exenteration may have to be performed based on the extent of disease.

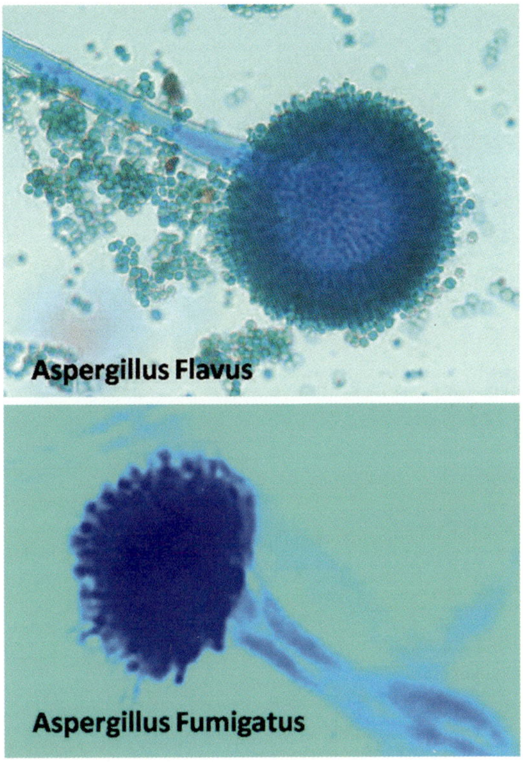


**Fig. 34.1** High-magnification photos of *Aspergillus flavus* and *A. fumigatus*

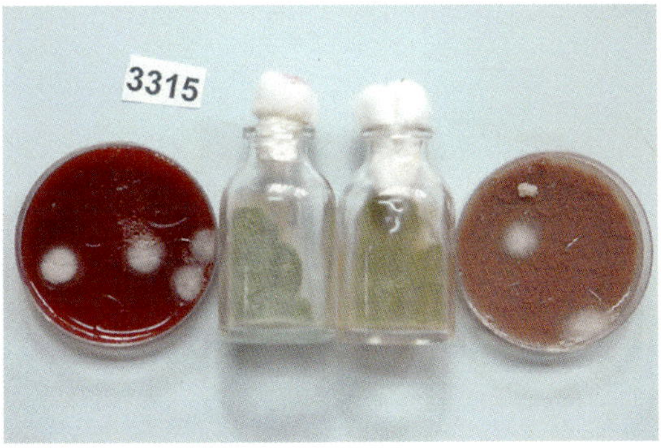


**Fig. 34.2** Fungal culture features of *A. flavus*

## Aspergillosis

*Aspergillus* is a deuteromycete fungus and is ubiquitous in nature. It has septate hyphae, and *Aspergillus flavus* and *A. fumigatus* are commonly implicated pathogenic species (Fig. 34.1). Although routinely harmless, it is an opportunistic pathogen, known to occur in immunocompromised status and in drug addicts. Disseminated aspergillosis is rare and is not known to involve the orbit, since mortality occurs much before it invades the orbit [16]. Localized invasive sino-orbital aspergillosis is more common and may present with proptosis, dystopia, and painful ophthalmoplegia with an occasional fistula formation and fungal abscess [22–24].Although slow growing, if untreated, it may lead to widespread local invasion with catastrophic complications and death [22]. Diagnosis is based on tissue biopsy for microbiological workup (smears and fungal culture, polymerase chain reaction for fungal DNA) and histopathological diagnosis (Figs. 34.2 and 34.3). CT scans may show the involved sinuses, breach of sino-orbital walls, mass lesions, and extent of spread. Once established, if widespread locally, a surgical debulking followed

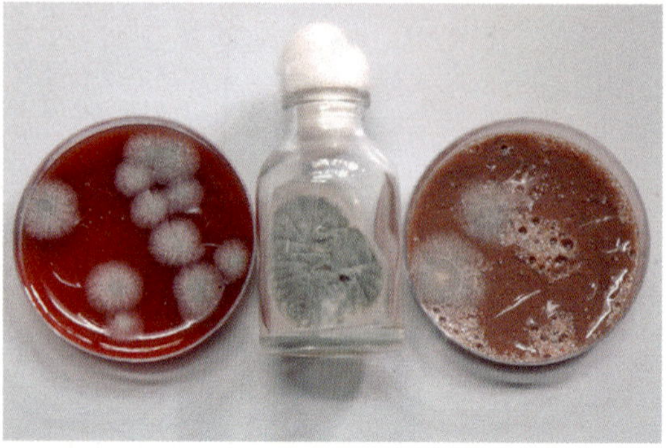

**Fig. 34.3** Fungal culture features of *A. fumigatus*

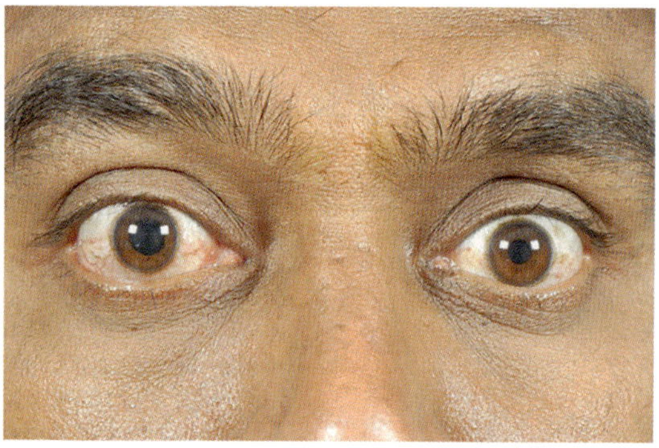

**Fig. 34.4** A case of orbital fungal infection presenting as a right-sided proptosis

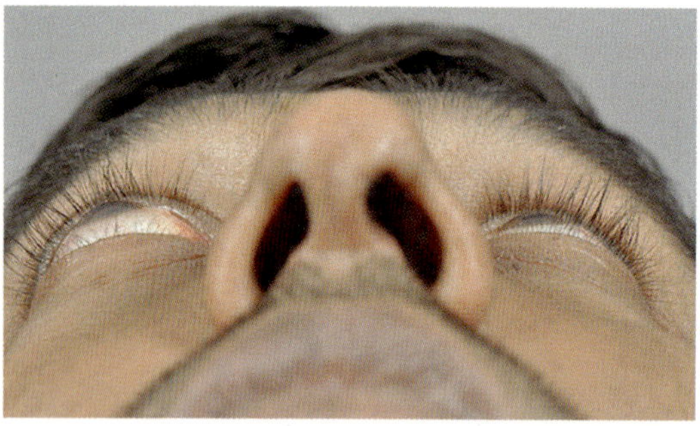

**Fig. 34.5** Same patient as in Fig. 34.4, worm's eye view showing right proptosis

by systemic antifungals like voriconazole for a prolonged duration (months) based on response should be initiated (Figs. 34.4, 34.5, 34.6, 34.7, 34.8, 34.9, and 34.10) [24].

Johnson et al. [22] studied invasive sino-orbital aspergillosis in patients with AIDS and found it to be a relentless, progressive, and fatal infection.

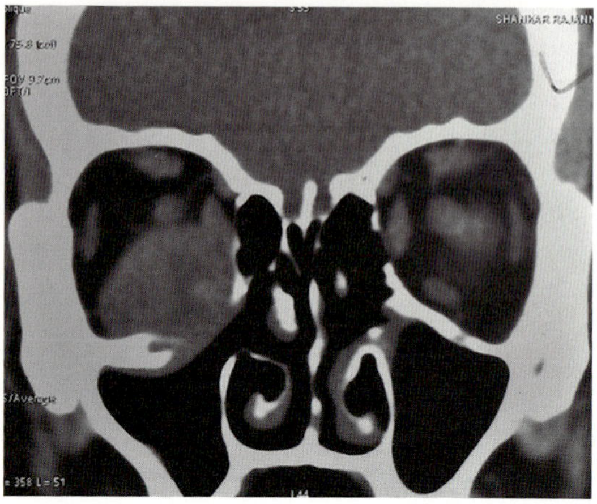

**Fig. 34.6** Coronal CT scan showing a large mass in the inferior quadrant with indistinct inferior rectus and orbital floor erosion

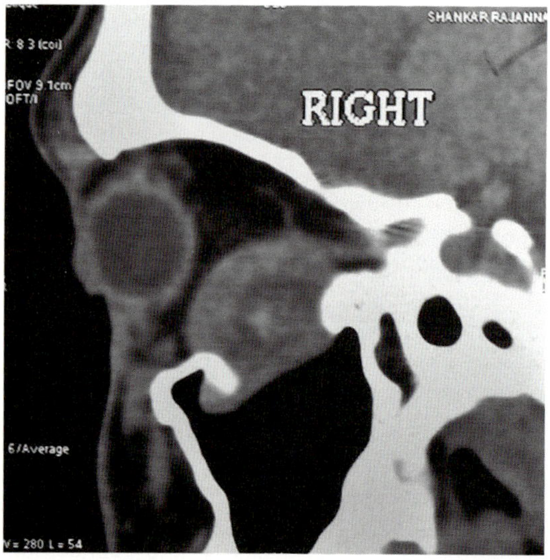


**Fig. 34.7** Sagittal reconstructed CT scan of the same patient showing the posterior extent of the mass

Unlike immunocompetent patients, this group may present with minimum external signs till late spread. Newer antifungals like protease inhibitors may help prolong the longevity in patients with advanced AIDS. The author of the current chapter and his group have published the largest series of orbital aspergillosis in immunocompetent patients, which is currently the focus of increasing interest [24]. They evaluated 35 patients with a mean age of 37.6 years (range 8–73 years). Proptosis and mass lesions were the most common presenting

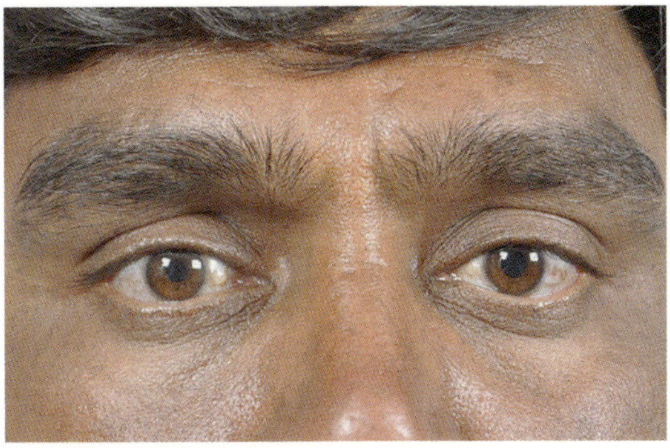

**Fig. 34.8** Same patient as in Figs. 34.4, 34.5, 34.6, and 34.7, following voriconazole therapy. Note the reduction of proptosis

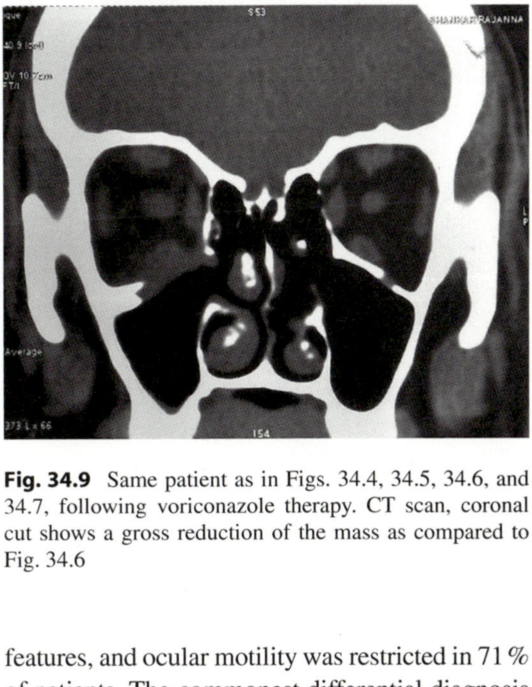


**Fig. 34.9** Same patient as in Figs. 34.4, 34.5, 34.6, and 34.7, following voriconazole therapy. CT scan, coronal cut shows a gross reduction of the mass as compared to Fig. 34.6

features, and ocular motility was restricted in 71 % of patients. The commonest differential diagnosis was nonspecific orbital inflammatory disorder and sino-orbital malignancies. Sixty-three percent of patients showed infiltrative lesions and sinus involvement with destruction of sino-orbital walls with 30 % having radiological evidence of intracranial extension. Biopsy revealed 86 % of the patients to be infected with *Aspergillus flavus* followed by *A. fumigatus* in the remaining 14 %. Fifty-one percent of the patients were managed medically and 49 % needed additional surgical debulking. At a mean follow-up of 37.6 months, 94 % survival was achieved in this study [24].

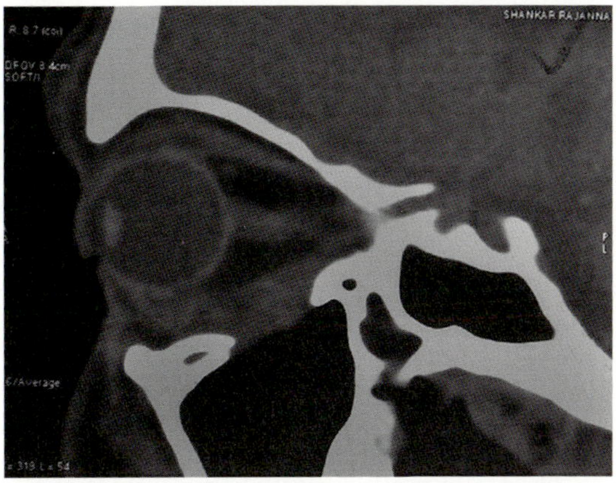


**Fig. 34.10** Sagittal reconstructed CT scan of the same patient as in Fig. 34.7, showing gross reduction in the mass following voriconazole therapy with minimal residual lesion

## Other Fungal Infections

Numerous other fungal species may cause orbital infection, although they are rare and vary based on regional epidemiology [25, 26]. Notably among them include rhinosporidiosis, candidiasis, blastomycosis, histoplasmosis, coccidioidomycosis, and sporotrichosis [16, 25, 26]. Diagnosis is predominantly biopsy based and includes microbial identification. Treatment depends on the organism isolated with local and systemic antifungals and surgical debridement where needed.

### Conclusion

This chapter described the most common clinical-radiological features and management of viral and fungal orbital infection with a brief review of literature. With newer techniques of diagnosis and newer drugs, early identification is possible, and with early institution of treatment, the outcomes can be satisfactory.

## References

1. Kanski JJ, Bowling B. Herpes zoster ophthalmicus. In: Kanski JJ, Bowling B, editors. Clinical ophthalmology – a systematic approach. London: Elsevier; 2011. p. 187–90.

2. Paraskevas GP, Anagnostou E, Vassilopoulou S, et al. Painful ophthalmoplegia with simultaneous orbital myositis, optic and oculomotor nerve inflammation and trigeminal nucleus involvement in a patient with herpes zoster ophthalmicus. BMJ Case Rep. 2012. (Epub).
3. Rozenbaum O, Rozenberg F, Charlotte F, et al. Catastrophic acute retinal necrosis associated with diffuse orbital cellulitis: a case report. Graefes Arch Clin Exp Ophthalmol. 2007;245:161–3.
4. Tornerup NR, Fomsgaard A, Nielsen NV. HSV-1 induced acute retinal necrosis syndrome presenting with severe inflammatory orbitopathy, proptosis and optic nerve involvement. Ophthalmology. 2000;107:397–401.
5. Lee MS, Cooney EL, Stoessel KM, et al. Varicella Zoster virus retrobulbar optic neuritis preceding retinitis in patients with acquired immunodeficiency syndrome. Ophthalmology. 1998;105:467–71.
6. Acharya PK, Venugopal KC, Karimsab DP, et al. Ocular manifestations in patients with HIV infection/AIDS who were referred from ART center, Hassan, Karnataka, India. J Clin Diag Res. 2012;6:1756–60.
7. Scheschonka A, Mosch M, Krieglsteiner S, et al. Pre and post treatment MR imaging in AIDS-related Kaposi sarcoma of the conjunctiva and lacrimal gland. Am J Neuroradiol. 2003;24:1327–9.
8. Perez-Blazquez E, Redondo MI, Gracia T. AIDS and ophthalmology: a contemporary view. An Sist Santi Navar. 2008;31:69–81.
9. Uchiyama T, Arai K, Yamamoto-Tabata T, et al. Generalized myositis mimicking polymyositis associated with chronic Epstein-Barr virus infection. J Neurol. 2005;252:519–25.
10. Jin R, Zhao P, Ma X, et al. Quantification of Epstein-Barr virus DNA in patients with idiopathic orbital inflammatory pseudotumor. PLoS One. 2013;8:e50812.
11. Sakata N, Toguchi N, Kimura M, et al. Development of Langerhans cell histiocytosis associated with chronic Epstein-Barr virus infection. Pediatr Blood Cancer. 2008;50:924–7.
12. Van Aalsburg R, de Pagter AP, Van Genderen PJ. Urticaria and periorbital edema as prodromal presenting signs of acute hepatitis B infection. J Travel Med. 2011;18:224–5.
13. Strianese D, Tranfa F, Finelli M, et al. Hepatitis C virus infection in ocular adnexal lymphoma. Arch Ophthalmol. 2010;128:1295–9.
14. Verma V, Shen D, Sieving PC, et al. The role of infectious agents in the etiology of ocular adnexal neoplasia. Surv Ophthalmol. 2008;53:312–31.
15. Shome D, Jaydeep W, Angshuman M. Orbital infections. In: Subrahmanyam M, editor. Surgical atlas of orbital diseases. New Delhi: Jaypee Medical Brothers Publishers; 2007. p. 120–7.
16. Rootman J. Inflammatory disorders. In: Rootman J, editor. Diseases of the orbit: a multidisciplinary approach. 2nd ed. Philadelphia: Lippincott William Wilkins; 2004. p. 467–81.
17. Ferry AP, Abedi S. Diagnosis and management of rhino-orbito-cerebral mucormycosis. A report of 16 personally observed cases. Ophthalmology. 1983;90:1096–104.
18. Lee FY, Mossad SB, Adal KA. Pulmonary mucormycosis: the last 30 years. Arch Intern Med. 1999;159:1301–9.
19. Gass JDM. Ocular manifestations of acute mucormycosis. Arch Ophthalmol. 1961;65:226–37.
20. Langford JD, McCartney DL, Wang RC. Frozen section-guided surgical debridement for management of rhino-orbital mucormycosis. Am J Ophthalmol. 1997;124:265–7.
21. Kohn R, Hepler R. Management of limited rhino-orbital mucormycosis without exenteration. Ophthalmology. 1985;92:1440–4.
22. Johnson TE, Casiano RR, Kronish JW, et al. Sino-orbital aspergillosis in acquired immunodeficiency syndrome. Arch Ophthalmol. 1999;117:57–64.
23. Sivak-Calcott JA, Livesly N, Nugent RA, et al. Localized invasive sino-orbital aspergillosis: characteristic features. Br J Ophthalmol. 2004;88:681–7.
24. Mody KH, Ali MJ, Vemuganti GK, et al. Orbital aspergillosis in immunocompetent patients. Br J Ophthalmol. 2014;98(10):1379–84.
25. Ajayi BG, Osuntokun B, Olurin O, et al. Orbital histoplasmosis due to *Histoplasma capsulatum*: successful treatment with Septrin. J Trop Med Hyg. 1986;89:179–87.
26. Vida L, Moel SA. Systemic North American blastomycosis with orbital involvement. Am J Ophthalmol. 1974;77:240–2.

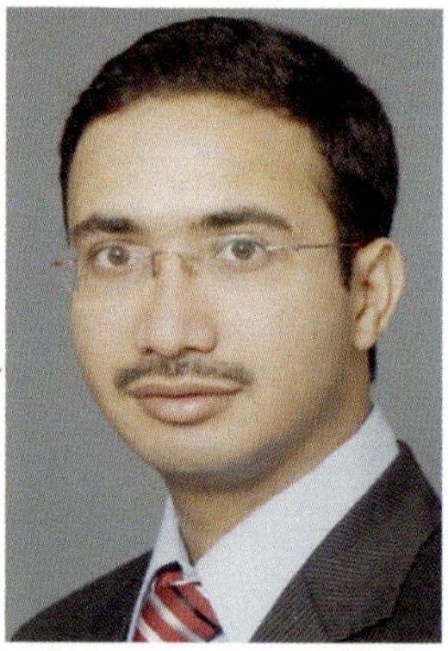

**Mohammad Javed Ali** Dr. Mohammad Javed Ali currently leads The Institute of Dacryology at the LV Prasad Eye Institute. Javed described two new diseases of the lacrimal system along with their classifications and clinicopathologic profiles. He is one among the rare recipients of The Experienced Researcher – Alexander Von Humbold Fellowship Award, one of the pinnacle awards in the research world. He was honored by the 2015 ASOPRS Merrill Reeh Award for his path-breaking work on etiopathogenesis of punctal stenosis. His textbook *Principles and Practice of Lacrimal Surgery* is considered to be the most comprehensive treatise on the subject. He is a section editor for 3 journals and reviewer for 16 major journals. He has to his credit a total of 203 publications, of which 141 are peer reviewed and 30 are non peer reviewed, 32 book chapters, 21 instruction courses, 3 keynote addresses, 214 conference presentations, 12 live surgical workshops, and 26 awards.

# Life-Threatening Infections

# 35

Akshay Gopinathan Nair and Milind N. Naik

## Introduction

Most ophthalmologists routinely treat clinical conditions that seldom have ramifications beyond the eye. An ophthalmologist commonly may come across conditions that may present as immediate threats to the visual system and can lead to permanent loss of visual function if left untreated. Such vision-threatening emergencies such as orbital hemorrhage, central retinal artery occlusion, and chemical burns require prompt action to salvage vision. However, it is uncommon for the ophthalmologist to come across emergencies, which if not treated immediately have the potential to become life-threatening conditions. The oculoplastic surgeon is the one who usually sees such conditions, and therefore it is important to know how to diagnose and treat these life-threatening infective emergencies in oculoplastic practice. In this chapter, cavernous sinus thrombosis, periocular necrotizing fasciitis, and invasive fungal sinusitis will be discussed in detail.

A.G. Nair, MBBS, DNB • M.N. Naik, MD (✉)
Ophthalmic Plastic Surgery, L. V. Prasad Eye Institute, 500034 Hyderabad, Telangana, India
e-mail: akshaygn@gmail.com; milind@drmilindnaik.com; milnaik@gmail.com

## Cavernous Sinus Thrombosis

Cavernous sinus thrombosis (CST) is defined as thrombophlebitis of the cavernous sinus. CST is a dramatic and potentially fatal condition which is seen commonly in children and young adults [1]. CST usually is seen as an indicator of an infectious process which is fast evolving and spreading, most commonly craniofacial in origin [1]. However, with the advent of broad-spectrum antibiotics, CST is not commonly encountered off late. Late recognition and delay in treatment can increase the risk of morbidity and mortality.

The venous drainage of the brain is a part of a unique system where all the dural sinuses, which are interconnected in a complex network, finally drain into the internal jugular vein [2]. The cavernous sinuses receive blood from the ophthalmic veins, the superficial middle and inferior cerebral veins, and the sphenoparietal and sphenoid sinuses. From the cavernous sinuses, the blood drains into the pterygoid plexus via emissary veins and also into the internal jugular vein via the inferior petrosal sinus and the sigmoid sinus through the superior sinus [2]. There are no directional valves in the cavernous sinus and its connections, therefore allowing bidirectional spread of infection and also leading to extensive thrombi throughout the network of sinuses [3].

Common facial infections that may potentially lead to CST include sinusitis, especially those that originate from the sphenoid, ethmoid,


B. Mukherjee, H. Yuen (eds.), *Emergencies of the Orbit and Adnexa*,
DOI 10.1007/978-81-322-1807-4_35

and frontal sinuses, superficial infections that arise from the middle one third of the face. Orbital cellulitis, dental abscesses, septic foci in the nose, tonsils, soft palate, and ears may constitute primary source of the infection that leads to CST.

### Clinical Features

The most common feature is headache, and it usually precedes fever and the cranial neuropathies. The classical clinical features seen include decrease or loss of vision, chemosis, proptosis, and paralysis of the cranial nerves that course through the cavernous sinus. Ptosis and mydriasis resulting from III nerve dysfunction may also be seen as the disease progresses [4].

### Diagnosis

In most cases, CST is usually a clinical diagnosis. Radiologically, MRI and MR venography are more sensitive compared to CT scans for diagnosis. Typically it may show a heterogeneous signal from the abnormal cavernous sinus along with deformity of the cavernous portion of the internal carotid artery and a hyperintense signal of thrombosed vascular sinuses [5]. Other features that may also be seen are dilated superior ophthalmic vein and proptosis on the ipsilateral side. Gallium scintigraphy has occasionally been used as a confirmatory tool in septic CST, demonstrating increased uptake in the cavernous sinus [6].

### Treatment

Immediate institution of broad-spectrum antibiotics that give coverage against gram-positive, gram-negative, and anaerobic bacteria is essential. Surgical management of the primary septic focus is recommended to reduce the bacterial load in cases such as nasal infections, necrotizing fasciitis. Empirical antimicrobial therapy usually depends on the antecedent clinical condition and must include coverage for methicillin-resistant *Staphylococcus aureus* (MRSA). An empirical combination, consisting of parenteral metronidazole, vancomycin, and ceftriaxone, will achieve reasonable CSF and brain penetration and will be active against *S. aureus* [7]. Microbiological testing to narrow down the spectrum and isolate the offending pathogen will help to choose the right antimicrobial agent. Once antibiotics show effect, authors have also reported beneficial use of intravenous steroids in reducing edema [8].

The role of anticoagulants is still controversial. There have been no controlled trials; however, it is reported that early institution (within 5–7 days) may help in reducing morbidity, but delayed use provides no benefits [2, 9]. The rationale behind anticoagulant therapy is to prevent thrombus propagation, recanalize occluded sinuses and cerebral veins, and prevent complications of deep vein thrombosis and pulmonary embolism [7]. This however has to weigh against the risk of an intracranial bleed and also tendency for sinus infarcts to become hemorrhagic even before anticoagulants have been administered [10].

Rare but potential complications include carotid thrombosis, brain abscess, and meningitis. However, with prompt treatment, the prognosis of septic CST has improved reducing mortality from near 100% to 20–30% [11]. Residual sequelae such as numbness, paresthesia, ptosis, and residual squint have been noted.

Cavernous sinus thrombosis is a rare but potentially fatal, rapidly progressive condition that requires a high clinical suspicion, immediate institution of intensive treatment primarily consisting of broad-spectrum antibiotics along with appropriate surgical drainage of the source of infection, anticoagulants, and possibly steroids.

## Periorbital Necrotizing Fasciitis

Necrotizing fasciitis (NF) is an infection of the subcutaneous tissue and superficial fascia accompanied with secondary necrosis of the skin. Although the periorbital tissue is not a common site, when affected, it is associated with a mortality rate ranging from 8 to 15% and 13.8% of the patients have resultant loss of vision [12]. Periorbital necrotizing fasciitis (PNF) is one of the few rare situations where an ophthalmologist deals with a potentially life-threatening entity.

### Triggering Factors

PNF most commonly has a history of preceding trauma. In many cases, the trauma is extremely trivial and the patient may not be able to recollect it. In an exhaustive review of available literature on PNF, Amrith et al. reported that in as many as 35 % cases, trauma was identified as the main triggering factor [13]. Recent surgery, immunosuppression, and chemotherapy were also noted; however in a substantial proportion of cases (27 %), no triggering factor was found [13]. Preexisting comorbidities that were noted in this review included alcoholism, diabetes mellitus, and collagen vascular diseases such as rheumatoid arthritis, systemic lupus, deep vein thrombosis, and cardiovascular diseases [14, 15].

### Microbiological Profile

Based on the microbiological profile, necrotizing fasciitis is broadly divided into two types. Type 1 NF is polymicrobial and caused by both aerobic and anaerobic organisms. A single organism, such as *Streptococcus* or *Staphylococcus*, or a combination of the two, causes type 2 NF. Type 1 NF is commonly seen in patients with immunocompromised status, as compared to patients with type 2 NF (more commonly seen in the periorbital area) often have no such immunodeficiency [13, 16]. The most commonly reported offending organism is gram-positive group A β-hemolytic *Streptococcus* (GABHS) closely followed by *Pseudomonas* species.

### Clinical Picture and Pathophysiology

PNF usually begins as an acutely presenting painful nonspecific erythematous rash with edema resembling preseptal cellulitis. The infection slowly progresses and the patient may complain a deep periorbital pain [16]. The vascular orbicularis muscle acts as a barrier between the superficial skin and the periorbita below. If untreated, it soon gains entry into the superficial and deep fascial planes, and the infection spreads rapidly [17]. The thin skin of the eyelids however allows clinical signs to be easily detectable early on in the course of the disease [18]. The dermis is attached firmly at the nasojugal fold medially and the malar fold laterally which is a firm attachment and prevents the spread of infection. However once the infection is able to overcome this anatomical hurdle, it quickly spreads following the path of least resistance across the nasal bridge and also into the deep fascial planes of the neck and face, probably accounting for the high number of bilateral cases [19]. It is extremely important to differentiate NF from orbital cellulitis as the clinical picture in both, eye pain, periorbital swelling, and/or fever, may be similar. This is mainly because in PNF, a far more aggressive approach that includes parenteral antibiotics and surgical debridement is necessary [16].

Systemically, a low- to medium-grade fever associated with tachycardia out of proportion to the temperature elevation is seen [20]. Over the next 48 h, a violaceous discoloration is noted along with bullae over the skin. As the disease progresses, the bacterial toxins released by the pathogens are responsible for angiothrombotic microbial invasion and liquefactive necrosis [21]. As the infection progresses deeper, the fascia are infiltrated by leukocytes, with thrombosis of nutrient vessels and occasional suppuration of the veins and arteries that pass through the fascia, causing black or avascular necrotic patches (Fig. 35.1) [22]. Subsequently the bacteria then proliferate within the destroyed fascia. Eventually, cutaneous gangrene develops within 96 h of the infection setting in. The skin sloughs to become gangrenous due to underlying suppuration by day 10 [16].

### Diagnosis

Radiological investigations such as CT and MRI may help in identifying the extent of the infection as well as the depth of the infection. CT, however, remains as the investigation of choice since it offers easy localization of the initial site of infection, extent of disease, presence of fluid-filled bullae and gas, and anatomical information which may help to guide surgical exploration [23]. That aside, the diagnosis of PNF is primarily clinical, and the treatment must not be delayed for the sake of investigations [16].

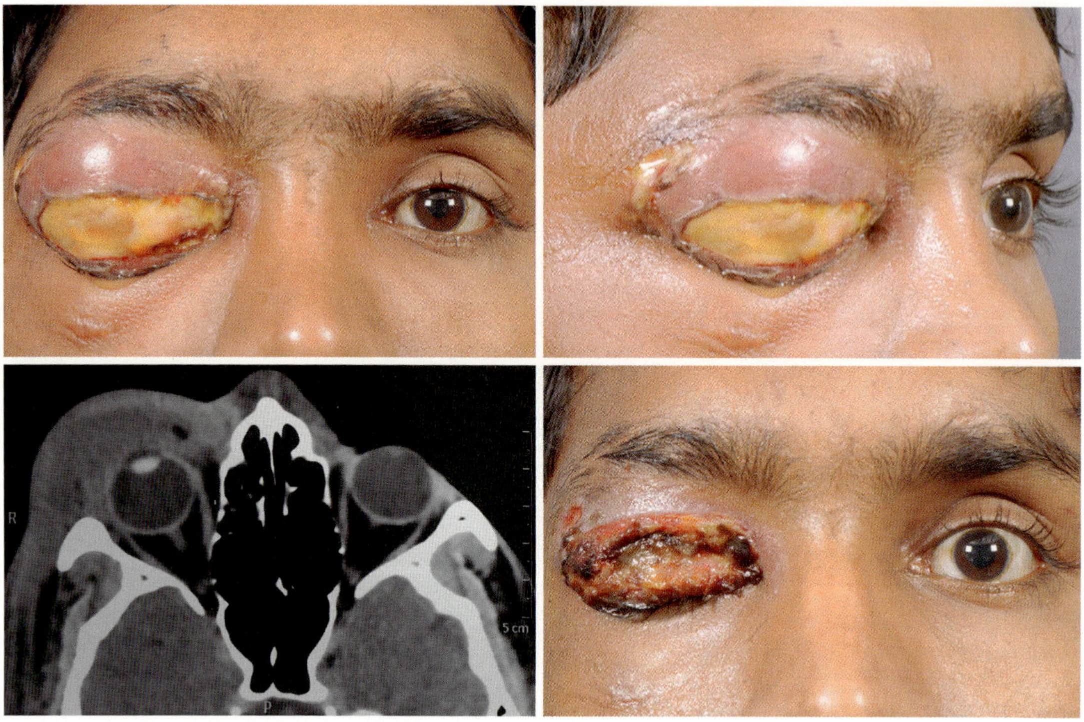


**Fig. 35.1** A young male with right periorbital necrotizing fasciitis following trauma to the upper eyelid. Note the white, avascular eschar and the surrounding cellulitis that rapidly spread within the subfascial planes

## Differential Diagnosis

The differentials that may be considered include blepharitis, conjunctivitis, preseptal cellulitis, orbital cellulitis, endophthalmitis, cavernous sinus thrombosis, and rhino-orbital mucormycosis [13, 15, 16]. The absence of the violaceous hue, bullae, crepitus, and subsequent necrosis can help to differentiate orbital cellulitis from PNF.

## Treatment

Early recognition, prompt diagnosis, aggressive medical therapy, and surgical debridement can help prevent fatal outcomes in PNF. The treatment largely rests on the institution of broad-spectrum antibiotics and surgical debridement. Hyperbaric oxygen has been shown to play a beneficial role in the treatment of NF. Empirical antimicrobial therapy should consist of beta-lactam antibiotics, such as penicillin or cephalosporin and clindamycin [24]. The selected broad-spectrum antibiotics should be effective against β-hemolytic *Streptococcus* [25].

However, once the diagnosis is established, regardless of whether antibiotics have been initiated, prompt and adequate operative debridement should be carried out at this time, whether necrotic tissue is already present or not [18]. Gradually as the antibiotics are administered, a clear zone of demarcation will appear over the next few hours which will permit further debridement to be done either at the bedside or in the operating room. The surgical exploration and debridement must ensure that all the necrotic tissue is completely excised. The aim of debridement is to remove all nonviable tissue; this reduced the bacterial load and the level of circulating toxins as well as halted the progression of infection. It may also be prudent to perform an exploratory incision over an area beyond the limits of debridement when it is uncertain whether necrosis is undermining viable skin [16, 18, 19].

It has been noted that in PNF, preserving viable skin and orbicularis oculi muscle promotes the action of antibiotics, which thus improves healing, preventing, or reducing morbidity and facial disfigurements [19]. Hyperbaric oxygen therapy has been shown to reduce mortality, but it has also been shown to improve the salvage of tissue viability [16]. Hyperbaric oxygen therapy leads to inhibition of exotoxin production, improved leukocyte function, attainment of sufficient tissue oxygen levels which kills strict anaerobes, and inhibition of growth of facultative anaerobes [26].

The possible sequelae of PNF that often causes vision loss are central retinal artery occlusion, orbital spread necessitating removal of orbital contents including eyeball [19, 27], or corneal perforation [28]. Lagophthalmos that leads to exposure keratopathy can also be one of the causes of vision loss. Reconstruction can only begin once the infection is resolved and the wound is clean and stable [16].

### Outcomes

The most critical factors for reducing mortality from NF remain early recognition and urgent operative debridement [29, 30]. NF involving the lower part of the face and cervical area (30 %) than that involving the upper and the middle areas of the face (10–12.5 %) [16] – primarily due to contiguous spread into important structures such as the mediastinum, chest, and carotid sheath – results in pulmonary complications and death. Other causes for mortality include systemic complications like septicemia, shock, and multi-organ failure [13]. The delay between hospital admission and initial debridement and broad-spectrum antibiotic therapy initiation should be considered as the most critical factor influencing morbidity and mortality [16].

In summary, the key to good outcomes in PNF lies in early diagnosis and institution of treatment. Multiple surgical debridement, if necessary, prevents escalation to toxic shock, which seems to precede all deaths reported in literature.

## Invasive Fungal Sinusitis

One more addition to the list of diseases presenting to the ophthalmologist that are potentially curable if identified and treated early, but fatal if detected late, is fungal sinusitis. Fungal sinusitis has two basic clinical forms: invasive and noninvasive. Based on the tempo of evolution, invasive fungal sinusitis can be classified as acute, subacute, or chronic [31–33].

Fungal sinusitis is known to occur when common saprophytes of the paranasal sinuses invade the paranasal sinus mucosa, frequently in the setting of an immunocompromised state [31, 34]. The invasive fungal sinusitis (IFS) gradually proceeds to extend from the paranasal sinuses into the orbit and then on to the orbital apex, from where it further spreads into the cavernous sinus and cavernous carotid artery, causing carotid occlusion, cerebral infarction, intracranial aneurysms and hemorrhage, meningitis, cerebral abscess, and eventually leading up to the inevitable consequence of this entity – death [31].

### Mucormycosis

Mucormycosis is an aggressive, fulminant fungal infection that usually affects immunocompromised patients [35]. The three genera that cause mucormycosis, *Mucor*, *Rhizopus*, and *Absidiu*, are ubiquitous fungi and are found in soil, fruits, and decomposing plant and animal matter and can be cultured from most body orifices and surface. While it can affect normal healthy individuals, mucormycosis is the most acutely fatal fungal infection of humans, and in most cases, the rhino-orbital-cerebral form of infection (ROCM) is the most common of infection [36].

### Aspergillosis

*Aspergillus* is a ubiquitous fungus found in soil and decaying vegetation. Three distinct pathologies may be seen in aspergillosis: allergic sinusitis, fungal granuloma in the sinuses, and invasive aspergillosis [37]. Unlike mucormycosis that occurs in patients debilitated by systemic illness, sino-orbital aspergillosis usually occurs in healthy patients [38]. *A. fumigatus* and *A. flavus* are the most common fungal contaminants of the sinuses and thus have the potential to infect the orbit secondarily, causing sino-orbital aspergillosis [39–42]. It is also important to note that orbital aspergillosis in an immunocompetent individual without paranasal sinus involvement is often diagnosed only late in the course of the disease [39].

## Clinical Features

Given the indolent clinical course, few patients present early with solely nasal symptoms such as nasal stuffiness, blocked nose, rhinitis, and epistaxis. Oftentimes patients with IFS present to the ophthalmologist when the disease has reached an advanced stage. They may present as chronic progressive decrease in vision, squint, proptosis which may be axial or abaxial, nasolacrimal duct obstruction, and optic neuropathy [43]. Other non-ocular symptoms may be facial pain with swelling, headache, fever, granular or purulent nasal discharge, and nasal ulceration [44]. In the setting of orbital apex syndrome, it is not uncommon to see patients present with multiple cranial nerve palsies (Fig. 35.2). In cases where there is intracranial extension of the mass lesion, patients may present with altered sensorium and even hemiplegia. The symptoms may range anywhere between a few days and several weeks. Orbital involvement is due to the spread of the disease from the paranasal sinuses; however, there may be no clinical involvement of the sinuses or the nose. The disease is usually unilateral and remains so in most cases, but bilateral cases do occur [44].

Patients with invasive fungal sinusitis may also present in an acute setting with a wide range or clinical presentation such as lid abscesses, ptosis, orbital cellulitis, orbital abscesses, fungal endophthalmitis, superior orbital fissure syndrome, superior ophthalmic vein thrombosis, orbital apex syndrome, external ophthalmoplegia (total or partial), involvement of multiple cranial nerves, diplopia, central retinal artery occlusion, internal carotid artery occlusion, and cavernous sinus thrombosis (CST) [44].

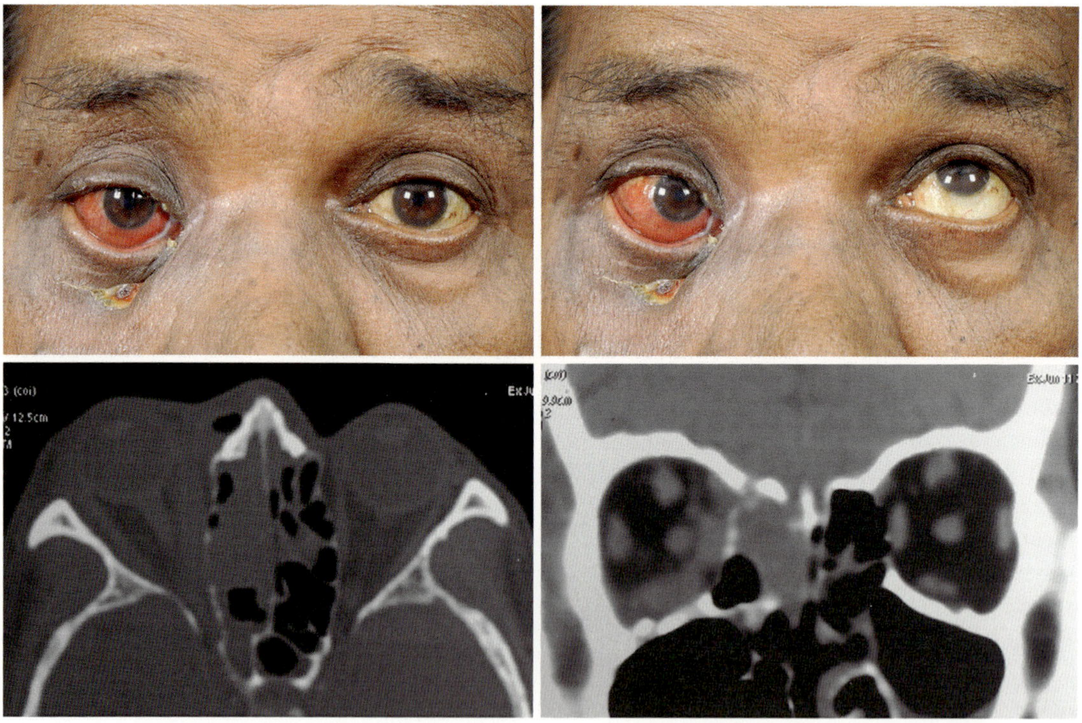

**Fig. 35.2** A 50-year-old male diabetic patient with recent onset right proptosis, motility restriction, and a lower eyelid discharging sinus. CT scan of the orbit showed an ill-defined soft-tissue mass within the infero-medial orbit, along with soft-tissue haze within the ethmoid sinuses. Endonasal biopsy proved this to be a case of sino-orbital mucormycosis, with eyelid skin involvement

## Risk Factors

Uncontrolled diabetes mellitus is the most common comorbidity reported in most cases of IFS. Ketoacidosis decreases the inflammatory response of the body and delays the local aggregation of granulocytes and fibroblasts. The sera of diabetics appear to lack a dialyzable antifungal inhibitory factor [36]. IFS may also rarely be seen in immunocompetent patients; however majority of the cases in literature have been either immunosuppressed, neutropenic, or diabetic. Hematological malignancies are also known to be a condition which predisposes to IFS. Certain conditions are known to produce favorable conditions for selected species of fungi: iron overload states and use of desferrioxamine are a known risk factor for mucormycosis [45]. Risk factors for invasive aspergillosis include neutrophil defects and corticosteroid use [42], and there is a predilection for *Scedosporium* infection in patients with hematological malignancies and in transplant recipients [46, 47].

## Diagnosis

An evaluation of the immune status of patients of suspected IFS is essential. CT scan often helps to delineate the soft-tissue involvement, mucosal thickening, bone erosion and necrosis (a late finding and a poor prognostic sign), and intracranial and cavernous sinus involvement, whereas MRI provides a better delineation of the blood vessel involvement and intracranial extension of the infection. More specifically, T2-weighted MRI studies and gadolinium (Gd)-enhanced T1-weighted images are also vital to properly assess the extent of disease. This is because of their high sensitivity for demonstrating meningeal and optic nerve involvement; however, CT is far superior to MRI in demonstrating destruction of cortical bone [48]. An ill-defined, irregular, iso- to hypodense mass lesion with its epicenter often in the maxillary or ethmoidal sinuses is the hallmark of invasive sino-orbital lesions (Fig. 35.3). Bony erosion, thinning of the bones, and intracranial extension with enhancement of the underlying dura are noted in advanced cases.

The presence of fungi must be microscopically confirmed to clinch the diagnosis, and a biopsy is required to do so. Based on the radiological evidence, the most accessible route that is associated with least morbidity must be chosen to procure the biopsy specimen. An orbitotomy may be required in some cases where an endoscopic route is preferred when the mass is more accessible through the nose. However, even if the sinus biopsies are negative and the clinical features are still suggestive of IFS, and in particular if the eye is already blind, then targeted biopsies from the orbital apex should be obtained to establish the diagnosis [49].

## Laboratory Studies

Once biopsied, the excised mass must be processed appropriately to optimize the probability of diagnosis.

I. Fresh tissue preparations utilizing 10–20 % potassium hydroxide are ideal for direct microscopic examinations. Hematoxylin and eosin, Grocott-Gomori methenamine silver, and periodic acid-Schiff are commonly used stains that can show nonseptate hyphae with right-angled branching quite vividly [44]. It is important to communicate to the pathologist in case a fungal etiology is suspected so that the pathologist is aware of the need to use special stains for fungal elements.
II. The culture media of choice in isolating fungi are brain-heart infusion broth, potato dextrose agar, and Sabouraud dextrose agar.
III. Polymerase chain reaction (PCR) is useful in molecular diagnosis in cases when the cultures may be negative.

## Management

Aggressive surgical debridement, amphotericin-soaked packs, and intravenous amphotericin B therapy are considered appropriate treatment for rhino-orbital-cerebral mucormycosis [50]. However, surgical debridement is easier when disease is limited to the paranasal sinuses.

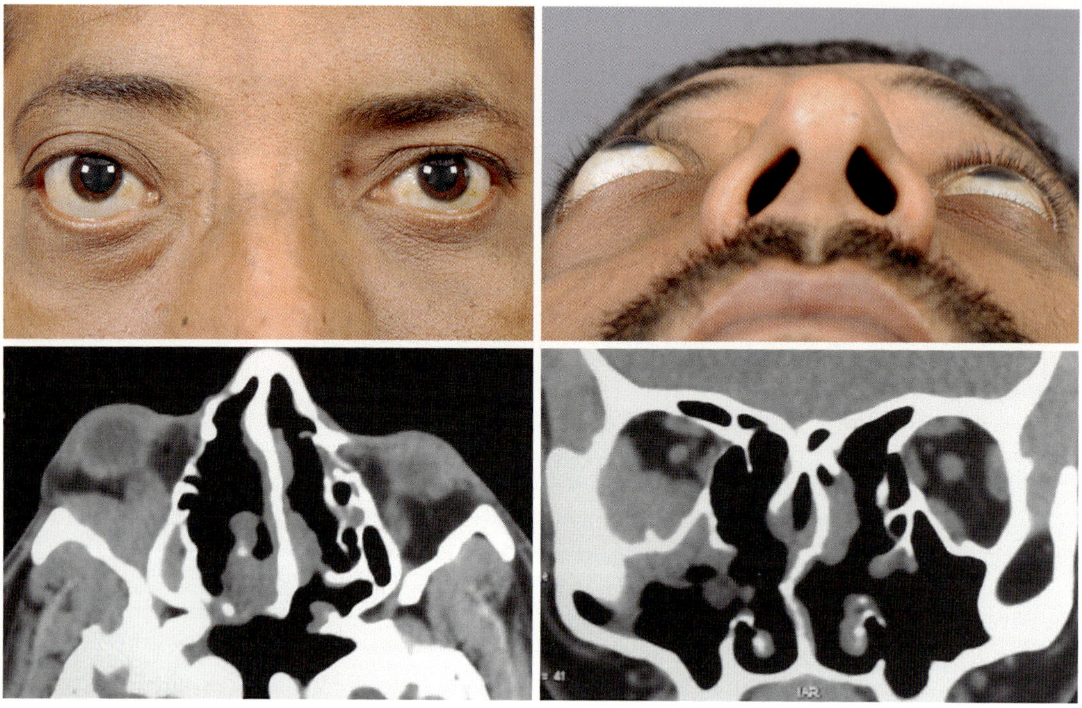

**Fig. 35.3** A 45-year-old immunocompetent nondiabetic male with a recurrent right proptosis. He had prior surgical removal of an ethmoid sinus mass through a medial orbitotomy. CT scan of the orbit showed an ill-defined soft-tissue mass involving the inferior orbit, along with the maxillary sinus. Ethmoid sinuses appeared clear. Sino-orbital debulking of the mass was performed and microbiological evaluation revealed *Aspergillus flavus*

In the orbit, surgical debridement is limited by many factors, namely:

I. Involvement of bone and blood vessels, through which the infection has extended into the orbit
II. Presence of vital structures
III. An inability to be sure of the extent of disease [38, 51]

When limited to the orbit, especially when the affected eye has no vision, orbital exenteration, though morbidly disfiguring, may offer a possible curative option.

Deciding which single drug or combination to use is difficult with reports suggesting different conclusions, but amphotericin B is usually considered the gold standard based on extensive experience. Therapy is often prolonged and can be complicated by adverse effects such as renal dysfunction [51]. Other drugs such as itraconazole and voriconazole have also shown to be effective and associate with lesser side effects. Administration of the maximum daily dose possible of the chosen medication is recommended, and after the disease is controlled, prolonged administration of oral itraconazole is also advised to ensure eradication [52]. Furthermore, medical treatment should continue well past any remaining signs of disease, and indefinite use should be considered in patients with immunosuppression [50–52]. A potential pitfall is that in some cases, optic nerve dysfunction with aspergillosis can transiently respond to corticosteroids. This can lead to delay in definitive diagnosis and subsequent progression of the infection [48, 49].

In summary, a clinician must have a high index of suspicion (especially with diabetics and immunocompromised patients), as delays in adequate diagnosis and treatment can lead to potentially devastating consequences [48].

## References


1. Berdai AM, et al. Cavernous sinus thrombophlebitis complicating sinusitis. Am J Case Rep. 2013;14:99–102.
2. Verma R, Junewar V, Singh RK, Ram H, Pal US. Bilateral cavernous sinus thrombosis and facial palsy as complications of dental abscess. Natl J Maxillofac Surg. 2013;4:252–5.
3. Kiddee W, Preechawai P, Hirunpat S. Bilateral septic cavernous sinus thrombosis following the masticator and parapharyngeal space infection from the odontogenic origin: a case report. J Med Assoc Thai. 2010;93:1107–11.
4. DiNubile MJ. Septic thrombosis of the cavernous sinuses. Arch Neurol. 1988;45(5):567–72.
5. Feldman DP, Picerno NA, Porubsky ES. Cavernous sinus thrombosis complicating odontogenic parapharyngeal space neck abscess: a case report and discussion. Otolaryngol Head Neck Surg. 2000;123:744–5.
6. Piazza G. Cerebral venous thrombosis. Circulation. 2012;125(13):1704–9.
7. Swaminath D, Narayanan R, Orellana-Barrios MA, Temple B. Necrotizing fasciitis of the nose complicated with cavernous sinus thrombosis. Case Rep Infect Dis. 2014;2014:914042.
8. Clarke M, Enuh H, Saverimuttu J, Nfonoyim J. Streptococcus group C meningitis with cavernous sinus thrombosis. Infect Drug Resist. 2013;6:79–81.
9. Ebright JR, Pace MT, Niazi AF. Septic thrombosis of the cavernous sinuses. Arch Intern Med. 2001;161:2671–6.
10. Saposnik G, Barinagarrementeria F, Brown Jr RD, Bushnell CD, Cucchiara B, Cushman M, de Veber G, Ferro JM, Tsai FY, American Heart Association Stroke Council, Council on Epidemiology and Prevention. Diagnosis and management of cerebral venous thrombosis: a statement for healthcare professionals from the American Heart Association/American Stroke Association. Stroke. 2011;42(4):1158–92.
11. Yarington Jr CT. Cavernous sinus thrombosis revisited. Proc R Soc Med. 1977;70:456–9.
12. Mehta R, Kumar A, Crock C, McNab A. Medical management of periorbital necrotising fasciitis. Orbit. 2013;32(4):253–5.
13. Amrith S, HosdurgaPai V, Ling WW. Periorbital necrotizing fasciitis – a review. Acta Ophthalmol. 2013;91(7):596–603.
14. Prendiville KJ, Bath PE. Lateral cantholysis and eyelid necrosis secondary to Pseudomonas aeruginosa. Ann Ophthalmol. 1988;20(5):193–5.
15. Scheepers MA, Keel S, Michaelides M. Bilateral necrotising fasciitis of the ocular adnexa secondary to Pseudomonas aeruginosa septicaemia in a HIV-positive child. Orbit. 2010;29(1):63–4.
16. Lazzeri D, Lazzeri S, Figus M, Tascini C, Bocci G, Colizzi L, Giannotti G, Lorenzetti F, Gandini D, Danesi R, Menichetti F, Del Tacca M, Nardi M, Pantaloni M. Periorbital necrotising fasciitis. Br J Ophthalmol. 2010;94(12):1577–85.
17. Bilyk JR. Periocular infection. Curr Opin Ophthalmol. 2007;18(5):414–23.
18. Luksich JA, Holds JB, Hartstein ME. Conservative management of necrotising fasciitis of the eyelids. Ophthalmology. 2002;109(11):2118–22.
19. Elner VM, Demirci H, Nerad JA, Hassan AS. Periocular necrotizing fasciitis with visual loss pathogenesis and treatment. Ophthalmology. 2006;113(12):2338–45.
20. Kronish JW, McLeish WM. Eyelid necrosis and periorbital necrotizing fasciitis. Report of a case and review of the literature. Ophthalmology. 1991;98(1):92–8.
21. Akamine M, Miyagi K, Uchihara T, Azuma M, Yara S, Higa F, Haranaga S, Tateyama M, Matsuzaki A, Nakayama T, Fujita J. Necrotizing fasciitis caused by Pseudomonas aeruginosa. Intern Med. 2008;47(6):553–6.
22. Stone L, Codere F, Ma SA. Streptococcal lid necrosis in previously healthy children. Can J Ophthalmol. 1991;26(7):386–90.
23. Henrich DE, Smith TL, Shockley WW. Fatal craniocervical necrotizing fasciitis in an immuno competent patient: a case report and review of the literature. Head Neck. 1995;17(4):351–7.
24. Committee on Infectious Diseases, American Academy of Pediatrics. Severe invasive group A streptococcal infections: a subject review. Pediatrics. 1998;101:136–40.
25. Carlisle RT, Fredrick GT. Preseptal and orbital cellulitis. Hosp Physician. 2006;42:15–9.
26. Brown DR, Davis NL, Lepawsky M, Cunningham J, Kortbeek J. A multicenter review of the treatment of major truncal necrotizing infections with and without hyperbaric oxygen therapy. Am J Surg. 1994;167:485–9.
27. Beerens AJ, Bauwens LJ, Leemans CR. A fatal case of craniofacial necrotising fasciitis. Eur Arch Otorhinolaryngol. 1999;256(10):506–9.
28. Steinkogler FJ, Huber-Spitzy V. Necrotising destruction of the ocular adnexa by Pseudomonas aeruginosa. J Craniomaxillofac Surg. 1988;16(1):28–30.
29. Doorenbos-Bot AC, Hooymans JM, Blanksma LJ. Periorbital necrotising fasciitis due to Cryptococcus neoformans in a healthy young man. Doc Ophthalmol. 1990;75:315–20.
30. Shindo ML, Nalbone VP, Dougherty WR. Necrotizing fasciitis of the face. Laryngoscope. 1997;107:1071–9.
31. Thurtell MJ, Chiu AL, Goold LA, Akdal G, Crompton JL, Ahmed R, Madge SN, Selva D, Francis I, Ghabrial R, Ananda A, Gibson J, Chan R, Thompson EO, Rodriguez M, McCluskey PJ, Halmagyi GM. Neuro-ophthalmology of invasive fungal sinusitis: 14 consecutive patients and a review of the literature. Clin Experiment Ophthalmol. 2013;41(6):567–76.
32. Epstein VA, Kern RC. Invasive fungal sinusitis and complications of rhinosinusitis. Otolaryngol Clin N Am. 2008;41:497–524.

33. Chakrabarti A, Das A, Panda NK. Controversies surrounding the categorization of fungal sinusitis. Med Mycol. 2009;47 Suppl 1:S299–308.
34. Arndt S, Aschendorff A, Echternach M, Daemmrich TD, Maier W. Rhino-orbital-cerebral mucormycosis and aspergillosis: differential diagnosis and treatment. Eur Arch Otorhinolaryngol. 2009;266:71–6.
35. Johnson TE. Fungal disease of the orbit. Ophthalmol Clin N Am. 2000;13:643–56.
36. Yohai R, Bullock J, Aziz A, Markert RJ. Survival factors in rhino-orbital-cerebral mucormycosis. Surv Ophthalmol. 1994;39(1):3–22.
37. Lee AG, Brazis PW. Systemic infections of neuro-ophthalmic significance. OphthalmolClin North Am. 2004;17(3):397–425.
38. Pushker N, Meel R, Kashyap S, Bajaj MS, Sen S. Invasive aspergillosis of orbit in immunocompetent patients: treatment and outcome. Ophthalmology. 2011;118(9):1886–91.
39. Decanini-Mancera A, Lessell S, Lee MS, Subramanian PS. Syphilis and the monk. Surv Ophthalmol. 2011;56(3):267–73.
40. Clancy CJ, Nguyen MH. Invasive sinus aspergillosis in apparently immunocompetent hosts. J Infect. 1998;37:229–40.
41. Green WR, Font RL, Zimmerman LE. Aspergillus of the orbit. Arch Ophthalmol. 1969;82:302–13.
42. Levin LA, Avery R, Shore JW, et al. The spectrum of orbital aspergillosis: a clinicopathological review. Surv Ophthalmol. 1996;41:142–54.
43. Mody KH, Ali MJ, Vemuganti GK, Nalamada S, Naik MN, Honavar SG. Orbital aspergillosis in immunocompetent patients. Br J Ophthalmol. 2014;98(10):1379–84.
44. Wali U, Balkhair A, Al-Mujaini A. Cerebro-rhino orbital mucormycosis: an update. J Infect Public Health. 2012;5(2):116–26.
45. Eucker J, Sezer O, Graf B, Possinger K. Mucormycosis. Mycoses. 2001;44:253–60.
46. Vagefi MR, Kim ET, Alvarado RG, Duncan JL, Howes EL, Crawford JB. Bilateral endogenous Scedosporium prolificans endophthalmitis after lung transplantation. Am J Ophthalmol. 2005;139:370–3.
47. Rodriguez-Tudela JL, Berenguer J, Guarro J, et al. Epidemiology and outcome of Scedosporium prolificans infection, a review of 162 cases. Med Mycol. 2009;47:359–70.
48. Dinowitz M, Leen JS, Hameed M, Wolansky L, Frohman L. Sudden painless visual loss. Surv Ophthalmol. 2001;46(2):143–8.
49. McNab AA. Invasive fungal sinusitis: ophthalmic emergency. Clin Experiment Ophthalmol. 2013;41(6):521.
50. Fairley C, Sullivan TJ, Bartley P, Allworth T, Lewandowski R. Survival after rhino-orbital-cerebral mucormycosis in an immunocompetent patient. Ophthalmology. 2000;107(3):555–8.
51. Sivak-Callcott JA, Livesley N, Nugent RA, et al. Localized invasive sino-orbital aspergillosis: characteristic features. Br J Ophthalmol. 2004;88:681–7.
52. Stevens DA, Kan VL, Judson MA. Practice guidelines for disease caused by aspergillus. Clin Infect Dis. 2000;30:696–709.

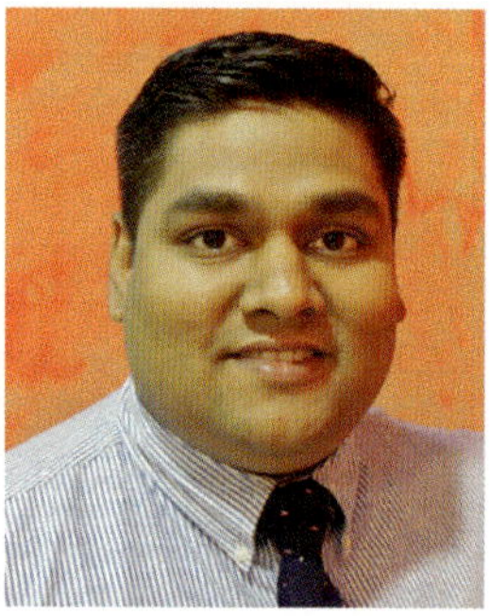

**Akshay Gopinathan Nair** Akshay Gopinathan Nair received his medical degree from Maharashtra University of Health Sciences, India, and completed his residency training in ophthalmology from Sankara Nethralaya in Chennai, India. Following this, he underwent fellowship training in ophthalmic plastic surgery, ocular oncology, and facial aesthetics at L V Prasad Eye Institute, Hyderabad, India, and New York Eye & Ear Infirmary of Mount Sinai, USA. Dr. Nair has over 50 peer-reviewed publications and 8 book chapters in ophthalmology. His areas of special interest are ocular surface and eyelid tumors, ophthalmic imaging, and neuroimaging. Dr. Nair is a faculty member at Lokmanya Tilak Municipal Medical College, Mumbai, India, and is also affiliated with Advanced Eye Hospital & Institute and Aditya Jyot Eye Hospital in Mumbai.

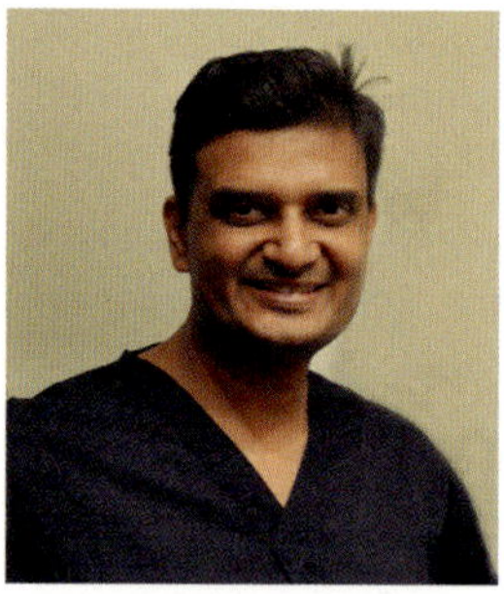

**Milind N. Naik** Dr. Milind Naik acquired his postgraduate training in Ophthalmology at the Christian Medical College, Vellore, India. He further completed his ophthalmic and facial plastic surgery fellowship at the prestigious University of California, Los Angeles, in the year 2006–2007. His areas of interest include aesthetic and facial plastic surgery, thyroid eye disease, and minimally invasive ophthalmic plastic surgery.

Dr. Naik has been awarded the Senior Achievement Award by the American Academy of Ophthalmology in the year 2015, and has served as the Vice President of the Asia Pacific Society of Ophthalmic Plastic and Reconstructive Surgery in the year 2010–2012.

Dr. Naik has over 100 peer-reviewed publications in international journals and lectures extensively across the globe in the field of ophthalmic plastic surgery and facial aesthetics. He currently heads the Ophthalmic Plastic Surgery Services at LV Prasad Eye Institute, Hyderabad, India. He also serves as Adjunct Associate Professor, Department of Ophthalmology and Visual Sciences, University of Rochester, New York, USA.

Dr. Naik's extracurricular interests include painting, 3D videography, and paperfolding.

Dr. Naik's better half, Dr. Vibhavari Naik is an anesthesiologist, and they have a 16-year-old daughter, Jaee.

# Fulminant Streptococcal Infections and Necrotizing Fasciitis

# 36

Stephanie Ming Young and Seah Lay Leng

## Introduction

Group A beta-hemolytic *Streptococcus* is one of the most common human pathogens [1]. It is a gram-positive bacterium responsible for a wide range of both invasive and noninvasive infections [1, 2]. They are known to cause three overlapping clinical presentations: toxic shock syndrome, necrotizing fasciitis, and bacteremia with no identifiable focus [2].

Necrotizing fasciitis is a rapidly progressing and potentially fatal infection that spreads along subcutaneous tissue planes and is associated with high morbidity and mortality [1]. Necrotizing fasciitis has also been referred to as hemolytic streptococcal gangrene, Meleney ulcer, acute dermal gangrene, hospital gangrene, suppurative fasciitis, and synergistic necrotizing cellulitis.

The frequency of necrotizing fasciitis has been on the rise because of an increase in immunocompromised patients with diabetes mellitus, cancer, alcoholism, vascular insufficiencies, organ transplants, HIV infection, or neutropenia. The estimated annual incidence of these infections is 3 cases per 100,000 people, with about 10,000 cases occurring each year in the United States [3, 4]. There may be an increased incidence in African and Asian countries; however, because of the lack of recorded cases, the true incidence is not known. Overall mortality is estimated to be from 10 to 15 % [4, 5].

While it usually involves the extremities, abdominal wall, and groin, about 10 % of cases may affect the head and neck region [4–6]. Necrotizing fasciitis may sometimes, although rarely, involve the eyelids, with approximately 65 well-documented case reports over the last 50 years [4, 5, 7–44]. Necrotizing fasciitis has a different clinical course in the eyelids than elsewhere in the body due to the thin eyelid skin with a rich blood supply harbored by the orbicularis oculi muscle, which lies superficial to the orbital septum fascia and fat. This allows the skin infection to become noticeable earlier, while spread occurs deep to the orbicularis oculi muscle. In addition, by behaving as a vascularized barrier between the skin and underlying infected tissues, the orbicularis oculi muscle also may act to preserve more skin to spare the eyelid margins from necrosis in most cases [4]. However, in all cases orbital involvement may lead to vision loss, and failure to recognize periocular necrotizing fasciitis can lead to severe ocular morbidity and even loss of life, if facial, cervical, or intracranial extension occurs [5].

S.M. Young, MBBS, MMed(Ophthalmology), FAMS, FRCOphth (✉)
Oculoplastics, Department of Ophthalmology, National University Hospital, Singapore, Singapore, 119228
e-mail: stephanieyoung83@gmail.com

S.L. Leng, MBBS, FRCS, FRCOphth, FAMS
Oculoplastics, Singapore National Eye Centre, Singapore, Singapore
e-mail: seah.lay.leng@snec.com.sg


B. Mukherjee, H. Yuen (eds.), *Emergencies of the Orbit and Adnexa*,
DOI 10.1007/978-81-322-1807-4_36

## Overview

### Classification

Different terms and classifications have been used to describe necrotizing infections of the skin and subcutaneous tissue. Historically, necrotizing infections were classified according to anatomical sites. Fournier gangrene (involving the perineum) and Ludwig angina (involving submandibular and sublingual spaces) are examples. These infections were named after the physicians who first described them. Other names which necrotizing fasciitis has been known by include synergistic necrotizing cellulitis, streptococcal myonecrosis, and gas gangrene. While many terms have been used to describe necrotizing soft-tissue infections, a few distinct necrotizing fasciitis syndromes should be recognized. The causative bacteria may be aerobic, anaerobic, or mixed flora [45]. Three most important types and their associated causative organisms are as follows:

1. Necrotizing fasciitis type I: Mixed anaerobes, gram-negative aerobic bacilli, enterococci
2. Necrotizing fasciitis type II: Group A *Streptococcus*
3. Necrotizing fasciitis type III or gas gangrene: Clostridial species (*C. perfringens*, *C. histolyticum*, *C. septicum*)

More detailed descriptions of the manifestations and a differential diagnosis of infections due to organisms other than group A *Streptococcus* are available elsewhere [46, 47]. For the purpose of this textbook chapter, we will concentrate on necrotizing fasciitis caused by group A *Streptococcus*.

### Etiology

Predisposing factors for the development of necrotizing fasciitis due to group A *Streptococcus* (*Streptococcus pyogenes*) include varicella, penetrating injuries, minor cuts, burns, splinters, surgical procedures, childbirth, blunt trauma, and muscle strain [1, 48]. Surgical procedures may cause local tissue injury and bacterial invasion, resulting in necrotizing fasciitis, as can intramuscular injections and intravenous infusions. Similarly, minor insect bites may set the stage for necrotizing infections as *Streptococci* are introduced into the wounds. Illnesses such as diabetes or cancer have been described in over 90 % of cases of progressive bacterial gangrene. Host defenses can be compromised by underlying systemic diseases favoring the development of these infections. In addition, local ischemia and hypoxia can occur in patients with systemic illnesses (e.g., diabetes) [1–3, 6, 7, 49]. Of patients with necrotizing fasciitis, 20–40 % are diabetic, a condition primarily affecting the microvascular circulation. Contact with an infected person may be associated with secondary infection, though such cases are uncommon. The patient's use of nonsteroidal anti-inflammatory agents may delay diagnosis by attenuating the cardinal manifestations of inflammation. Furthermore, because such agents impair phagocytic function and alter the host's humoral immune responses, a minor infection may develop into a fulminant one [48, 50, 51]. It has also been reported that patients with invasive streptococcal infections are prone to them because they have low antibody titers directed to the bacterial exotoxins or membrane M proteins [52].

## Presentation

### History

Diagnosis of necrotizing fasciitis can be difficult and requires a high degree of suspicion. Risk factors described above should be identified. Outcome depends on prompt recognition and early treatment. Delayed diagnosis and treatment are associated with higher morbidity and mortality.

Patients with necrotizing fasciitis present with the history of acute periorbital swelling associated with severe pain. The overlying skin is initially red, tense, and swollen. The hallmark symptom of necrotizing fasciitis is intense pain and tenderness over the involved skin and underlying muscle, as the infection spreads subcutaneously along fascial planes [4, 53]. This severe pain may frequently present before the patient develops systemic features (high fever, chills, rigors, sweating), and the pain may be out of proportion to physical findings. As it is a rapidly progressive condition, the skin may become cyanotic and blue gray within 1–2 days, with irregular erythematous borders [2, 21]. Within 4–5 days, frank cutaneous gangrene usually develops, followed by sloughing of the skin due to underlying suppuration by 8–10 days [2, 21, 22] (Fig. 36.1). In the later stages, the area involved becomes anesthetic from the destruction of the cutaneous nerves [54, 55]. The patient may be toxic and in later stages may have signs of multi-organ failure or disseminated intravascular coagulation [54].

## Physical Examination

Physical findings may not be commensurate with the degree of patient discomfort. Early in the disease course, the patient may look deceptively well; unfortunately, this may interfere with early detection, which is key to a favorable outcome. Soon, however, the patient will usually begin to appear moderately to severely toxic.

The infection begins with swelling and redness over the periocular region. The skin over the swelling appears erythematous and can be mistaken for erysipelas. The redness quickly spreads, and its margins move out into normal skin without being raised or sharply demarcated. As the infection progresses, the skin near the site of insult develops a dusky or purplish discoloration. The disease progresses rapidly, and the lesion may turn gangrenous within 24 h [55]. At this stage, the skin shows violaceous discoloration, and fluid-filled bullae appear on the skin, which helps to distinguish it from preseptal cellulitis. The initial necrosis appears as a massive undermining of the skin and subcutaneous layer (Fig. 36.2). If the skin is open, gloved fingers can pass easily between the two layers and may reveal yellowish-green necrotic fascia. The nor-

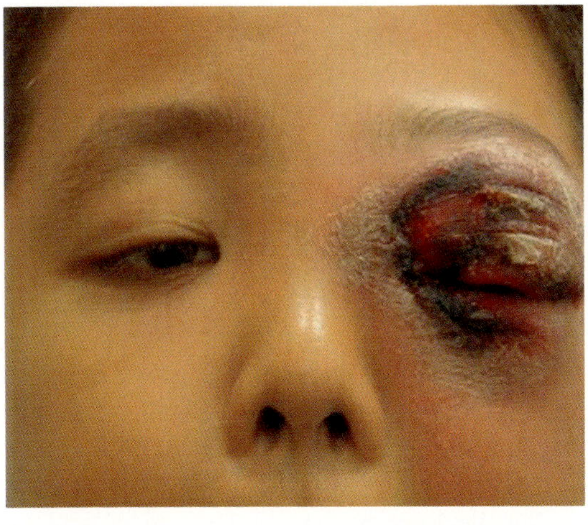

**Fig. 36.1** Young boy presenting with *left* periorbital necrotizing fasciitis. The periorbital skin is erythematous, edematous, and tender. There is also evidence of cutaneous gangrene and sloughing of skin, signs that should alert the physician to an ongoing necrotizing process

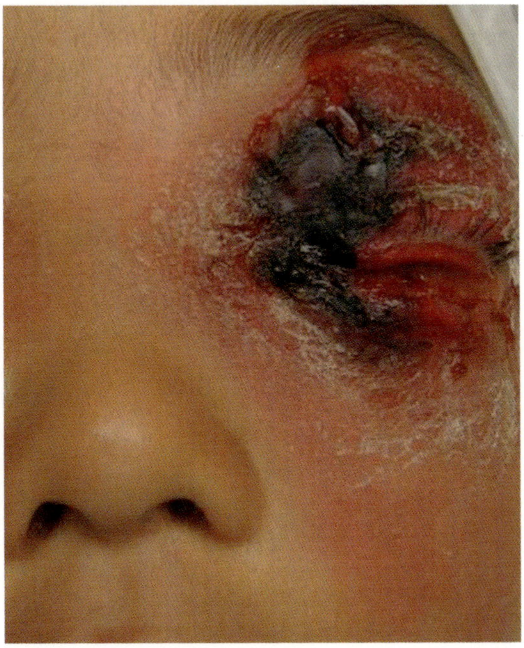

**Fig. 36.2** Patient with fulminant periorbital necrotizing fasciitis. On examination there is significant periorbital swelling and erythema, sometimes (as in this case) extending to the *lower* cheek and face. There is sloughing of the preseptal and pretarsal skin, with areas of necrosis and eschar formation. The violaceous to blackish skin discoloration and fluid-filled bullae help to distinguish it from preseptal cellulitis

mal skin and subcutaneous tissue become loosened from the rapidly spreading deeper necrotic fascia that may be some distance away from the initiating wound. The subcutaneous tissue involvement is more extensive than the involved overlying skin. In the later stages, the area involved becomes anesthetic, caused by thrombosis of the subcutaneous blood vessels, leading to necrosis of nerve fibers [54]. There can be crepitus on palpation, which may be seen as air in the soft tissue on X-ray [56]. Without treatment, secondary involvement of deeper muscle layers may occur, resulting in myositis or myonecrosis. Normally, however, the muscular layer remains healthy red with normal bleeding muscle under the yellowish-green fascia. In summary, the most important signs are tissue necrosis, putrid discharge, bullae, severe pain, gas production, rapid burrowing through fascial planes, and lack of classical tissue inflammatory signs. The patient may be toxic and in later stages may have signs of multi-organ failure or disseminated intravascular coagulation [54, 55].

## Clinical Course

As mentioned above, necrotizing fasciitis has a different clinical course in the eyelids than elsewhere in the body due to the thin eyelid skin with a rich blood supply harbored by the orbicularis oculi muscle, which lies superficial to the fascia of the orbital septum and fat. This allows the skin infection to become noticeable, usually less than 3 days from onset of symptoms [4]. The necrosis of the skin occurs rapidly, and as a result, the lids are unlikely to harbor the smoldering nidus of infection [41]. In addition, the orbicularis oculi muscle contains the eyelid marginal arterial arcades, whose perfusion serves to spare the eyelid margins from necrosis in most cases, even in cases of deep orbital involvement [4]. Lastly, the dermis is attached firmly at the nasojugal fold medially and to the malar fold laterally, forming a firm adhesion that prevents the spread of inflammation. Of reported cases of periorbital necrotizing fasciitis, 45 % had bilateral involvement and 55 % had unilateral involvement [5, 7–44]. The reason that necrotizing fasciitis may involve both eyes is because of the little resistance provided by the subcutaneous tissue over the nose to the spread of infection.

Necrotizing fasciitis of the eyelids has a reported mortality rate of 8.5–14.2 % and is attributable to systemic complications like septicemia, shock, and multi-organ failure [55]. This reported rate is lower than that of other body site involvement (28–32 %) [3, 5, 55]. This may be due to earlier recognition and treatment of infection in this area, compared to infection of the lower half of the face, with the latter having a higher risk of spread to the vital structures of the neck and thoracic cavity.

However, periocular necrotizing fasciitis has a high morbidity especially in cases of orbital involvement with vision loss [4, 28, 57]. It can cause deep orbital involvement by spread of the infection along the orbital fibrous septae and blood vessels, resulting in arterial occlusion and blindness [4]. Development of retinal artery occlusion is due to severe perivascular involvement causing thrombosis, which may be accentuated by systemic hypercoagulability, increased fibrin deposition, and fibrinolysis in patients with necrotizing fasciitis [58, 59]. In addition, increased intraorbital pressure due to severe inflammation and edema of the periorbital tissues may also contribute to ischemic necrosis and development of arterial occlusion.

## Differential Diagnosis

Differential diagnoses of periorbital necrotizing fasciitis would include any infectious or inflammatory processes affecting the eyelids, eye, and orbit [60]. Infectious possibilities (in increasing degree of severity) include blepharitis, conjunctivitis, preseptal cellulitis, orbital cellulitis, endophthalmitis, cavernous sinus thrombosis, and rhino-orbital mucormycosis [34, 44]. In particular, necrotizing fasciitis may be difficult to distinguish from preseptal or orbital cellulitis. However the former will show signs of rapid progression and subsequent cyanosis of involved tissue and formation of serious fluid-filled bullae, which will not be found in the more common non-necrotizing cellulitis [60–64].

Noninfectious differentials would include orbital pseudotumor, rapidly growing orbital tumor, Graves' disease, and subperiosteal hematomas [60–64]. However, fever would typically be absent for most of these entities. Similar to the infectious differentials, these entities would not show presence of bullae and violaceous discoloration and necrosis of the skin, which would point toward the diagnosis of necrotizing fasciitis [55, 65].

## Workup

The diagnosis of necrotizing fasciitis is mostly made on the basis of clinical features. Laboratory tests, along with appropriate imaging studies, may facilitate the diagnosis of necrotizing fasciitis [66].

### Laboratory Investigations

A complete laboratory evaluation should include the following: complete blood count with differential, serum chemistry studies, arterial blood gas measurement, urinalysis, as well as blood and tissue cultures. Numerous parameters have been shown to relate significantly to the severity of NF and subsequent death [67–72]: white cell count over 15,000/μl or less than 4,000/μl, more than 10 % neutrophils, platelet count below 100,000/μl, abnormal coagulation (activated partial thromboplastin time over 60s, international normalized ratio more than 1.5), serum creatinine concentration over 2.0 mg/dl, raised liver enzyme levels, C-reactive protein concentration exceeding 13 mg/dl, and creatinine kinase level over 700 units/l.

### Imaging

The presence of gas in the soft tissue on plain radiographs has been reported, but has been found to have no value in the diagnosis of necrotizing infections and may even hinder the diagnosis with consequent increased morbidity and mortality [73–75].

Bedside ultrasonography may be useful in patients with necrotizing fasciitis, as it may reveal subcutaneous emphysema spreading along the deep fascia, swelling, and increased echogenicity of the overlying fatty tissue with interlacing fluid collections [76, 77].

Computer tomography (CT) scan and magnetic resonance imaging (MRI) are extremely useful in making an early diagnosis and can serve as a guide to surgical debridement [69] (Fig. 36.3). Both modalities can detect the extent of necrotizing fasciitis and identify soft-tissue edema infiltrating the fascial planes many hours prior to the appearance of cutaneous signs. The characteristic CT findings of necrosis with asymmetric fascial thickening and the presence of gas in tissues help to differentiate necrotizing fasciitis from cellulitis, myonecrosis, and phycomycosis [68]. MRI is useful in detecting soft-tissue infection with its unsurpassed spatial resolution, multiplanar capabilities, and soft-tissue contrast and sensitivity in detecting soft-tissue fluid [78–80]. Absence of gadolinium contrast enhancement in T1-weighted images reliably detects fascial necrosis in patients requiring operative debridement, while T2-weighted images may show well-defined regions of high signal intensity in the deep tissues.

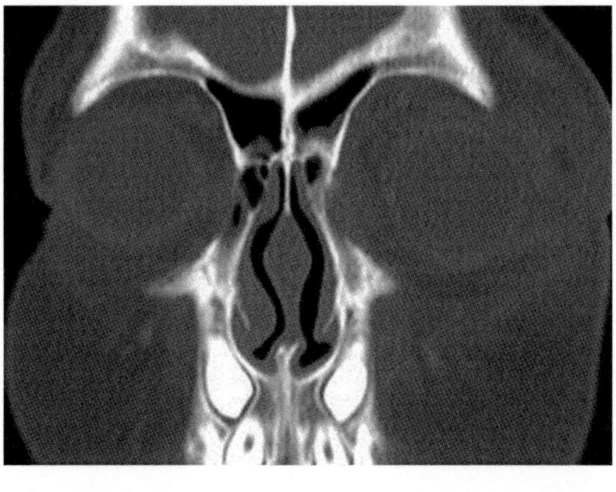

**Fig. 36.3** Computer tomography (*CT*) findings of necrosis with asymmetric fascial thickening and the presence of gas in tissues correlate with the picture of necrotizing fasciitis seen in Fig. 36.1

## Microbiology

In a systematic review by Goh et al., the overall rates of positive wound and blood cultures were 76.5 % and 36.2 %, respectively, in patients with necrotizing fasciitis [72]. Organisms common in polymicrobial infections were *Staphylococcus* spp., *Streptococcal* spp., *Bacteroides*, and *Escherichia coli* [81–85]. Organisms found in monomicrobial infections were *Streptococcus pyogenes* and *Staphylococcus aureus* [71, 86]. Marine bacteria (*Vibrio* spp., *Aeromonas* spp., and *Shewanella* spp.) were causal organisms in several studies from Korea and Taiwan, which have extensive coastal areas where these marine bacteria thrive in [70, 71, 87].

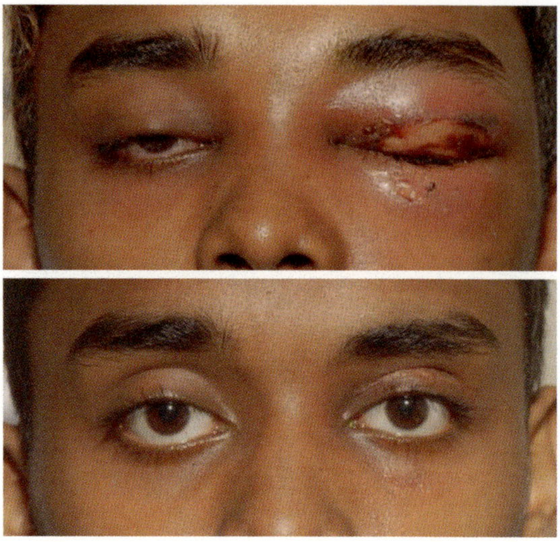

**Fig. 36.4** Patient on admission (*above*) and at 5 months after treatment (*below*), after skin reconstructive surgery was carried following resolution of acute infection. This patient showed marked clinical and cosmetic improvement with intravenous antibiotic therapy alone, suggesting that selected cases of uncomplicated eyelid necrotizing fasciitis can be treated conservatively with good results

## Treatment

Once the diagnosis of necrotizing fasciitis is confirmed, treatment must be initiated without delay. Because of the complexity of this disease, aggressive multidisciplinary treatment is mandatory to avoid morbidity (e.g., severe permanent disfigurement, loss of vision, exenteration) and mortality linked to misdiagnosis or delay in diagnosis [82]. Hemodynamic parameters should be closely monitored and aggressive resuscitation initiated immediately if needed to maintain hemodynamic stability. The patient should ideally be admitted to a surgical intensive care unit where the surgical staff is skilled in performing extensive debridement and reconstructive surgery.

Early recognition and initiation of high-dose antibiotics combined with tissue debridement help to decrease the mortality. There has been literature documenting successful nonsurgical management of group A *Streptococcus* eyelid necrotizing fasciitis [41, 88–90] (Fig. 36.4). However, while milder cases may respond to antibiotic therapy alone, because of the thrombosis of the blood vessels, antibiotics may not reach the infected site. Therefore, antibiotic therapy has to be combined with prompt surgical debridement of the affected tissue. By decreasing bacterial load and hyaluronic acid production, surgical debridement limits bacterial dissection through connective tissue and decreases the production of pyogenic exotoxins [4, 89].

Intravenous antimicrobial therapy is indicated in all patients with necrotizing fasciitis. The broad-spectrum antibiotics initiated should be effective against beta-hemolytic *Streptococcus* (principally *S. pyogenes*) and other organisms that may be involved in the pathogenesis of necrotizing fasciitis of the eyelids [60]. Although *S. pyogenes* is the bacterium most frequently involved in periorbital necrotizing fasciitis, the microbiology of the infection cannot often be predicted accurately before final identification of organism on wound culture. Hence, empirical antimicrobial therapy should consist of beta-lactam antibiotics, such as penicillin or cephalosporin and clindamycin [2, 3, 91, 92]. Penicillin is effective against group A beta-hemolytic *Streptococcus*. Addition of protein synthesis inhibiting antibiotics like clindamycin has a favorable outcome. It decreases the production of streptococcal toxins and enzymes even at subinhibitory concentration [93]. Type 1 necrotizing fasciitis (polymicrobial) requires the addition of aminoglycosides and/or metronidazole.

It has also been reported anecdotally that topical application of clindamycin may be effective in treating periocular necrotizing fasciitis. Clindamycin 2% ointment is applied on the infected tissue, which is kept covered with regular irrigation of clindamycin fluid. Clindamycin is known to act by inhibiting bacterial protein synthesis at the level of the 50S ribosome, hence exerting a prolonged postantibiotic effect and reducing the production of toxins. However, while topical use alone may suffice for milder skin infections, it should be used in adjunct with systemic antibiotics for more severe skin infections like necrotizing fasciitis.

Surgical debridement remains one of the most critical factors for reducing mortality from necrotizing fasciitis [4, 5, 28, 34, 39, 94] (Fig. 36.5). Aggressive, widespread debridement of all apparent necrotic and infected tissue is essential, as necrotic tissue serves as a nidus for infection (Fig. 36.6). Since the degree of subcutaneous necrosis typically is of a greater extent than suggested by changes in the overlying skin, debridement should be continued until viable tissue is observed. Good blood supply of the eyelids spares the lid margin from necrosis. It has been suggested that surgical debridement should involve mainly the subcutaneous tissue that harbors the infection without extensive skin resection in necrotizing fasciitis involving the head and neck [23]. Retention of maximum amount of viable skin and orbicularis oculi permits rapid healing, assists in antibiotic delivery, and reduces facial disfigurement. Re-exploration should be routinely performed within 24–36 h to ensure that all necrotic tissue has been debrided. Debridement is repeated as necessary until the infection is controlled [60]. After debridement, the exposed areas can be covered with sterile 0.9% normal saline wet-to-dry dressings. The dressing changes can be continued by the bedside with sufficient analgesia once the infection has been controlled and debridement is no longer necessary.

Once the acute phase is taken care of, reconstructive surgery can be planned at a later date. The choice of reconstructive procedure depends mainly on the extent of the defect. In periorbital necrotizing fasciitis, split- or full-thickness skin grafts are usually satisfactory for coverage of periorbital skin defect. Fasciocutaneous free flap should be considered in extended cases to cover a large skin defect and restore the facial contour. A full-thickness skin graft, accompanied by delayed placement of cartilage for soft-tissue support, is an ideal way to restore eyelid defects and prevent postsurgical complications, including ectropion and lagophthalmos [60, 95].

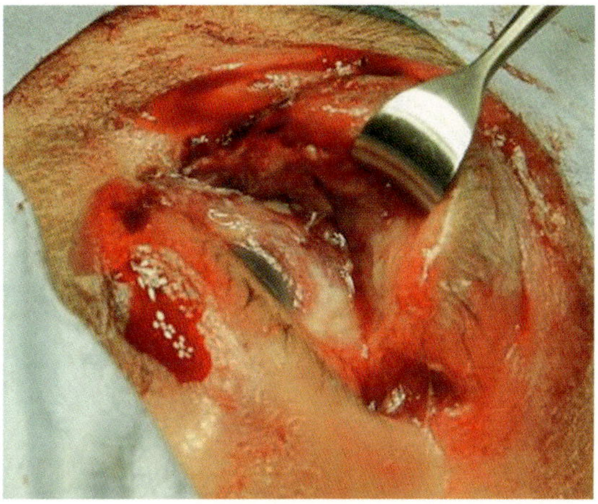

**Fig. 36.5** Surgical debridement remains one of the most critical factors for reducing mortality from necrotizing fasciitis

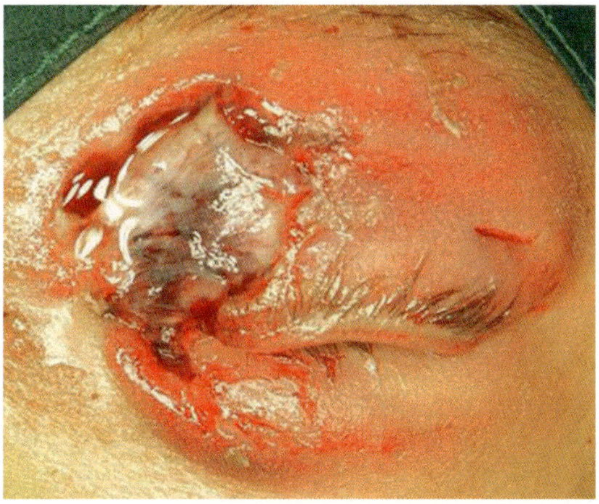

**Fig. 36.6** Surgical removal of any apparent infected or gangrenous tissue is essential, as necrotic tissue serves as a nidus for infection

The role of hyperbaric oxygen therapy in the management of necrotizing fasciitis is controversial. It may help to limit the ischemic tissue affected by necrotizing fasciitis by inhibition of exotoxin production, improving leukocyte function, and killing strict anaerobes and inhibiting growth of facultative anaerobes [96]. While some reports support the use of hyperbaric oxygen as an adjunctive treatment measure in patients with necrotizing fasciitis, operative debridement should not be delayed to accommodate hyperbaric oxygen therapy [5, 30, 34, 60, 97, 98].

## Conclusions

Necrotizing fasciitis is a severe infection characterized by widespread necrosis of the fascia and subcutaneous tissue. Periorbital necrotizing fasciitis is uncommon because of the excellent blood supply to the area; nevertheless, when it occurs it can lead to deep orbital extension and associated complications of blindness and even death. Outcome depends on prompt recognition and early treatment. Physicians must maintain a high index of suspicion for necrotizing fasciitis, which demands emergent ophthalmologic consultation, hospital admission, broad-spectrum systemic antibiotic therapy, and surgical debridement of necrotic tissue.

## References


1. Bisno AL, Stevens DL. Streptococcal infections of skin and soft tissues. N Engl J Med. 1996;334(4): 240–5.
2. Committee on Infectious Diseases, American Academy of Pediatrics. Severe invasive group A streptococcal infections: a subject review. Pediatrics. 1998;101:136–40.
3. Childers BJ, Potyondy LD, Nachreiner R, et al. Necrotizing fasciitis: a fourteen-year retrospective study of 163 consecutive patients. Am Surg. 2002;68:109–16.
4. Elner VM, Demirci H, Nerad JA, Hassan AS. Periocular necrotizing fasciitis with visual loss – pathogenesis and treatment. Ophthalmology. 2006;113:2338–45.
5. Kronish JW, McLeish WM. Eyelid necrosis and periorbital necrotizing fasciitis: report of a case and review of the literature. Ophthalmology. 1991;98:92–8.
6. Beall B, Facklam RR, Hoenes T, Schwartz B. Survey of emm gene sequences and T-antigen types from systemic Streptococcus pyogenes infection isolates collected in San Francisco, California; Atlanta, Georgia; and Connecticut in 1994 and 1995. J Clin Microbiol. 1997;35:1231–5.
7. Moore JR, Gerrie J, Elliott H. Massive cellulitis of the scalp in persons with diabetes. Arch Surg. 1950;60: 897–905.
8. Schott EG. Gangrene of the eyelids. Ind Med Surg. 1966;35:27–9.
9. Beathard GA, Guckian JC. Necrotizing fasciitis due to group A beta-hemolytic streptococci. Arch Intern Med. 1967;120:63–7.
10. Buchanan CS. Necrotizing fasciitis due to group A betahemolytic streptococci. Arch Dermatol. 1970;101:664–8.
11. Ross J, Kohlhepp PA. Gangrene of the eyelids. Ann Ophthalmol. 1973;5:84–8.
12. Carruthers A, Carruthers J, Wright P. Necrotizing fasciitis with polymyositis. Br Med J. 1975;3:355–6.
13. Klabacha ME, Stankiewicz JA, Clift SE. Severe soft tissue infection of the face and neck: a classification. Laryngoscope. 1982;92:1135–9.
14. Einarsson OJ, Pers M. Streptococcal gangrene of the eyelids: case reports. Scand J Plast Reconstr Surg. 1986;20:331–5.
15. Holliman RE, Catford GV. Periorbital necrotising fasciitis with loss of vision. J Infect. 1986;13:35–6.
16. Lloyd RE. Necrotizing fasciitis of the orbit. Br J Oral Maxillofac Surg. 1987;25:323–7.
17. Rosenthal WN, Gore HL, Insler MS. Periorbital necrotizing fasciitis. Ann Ophthalmol. 1987;19:426–7.
18. Balcerak RJ, Sisto JM, Bosack RC. Cervicofacial necrotizing fasciitis: report of three cases and literature review. J Oral Maxillofac Surg. 1988;46:450–9.
19. Walters R. A fatal case of necrotizing fasciitis of the eyelid. Br J Ophthalmol. 1988;72:428–31.
20. Doorenbos-Bot AC, Hooymans JM, Blanksma LJ. Periorbital necrotizing fasciitis due to Cryptococcus neoformans in a healthy young man. Doc Ophthalmol. 1990;75:315–20.
21. Stone L, Codere F, Ma SA. Streptococcal lid necrosis in previously healthy children. Can J Ophthalmol. 1991;26:386–90.
22. Rose GE, Howard DJ, Watts MR. Periorbital necrotizing fasciitis. Eye. 1991;5:736–40.
23. Williams SR, Carruth JA, Brightwell AP. Necrotizing fasciitis of the face without significant trauma. Clin Otolaryngol Allied Sci. 1992;17:344–50.
24. Kiely PD, Gilvarry A. Periorbital necrotizing fasciitis: trivial facial injury resulting in cardiac arrest. Br J Clin Pract. 1993;47:169–70.
25. Suharwardy J. Periorbital necrotizing fasciitis. Br J Ophthalmol. 1994;78:233–4.
26. Sabb PC, Sires BS, Lemke BN, Goldstein JA. Orbital involvement of cervicofacial necrotizing fasciitis [letter]. Arch Ophthalmol. 1995;113:1571.
27. Kent D, Atkinson PL, Patel B, Davies EW. Fatal bilateral necrotizing fasciitis of the eyelids. Br J Ophthalmol. 1995;79:95–6.
28. Shayegani A, MacFarlane D, Kazim M, Grossman ME. Streptococcal gangrene of the eyelids and orbit. Am J Ophthalmol. 1995;120:784–92.

29. Ingraham HJ, Ryan ME, Burns JT, et al. Streptococcal preseptal cellulitis complicated by the toxic Streptococcus syndrome. Ophthalmology. 1995;102: 1223–6.
30. Ray AM, Bressler K, Davis RE, et al. Cervicofacial necrotizing fasciitis: a devastating complication of blepharoplasty. Arch Otolaryngol Head Neck Surg. 1997;123:633–6.
31. Marshall DH, Jordan DR, Gilberg SM, et al. Periocular necrotizing fasciitis: a review of 5 cases. Ophthalmology. 1997;104:1857–62.
32. Anzai S, Sato T, Takayasu S, Tatsukawa T. Periorbital necrotizing cellulitis [letter]. Int J Dermatol. 1998;37:799.
33. Jordan DR, Mawn L, Marshall DH. Necrotizing fasciitis caused by group A streptococcus infection after laser blepharoplasty. Am J Ophthalmol. 1998;125: 265–6.
34. Knudtson KJ, Gigantelli JW. Necrotizing fasciitis of the eyelids and orbit. Arch Ophthalmol. 1998;116: 1548–9.
35. Barapouti FG, Kamel OR, Sampath R. Periorbital necrotizing fasciitis in a child [letter]. Eye. 1999;13:676–8.
36. Beerens AJ, Bauwens LJ, Leemans CR. A fatal case of craniofacial necrotizing fasciitis. Eur Arch Otorhinolaryngol. 1999;256:506–9.
37. Suner JI, Meldrum ML, Johnson TE, Tse DT. Necrotizing fasciitis after cosmetic blepharoplasty. Am J Ophthalmol. 1999;128:367–8.
38. Gates RL, Cocke WM, Rushton TC. Invasive streptococcal infection of the periorbita and forehead. Ann Plast Surg. 2001;47:565–7.
39. Pal B, Evans S, Walters RF. Necrotising fasciitis of the periorbital region [letter]. Eye. 2001;15:676–7.
40. Puri P, Innes JR. Necrotising fasciitis of the orbit: early recognition and treatment a key to success. Eur J Ophthalmol. 2001;11:180–2.
41. Luksich JA, Holds JB, Hartstein ME. Conservative management of necrotizing fasciitis of the eyelids. Ophthalmology. 2002;109:2118–22.
42. Goldberg RA, Li TG. Postoperative infection with Group A beta-hemolytic streptococcus after blepharoplasty. Am J Ophthalmol. 2002;134:908–10.
43. Lin PW, Lin HC. Facial necrotizing fasciitis following acute dacryocystitis. Am J Ophthalmol. 2003;136: 203–4.
44. Jensen SL, Amato JE, Hartstein ME, Breer WA. Bilateral periorbital necrotizing fasciitis. Arch Dermatol. 2004;140:664–6.
45. Kihiczak GG, Schwartz RA, Kapila R. Necrotizing fasciitis: a deadly infection. J Eur Acad Dermatol Venereol. 2006;20:365–9.
46. Swartz MN. Cellulitis and subcutaneous tissue infections. In: Mandell GL, Bennett JE, Dolin R, editors. Mandell, Douglas and Bennett's principles and practice of infectious diseases. 4th ed. New York: Churchill Livingstone; 1995. p. 909–29.
47. *Idem.* Myositis. In: Mandell GL, Bennett JE, Dolin R, editors. Mandell, Douglas and Bennett's principles and practice of infectious diseases. 4th ed. New York: Churchill Livingstone; 1995. p. 929–36.
48. Stevens DL. Invasive group A streptococcus infections. Clin Infect Dis. 1992;14:2–11.
49. Gürlek A, Firat C, Oztürk AE, Alaybeyoğlu N, Fariz A, Aslan S. Management of necrotizing fasciitis in diabetic patients. J Diabetes Complications. 2007;21:265–71.
50. Stevens DL, Tanner MH, Winship J, et al. Severe group A streptococcal infections associated with a toxic shock–like syndrome and scarlet fever toxin A. N Engl J Med. 1989;321:1–7.
51. Stevens DL. Invasive group A streptococcal infections: the past, present and future. Pediatr Infect Dis J. 1994;13:561–6.
52. Basma H, Norrby-Teglund A, Guedez Y, et al. Risk factors in the pathogenesis of invasive group A streptococcal infections: role of protective humoral immunity. Infect Immun. 1999;67:1871–7.
53. Olafsson EJ, Zeni T, Wilkes DS. A 46-year-old man with excruciating shoulder pain. Chest. 2005;127: 1039–44.
54. Hu V, Turner S, Robinson F. Nonprogressive periorbital necrotising fasciitis. Orbit. 2008;27:59–62.
55. Amrith S, Hosdurga Pai V, Ling WW. Periorbital necrotizing fasciitis: a review. Acta Ophthalmol. 2013;91: 596–603.
56. Wilson B. Necrotising fasciitis. Am Surg. 1952;18: 416–31.
57. Nallathambi MN, Ivatury RR, Rohman M, et al. Craniocervical necrotizing fasciitis: critical factors in management. Can J Surg. 1987;30:61–3.
58. Bryant AE. Biology and pathogenesis of thrombosis and procoagulant activity in invasive infections caused by group A streptococci and Clostridium perfringens. Clin Microbiol Rev. 2003;16:451–62.
59. Hammar H, Sverdrup B, Borglund E, Blomback M. Coagulation and fibrinolytic systems during the course of erysipelas and necrotizing fasciitis and the effect of heparin. Acta Derm Venereol. 1985;65: 495–503.
60. Lazzeri D, Lazzeri S, Figus M, Tascini C, Bocci G, Colizzi L, Giannotti G, Lorenzetti F, Gandini D, Danesi R, Menichetti F, Tacca MD, Nardi M, Pantaloni M. Periorbital necrotising fasciitis. Br J Ophthalmol. 2010;94:1577–85.
61. Lessner A, Stern GA. Preseptal and orbital cellulitis. Infect Dis Clin North Am. 1992;6:933–52.
62. Howe L, Jones NS. Guidelines for the management of periorbital cellulitis/abscess. Clin Otolaryngol Allied Sci. 2004;29:725–8.
63. Carlisle RT, Fredrick GT. Preseptal and orbital cellulitis. Hosp Physician. 2006;42:15–9.
64. Haufschild T, Weber P, Nuttli I, et al. Idiopathic isolated abscess in an extraocular muscle in a child. Arch Ophthalmol. 2004;122:1233–4.
65. Shimuzu T, Tokuda Y. Necrotising fasciitis. Intern Med. 2010;49:1051–7.
66. Simonart T, Simonart JM, Derdelinckx I, et al. Value of standard laboratory tests for the early recognition

of group A beta-hemolytic streptococcal necrotizing fasciitis. Clin Infect Dis. 2001;32:E9–12.
67. Wong CH, Khin LW, Heng KS, et al. The LRINEC (laboratory risk indicator for necrotising fasciitis) score: a tool for distinguishing necrotising fasciitis from other soft tissue infections. Crit Care Med. 2004; 32:1535–41.
68. Wysoki MG, Santora TA, Shah RM, et al. Necrotising fasciitis: CT characteristics. Radiology. 1997;203: 859–63.
69. Saldana M, Gupta D, Khandwala M, Weir R, Beigi B. Periorbital necrotizing fasciitis: outcomes using a CT-guided surgical debridement approach. Eur J Ophthalmol. 2010;20:209–14.
70. Hsiao C, Weng H, Yuan Y, Chen C, Chen I. Predictors of mortality in patients with necrotizing fasciitis. Am J Emerg Med. 2008;26:170–5.
71. Huang KF, Hung MH, Lin YS, Lu CL, Liu C, Chen CC, et al. Independent predictors of mortality for necrotizing fasciitis: a retrospective analysis in a single institution. J Trauma. 2011;71:467–73.
72. Goh T, Goh LG, Ang CH, Wong CH. Early diagnosis of necrotizing fasciitis. Br J Surg. 2014;101:e119–25.
73. Drake DB, Woods JA, Bill TJ, et al. Magnetic resonance imaging in the early diagnosis of group A beta streptococcal necrotizing fasciitis: a case report. J Emerg Med. 1998;16:403–7.
74. Namias N, Martin L, Matos L, Sleeman D, Snowdon B. Symposium: necrotizing fasciitis. Contemp Surg. 1996;49:167–78.
75. Lille ST, Sato TT, Engrav LH, Foy H, Jurkovich GJ. Necrotizing soft tissue infections: obstacles in diagnosis. J Am Coll Surg. 1995;182:7–11.
76. Ramirez-Schrempp D, Dorfman DH, Baker WE, Liteplo AS. Ultrasound soft-tissue applications in the pediatric emergency department: to drain or not to drain? Pediatr Emerg Care. 2009;25:44–8.
77. Wronski M, Slodkowski M, Cebulski W, Karkocha D, Krasnodebski IW. Necrotizing fasciitis: early sonographic diagnosis. J Clin Ultrasound. 2011;39:236–9.
78. Beltran J, McGhee RB, Shaffer PB, et al. Experimental infections of the musculoskeletal system: evaluation with MR imaging and Tc-99m MDP and Ga-67 scintigraphy. Radiology. 1988;167:167–72.
79. Tang JS, Gold RH, Bassett LW, Seeger LL. Musculoskeletal infection of the extremities: evaluation with MR imaging. Radiology. 1988;166:205–9.
80. Rahmouni A, Chosidow O, Mathieu D, et al. MR imaging in acute infectious cellulitis. Radiology. 1994;192:493–6.
81. Elliott DC, Kufera JA, Myers RA. Necrotizing soft tissue infections. Risk factors for mortality and strategies for management. Ann Surg. 1996;224:672–83.
82. Frazee B, Fee C, Lynn J, Wang R, Bostrom A, Hargis C, Moore P. Community-acquired necrotising soft tissue infections: a review of 122 cases presenting to a single emergency department over 12 years. J Emerg Med. 2008;34:139–46.
83. Dworkin M, Westercamp M, Park L, McIntyre A. The epidemiology of necrotising fasciitis including factors associated with death and amputation. Epidemiol Infect. 2009;137:1609–14.
84. Wong C, Chang H, Pasupathy S, Khin L, Tan J, Low C. Necrotizing fasciitis: clinical presentation, microbiology, and determinants of mortality. J Bone Joint Surg Am. 2003;85-A:1454–60.
85. Singh G, Sinha S, Adhikary S, Babu K, Ray P, Khanna S. Necrotising infections of soft tissues – a clinical profile. Eur J Surg. 2002;168:366–71.
86. Nisbet M, Ansell G, Lang S, Taylor S, Dzendrowskyj P, Holland D. Necrotising fasciitis: review of 82 cases in South Auckland. Intern Med J. 2011;47:543–8.
87. Park K, Jung S, Jung Y, Shin J, Hwang J. Marine bacteria as a leading cause of necrotising fasciitis in coastal areas of South Korea. Am J Trop Med Hyg. 2009;80:646–50.
88. Balaggan KS, Goolamali SI. Periorbital necrotising fasciitis after minor trauma. Graefes Arch Clin Exp Ophthalmol. 2006;244:268–70.
89. Lee Hooi L, Hou BAC, Lay LS. Group A streptococcus necrotising fasciitis of the eyelid: a case report of good outcome with medical management. Ophthal Plast Reconstr Surg. 2012;28:e13–5.
90. Shome D, Jain V, Jayadev C, et al. Periocular necrotizing fasciitis associated with kerato-conjunctivitis and treated with medical management: a case report. Indian J Ophthalmol. 2008;56:231–2.
91. McHenry CR, Compton CN. Soft tissue infections. In: Malangoni MH, Soper NJ, editors. Problems in general surgery. Philadelphia: Lippincott Williams & Wilkins; 2002. p. 7.
92. Elliott D, Kufera JA, Myers RA. The microbiology of necrotizing soft tissue infections. Am J Surg. 2000;179:361–6.
93. Seal DV. Necrotising fasciitis. Curr Opin Infect Dis. 2001;14:127–32.
94. Shindo ML, Nalbone VP, Dougherty WR. Necrotizing fasciitis of the face. Laryngoscope. 1997;107:1071–9.
95. Elwood ET, Sommerville DN, Murray JD. Periorbital necrotizing fasciitis. Plast Reconstr Surg. 2007;120: 107–11.
96. Brown DR, Davis NL, Lepawsky M, et al. A multicenter review of the treatment of major truncal necrotizing infections with and without hyperbaric oxygen therapy. Am J Surg. 1994;167:485–9.
97. Hirschbein MJ, LaBorwit SE, Karesh JW. Streptococcal necrotizing fasciitis complicating a conjunctival dacryocystorhinostomy. Ophthal Plast Reconstr Surg. 1998;14:281–5.
98. Costet-Fighiera C, Lagier J, Bastiani-Griffet F, et al. Necrotizing fasciitis of the eyelids and orbit: a life-threatening ophthalmological emergency. J Fr Ophtalmol. 2002;25:375–8.

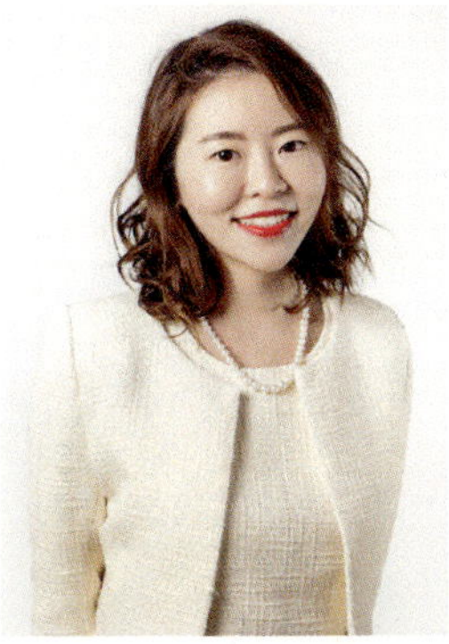

**Stephanie Ming Young** Stephanie Ming Young received her Bachelor of Medicine and Bachelor of Surgery degrees from the National University of Singapore (NUS). She completed her basic and advanced ophthalmology training in National University Hospital and Singapore National Eye Centre, and went on to subspecialize in ophthalmic plastic and reconstructive surgery. She won the Gold Medal and Book Prize in Ophthalmology and received a Distinction Award for Ophthalmology-related research for her Undergraduate Research Opportunities Program in medical school. Since then, she has won several ophthalmology-related awards and grants, as well as published various papers on the subject in peer-reviewed journals. Aside from clinical work and research, Dr. Young is a clinical lecturer with the NUS Clinical Faculty Scheme and teaches medical students as well as junior doctors. She strongly believes in giving back actively to society and sits on the executive committee of Singapore Women's Association, where she runs monthly free eye screening events for the community as part of the Singapore Visioncare Programme. She has also participated in many cataract and Oculoplastic trips to remote areas in need of eye care in various countries around the world.

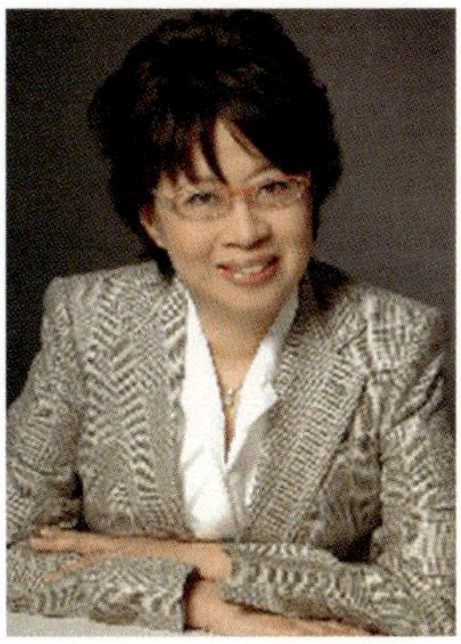

**Seah Lay Leng** Professor Seah is one of the few pioneers in the Oculoplastic and Orbit sub-specialty. She is recognized for her contribution to the establishment and the development of the Oculoplastic Department, Orbit and Ophthalmic Prosthetic departments in the Singapore National Eye Center and Pediatric Oculoplastic in the Kandan Kabau Women' and Children's Hospital in Singapore. She received her fellowship training in Oculoplastic Surgery at the London Moorfield's Eye Hospital, UK and Orbital Surgery Centre at the Vancouver Eye Center in Canada. In recognition of her contribution to the development of Orbit sub specialty at the Singapore National Eye Center and the region, she was elected to be a member of the "Orbit Society" in 2008 organized by the International Orbital Surgeons. She is also a board member of the prestigious International Thyroid Eye Disease Society (ITEDS).

Professor Seah is particularly active in medical education for undergraduate and post-graduate medical students of the National University of Singapore and has been a mentor for many local and overseas fellows for advanced fellowship training in Oculoplastic Surgery. Her international participation includes numerous presentations as an invited speaker. She had held the chair in regional and international conferences and the chair of organizing committee of regional and international orbital symposia and oculoplastic workshops

# 37 Viral Keratitis

Bhaskar Srinivasan, Geetha Iyer, Mamta Agarwal, and Shweta Agarwal

## Introduction

Herpetic infections are one of the commonest cause of infectious corneal blindness in the world with United States alone accounting for 50,000 new and recurrent cases of herpes simplex virus (HSV) infections every year [1–3].

## HSV Keratitis

Herpes simplex viruses are ubiquitous human pathogens that can cause subclinical or active disease. HSV-1 is primarily responsible for ophthalmic and orofacial manifestations, and HSV-2 is responsible for genital infections, the exception being neonatal HSV infections where HSV-2 is the causative agent in 75 % cases [3, 4].

## Pathophysiology

Humans are the only known host for the virus, and transmission is by close personal contact via salivary droplets or mucosal secretions. The incubation period is 1–28 days. Primary infection mostly result in a subclinical disease, and the virus travels via retrograde axonal transport to establish a dormant state in trigeminal root ganglion. Active disease is mostly due to recurrence of the infection in the same or new end organ or an inflammatory host response to the presence of viral antigens in the target tissue. There are reports of dormant HSV even in corneal tissue causing episodes of recurrent keratitis [4, 5].

## Clinical Types

### Primary Disease

It is usually seen in children or adolescents. In neonates in addition to causing ophthalmic manifestation, it can cause encephalitis and is life threatening. A viral prodromal phase with fever and malaise may accompany lymphadenopathy and periocular vesicles. Ophthalmic manifestations are mostly unilateral and consist of blisters involving the lids, blepharitis, follicular conjunctivitis, and dendritic conjunctivitis. Corneal involvement is in the form of punctuate epithelial keratitis and corneal microcyst which break down

B. Srinivasan, MS(Ophthalmology) (✉) • G. Iyer, FRCS • S. Agarwal, MS(Ophthalmology)
Cornea, Refractive Surgery & Ocular Surface, Sankara Nethralaya, Chennai, Tamil Nadu 600006, India
e-mail: drbhaskar@hotmail.com; drgeethaiyer@gmail.com; Swe20@yahoo.com

M. Agarwal, MBBS, DNB(Ophthalmology)
Uvea & Cornea, Sankara Nethralaya, Chennai, Tamil Nadu, India


B. Mukherjee, H. Yuen (eds.), *Emergencies of the Orbit and Adnexa*,
DOI 10.1007/978-81-322-1807-4_37

to form small dendrites without any stromal involvement. Prognosis is good but it leads to a state of latency and can cause recurrent infections.

## Recurrent Disease

Most active disease in adults are due to recurrences, and the rates are about 36 % at 5 years and 63 % at 20 years after a primary episode. After a second episode, 70–80 % of patients had another recurrence within 10 years [4, 5]. The lesions in a recurrent disease are:

Blepharitis and dacryoadenitis – There can be focal pinhead-sized vesicular lesion which erupts in crops and contains serous fluid. The vesicles rupture with crusting and heal without scar formation unlike the lesions of zoster. Eyelid lesions may masquerade as edema/eschar in rare cases. The lid margin involvement might not show the typical blisters as they get ruptured during blinking and are called as weeping ulcers. Immune competent patients with blepharitis shed virus only for 2–3 days and heal in a week's time. Rarely involvement of the lacrimal system with resultant scarring results in epiphora which is normally amenable to probing and syringing. A rare case of herpetic dacryoadenitis in an immunocompromised individual which required treatment with high-dose acyclovir has also been reported [4, 5].

Blepharoconjunctivitis/conjunctivitis – Conjunctiva shows congestion, follicular reaction, and dendritic lesions very similar to lesions in primary disease.

Keratitis – Recurrent keratitis can be of various types:

1. Infectious epithelial keratitis
2. Neurotrophic keratitis
3. Immune stromal keratitis
4. Necrotizing stromal keratitis
5. Endothelitis

## Infectious Epithelial Keratitis

This could start as superficial punctuate lesion which then evolve to form corneal vesicles which stain negatively with fluorescein. These vesicles are virus-laden cells which then lyse to form the classical dendritic corneal ulcer as depicted in Fig. 37.1. The base of the ulcer stains with fluorescein and the edges with rose bengal. If not treated appropriately or in patients inadvertently started on steroids, the dendrite may progress to an amoeboid or geographic ulcer pattern as seen in Fig. 37.2. A form of epithelial keratitis involves localized limbal vascularization, anterior stromal infiltration, and dendritic lesion close to limbus; this entity is called as herpes marginal epithelial keratitis, and the patients are more asymptomatic as compared to the other epithelial keratitis. This marginal keratitis needs to be differentiated from staphylococcal immune keratitis which preferentially occurs at the two and ten or four and eight o'clock meridian with a lucid interval and intact overlying epithelium to begin with, whereas the herpetic marginal keratitis can occur at any sector and has dendritic epithelial defect, and vessels cross the limbus to reach the anterior stroma near the dendrite. Sometimes after the epithelial keratitis heals, a faint sub-epithelial dendrite-like lesion is seen in the anterior stroma called as footprints or ghost figures; these are telltale signs of previous herpetic keratitis [6–8].

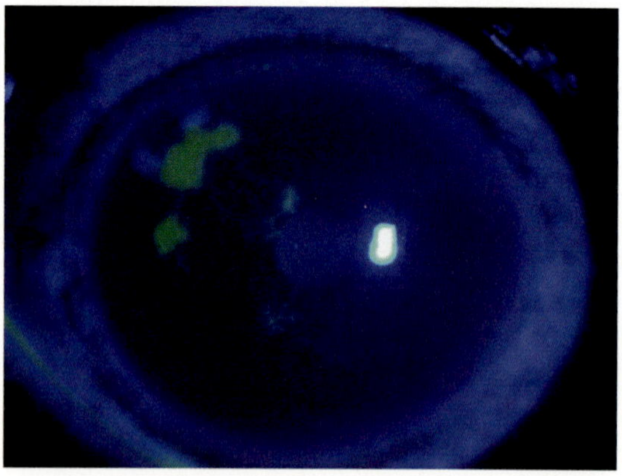

**Fig. 37.1** Classical dendritic lesion stained with fluorescein dye

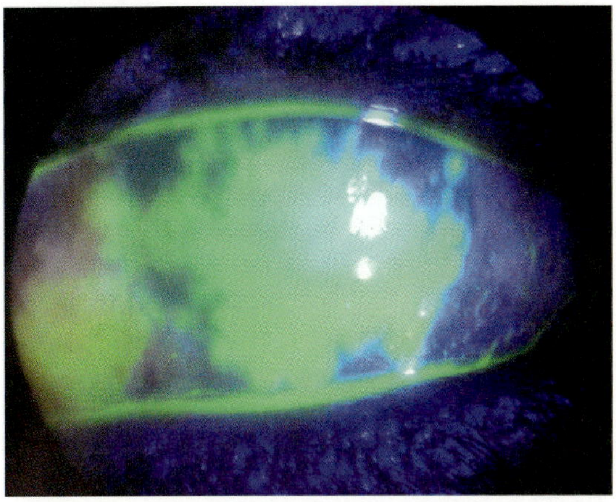

**Fig. 37.2** Conjunctival and corneal geographic ulceration in a patient on systemic immune suppression

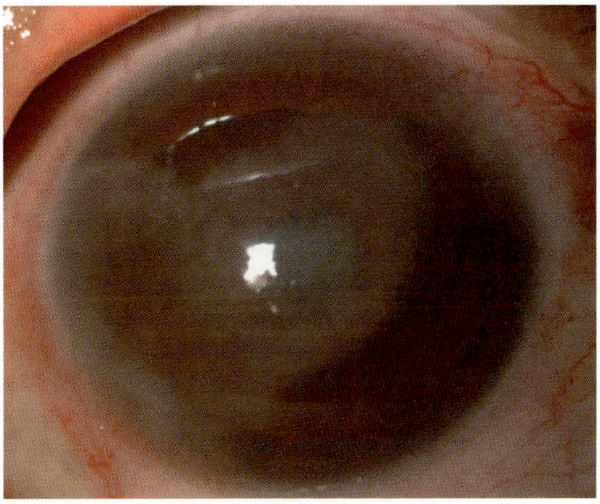

**Fig. 37.3** Non-necrotizing stromal keratitis

## Neurotrophic Keratitis

Decreased corneal sensations and the relative dry eye state predisposes to neurotrophic corneal ulceration that needs to be differentiated from geographic ulcer which is an infective state. The typical neurotrophic ulcer is an oval-shaped ulcer in the exposed area that has a dry irregular hazy base and smooth rolled edges with heaped up epithelium. Corneal stromal melting, scarring vascularization, and secondary infections are possible complications of neurotrophic ulcer [6–8].

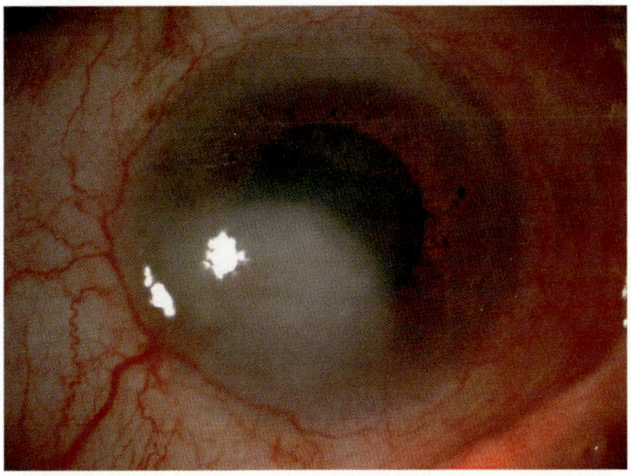

**Fig. 37.4** Limbal immune stromal keratitis

## Immune Stromal Keratitis

This is due to antigen-antibody reaction, and clinically there is single or multiple punctate stromal opacities associated with surrounding corneal haze due to inflammation and stromal edema. Edema is secondary to stromal inflammation rather than endothelial dysfunction. As shown in Figs. 37.3 and 37.4, there can be minimal anterior chamber reaction and ciliary flush. Repeated attacks of stromal keratitis and severity of each attack can predispose to corneal vascularization, lipid deposition, and scarring as depicted in Figs. 37.5 and 37.6 [6–8].

## Necrotizing Stromal Keratitis

This is due to active viral invasion of the stroma with accompanying inflammatory reaction. Clinically there is an epithelial defect with ulceration and intense inflammatory infiltration of the stroma as seen in Fig. 37.7. Clinical appearance can mimic bacterial/fungal keratitis, and scarping needs to be done in suspicious cases to confirm the same. This can very often progress to corneal melt and perforation [6–8].

## Endotheliitis

This manifests as stromal edema without any evidence of stromal inflammation. There is presence of keratic precipitates and anterior chamber reaction and iritis. The commonest type is called disciform endotheliitis which results in a disc-shaped area of corneal edema with underlying keratic precipitates remaining in the cornea that is clear. Diffuse endotheliitis involves the entire endothelium with diffuse stromal edema and epithelial

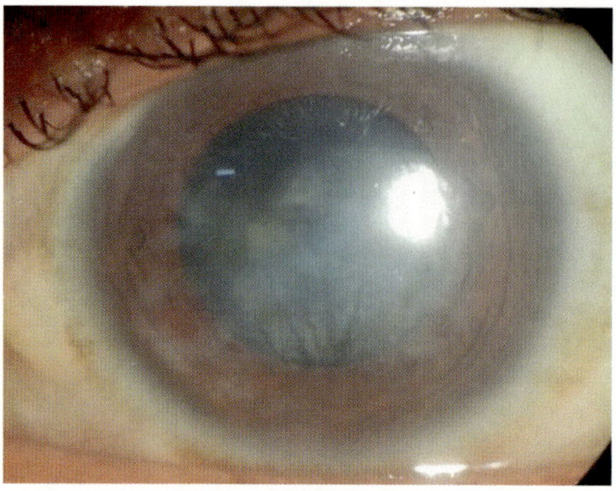

**Fig. 37.5** Long-term sequelae of viral stromal keratitis with ghost vessels and lipid keratopathy

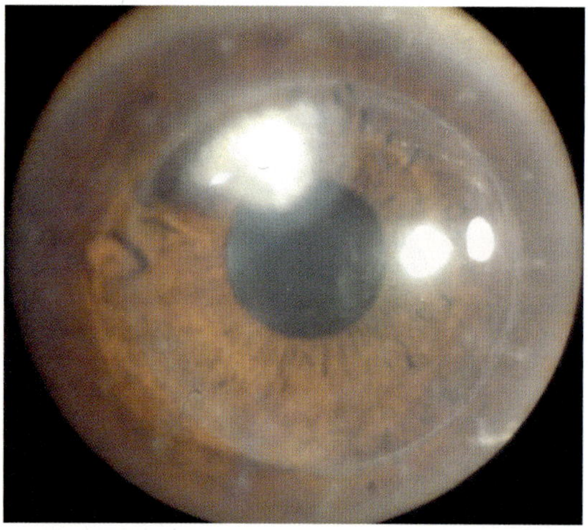

**Fig. 37.6** Deep anterior lamellar keratoplasty for a viral keratitis with vascularization with lipid keratopathy

edema as seen in Fig. 37.8. Linear endothelitis refers to localized endothelitis occurring along a line extending from the limbus across the cornea very much like the Khodadoust line in graft rejection with corneal edema peripheral to the line; this carries the worst prognosis [6–8].

### Iridocyclitis

This presents as anterior chamber flare and cells with keratic precipitates as seen in Fig. 37.9. Intra-ocular pressure can increase due to associated trabeculitis; sectoral iris atrophic patches can be seen. It normally occurs along with immune stroma keratitis or endothelitis [6–8].

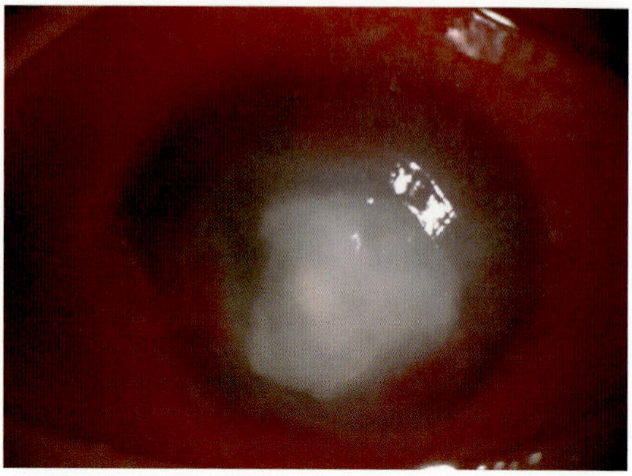

**Fig. 37.7** Necrotizing stromal keratitis

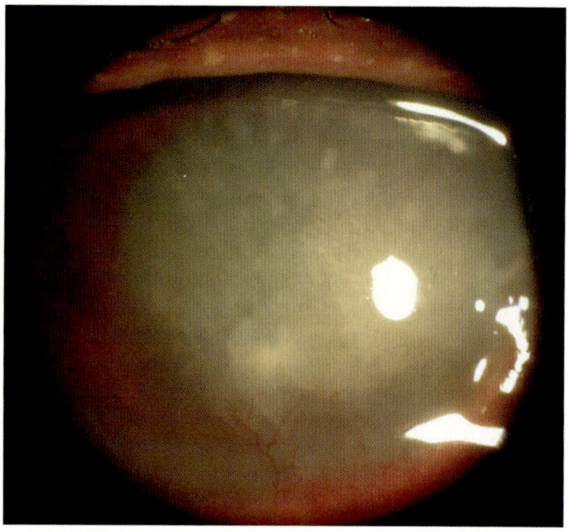

**Fig. 37.8** Diffuse endotheliitis

## Diagnosis

It is primarily by clinical features and cell culture studies, and polymerase chain reaction can be used in certain situations for confirmation or for research.

### Treatment

Blepharitis: Treatment is supportive in immune competent patients, and most lesions resolve by a 2-week period. In extensive lesions systemic acyclovir 400 mg five times a day can be used for 10 days till skin lesions heal. Topical

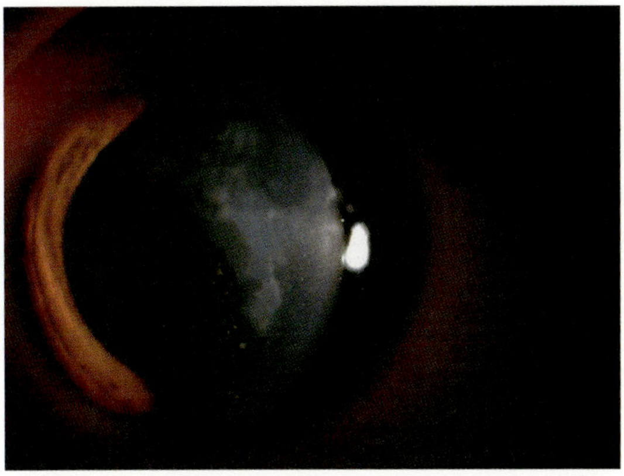

**Fig. 37.9** Viral keratouveitis

broad-spectrum antibiotic ointment can be applied to the skin lesion to prevent superadded bacterial infection.

Infectious epithelial keratitis: Antiviral agents like acyclovir 3 % ointment five times a day or ganciclovir 0.15 % gel five times a day or trifluridine drops 1 % nine times a day till infection heals are the primary treatment modality [6–10]. If the lesion does not respond to treatment by 2 weeks, then other causes need to be ruled out especially neurotrophic ulceration secondary to toxic medicamentosa. The other possibility is resistance to the antiviral, in which case shift from acyclovir or trifluridine that use viral thymidine kinase to get activated to a drug not using the same enzyme like vidarabine. Systemic antiviral acyclovir 400 mg five times a day can be used in certain situation in lieu of topical application especially in patient with ocular surface disease. Systemic acyclovir results in increased concentration of the drug inside the eye and even in the cornea and tear film.

Neurotrophic keratitis: Stop all offending medications and use artificial preservative-free lubricants. Bandage contact lens can be used to facilitate healing. Vitamin C and systemic doxycycline can help prevent corneal melts.

Necrotizing stromal keratitis: Topical antiviral frequency is similar to infective epithelial disease. Judiciously use topical steroids after starting antiviral to control the inflammatory responses.

Immune stromal keratitis: Topical steroids form the mainstay of treatment along with topical antiviral (dose for dose) to prevent an epithelial disease [6–10]. In some patients a very low dose of topical steroids might be required for a long time to control inflammation; in this respect the treatment is based on the concept of a flare dose of steroids (the minimum required to keen the disease in remission).

Endothelitis: Topical steroids and topical antiviral (dose for dose) along with systemic antiviral acyclovir 400 mg five times a day for a couple of weeks might be needed in severe diffuse endotheliitis and linear endotheliitis [6, 7].

The dosage of systemic acyclovir in active disease is 400 mg five times a day. As prophylaxis a maintenance dose of 400 mg BD is used to reduce the number or epithelial and stromal recurrences in patients with multiple recurrences and in post-keratoplasty state [11–16].

### Surgical Measures

Tectonic surgeries like amniotic membrane/patch grafts/full-thickness grafts/conjunctival flaps might be required for persistent epithelial defect and corneal melts. In certain situations, temporary/permanent tarsorrhaphy or botulinum toxin (Botox)-assisted ptosis may be attempted to facilitate healing.

In patients with significant corneal scarring causing loss of vision, penetrating keratoplasty or anterior lamellar keratoplasty can be attempted [17]. In select cases of failed high risk graft as seen in Fig. 37.10, Boston keratoprosthesis might help to restore vision [18].

## Herpes Zoster Infection

Introduction: varicella zoster virus (herpes type 3 virus) causes varicella or herpes zoster infection.

## Varicella

Varicella is due to primary infection with the virus and manifests as either congenital varicella syndrome due to intrauterine infection in first and

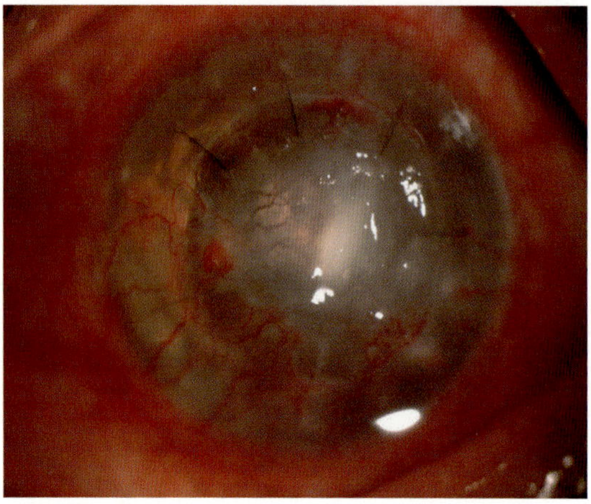

**Fig. 37.10** Failed graft with vascularization

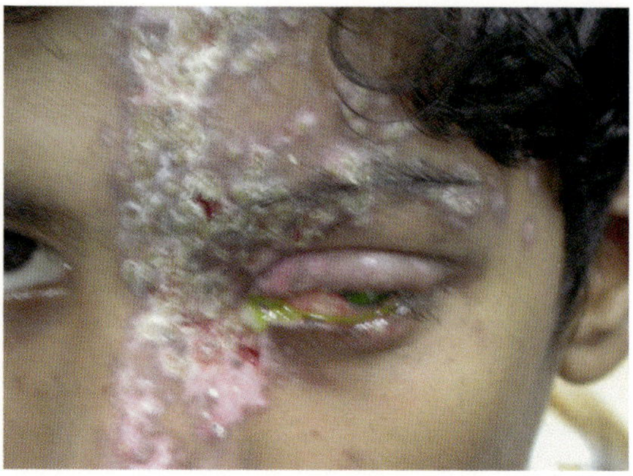

**Fig. 37.11** Hutchinson sign

second trimester or disseminated varicella with fever and maculopapular, vesicular rash on the skin that erupts in crops. Ophthalmic involvement is rare. Lid involvement is characterized by non-grouped vesicular lesions. The presence of lid lesions should prompt one to examine the conjunctiva for any ulcerations and cornea for superficial keratitis, dendritic figures, or disciform keratitis [18].

## Herpes Zoster

Herpes zoster is due to recurrence of varicella infection and is more often seen in elderly patients and in those with decreased cell-mediated immunity. This occurs due to viral replication at the dorsal root ganglion and its spread to the neuronal dermatome. In addition systemic viremia can cause involvement of organs other than those involved by the neuronal spread.

Involvement of the trigeminal ganglion results in ophthalmic involvement (herpes zoster ophthalmicus (HZO)). Ten to twenty percent zoster patients develop involvement of ophthalmic division, and 20–70 % of these develop HZO. The extensive ocular involvement of the eye is due to the involvement of the nasociliary branch of the frontal division of ophthalmic division of the trigeminal nerve [6, 7].

## Clinical Features

The patient can present with fever, malaise, and myalgia which may precede the development of the classical pruritic maculopapular, vesicular eruptions with tingling and pain. The vesicles follow a strict dermatomal distribution, are unilateral, do not cross the midline, and heal with scar formation. Involvement of tip of the nose increases likelihood of ophthalmic involvement and is called Hutchinson sign as shown in Fig. 37.11. Systemic viremia can cause pneumonitis, hepatitis, nephritis, and even central nervous system involvement.

Ophthalmic manifestation: Patients may present with redness, pain, decrease in vision, and photophobia. Lid involvement can occur in the form of edema and vesicular eruption which heals with scar formation resulting in ptosis as shown in Fig. 37.12; other findings are entropion, ectropion, lash loss, aberrant lashes, punctual and canalicular stenosis, lid retraction, and in rare cases necrosis with subsequent exposure keratitis. There can be follicular conjunctivitis, sectoral or nodular scleritis, and episcleritis. Corneal involvement is in the form of superficial punctate keratitis, pseudo dendrites, delayed mucus plaques, anterior stromal keratitis, disciform keratitis, interstitial keratitis, exposure keratitis, neurotrophic keratitis, and peripheral ulcerative keratitis. Hypoesthesia occurs in 60 % patients and can lead to non-healing epithelial defect with subsequent scaring and melt.

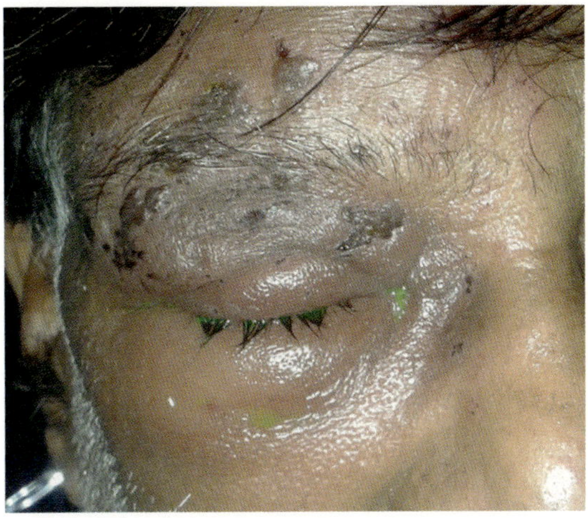

**Fig. 37.12** Herpes zoster skin lesions

Other manifestations are uveitis, sectoral iris atrophy, choroiditis, acute retina necrosis, optic neuritis, retrobulbar neuritis, cranial nerve palsies, and exophthalmos. The loss of vision can occur due to corneal complications, cataract, secondary glaucoma, retinitis, and optic neuritis sequelae.

Herpes sine herpete is the presence of features of herpes infection without the characteristic skin rash.

Post-herpetic neuralgia is a neuropathic condition with paresthesia/neuralgic pain persisting beyond 3 months of the infection [19–21].

## Treatment

Skin involvement: The patient needs to be started immediately on oral acyclovir 800 mg five times a day or valacyclovir 1 g three times a day for 7–10 days [22–24]. An antiseptic skin ointment can be applied to skin lesions to prevent superadded bacterial infections. Cold compress with saline or aluminum sulfate and calcium acetate solution improves patient comfort.

### Ophthalmic Manifestation

Conjunctivitis requires only symptomatic relief with lubricants in addition to the systemic antiviral the patient is on for the skin lesion.

Episcleritis and scleritis – Mild cases respond to lubricants, cycloplegics, or topical steroids. In severe cases systemic steroids or nonsteroidal anti-inflammatory agents might be required.

Keratitis – Topical antiviral like acyclovir ointment 3 % can be used for epithelial keratitis. For stromal or immune keratitis, topical steroids might be required. Neurotrophic keratitis is treated as elucidated for HSV keratitis.

Iritis/uveitis is treated with cycloplegics and topical steroids and anti-glaucoma medications as required.

Retinitis/choroiditis/optic neuritis are emergency situations and need intravenous acyclovir and oral steroids.

Post-herpetic neuralgia is difficult to treat. Local application like capsaicin can be tried; if it does not relieve the pain, systemic medications like tricyclic antidepressants or gabapentin in consultation with a neurologist can be given.

### Surgical Treatment

In case of HZO, surgical treatment is primarily for exposure keratitis or neurotrophic keratopathy. In either situation tarsorrhaphy will help the epithelium to heal. In case of loss of tissue due to necrosis, swinging flaps might be required.

Corneal thinning might need amniotic membrane transplant or conjunctival hooding or cyanoacrylate glue application. In case of corneal perforations, a tectonic keratoplasty might be required.

Visual rehabilitation might require a penetrating keratoplasty, but the success rate is limited by the anesthetic cornea. Recently Boston keratoprosthesis has also been used to restore vision in these patients with reasonable success [25, 26].

## References

1. Liesegang TJ, Melton III LJ, Dally PJ, Llstrup DM. Epidemiology of ocular herpes simplex. Incidence in Rochester Minn, 1950 through 1982. Arch Ophthalmol. 1989;107:1155–9.
2. Liesegang TJ, Melton III LJ, Dally PJ, Llstrup DM. Epidemiology of ocular herpes simplex. Natural

history in Rochester Minn, 1950 through 1982. Arch Ophthalmol. 1989;107:1160–5.
3. Pavan-Langston D, et al. In: Foster S, Azar D, Dohlman C, editors. Viral disease of the ocular anterior segment: basic science and clinical disease. Philadelphia: Lippincott, Williams & Wilkins; 2005. p. 297–397.
4. Egerer U-D, Stary A. Erosive-ulcerative herpes simplex blepharitis. Arch Ophthalmol. 1980;98:1760.
5. Foster Jr WJ, Kraus MD, Custer PL. Herpes simplex virus dacryoadenitis in an immunocompromised patient. Arch Ophthalmol. 2003;121:911–3.
6. Holland EJ, Schwartz GS, Neff KD. Herpes simplex keratitis chapter 79 In: Krachmer, Cornea 3rd edition, Elseiver 2011, Volume 1 chapter 79, 953–984.
7. Coepland Jr R, Afshari NA. Viral keratitis. Chapter 23 in principles and practice of Cornea. vol 1, 1st ed. 2013: p. 265–83.
8. Pavan-Langston D. In: Albert D, Jakobiec F, editors. Viral disease of the cornea and external eye. Philadelphia: WB Saunders; 2000. p. 846–93.
9. Barron BA, Gee L, Hauck WW, et al. Herpetic eye disease study. A controlled trial of oral acyclovir for herpes simplex stromal keratitis. Ophthalmology. 1994;101:1871–82.
10. HEDS. Oral acyclovir for herpes simplex virus eye disease. Effect on prevention of epithelial keratitis and stromal keratitis. Herpetic Eye Disease Study Group. Arch Ophthalmol. 2000;118:1030–6.
11. HEDS. A controlled trial of oral acyclovir for the prevention of stromal keratitis or iritis in patients with herpes simplex virus epithelial keratitis. The epithelial keratitis trial. The Herpetic Eye Disease Study Group. Arch Ophthalmol. 1997;115:703–12.
12. HEDS. Acyclovir for the prevention of recurrent herpes simplex virus eye disease. Herpetic Eye Disease Study Group. N Engl J Med. 1998;339:300–6.
13. Khan BF, Pavan-Langston D. Clinical manifestations and treatment modalities in herpes simplex virus of the ocular anterior segment. Int Ophthalmol Clin. 2004;44:103–33.
14. Simon AL, Pavan-Langston D. Long-term oral acyclovir therapy. Effect on recurrent infectious herpes simplex keratitis in patients with and without grafts. Ophthalmology. 1996;103:1399–405.
15. van Rooij J, Rijneveld WJ, Remeijer L, et al. Effect of oral acyclovir after penetrating keratoplasty for herpetic keratitis: a placebo controlled multicenter trial. Ophthalmology. 2003;110:1916.
16. Scott G, Stones DU, James C. Evidence-based treatment of herpes simplex virus keratitis: a systematic review. Ocul Surf. 2007;5(3):240–50.
17. Langston RH, Pavan-Langston D. Penetrating keratoplasty for herpetic keratitis: decision-making and management. Int Ophthalmol Clin. 1975;15:125–40.
18. Kahn B, Aqualvella J, Harissi-Dagher M, et al. The Boston keratoprosthesis in herpetic keratitis. Arch Ophthlamol. 2007;125:745–9. Wilson FI. In: Tabbara K, Hyndiuk R, editors. Varicella and Herpes zoster ophthalmicus. Boston: Little, Brown; 1996. p. 387–400.
19. Liesegang TJ. Herpes zoster ophthalmicus. Natural history, risk factors, clinical presentation, and morbidity. Ophthalmology. 2008;115:S3–12.
20. Liesegang TJ. Diagnosis and therapy of herpes zoster ophthalmicus. Ophthalmology. 1991;98:1216–29.
21. Lee WB, Liesegang TJ. Herpes zoster keratitis. In: Krachmer, Cornea 3rd edition, Elseiver 2011: Volume 1, chapter 80, 985–1000.
22. Herbort CP. Acyclovir in herpes zoster ophthalmicus. Br J Ophthalmol. 1991;75(9):542–6.
23. Hoang-Xuan T, Büchi ER, Herbort CP, Denis J, Frot P, Thénault S, Pouliquen Y. Oral acyclovir for herpes zoster ophthalmicus. Ophthalmology. 1992;99(7):1062–70.
24. Colin J, Prisant O, Cochener B, Lescale O, Rolland B, Hoang-Xuan T. Comparison of the efficacy and safety of valaciclovir and acyclovir for the treatment of herpes zoster ophthalmicus. Ophthalmology. 2000;107(8):1507–11.
25. Soong HK, Schwartz AE, Meyer RF, Sugar A. Penetrating keratoplasty for corneal scarring due to herpes zoster ophthalmicus. Br J Ophthalmol. 1989;73:19–21.
26. Pavan-Langston D, Dohman CH. Boston keratoprosthesis treatment of herpes zoster neurotrophic keratopathy. Ophthalmology. 2008;115:S21–3.

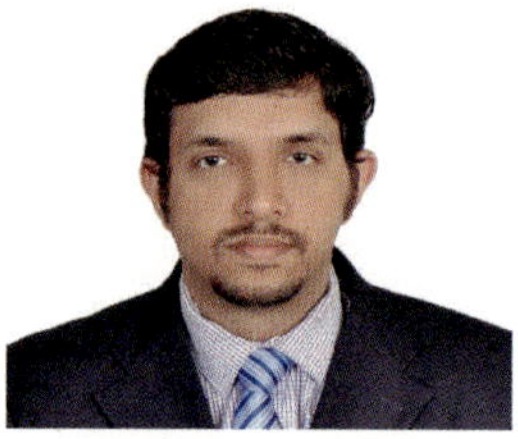

**Bhaskar Srinivasan** Dr. Bhaskar Srinivasan finished his graduation from Topiwala National Medical College, Mumbai, in 1997 and his masters in Ophthalmology (MS Ophthalmology) from Armed Forces Medical College, Pune, in 2002. He did his fellowship in cornea and external eye disease at Sankara Nethralaya, Chennai, following which he joined the same as faculty and is currently Senior Consultant Cornea and Refractive Services. His special interest is in managing various ocular surface diseases especially treating chemical injuries and Stevens–Johnson syndrome. He has experience with different kinds of keratoprosthesis and is a part of the ocular surface clinic at Sankara Nethralaya, a one of its kind in the world dealing with both ocular surface stem cell and various keratoprosthesis-based treatments. He is well versed in various kinds of corneal transplants (PK/DSEK/DALK), refractive surgery, and management of ocular surface tumors. He has 30 publications in peer-reviewed literature and has served as a faculty in various national and international conferences.

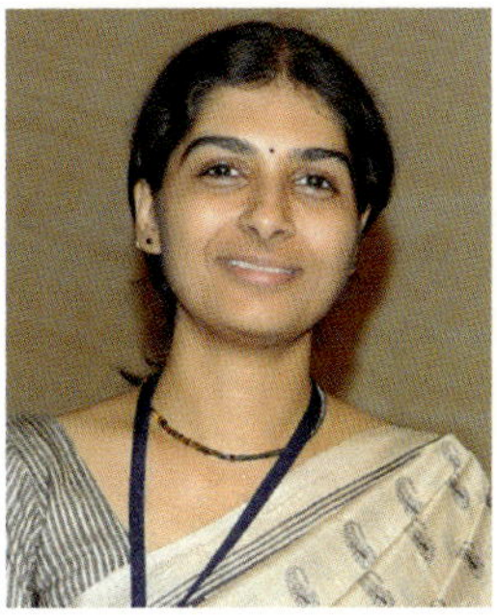

**Geetha Iyer** Dr. Geetha Iyer, FRCS (Glasgow), completed her basic medical training in 1999. She did her postgraduate training in Ophthalmology and fellowship in cornea and external disease from Sankara Nethralaya, Chennai, India. She was awarded the best postgraduate student following completion of her ophthalmology training at Sankara Nethralaya and has been adjudged twice as the Best Associate Consultant during the early years of her tenure. She has been the recipient of awards for the Best Cornea Paper at both regional and national conferences. She has done a short-term observership in Ocular Surface Disorders with Dr. Scheffer C G Tseng, Miami, USA, in October 2006 and in Boston Type 1 keratoprosthesis with Dr. Claes H Dohlman in November 2006. She was trained and is being guided by Prof. Giancarlo Falcinelli in performing the MOOKP procedure. She has so far done more than 100 keratoprosthesis surgeries (MOOKP, Boston Type 1 and 2 Kpro).

Dr. Geetha Iyer has to her credit publications in peer-reviewed journals and has conducted courses and presented papers in national and international meetings. She is actively involved in the management of ocular surface disorders and is currently working as Senior Consultant at the Ocular Surface Clinic and the Cornea Services, Sankara Nethralaya. Her areas of interest include pediatric penetrating keratoplasty, ocular surface tumors, ocular surface disorders including chemical injuries, stem cell transplants, keratoprosthesis, and in particular Stevens–Johnson Syndrome.

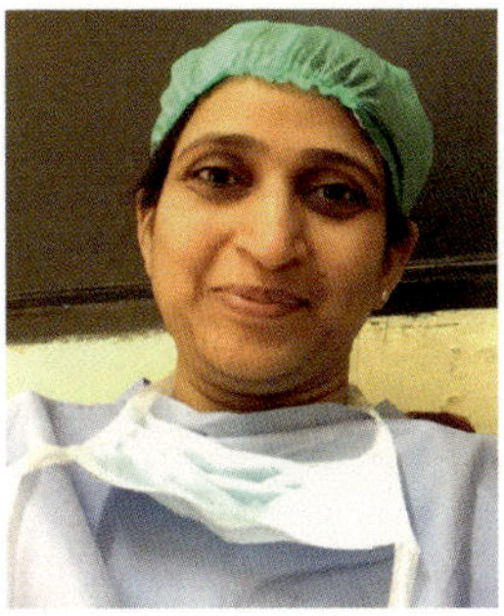

**Mamta Agarwal** Dr. Mamta Agarwal completed her medical graduate degree from Government Medical College, Amritsar, India, in 1996. She passed Diplomate in National Board of Examination (DNB) at Sankara Nethralaya, Chennai, in 2002. She specialized in uveitis and intraocular inflammation at Medical Research Foundation, Sankara Nethralaya, Chennai (2002–2004). Further, she pursued an international fellowship in 'Cornea, external diseases and uveitis' at Francis I. Proctor Foundation, University of California, San Francisco, USA (2010–2011). She currently works as a Senior Consultant in Uveitis and Cornea services at Medical Research Foundation, Chennai. She has presented several papers at national and international conferences. She was also a grant winner for IUSG 2009 Venice course in Uveitis. She has authored Atlas of Uveitis and Scleritis published in 2005. She is a member of All India Ophthalmological Society, Uveitis Society of India, Cornea Society of India, American Uveitis Society (AUS), and Intraocular inflammation Society (IOIS). Her areas of interest include management of uveitis, scleritis, corneal infections, and ocular surface diseases.

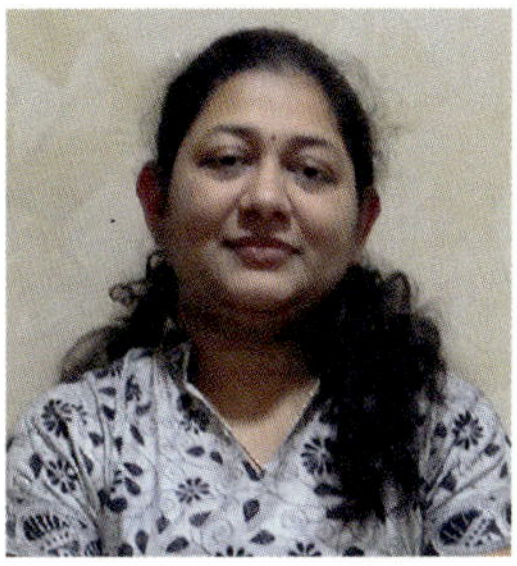

**Shweta Agarwal** Dr. Shweta Agarwal, D.O, a gold medalist from Pune university, completed her cornea fellowship from Sankara Nethralaya Chennai in 2009. She was awarded the Dr. D.S.Sardesai ophthalmology award from Pune university. She has quite a few publications in national and international journals and also a chapter on dry eyes in post graduate textbook of ophthalmology. She has been a primary investigator in two studies and a co-investigator in many studies related to cornea and ocular surface disorders funded by national agencies. She has been invited as a faculty in several national and international conferences. She was awarded the Best Cornea Free Paper in AIOC 2012. Her areas of interest are corneal diseases, ocular surface disorders, stem cells, and keratoprosthesis.

# Dacryoadenitis

# 38

Gangadhara Sundar

## Introduction

Inflammation of the lacrimal gland is a relatively common orbital inflammatory disorder, both in children and adults. Like in most clinical inflammatory syndromes, differentiation between an infectious and noninfectious etiology is important as both the treatment and the prognosis depend on the same. We shall herewith cover the various aspects of diagnostic and therapeutic challenges in the management of dacryoadenitis.

## Definition

Dacryoadenitis is any acute, subacute, or chronic inflammatory condition of the lacrimal gland [1]. While it is commonly attributed to the main lacrimal gland, the accessory lacrimal glands may also be affected. Inflammations may be either of infectious or noninfectious etiology, and when both have been ruled out, infiltrative and masquerade syndromes have to be considered.

## Applied Anatomy

The lacrimal secretory system is comprised of the main and accessory lacrimal glands. Rarely, ectopic cell rests of the lacrimal gland may also be present which may be a source of lacrimal secretory pathology. The main lacrimal gland is an almond-shaped structure resting in the lacrimal gland fossa of the frontal bone along the superotemporal quadrant of the orbit behind the orbital rim [2]. The palpebral lobe extends anteriorly towards the upper and outer quadrant of the upper eyelid and separated from the orbital lobe by the lateral horn of the aponeurosis of the levator palpebrae superioris. The main lacrimal gland drains into the superotemporal and lateral fornix through 10–15 ductules, which can be identified on slit-lamp examination. The accessory lacrimal glands are mainly comprised of the glands of Krause and Wolfring. The glands of Krause are present primarily along the superior fornix (approximately 42 in number) and minimally along the inferior fornix (around eight), draining directly into the fornices mainly laterally. The glands of Wolfring are present along the superior and inferior tarsal margins (5–10). Accessory lacrimal glands may also be present in the caruncle and the lateral forniceal areas.

G. Sundar, DO, FRCSEd, FAMS, AB Ophth(USA)
Department of Ophthalmology, National University of Singapore Head and Senior Consultant, Orbit and Oculofacial Surgery, 119228, Singapore

Department of Ophthalmology, National University Hospital, 119228, Singapore
e-mail: gsundar1@yahoo.com, Gangadhara_sundar@nuhs.edu.sg


B. Mukherjee, H. Yuen (eds.), *Emergencies of the Orbit and Adnexa*, DOI 10.1007/978-81-322-1807-4_38

## Etiology and Classification

Most inflammatory conditions of the lacrimal gland are either of viral etiology or of nonspecific etiology [3]. Acute suppurative infection of the lacrimal gland is rare and, when present, should prompt a search for an underlying systemic etiology, significant systemic immunocompromise, or in endemic areas tuberculosis as well. Isolated fungal infections are extremely rare and may be seen only in the immunocompromised patients. Parasitic infestations are not uncommon in endemic areas, the most common being cysticercosis and rarely hydatidosis. When infectious etiologies are presumed less likely or have been ruled out, noninfectious causes of lacrimal gland inflammation should be considered. As a general rule, all noninfectious inflammations of the lacrimal gland are of "specific" etiology until proven otherwise. When chronic or recurrent dacryoadenitis is present, either unilateral or bilateral, a tissue diagnosis is often useful especially in ruling out lymphoproliferative disorders and other rare pathologic entities.

An outline of the various etiologies is shown in Table 38.1.

## Clinical Presentation

Viral dacryoadenitis presents typically in a child or young adult [5] with either a unilateral or bilateral acute onset of swelling, redness, and induration with pain on palpation over the upper outer eyelid (Fig. 38.1). Fever, malaise, or other constitutional signs and symptoms from systemic viral infection may be present. Although symptoms may be unilateral, not infrequently patients may have bilateral features either clinically or radiologically. Overlying preseptal swelling and underlying orbital signs of limitation of ocular motility and chemosis with mucoid discharge may be present. In the pre-MMR (Measles, Mumps, Rubella) universal vaccination era, associated features of parotitis were not uncommon

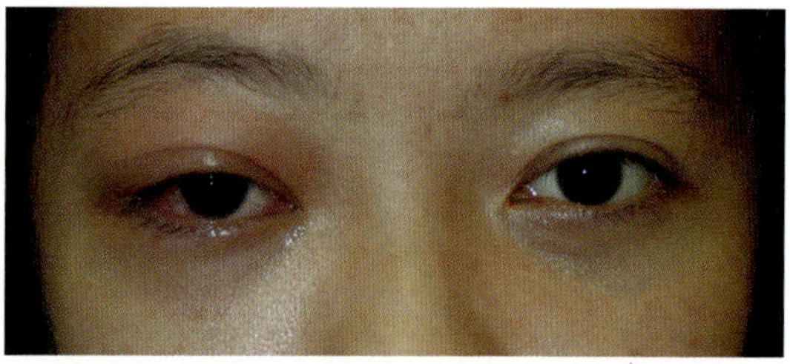

**Fig. 38.1** Typical presentation of viral dacryoadenitis in a young adult

**Table 38.1** Etiological classification of dacryoadenitis

| Infectious | Noninfectious | Masquerades |
|---|---|---|
| Viral, e.g., mumps, EBV (Epstein-Barr Virus), infectious mononucleosis [4–8] | Thyroid eye disease [16] | Lymphoproliferative disorders [29] |
| Bacterial, e.g., staphylococcus [9], streptococcus, gonococcus, Lyme disease [10], mycobacterial – typical and atypical [11–13] | IgG 4-related disease [17, 18] | Malignant lacrimal gland tumors, e.g., adenoid cystic carcinoma, mucoepidermoid carcinoma |
| Fungal | Sarcoidosis [19] | Metastasis |
| Parasitic, e.g., cysticercosis [14], hydatidosis, schistosomiasis | Autoimmune disorders: Sjogren's syndrome [20], systemic lupus erythematosus [21] | |
| Protozoan, e.g., acanthamoeba [15] | ANCA-associated vasculitides: granulomatosis with polyangiitis (Wegener's) [22], polyarteritis nodosa, Crohn's disease [23–26], Churg-Strauss syndrome [27, 28], etc. | |
| | Nonspecific orbital inflammatory syndrome (idiopathic dacryoadenitis) | |

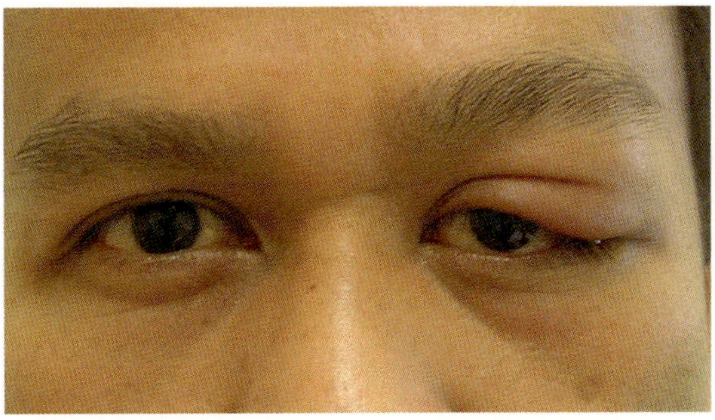

**Fig. 38.2** Bacterial dacryoadenitis of the left orbit

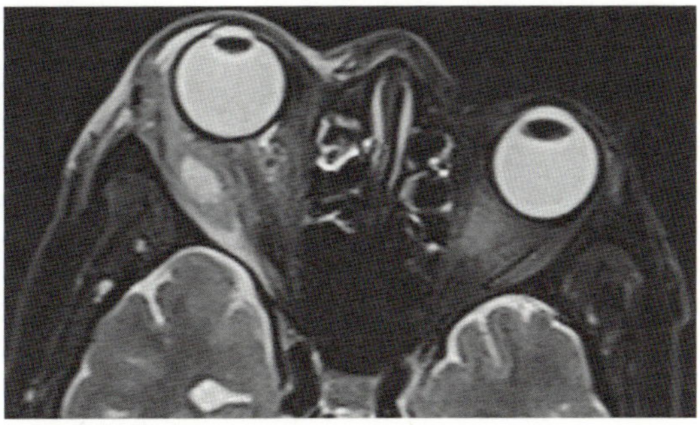

**Fig. 38.3** T2-weighted MR image showing cysticercosis of the right lacrimal gland

pointing towards mumps virus as a possible etiological agent.

Bacterial dacryoadenitis may have a similar presentation but usually unilateral with much more severe pain, chemosis, and limitation of ocular motility (Fig. 38.2). Commonly caused by staphylococcus aureus or streptococcus, the typical patient is an elderly or immunocompromised patient with systemic bacteremia as the infection is often endogenous. More commonly, spread from an overlying preseptal cellulitis (scratch wound infections or hordeolum internum or externum) may occur in immunocompetent children and young adults. A high degree of suspicion for atypical infections including tuberculosis (typical or atypical mycobacteria) should be considered in subacute and in high-risk cases. Rarely, they may progress towards an abscess formation [30] with a throbbing sensation, mass effect, and loculation seen on orbital imaging.

Parasitic infestations are not uncommon in the South Asian, African, and South American continents where they may be endemic. Cysticercosis is one of the most common orbital inflammatory diseases which may present as a dacryoadenitis, and usually unilateral (Fig. 38.3). It is only upon clinical suspicion, serological testing, and typical findings of a localized inflammation with a central cystic space and a scolex when present that helps clinch a diagnosis [31]. Hydatidosis may present as large multiloculated thick-walled cystic lesions involving any part of the orbit and has classic radiological features with absent systemic disease.

By far, the most common of all noninfectious inflammatory lesions of the lacrimal gland are "nonspecific dacryoadenitis" and often form a distinct subsect of nonspecific orbital inflammatory syndromes (NSOIS), previously termed "pseudotumor" or "idiopathic dacryoadenitis" [32]. However, they are diagnoses of exclusion, only after a complete workup for possible underlying systemic autoimmune and vasculitic disorders has been ruled out. Whenever possible a tissue diagnosis should be performed to confirm the diagnosis. Nonspecific dacryoadenitis may present in all age groups (Fig. 38.4a, b) and may be either unilateral or bilateral, typically with pain and the absence of systemic signs of either bacterial or viral infection. Not infrequently they may present as recurrent dacryoadenitis or a chronic inflammatory lesion with or without a mass effect. More commonly they are diagnosed based on limited or poor response to conventional treatment with antibiotics or anti-inflammatory agents and a dramatic response to systemic corticosteroids.

Lymphoproliferative disorders may also present as "nonspecific" inflammation, with recurrent attacks of unilateral or bilateral swelling in the region of the lacrimal gland [33] (Fig. 38.5a–c). Hence all patients presenting with dacryoadenitis or orbital inflammatory disease should be presumed to have a specific inflammatory or infiltrative pathology until proven otherwise. Such patients may also have regional or systemic lymphadenopathy which may raise level of suspicion.

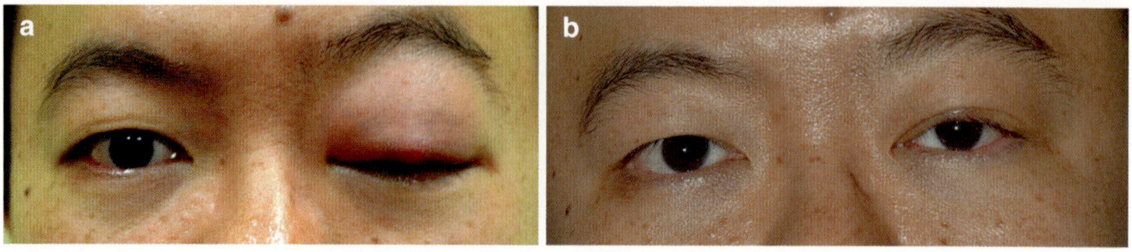


**Fig. 38.4** (a) Idiopathic dacryoadenitis pretreatment. (b) Idiopathic dacryoadenitis post-treatment

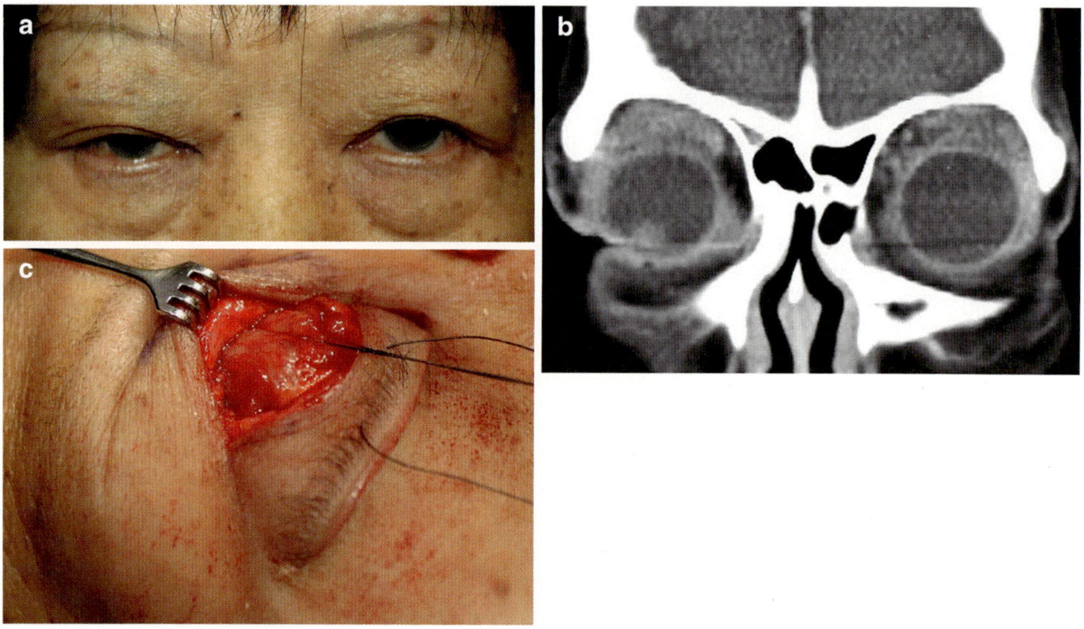


**Fig. 38.5** (a) Bilateral lacrimal gland enlargement from B-cell lymphoma in a patient referred for ptosis correction. (b) Bilateral lacrimal gland enlargement on CT scan. (c) Lacrimal gland biopsy

## Differential Diagnosis

Common differential diagnosis include the following:

Preseptal cellulitis secondary to underlying hordeolum internum (acute meibomitis) or hordeolum externum (stye)
Early orbital cellulitis
Myositis
Ruptured dermoid cyst
Thyroid eye disease
Lymphoproliferative disorder
Primary lacrimal gland neoplasms: pleomorphic adenoma [34], adenoid cystic carcinoma, mucoepidermoid carcinoma, and ductal carcinoma (Fig. 38.6a, b)
Metastasis

## Investigations

Diagnosis of dacryoadenitis is essentially based on a high level of clinical suspicion based on the history, review of systemic symptoms, and clini-

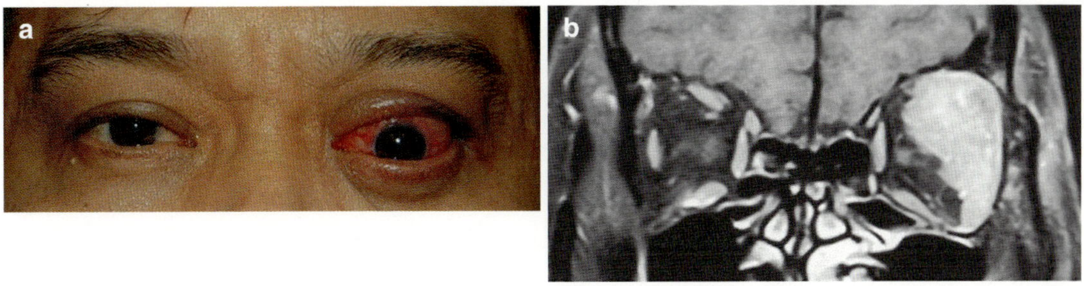


**Fig. 38.6** (**a**) Ductal carcinoma of lacrimal gland simulating dacryoadenitis and orbital inflammation. (**b**) Coronal MRI showing enhancing lesion of the left lacrimal gland

cal examination. Investigations are performed either to confirm or rule out the possible diagnosis and other differential diagnosis as listed above.

**Laboratory investigations**: A conjunctival swab of the discharge may help with early detection of bacterial infection and thus direct specific treatment. Bacterial sensitivity for antibiotic resistance may be important. Basic tests should include a complete blood count, erythrocyte sedimentation rate (ESR), C-reactive protein (CRP), syphilitic titres (VDRL, TPHA), chest x-ray (TB, sarcoidosis, etc.), and Mantoux testing. When bacterial dacryoadenitis is suspected especially with systemic symptoms, a blood culture with sensitivity to antibiotics [35] may also be useful. When parasitic infestations are suspected, anti-cysticercosis antibodies may complement imaging findings.

When a noninfectious etiology is suspected, a complete inflammatory workup is often indicated. Based on level of suspicion of underlying specific autoimmune vasculitic disorders, the following investigations may be considered: rheumatoid factor (RF), anti-nuclear antibody (ANA), Sjogren's antibody testing (anti-SS-A and anti-SS-B, as a part of an extractable nuclear antibodies (ENA) panel), anti-alpha-fodrin antibody (in juvenile Sjogren's syndrome), anti-neutrophilic cytoplasmic antibody (ANCA), and anti-proteinase 3 (anti-PR3 antibodies). Tests for sarcoidosis include serum amyloid A (SAA), soluble interleukin-2 receptor (sIL-2R), lysozyme, angiotensin-converting enzyme (ACE), and glycoprotein KL-6.

Associated comorbidities including systemic hypertension, diabetes mellitus, and other immunosuppressive disorders like HIV infections should be ruled out as well when suspected.

## Imaging

Orbital imaging should be performed in all patients, partly to confirm the diagnosis, to identify bilaterality, and more importantly to rule out space occupying lesions, masquerade syndromes, and associated pathology of adjacent tissue spaces (paranasal sinuses, intracranial cavity, overlying temporal bone).

Ultrasound examination of the orbit may be useful when cysticercosis is suspected and serial imaging is performed following medical treatment. However, given its limitations of technician dependence, inability to compare with contralateral orbit, and inability to visualize structures closer to the bone and apex of the orbit, it has a limited role in most patients.

The investigation of choice for most patients is a computed tomography (CT) of the orbits and face, with contrast enhancement [36, 37]. Advantages of a CT scan include easy accessibility, low cost, a short image acquisition time, and ability to identify calcification. More importantly, as orbital fat acts as a natural contrast, the lacrimal gland, extraocular muscles, and the overlying bone can be studied well with and without contrast. Axial, coronal, and sagittal images with soft tissue and bone windows should be thoroughly studied. Radiological features typically seen include a well-delineated or poorly delineated enlargement of the lacrimal gland (Fig. 38.7a, b), enhanced with contrast.

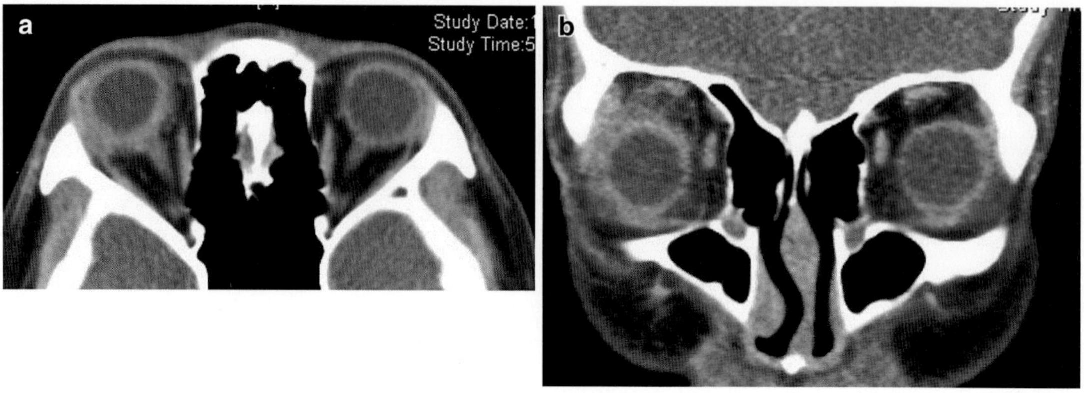


**Fig. 38.7** (**a**) Axial CT showing lacrimal gland enlargement with adjacent orbital inflammation. (**b**) Coronal CT showing lacrimal gland enlargement with adjacent tissue involvement

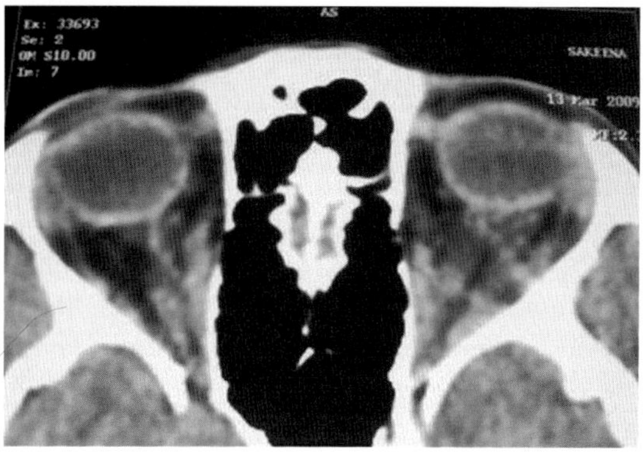

**Fig. 38.8** Orbital fat infiltration on CT scan

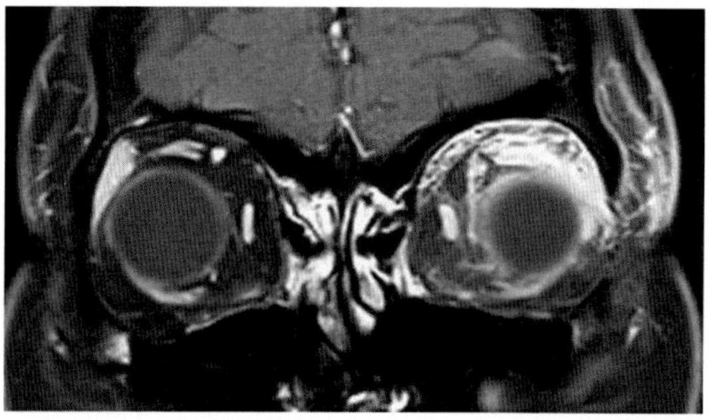

**Fig. 38.9** Coronal MRI showing infiltrative lesion of the left lacrimal gland

Underlying lateral rectus and overlying eyelid and temporal tissue may also enhance. Not infrequently bilateral lacrimal gland enlargement may be seen. Caution should be exercised in interpreting a prolapsed lacrimal gland as enlarged lacrimal gland. Other radiological signs may include "feathering or fat stranding" of the orbital soft tissues (Fig. 38.8), loculation within the lacrimal gland, and lacrimal ductal cyst or dacryops.

Other pathologic entities should be suspected when any of the following signs are present: indentation or erosion of the overlying frontal bone, calcification, radiolucency (foreign body), cystic lesion with central scolex, diffuse orbital fat infiltration, enlarged extraocular muscles beyond the lateral rectus, and other infiltrative lesions within the orbit, intracranial cavity, or paranasal sinuses.

An MRI may also be useful when isolated soft tissue pathology is suspected (Fig. 38.9), e.g., lymphoproliferative disorders, metastasis, or when repeated imaging is indicated. MRI may however miss calcification and early bony erosion or result in poor images secondary to motion artifacts.

An incisional biopsy (Fig. 38.10a, b) may be considered when all investigations are noncontributory, or the patient's condition is only partly or completely unresponsive to medical management to aid identify a "specific" inflammatory or neoplastic etiology.

## Management

Management of the patient is dependent upon the specific diagnosis.

When viral dacryoadenitis is suspected, symptomatic anti-inflammatory treatment with

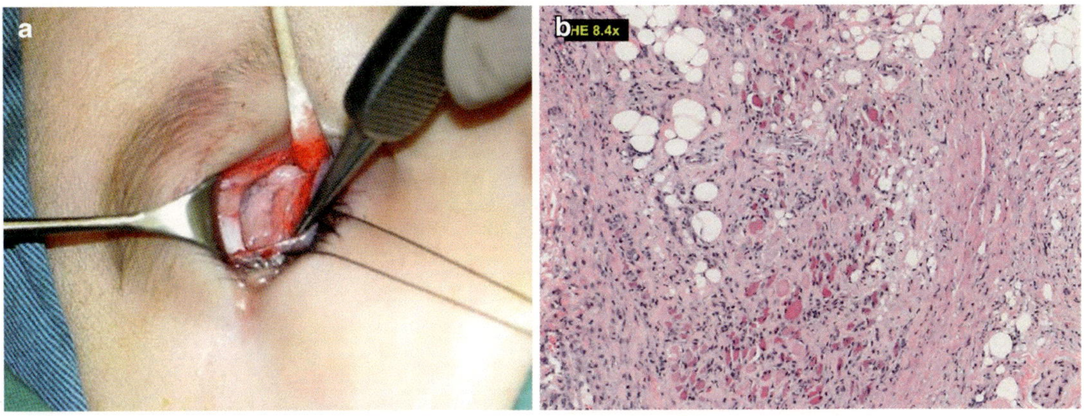


**Fig. 38.10** (**a**) Lacrimal gland biopsy through upper eyelid crease incision – intraoperative view. (**b**) Histopathology of lacrimal gland showing patchy fibrosis with acute or chronic inflammation

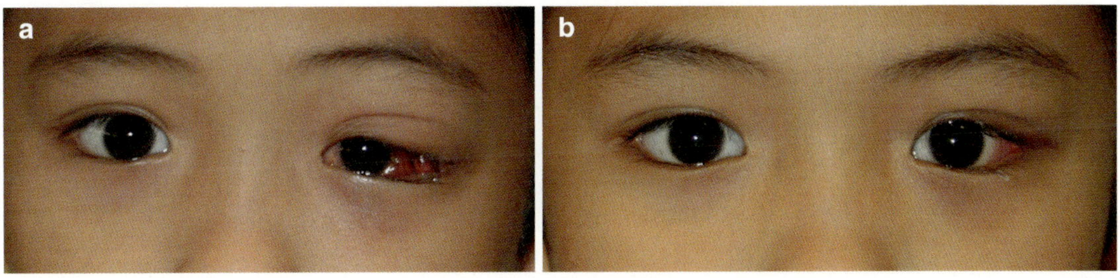


**Fig. 38.11** (**a**) Viral dacryoadenitis pretreatment. (**b**) Viral dacryoadenitis post-treatment

non steroidals may be all that is indicated [4]. Most patients show dramatic response within 24–48 h (Fig. 38.11a, b) and may not require long-term follow-up.

When bacterial dacryoadenitis is suspected, systemic antibiotics should be commenced. While healthy patiens may be followed up closely as outpatients, those with significant comorbidities or vision threatening inflammation should receive parenteral antibiotics and monitored as an inpatient. A broad-spectrum antibiotic (amoxicillin-clavulanate) is often useful along with anti-inflammatory medications. Associated bacterial conjunctivitis may be treated with topical antibiotics.

When cysticercosis is suspected based on epidemiology, clinical presentation, and radiologic features, oral albendazole (15 mg/kg/day in two divided doses for 3–7 days) or praziquantel with or without oral corticosteroids should be started [38, 39]. Monitoring response to treatment with complete course of treatment is warranted. Neuroimaging should be performed to rule out intracranial lesions prior to definitive anti-cysticercosis treatment to anticipate and prevent life-threatening seizures.

Hydatid cysts of the orbit often require a lateral orbitotomy with complete surgical removal of the cysts.

Tuberculosis is commonly a systemic disease that is increasingly globally prevalent especially in endemic geographic areas, sometimes seen in patients with chronic immunosuppressive disorders and other conditions requiring immunosuppressant treatment. Following high clinical suspicion supported by tissue culture (Fig. 38.12a, b), antituberculous therapy with multidrug therapy is warranted [11] in consultation with an infectious disease specialist. Multidrug resistant tuberculosis should be kept in mind, and sensitivities may help direct specific treatment regimen.

As stated earlier, all non infectious dacryoadenitis should be considered to be of "specific" etiology

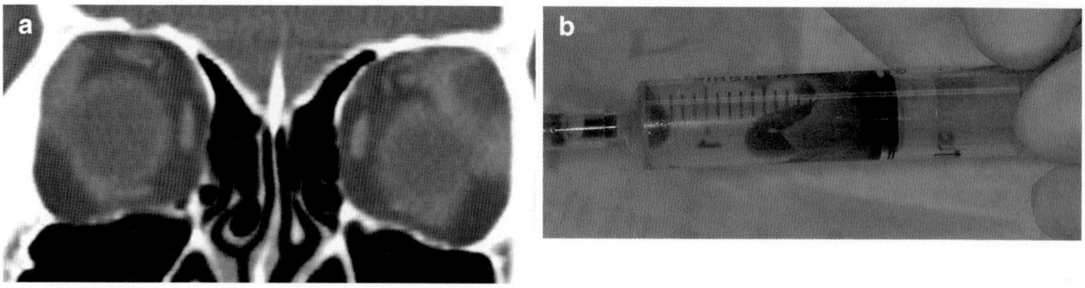

Fig. 38.12 (a) Tuberculous dacryoadenitis with abscess. (b) Abscess aspirate

until proven otherwise. If laboratory investigations are supportive of a specific clinical diagnosis, e.g., granulomatosis with polyangiitis (Wegener's), Sjogren's syndrome, and thyroid orbitopathy, specific treatment should be aimed at the primary condition. Whenever possible, an incisional biopsy of the lacrimal gland [40] should be considered in all such cases, unless contraindicated. Relative contraindications for biopsy include unwilling patients or parents of children and severe systemic comorbidity precluding sedation or general anesthesia.

Principles of management of nonspecific orbital inflammatory syndromes are outlined below. In general keep a low threshold for incisional biopsy [41, 42]. Once specific conditions are ruled out, systemic corticosteroids are the initial modality of treatment. When refractory or if disease recurs following tapering of steroids, steroid-sparing disease-modifying anti-rheumatic drugs (DMARDs), targeted anti-B-cell therapy (rituximab), and, in extreme cases, surgical excision of a localized inflammation [43] or even radiation may be indicated.

Specific conditions when tissue diagnosis is useful include the spectrum of lymphoproliferative disorders (reactive lymphoid hyperplasia, atypical lymphoid hyperplasia, and lymphoma), primary lacrimal gland neoplasms, metastatic disease, and IgG4-related dacryoadenitis. While the treatment for the above conditions are directed at the underlying condition based on systemic evaluation [44], IgG4 related inflammation may require systemic symptomatic treatment with or without steroids with need for long-term follow-up for evolution towards lymphoma.

## Summary

Dacryoadenitis is a common condition that should be considered as a differential diagnosis in all orbital inflammatory disorders. Both infectious and noninfectious etiologies should be considered, as should masquerade syndromes when a low threshold for incisional biopsy is indicated. After ruling out related systemic conditions, specific treatment approaches based on the underlying condition are recommended.

## References

1. Kanski JJ. Acute dacryoadenitis. In: Clinical ophthalmology. A systematic approach. 6th ed. Butterworth-Heineman, Elsevier; 2008. p. 178–9.
2. Bron AJ, Tripathi RC, Tripathi BJ. Wolff's anatomy of the eye and orbit. 8th ed. London: Chapman & Hall Medical; 1997.
3. Bosniak S. Principles and practice of ophthalmic plastic and reconstructive surgery, vol. II. Philadelphia: WB Saunders Company; 1996.
4. Galpine JF, Waikowski J. A case of mumps with involvement of the lacrimal glands. Br Med J. 1952; 1(4767):1069–70.
5. Rhem MN, Wilhelmus KR, Jones DB. Epstein-Barr virus dacryoadenitis. Am J Ophthalmol. 2000;129: 372–5.
6. Foster Jr WJ, Kraus MD, Custer PL. Herpes simplex virus dacryoadenitis in an immunocompromised patient. Arch Ophthalmol. 2003;121:911–3.
7. Obata H, Yamagami S, Saito S, et al. A case of acute dacryoadenitis associated with herpes zoster ophthalmicus. Jpn J Ophthalmol. 2003;47:107–9.
8. Aburn NS, Sullivan TJ. Infectious mononucleosis presenting with dacryoadenitis. Ophthalmology. 1996; 103:776–8.
9. Goold LA, Madge SN, Au A, Leibovitch I, McNab A, Tumuluri K, Selva D. Acute suppurative bacterial

dacryoadenitis: a case series. Br J Ophthalmol. 2013;97(6):735–8.
10. Nieto JC, Kim N, Lucarelli MJ. Dacryoadenitis and orbital myositis associated with Lyme disease. Arch Ophthalmol. 2008;126:1165–6.
11. Bansal RK, Malhotra C, Bhatia R, Chhabra S, Sood S. Tubercular dacryoadenitis – a case report and review of literature. Indian J Pathol Microbiol. 2006;49(3):385–7.
12. Chakraborti C, Biswas R, Mondal M, Mukhopadhya U, Datta J. Tuberculous dacryoadenitis in a child. Nepal J Ophthalmol. 2011;3(2):210–3.
13. Sen DK. Tuberculosis of the orbit and lacrimal gland. A clinical study of 14 cases. J Pediatr Ophthalmol Strabismus. 1980;17(4):232–8.
14. Sen DK. Acute suppurative dacryoadenitis caused by cysticercosis cellulosae. J Pediatr Ophthalmol Strabismus. 1982;19(2):100–2.
15. Tomita M, Shimmura S, Tsubota K, Shimazaki J. Dacryoadenitis associated with Acanthamoeba keratitis. Arch Ophthalmol. 2006;124(9):1239–42.
16. Safonova TN, Likhvantseva VG, Kuz'min KA, Gontiurova OA, Rudenko EI. Morphological changes in autoimmune dacryoadenitis associated with thyroid eye disease. Vestn Oftalmol. 2012;128(6):15–9.
17. Lee FJ, Varikatt W, Kairaitis K, D'Souza F, Lin MW. IgG4-related dacryoadenitis. Ophthalmology. 2010;117(2):398.e3–4.
18. Kakuchi Y, Yamada K, Suzuki Y, et al. IgG4-related skin lesions in a patient with IgG4-related chronic sclerosing dacryoadenitis and sialoadenitis. Intern Med. 2011;50(14):1465–9.
19. Gutman J, Shinder R. Orbital and adnexal involvement in sarcoidosis: analysis of clinical features and systemic disease in 30 cases. Am J Ophthalmol. 2011;152(5):883.
20. Parkin B, et al. Lymphocytic infiltration and enlargement of lacrimal glands. A new subtype of primary Sjogren's syndrome? Ophthalmology. 2005;112: 2040–7.
21. Al-Busaidi T, Wali U, Al-Shirawi A, Al-Mujaini. Dacryoadenitis as first presenting feature in systemic lupus erythematosus. Lupus. 2013;22(13):1431–2.
22. Kirati H, Sekerogly A, Soylemezoglu F. Unilateral dacryoadenitis as the sole presenting signs of Wegener's Granulomatosis. Orbit. 2008;27(3):157–60.
23. Wong JC, Rossman D, Bressler B. Dacryoadenitis, an extra-intestinal manifestation of Crohn's disease. Am J Gastroenterol. 2010;105(8):1904–6.
24. Dutt S, Cartwright MJ, Nelson CC. Acute dacryoadenitis and Crohn's disease. Findings and management. Ophthal Plast Reconstr Surg. 1992;8:295–9.
25. Hwang IP, Jordan DR, Acharya V. Lacrimal gland inflammation as the presenting sign of Crohn's disease. Can J Ophthalmol. 2001;36:212–3.
26. Boukouvala S, Giakoup-Oglou I, Puvanachandra N, Burton BJ. Sequential right then left acute dacryoadenitis in Crohn's disease. BMJ Case Rep. 2012;9:2012.
27. Khandwala MA, Vayalambrone D, Ong J, Beigi B. Dacryoadenitis as a presenting feature of the Churg-Strauss syndrome. Eye (Lond). 2010;24(2):385–6. doi:10.1038/eye.2009.109. Epub 2009 May 15.
28. Jordan N, Verma H, Ekbote A, Sangle S, D'Cruz D. Dacryoadenitis and diffuse orbital inflammation: unusual first presentations of Churg-Strauss syndrome. Orbit. 2011;30(3):160–1.
29. Amin S, Ramsay A. Orbital and lacrimal gland progressive transformation of germinal centres – an underdiagnosed entity? Br J Ophthalmol. 2012;96(9): 1242–5.
30. Harris GJ, Snyder TW. Lacrimal gland abscess. Am J Ophthalmol. 1987;104:193–4.
31. Pushker N, Bajaj MS, Betharia SM. Orbital and adnexal cysticercosis. Clin Experiment Ophthalmol. 2002;30(5):322–33.
32. Bijlsma WR, Van't Hullenaar FC, Mourits MP, Kalmann R. Evaluation of classification systems for nonspecific idiopathic orbital inflammation. Orbit. 2012;31(4):238–45.
33. Rasmussen P, Ralfkiaer E, Prause JU, et al. Malignant lymphoma of the lacrimal gland: a nation based study. Arch Ophthalmol. 2011;129(10):1275–80.
34. Halhal M, Meyer A, Morel X, et al. Pleomorphic adenoma mimicking dacryoadenitis. J Fr Ophthalmol. 2004;27(10):1200–3.
35. Kubal A, Garibaldi DC. Dacryoadenitis caused by methicillin-resistant Staphylococcus aureus. Ophtalmol Plast Reconstr Surg. 2008;24(1):50–1.
36. Jakobiec FA, et al. Combined clinical and computed tomographic diagnosis of primary lacrimal fossa lesions. Am J Ophthalmol. 1982;94:785–807. 387–395.
37. Goh PS, Gi MT, Charlton A, et al. Review of orbital imaging. Eur J Radiol. 2008;66(3):387–95.
38. Del Brutto OH. Clinical management of neurocysticercosis. Expert Rev Neurother. 2014;14(4):389–96.
39. Chaudhary V, Bano S, Parmar PR, et al. Extraocular muscle cysticercosis mimicking as pseudotumor orbit. A clinical dilemma. Neurol India. 2013;61(6): 665–7.
40. Tang SX, Lim RP, Al-Dahmash S, et al. Bilateral lacrimal gland disease: clinical features of 97 cases. Ophthalmology. 3 Jun 2014. Pii S0161-6420(14)00365-0.
41. Andrew NH, McNab AA, Selva D. Review of 268 lacrimal gland biopsies in an Australian cohort. Clin Experiment Ophthalmol. 2014;43:5–11. doi:10.111/ceo.12371.
42. Cheuk W, Yuen HK, Chan AC, et al. Ocular adnexal lymphoma associated with IgG4+ chronic sclerosing dacryoadenitis: a previously undescribed complication of IgG4-related sclerosing disease. Am J Surg Pathol. 2008;32(8):1159–67.
43. Mombaerts I, Cameron JD, Chanlalit W, Garrity JA. Surgical debulking for idiopathic dacryoadenitis: a diagnosis and a cure. Ophthalmology. 2014; 121(2):603–9.
44. Toledano N, Tit-Liviu Stoica B, Genol Saavedra I, Garcia Saenz S, Conde E. Tuberculous dacryoadenitis unveils HIV infection. Can J Ophthalmol. 2013;48(5): e128–30.

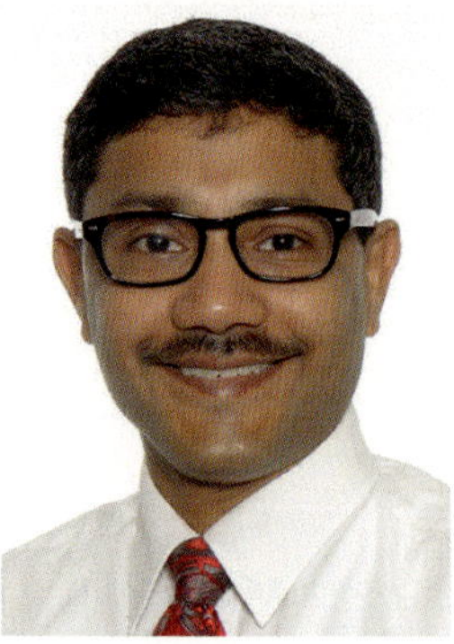

**Gangadhara Sundar**
Dr. Sundar graduated from the Madras Medical College. Following his basic ophthalmology training in India, he received his postgraduate ophthalmology residency and fellowship training in Ophthalmic Plastic & Reconstructive Surgery and Ocular Oncology at the Henry Ford Hospital, Detroit. With an extensive multinational multiethnic multispeciality practice exposure and patient experience, he currently serves as Head, Orbit & Oculofacial Surgery, Ophthalmic Oncology at the National University Hospital, Singapore, committed to clinical research, education of residents and fellows with national, regional, and international outreach. His interests include orbital inflammatory diseases including thyroid eye disease; minimally invasive orbital, lacrimal, and oculofacial surgery; orbito-facial trauma in addition to aesthetic oculofacial surgery and is a strong proponent of multidisciplinary approaches to complex orbito-facial disorders.

# Dacryocystitis

# 39

Gangadhara Sundar

## Introduction and Overview

Dacryocystitis is a common condition of bacterial etiology that ophthalmologists and oculoplastic surgeons face. Although typically seen in the middle aged and elderly [1], it may be seen in any age group. The diagnosis is often missed by the general ophthalmologist when the symptoms are either minimal or chronic. We shall discuss the presentation, diagnosis, and management in the section below.

## Definition

Dacryocystitis is an acute, subacute, or chronic suppurative infection of the lacrimal sac and proximal nasolacrimal duct [2], secondary to underlying nasolacrimal duct obstruction. The obstruction may be due to developmental dysgenesis or acquired in origin. Acute fulminant or chronic infections may also involve the lacrimal sac walls and perisaccal tissues, resulting in a lacrimal sac abscess, an overlying facial cellulitis, or even orbital cellulitis [3].

## Etiology

Most infections are of bacterial origin secondary to an underlying nasolacrimal duct obstruction. The bacteria may be native to the lacrimal sac and nasolacrimal duct or from the ocular surface. While most acute suppurative infections are caused by gram-positive organisms [4], chronic or partially treated infections are often polymicrobial, gram-positive and gram-negative organisms, sometimes even multidrug resistant [5]. Anaerobic infections, fungal infections, and parasitic infestations are extremely rare.

Nasolacrimal duct obstructions may either be due to developmental dysgenesis from failure of canalization of the nasolacrimal duct [6] (congenital nasolacrimal duct obstruction CNLDO), primary acquired nasolacrimal duct obstruction (PANDO) [7] or secondary acquired nasolacrimal duct obstruction (SANDO) from foreign bodies [8], trauma (midfacial or naso-orbital ethmoidal (NOE) fractures) [9], growths or tumors within the lacrimal sac, nasolacrimal duct or nasal cavity or rarely from disruption of the nasolacrimal duct during endonasal surgeries [10].

G. Sundar, DO, FRCSEd, FAMS, AB Ophth(USA)
Asst Professor, Dept of Ophthalmology,
National University of Singapore,
Head & Senior Consultant, Orbit & Oculofacial Surgery, Dept of Ophthalmology,
National University Hospital,
Singapore
e-mail: gsundar1@yahoo.com;
Gangadhara_sundar@nuhs.edu.sg


B. Mukherjee, H. Yuen (eds.), *Emergencies of the Orbit and Adnexa*,
DOI 10.1007/978-81-322-1807-4_39

## Types

Hyperacute: Uncommon, it is typically seen in the elderly and immunocompromised.

Acute: Typically unilateral, it is a more common presentation, seen in middle-aged and elderly females (Fig. 39.1), although it may be seen in all age groups. Affected patients present with pain, redness, and swelling in the region of the medial canthus, with purulent discharge and an injected eye. Less commonly it may be seen in the newborn, young adult males and may be bilateral (Fig. 39.2).

Chronic: The most common presentation, especially in adults and young children (Fig. 39.3) who are known to have an underlying nasolacrimal duct obstruction, with waxing and waning symptoms. Not infrequently these patients would have been managed as chronic conjunctivitis with intermittent topical antibiotic treatment [11].

Incidental: Typically diagnosed in patients undergoing routine preoperative lacrimal irrigation prior to intraocular surgery, a common practice in some developing nations, when mucoid or mucopurulent regurgitation is observed [12].

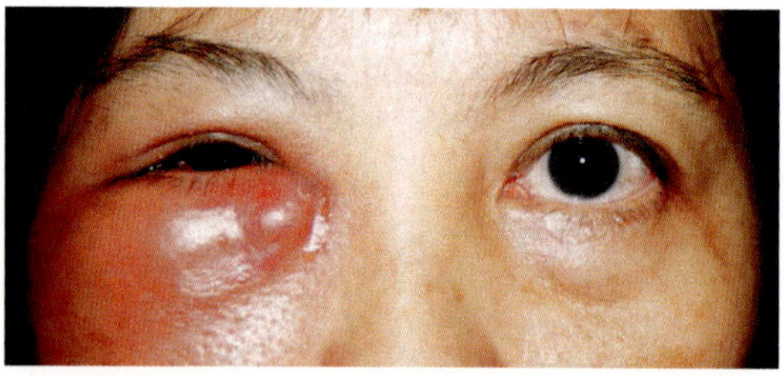

**Fig. 39.1** Right acute dacryocystitis in middle-aged female

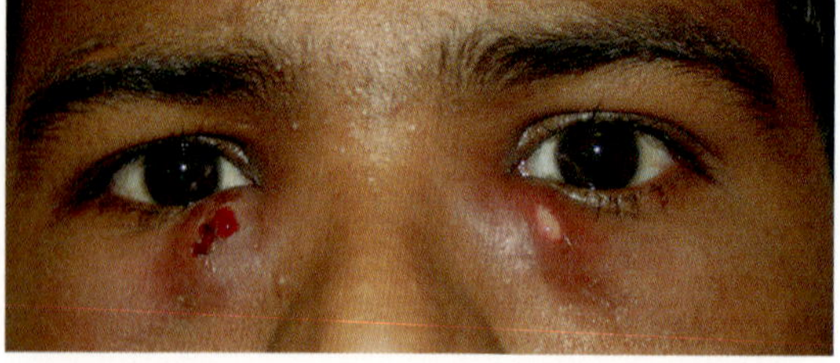

**Fig. 39.2** Bilateral acute dacryocystitis in young adult male

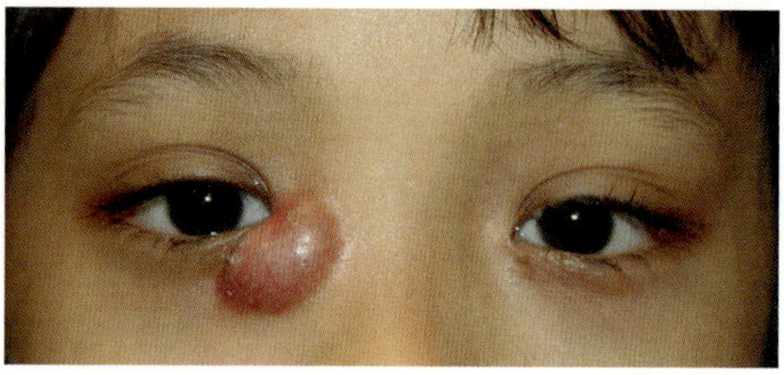

**Fig. 39.3** Chronic dacryocystitis in child from untreated congenital nasolacrimal duct obstruction

Secondary: These may be as a result of intraluminal foreign bodies (migrated punctal/intracanalicular plugs), long-term indwelling migrated lacrimal stents, or secondary infection with lacrimal sac tumors.

## Clinical Presentation

Dacryocystitis may be diagnosed in all age groups. Symptoms and signs are dependent upon the age, duration, underlying immune status, and previous treatment if any. Typical symptoms and signs are described below. Occasionally atypical presentations may also occur.

Symptoms: Most patients with acute dacryocystitis present with unilateral severe throbbing pain, redness, and swelling below the medial canthus with ipsilateral tearing and discharge from that eye for months or years. Rarely, they may present with fever, malaise, and loss of appetite, especially when there is overlying facial cellulitis (Fig. 39.4). In the partially treated patient, symptoms may be minimal. These include overlying erythema and induration without tenderness or swelling below the medial canthus alone.

Signs: Classic signs of acute inflammation are usually present. These include erythema, warmth, swelling with or without induration, pain or tenderness, and regurgitation on pressure over the lacrimal sac below the medial canthal tendon (Fig. 39.5). A patient with chronic infection may present with minimal signs except for mucoid or mucopurulent regurgitation on lacrimal sac irrigation, swelling with induration below the medial canthal tendon (mass lesion),

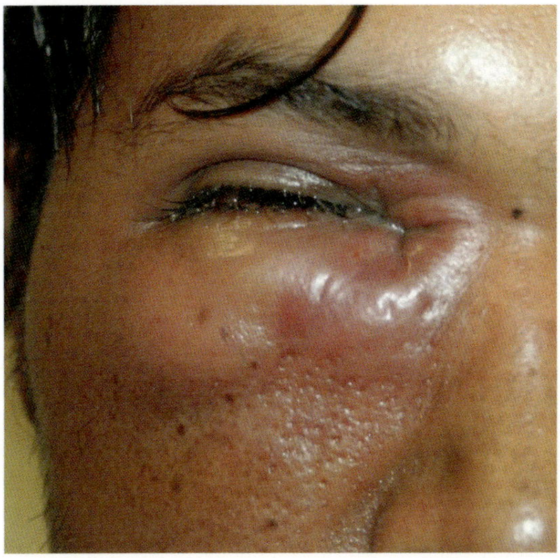

**Fig. 39.4** Right acute on chronic dacryocystitis with facial cellulitis

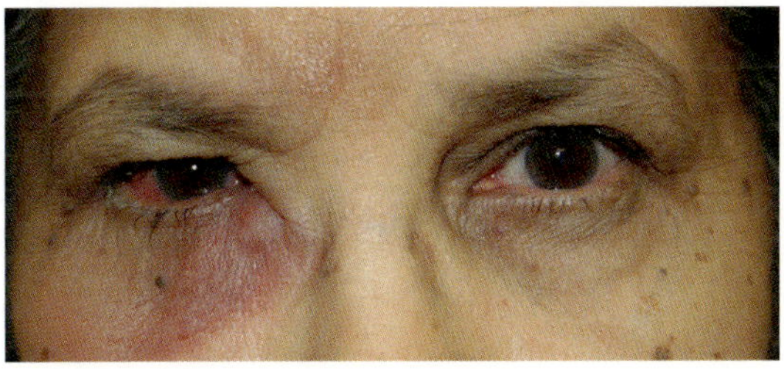

**Fig. 39.5** Chronic dacryocystitis

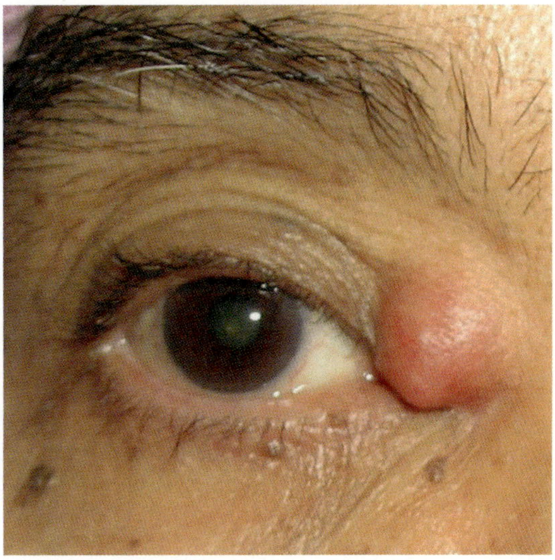

**Fig. 39.6** Right medial canthal neurofibroma

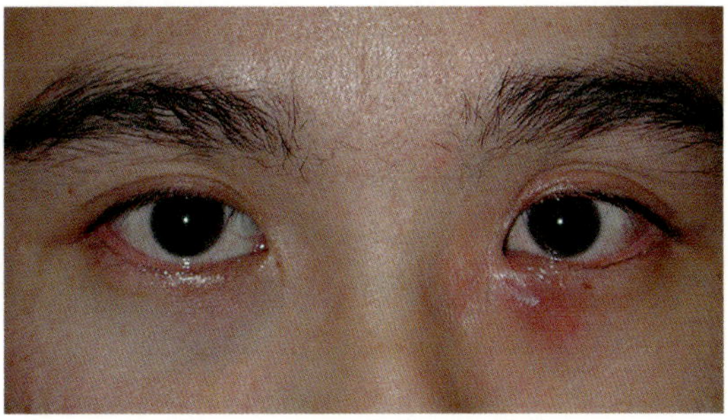

**Fig. 39.7** Infected lacrimal anlage (fistula)

or slightly raised tear meniscus with debris on slit lamp examination.

Based on the above, a subcutaneous inflammatory mass lesion below the medial canthal tendon is a dacryocystitis until proven otherwise. When a mass lesion presents above the medial canthal tendon, other conditions like a lacrimal sac tumor, medial orbital tumor, or intracranial space-occupying lesion with extension should be considered and thus imaging is warranted.

## Differential Diagnosis

In most cases, the diagnosis is straightforward and obvious. However there are special situations that one should be aware of and are listed below:

Medial canthal skin tumors (Fig. 39.6). Differentiating features include chronicity, inability to pinch the skin, and complete mobility from the underlying tissues.

Subcutaneous extrasaccal medial canthal tumors and infection. These are more difficult to diagnose and usually proven by patency of nasolacrimal duct on irrigation. Rarely an infected diverticulum of the lacrimal sac or canaliculus may present like a dacryocystitis (Fig. 39.7).

Lacrimal sac/drainage system tumors [13] (Fig. 39.8 a, b). Diagnosed based on high degree of clinical suspicion, findings on imaging (CT scan or MRI, dacryocystography), and rarely intraoperatively.

Medial orbital tumors. This is suspected based on posterior extension of the lesion, lateral

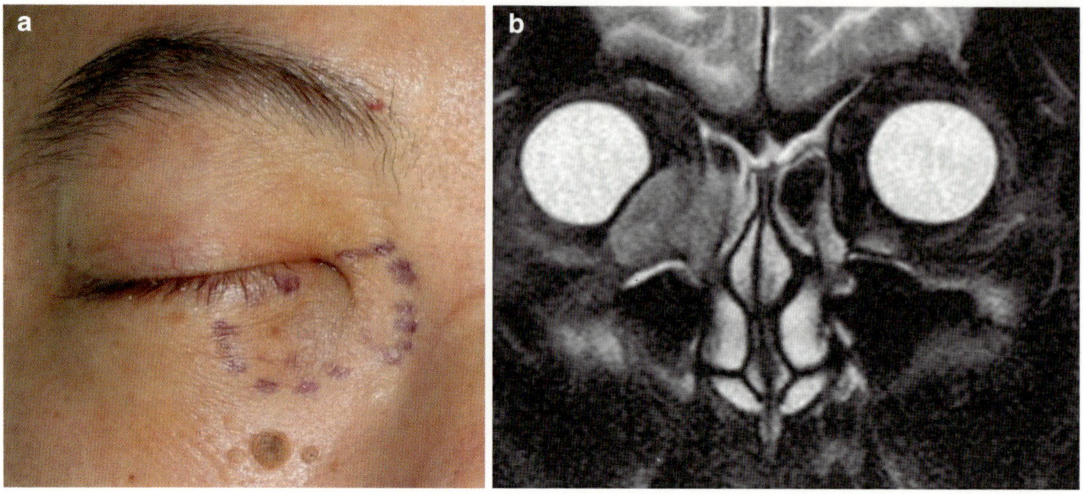


**Fig. 39.8** (**a**) Carcinoma of right lacrimal sac and nasolacrimal duct. (**b**) MRI showing infiltration of the right lacrimal drainage apparatus with globe displacement

displacement of the globe with or without ocular motility problems.

Nasal tumors.

Intracranial tumors.

In most situations, a good history including the duration of symptoms, previous medical and surgical interventions, clinical examination, and ancillary clinical investigations are sufficient to make a reliable diagnosis.

## Examination

All patients should undergo a complete ophthalmic examination of both eyes. Specific attention should be paid to the resting tear meniscus (height, debris, and discharge), laxity of the lower eyelid, position, size and tone of the lacrimal puncta, and microscopic or macroscopic regurgitation on pressure over the lacrimal sac (ROPLAS) [12]. Inspection of the overlying skin of the medial canthus for inflammation, induration, preexisting skin creases (relaxed skin tension line), epicanthal fold, previous scars of abscess drainage or external dacryocystorhinostomy, should be performed. Lacrimal irrigation is contraindicated in all cases of suspected acute dacryocystitis.

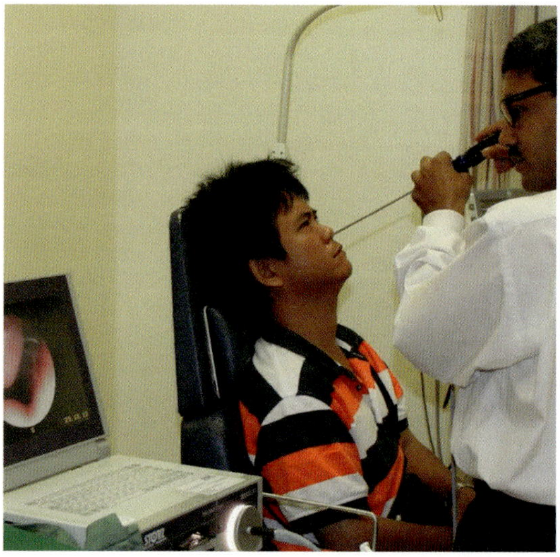

**Fig. 39.9** Office nasal endoscopy

However it may be performed gently in subacute or chronic cases especially when alternative differential diagnoses are being considered [14]. All patients with lacrimal system infections and obstructions should undergo a nasal endoscopic examination [15] under topical anesthesia and vasoconstrictors (Fig. 39.9). Specific attention should be paid to the inferior meatus under the inferior turbinate for the presence of tumors and adhesions and to the middle meatus (Fig. 39.10), scarring from previous surgery (Fig. 39.11a), or the presence of foreign bodies from previous facial trauma reconstruction (Fig. 39.11b). Any abnormal pathology should be documented and biopsy considered for suspicious lesions. Regional examination for lymphadenopathy (preauricular, submandibular, submental) and general systemic examination of the patient's overall well-being complemented by detailed medical history, medications taken including antiplatelet agents, fitness for locoregional, or general anesthesia should also be performed.

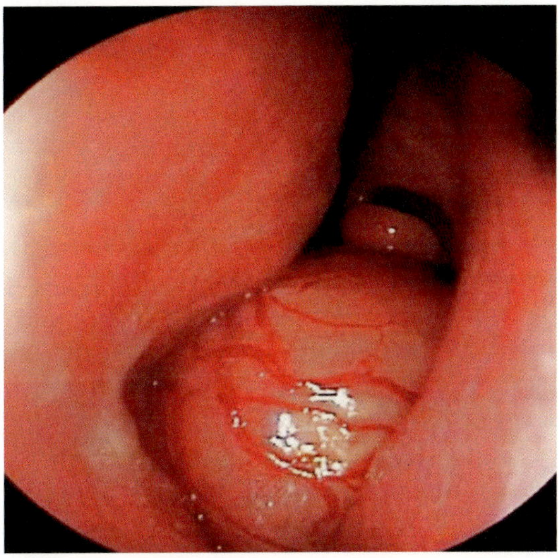

**Fig. 39.10** Tumor of nasal cavity on endoscopy

## Investigations

In most cases of suspected dacryocystitis, laboratory investigations may not be necessary to confirm the diagnosis.

A smear of the conjunctival discharge or mucopurulent regurgitant on lacrimal sac pressure may be sent for Gram and Giemsa stains and routine bacterial cultures and antibiotic sensitivity. This may help guide antibiotic coverage in chronic infections not responding to conventional systemic antibiotics. A negative smear in patients who have been treated with antibiotics however may not be reliable.

Systemic investigations including complete blood count (CBC) may be useful in patients with systemic symptoms and hospitalized patients with multiple systemic comorbidities. An erythrocyte sedimentation rate (ESR) and C-reactive protein (CRP) may also serve as a surrogate inflammatory marker. Blood cultures

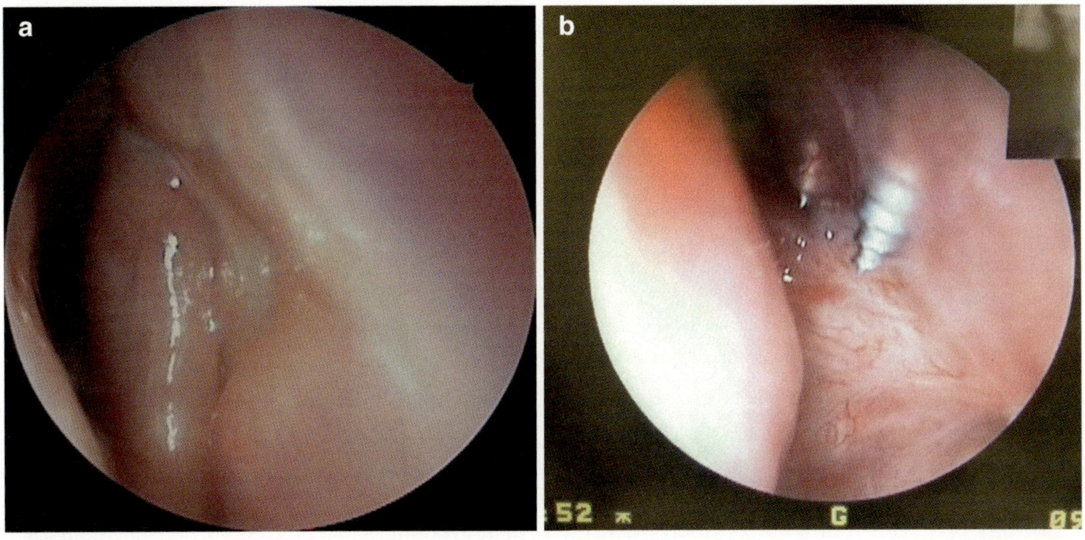


**Fig. 39.11** (**a**) Scar at the site of previous DCR. (**b**) Nasal endoscopy showing miniplate and screws in the region of lacrimal sac fossa causing obstruction

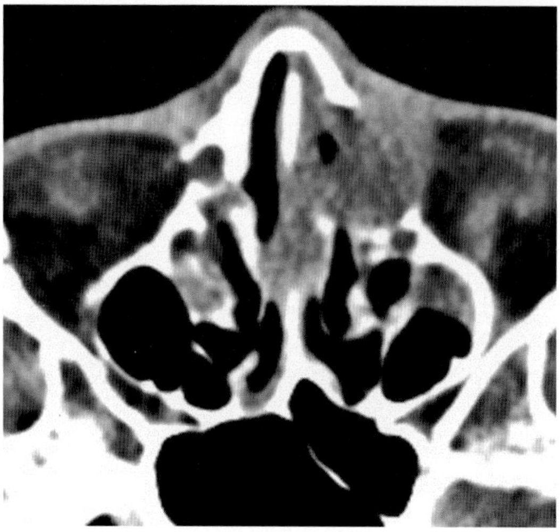

**Fig. 39.12** CT scan axial view showing tumor infiltration of left lacrimal sac fossa (inverted papilloma)

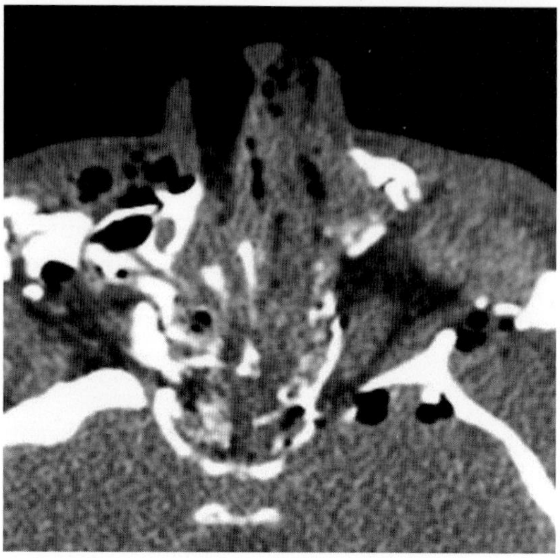

**Fig. 39.13** CT axial view showing disruption of lacrimal sac fossa from trauma

for aerobic and anaerobic organisms may also be performed in patients with fulminant infections, systemic symptoms, or immune compromise.

Imaging is not generally required for most cases of dacryocystitis prior to surgery. Indications for imaging include suspected lacrimal drainage tumors and previous history of facial or orbital trauma especially when surgery with internal fixation was performed or when diagnosis is in doubt. When indicated, CT scan [16, 17] of the face and orbits with axial, coronal, and sagittal sections with soft tissue and bone windows, with contrast, may be performed. This provides adequate visualization of the soft tissue and bony structures (Figs. 39.12 and 39.13), adjacent paranasal sinuses, and nasal cavity including any implants and deformities that may be present. An MRI may be considered when lacrimal or nasal cavity tumors are suspected or in medial canthal masses where an intracranial lesion (meningocele, encephalocele) is suspected. Dacryocystography (Fig. 39.14) is rarely indicated to rule out intraluminal space-occupying lesions and localize the level of obstruction. This may be performed with routine X-ray, CT scan [18], or MRI [19].

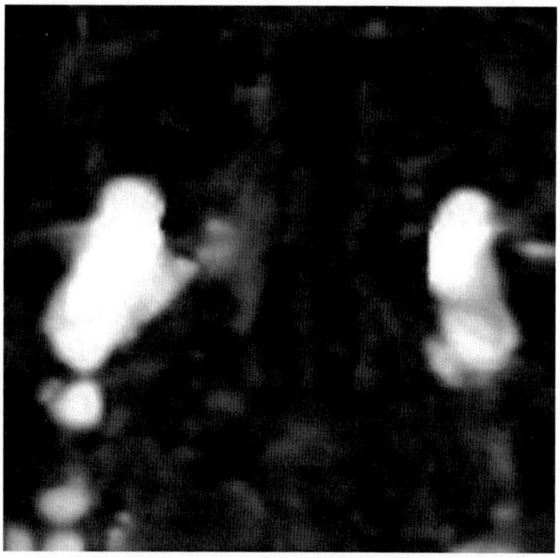

**Fig. 39.14** Dacryocystography showing obstruction of left proximal nasolacrimal duct compared to right side

## Prevention

In infants, prompt management of congenital nasolacrimal duct obstruction by lacrimal massages (Fig. 39.15) and, when ineffective, lacrimal irrigation and probing [20, 21] (Fig. 39.16), is effective in preventing a dacryocystitis. Older infants and young children may also benefit from lacrimal

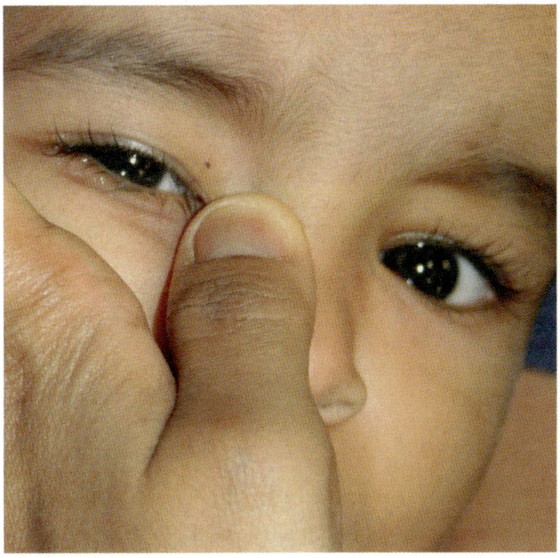

**Fig. 39.15** Lacrimal sac massage for congenital nasolacrimal duct obstruction

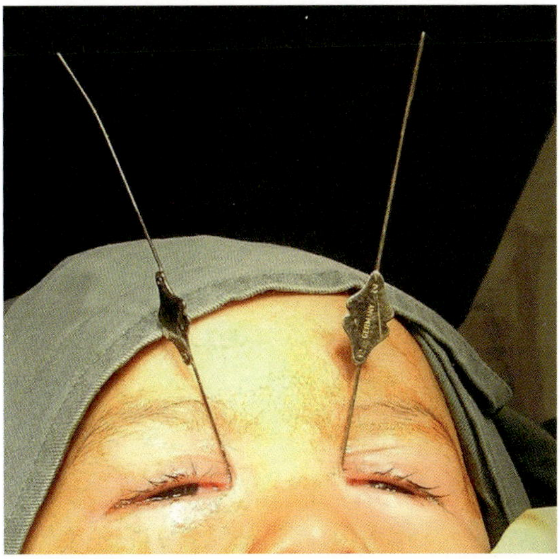

**Fig. 39.16** Probing for bilateral congenital nasolacrimal duct obstruction

intubation or balloon dacryoplasty causing resolution of symptoms and preventing a dacryocystitis.

In adults, a thorough evaluation of the lacrimal system to identify nasolacrimal duct obstruction and prompt restoration of patency by endoluminal lacrimal duct recanalization (ELDR) [22] (Fig. 39.17) or dacryocystorhinostomy also may help prevent acute or chronic dacryocystitis. This is especially imperative in elderly patients prior to cataract, glaucoma, and other intraocular surgeries [23]. In patients with midfacial and naso-orbital ethmoidal (NOE) fractures with involvement of the nasolacrimal duct (Fig. 39.18), prophylactic bicanalicular intubation [24] may also help prevent a complete nasolacrimal duct obstruction and dacryocystitis.

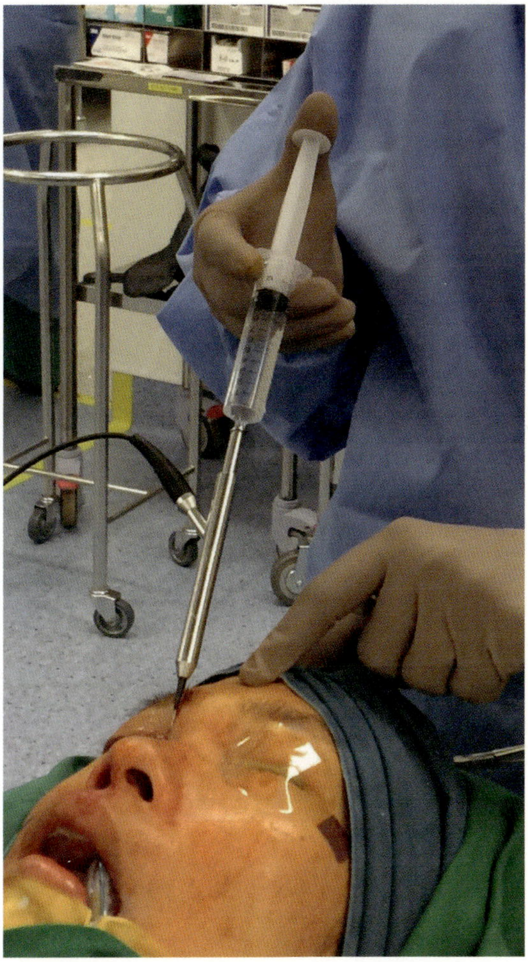

**Fig. 39.17** Dacryoendoscopy with Endoluminal duct recanalization

## Management

Management depends upon whether the underlying condition is a congenital nasolacrimal duct obstruction in infants or young children, older

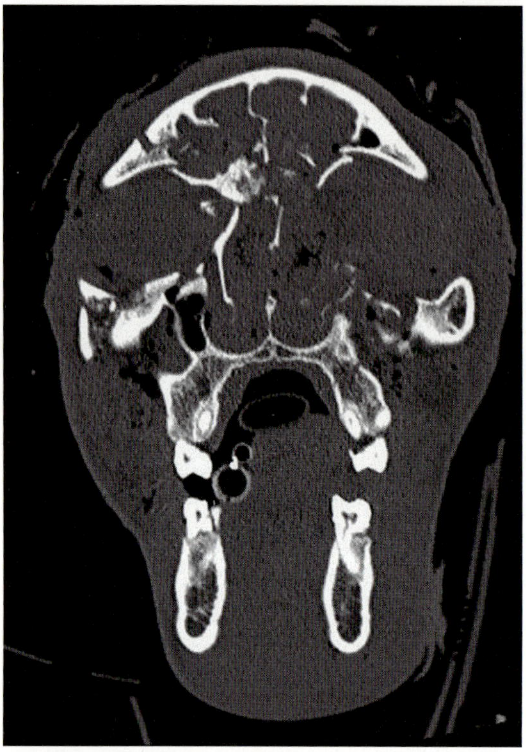

**Fig. 39.18** Coronal CT showing disruption of left nasolacrimal duct from blast injury

children, young adults, or the elderly. General principles of management are shown in Table 39.1.

A general outline of various treatment options for dacryocystitis is discussed below:

- Infantile dacryocystitis
  - Topical and systemic antibiotics with trial of lacrimal sac massages. If refractory, early probing of the nasolacrimal duct with nasal endoscopy to rule out intranasal cysts.
- Pediatric dacryocystitis
  - Acute: Medical treatment followed by early endonasal dacryocystorhinostomy
  - Chronic dacryocystitis: Attempt lacrimal syringing, probing with or without intubation, and balloon dacryoplasty. Endonasal dacryocystorhinostomy in refractory cases
- Adult dacryocystitis
  - Acute: Medical treatment (systemic and topical antibiotics) followed by early endonasal dacryocystorhinostomy or late external dacryocystorhinostomy

**Table 39.1**

| | |
|---|---|
| Infantile dacryocystitis young children (<5 years) | Medical treatment followed by lacrimal irrigation and probing with or without bicanalicular silicone intubation |
| | Alternative: Balloon dacryoplasty (Fig. 39.19) with or without bicanalicular silicone intubation |
| Older children, young adults | Consider lacrimal irrigation, probing, balloon dacryoplasty with/without bicanalicular silicone intubation as primary procedure |
| | Mechanical endonasal endoscopic dacryocystorhinostomy |
| Older adults | Elderly patients with skin creases, high risk for general anesthesia: external dacryocystorhinostomy with or without silicone intubation |
| | Younger adults without prominent skin creases, shallow nasal bridge, low risk for general anesthesia, and roomy nasal cavity: mechanical endoscopic endonasal dacryocystorhinostomy with or without silicone intubation |

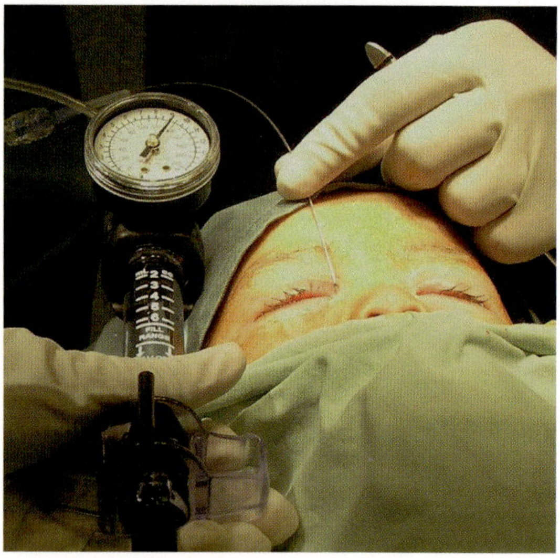

**Fig. 39.19** Balloon dacryoplasty

  - Chronic: External dacryocystorhinostomy or endonasal dacryocystorhinostomy. endoluminal lacrimal duct recanalization for patients unwilling for primary dacryocystorhinostomy or with lower nasolacrimal duct obstruction only

Acute dacryocystitis is managed medically in an ambulatory setting [25]. Empirical therapy is begun with an orally administered broad-spectrum antibiotic, e.g., amoxicillin – clavulanate, especially when the patient has associated sinusitis. Patients with penicillin allergy may be started on macrolides: erythromycin or clarithromycin. Topical antibiotics instilled into the conjunctival sac may be added for synergistic effect. Underlying chronic rhinosinusitis or nasal congestion should be managed appropriately with nasal decongestants. Systemic steroids are usually contraindicated unless the active acute infection is under control. Topical nasal steroids may occasionally be considered in the presence of persistent nasal congestion or inflammation with caution. Evacuating contents of the lacrimal sac either by progressive pressure over the lacrimal sac or in patients with fluctuation over the lacrimal sac, a large-bore needle aspiration of sac contents may help hasten recovery from the acute infection complemented by systemic antibiotics. Systemically ill patients, especially with severe comorbidities, e.g., uncontrolled diabetes, renal dysfunction, and immunocompromised, may require hospital admission and parenteral antibiotics to manage the acute infection until definitive surgical management. In some patients with recent onset intermittent or persistent dacryocystitis or where patients have multiple comorbidities precluding a conventional external or endonasal DCR or unwilling for the same, lacrimal endoscopy to identify intraluminal pathology and level of obstruction, followed by Endoluminal duct recanalization (ELDR) with balloon dacryoplasty (DCP) and standard or large diameter lacrimal stenting may be considered (Fig. 39.20).

Surgery is the most definitive management for all cases of nasolacrimal duct obstruction with or

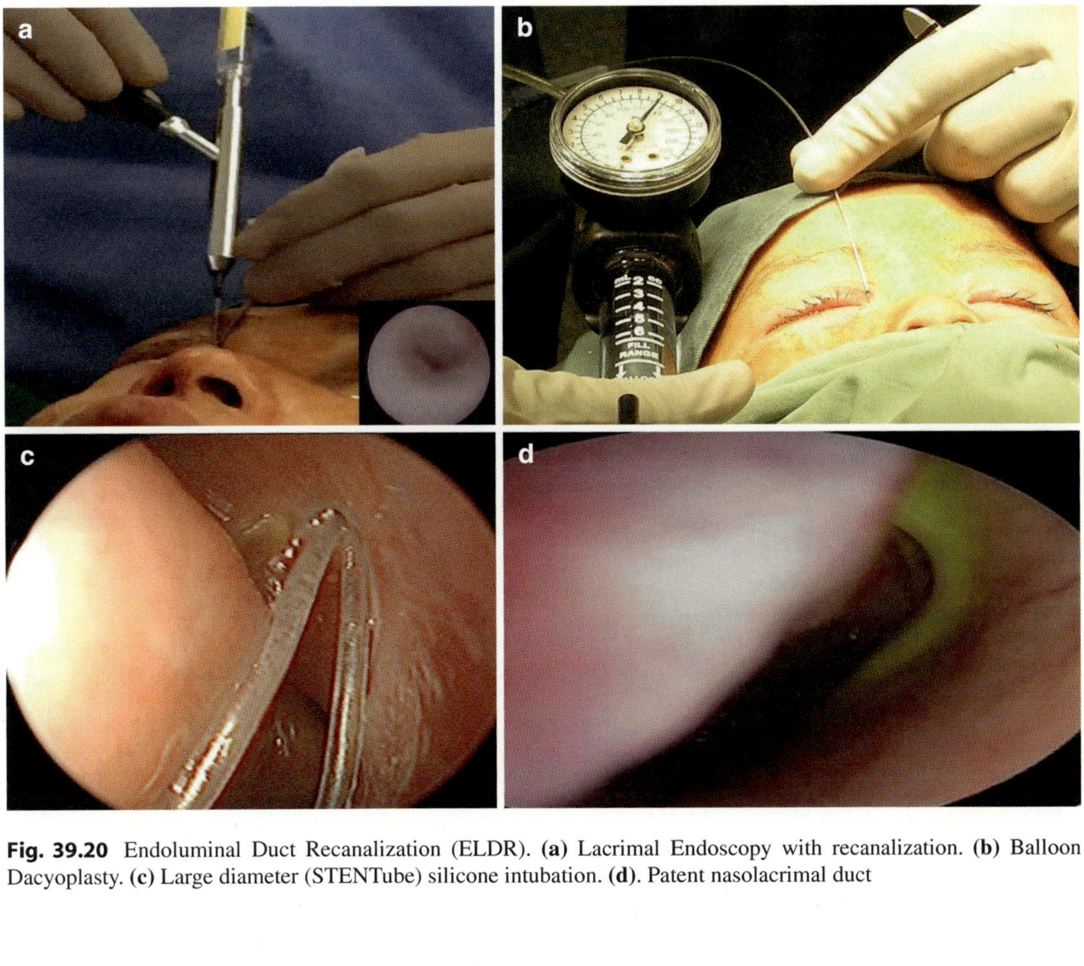

**Fig. 39.20** Endoluminal Duct Recanalization (ELDR). **(a)** Lacrimal Endoscopy with recanalization. **(b)** Balloon Dacyoplasty. **(c)** Large diameter (STENTube) silicone intubation. **(d)**. Patent nasolacrimal duct

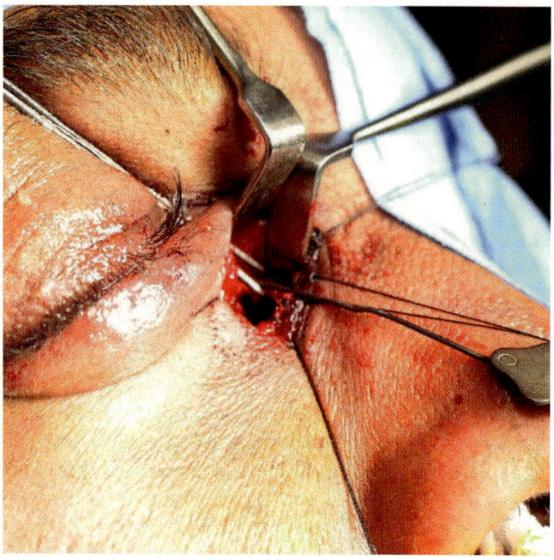

**Fig. 39.21** External DCR with intubation

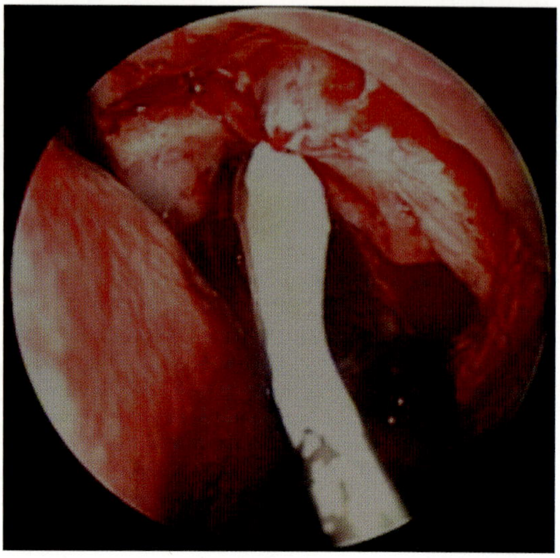

**Fig. 39.22** Endonasal DCR

without dacryocystitis, both in the children and adults. In patients with a lacrimal abscess not responding to conventional antibiotic therapy, a large-bore needle aspiration may help hasten recovery in association with systemic and topical antibiotics. Rarely a decompression of the lacrimal sac abscess by an incision and drainage may be indicated. Advantages of the procedure include hastening of recovery following an acute lacrimal abscess. Disadvantages, however, include the inability to sufficiently anesthetize the area of drainage resulting in severe pain and predisposition to a lacrimal sac fistula [26], especially if it is not followed up with an early dacryocystorhinostomy [27, 28] or lacrimal duct recanalization (ELDR) [22] procedure.

Once the acute infection is brought under control, the underlying nasolacrimal duct obstruction has to be addressed.

Most adult patients will benefit either from a conventional external dacryocystorhinostomy (Ex-DCR) [29] (Fig. 39.21) or a mechanical endoscopic endonasal dacryocystorhinostomy (Fig. 39.22) (MENDCR) [30, 31]. Typical indications for an external DCR include completely resolved acute dacryocystitis or chronic dacryocystitis, especially in the elderly with preexisting eyelid/medial canthal creases or skin folds, severe crowded nasal cavity/deviated nasal septum, patients with midfacial fractures with hyperostosis or hardware in the lacrimal fossa area, unavailability of endoscopic DCR service, patient choice, and local anesthesia (patient choice or high risk for general anesthesia). Typical indications for endonasal DCR include persistent medial canthal inflammation with skin involvement, young patient desirous of avoiding a potential medial canthal scar, well-trained endoscopic surgeon, and acute/subacute infections. When bilateral dacryocystitis is present, either a sequential DCR or simultaneous bilateral DCR may be performed with good results enabling early recovery and reduced anesthetic morbidity as well. In special situations where patients have multiple comorbidities, unfit for prolonged surgery, or unwilling for incisional procedures, various forms of endoluminal duct recanalization (ELDR) with or without balloon dacryoplasty (DCP) [32] and intubation may be considered.

In exceptional cases, when there's a lack of expertise in performing either an external or endonasal dacryocystorhinostomy, the patient is unfit for prolonged surgical procedure, has severe dry eyes (e.g., severe rheumatoid arthritis), or an early intraocular surgery is indicated, a dacryocystectomy (DCT) may also be considered [33]. However, a complete and meticulous surgical procedure is essential to prevent recurrent dacryocystitis from remnants of the sac structure. The patients should be counseled regarding the justification for the procedure and about the possibility of postoperative persistent epiphora.

Prior to all surgical procedures, optimization of the patient's medical status, temporary withdrawal of antiplatelet or antithrombotic agents (aspirin, warfarin, clopidogrel, heparin, etc.), and treatment of underlying rhinosinusitis are essential. While surgical outcomes are generally excellent when a DCR is performed in patients with subacute or chronic dacryocystitis, persistent inflammation may result in excessive flap inflammation, granuloma formation with scarring justifying early intervention in symptomatic patients prior to developing dacryocystitis. Rarely a revision DCR may be indicated in such patients, underlying the need for postoperative wound healing modulation as indicated.

## Summary

In summary, while acute dacryocystitis is commonly managed medically, definitive treatment for both acute and dacryocystitis is surgical intervention by various forms of lacrimal drainage surgery. Most acute infections in children and adults are preventable by prompt identification of complete nasolacrimal duct obstruction and early intervention. Novel techniques of balloon dacryoplasty and endoluminal lacrimal duct recanalization may play a role in selected patients who are not desirous of an open-invasive procedure or as an initial procedure as they are minimally invasive.

## References

1. AAO Basic and Clinical Science Course (BCSC), Section 7, 2014–2015.
2. Nerad JA. Oculoplastic surgery – the requisites in ophthalmology. St.Louis: Mosby; 2001.
3. Kikkawa DO, Heinz GW, Martin RT, Nunery WN, Eiseman AS. Orbital cellulitis and abscess secondary to dacryocystitis. Arch Ophthalmol. 2002;120(8):1096–9.
4. AVP, Patil SS, Koti SV, J S A, Garag SS, Hegde JS. Clinico-bacteriological study of chronic dacryocystitis cases in Northern Karnataka. India J Clin Diagn Res. 2013;7(11):2502–4.
5. Amato M, Pershing S, Walvick M, Tanaka S. Trends in ophthalmic manifestations of methicillin-resistant Staphylococcus aureus (MRSA) in a northern California pediatric population. J AAPOS. 2013;17(3):243–7.
6. Schnall BM. Pediatric nasolacrimal duct obstruction. Curr Opin Ophthalmol. 2013;24(5):421–4.
7. Linberg JV, McCormick SA. Primary acquired nasolacrimal duct obstruction. A clinicopathologic report and biopsy technique. Ophthalmology. 1986;93(8):1055–63.
8. Rumelt S, Remulla H, Rubin PA. Silicone punctal plug migration resulting in dacryocystitis and canaliculitis. Cornea. 1997;16(3):377–9.
9. Ali MJ, Gupta H, Honavar SG, Naik MN. Acquired nasolacrimal duct obstructions secondary to naso-orbito-ethmoidal fractures: patterns and outcomes. Ophthal Plast Reconstr Surg. 2012;28(4):242–5.
10. Cohen NA, Antunes MB, Morgenstern KE. Prevention and management of lacrimal duct injury. Otolaryngol Clin North Am. 2010;43(4):781–8.
11. Pinar-Sueiro S, Sota M, Lerchundi TX, Gibelalde A, Berasategui B, Vilar B, Hernandez JL. Dacryocystitis: systematic approach to diagnosis and therapy. Curr Infect Dis Rep. 2012.
12. Thomas R, Thomas S, Braganza A, Muliyil J. Evaluation of the role of syringing prior to cataract surgery. Indian J Ophthalmol. 1997;45(4):211–4.
13. Low JR, Bian Ng S, Sundar G. Undifferentiated carcinoma of the lacrimal sac: case report and review of literature. Orbit. 2011;30(6):293–6.
14. Nerad JA. Techniques in ophthalmic plastic surgery. London: Elsevier; 2010.
15. Golan S, Leibovitch I, Landsberg R. Unexpected pathologies in patients referred for endoscopic DCR. Eur Arch Otorhinolaryngol. 2014; 271(11):3053–8.
16. Weber AL, Rodriguez-DeVelasquez A, Lucarelli MJ, Cheng HM. Normal anatomy and lesions of the lacrimal sac and duct: evaluated by dacryocystography, computed tomography, and MR imaging. Neuroimaging Clin N Am. 1996;6(1):199–217.
17. Francis IC, Kappagoda MB, Cole IE, Bank L, Dunn GD. Computed tomography of the lacrimal drainage system: retrospective study of 107 cases of dacryostenosis. Ophthal Plast Reconstr Surg. 1999;15(3):217–26.
18. Tschopp M, Bornstein MM, Sendi P, Jacobs R, Goldblum D. Dacryocystography using cone beam CT in patients with lacrimal drainage system obstruction. Ophthal Plast Reconstr Surg. 2014;30(6):486–91.
19. Coskun B, Ilgit E, Onal B, Konuk O, Erbas G. MR dacryocystography in the evaluation of patients with obstructive epiphora treated by means of interventional radiologic procedures. AJNR Am J Neuroradiol. 2012;33(1):141–7.
20. Kapadia MK, Freitag SK, Woog JJ. Evaluation and management of congenital nasolacrimal duct obstruction. Otolaryngol Clin North Am. 2006;39(5):959–77.

21. Paul TO, Shepherd R. Congenital nasolacrimal duct obstruction: natural history and the timing of optimal intervention. J Pediatr Ophthalmol Strabismus. 1994;31(6):362–7.
22. Javate RM, Pamintuan FG, Cruz Jr RT. Efficacy of endoscopic lacrimal duct recanalization using microendoscope. Ophthal Plast Reconstr Surg. 2010;26(5):330–3.
23. Song A, Scott IU, Flynn Jr HW, Budenz DL. Delayed-onset bleb-associated endophthalmitis: clinical features and visual acuity outcomes. Ophthalmology. 2002;109(5):985–91.
24. Spinelli HM, Shapiro MD, Wei LL, Elahi E, Hirmand H. The role of lacrimal intubation in the management of facial trauma and tumor resection. Plast Reconstr Surg. 2005;115(7):1871–6.
25. Thompson CJ. Review of the diagnosis and management of acquired nasolacrimal duct obstruction. Optometry. 2001;72(2):103–11.
26. Barrett RV, Meyer DR, ASOPRS Acquired Lacrimal Fistula Study Group. Acquired lacrimal sac fistula after incision and drainage for dacryocystitis: a multicenter study. Ophthal Plast Reconstr Surg. 2009;25(6):455–7.
27. Lombardi D, Mattavelli D, Accorona R, Turano R, Semeraro F, Bozzola A, Nicolai P. Acute dacryocystitis with empyema of the lacrimal sac: is immediate endoscopic dacryocystorhinostomy justified? Otolaryngol Head Neck Surg. 2014;150(6):1071–7.
28. Madge SN, Chan W, Malhotra R, Ghabrial R, Floreani S, Wormald PJ, Tsirbas A, Selva D. Endoscopic dacryocystorhinostomy in acute dacryocystitis: a multicenter case series. Orbit. 2011;30(1):1–6.
29. Lieberman SM, Casiano RR. Is an endoscopic approach superior to external dacryocystorhinostomy for nasolacrimal obstruction? Laryngoscope. 2014. doi:10.1002/lary.24734.
30. Tsirbas A, Wormald PJ. Mechanical endonasal dacryocystorhinostomy with mucosal flaps. Br J Ophthalmol. 2003;87(1):43–7.
31. Ali MJ, Psaltis AJ, Bassiouni A, Wormald PJ. Long-term outcomes in primary powered endoscopic dacryocystorhinostomy. Br J Ophthalmol. 2014. doi:10.1136/bjophthalmol-2014-305510. pii: bjophthalmol-2014-305510.
32. Yakopson VS, Flanagan JC, Ahn D, Luo BP. Dacryocystorhinostomy: history, evolution and future directions. Saudi J Ophthalmol. 2011;25(1): 37–49.
33. Ali MJ. Dacryocystectomy: goals, indications, techniques and complications. Ophthal Plast Recosntr Surg. 2014;30(6):512–6.

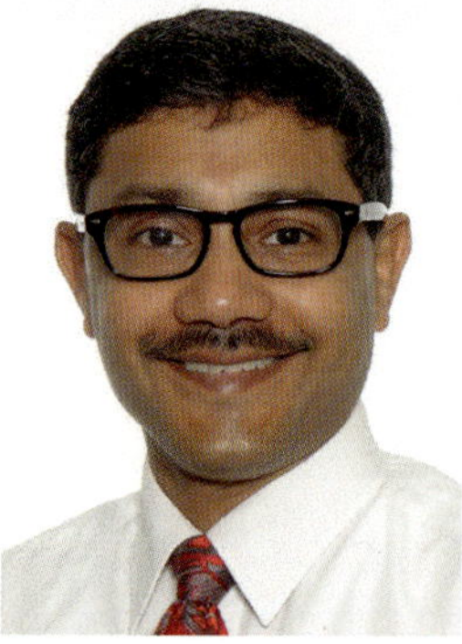

**Gangadhara Sundar** Dr. Sundar graduated from the Madras Medical College. Following his basic ophthalmology training in India, he received his post-graduate ophthalmology residency and Fellowship training in Ophthalmic Plastic & Reconstructive Surgery and Ocular Oncology at the Henry Ford Hospital, Detroit. With an extensive multinational multiethnic multispeciality practice and patient experience, he currently serves as Head, Orbit & Oculofacial Surgery, Ophthalmic Oncology at the National University Hospital, Singapore and is committed to clinical research, education of residents & fellows with national, regional and international outreach. His interests include orbital inflammatory diseases including Thyroid Eye Disease, minimally invasive orbital, lacrimal and oculofacial surgery, orbitofacial trauma and esthetic oculofacial surgery. He is a strong proponent of multidisciplinary approaches to complex orbito-facial disorders.

# 40 Canaliculitis and Intracanalicular Foreign Bodies

Mohammad Javed Ali

## Introduction

The canaliculi and the lacrimal sac are the regions of lacrimal drainage system, which are prone for infections. Canaliculitis is an infection of the canalicular part of lacrimal drainage system (Fig. 40.1) [1]. This chapter would describe the epidemiology, etiology, clinical presentations, microbiological profiles, diagnosis, management, and outcomes of canaliculitis along with a brief discussion on intracanalicular foreign bodies.

## Epidemiology

It accounts for only 2 % of all patients with lacrimal diseases [2]. Canaliculitis affects the lower eyelid more than the upper eyelid and women more than men [3]. This female preponderance is thought to be partly due to physiological or hormonal changes during menopause, which may cause decreased tear production and reduced protection against infections [4]. Furthermore, cosmetic products may occlude the canaliculus and promote bacterial growth, predisposing to canaliculitis [5].

## Etiology

Most of the cases are idiopathic in nature. Few rare predisposing factors include diverticulum or obstruction of the canaliculus which promote anaerobic bacterial growth secondary to stasis of tear and use of cosmetics.

## Microbiological Profile

Most published case series report *Actinomyces* and *Nocardia* species, prominent among them being *Actinomyces israelii* and *Nocardia asteroides* as the common pathogenic organisms [6–16]. There are only isolated case reports of canaliculitis due to other various organisms like *Mycobacterium chelonae*, *Lactococcus lactis*, *Eikenella corrodens*, *Enterobacter cloacae*, *Fusobacterium*, and *Kocuria rosea*, viruses like *Herpes simplex*, and fungal organisms like *Pityrosporum pachydermatis and Candida albicans* [17–25]. However, in one of the largest studies in literature from the author's institution, the culture-positive rates were 91 % with *Staphylococcus* species being the most common isolate (39 %) (Fig. 40.2) followed by *Streptococcus* species (29 %) and *Actinomyces* (10 %) [3].

M.J. Ali, FRCS, FRCGP
Ophthalmic Plastic Surgery, L.V. Prasad Eye Institute, Road No 2, Banjara Hills, Hyderabad-34, Hyderabad, Telangana 50034, India
e-mail: drjaved007@gmail.com


B. Mukherjee, H. Yuen (eds.), *Emergencies of the Orbit and Adnexa*,
DOI 10.1007/978-81-322-1807-4_40

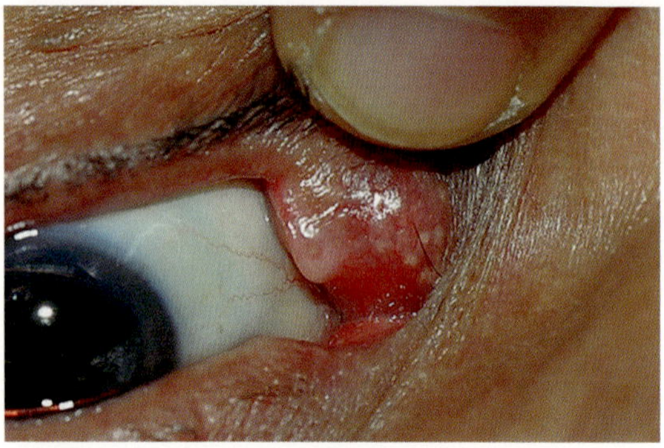

**Fig. 40.1** Clinical presentation of canaliculitis

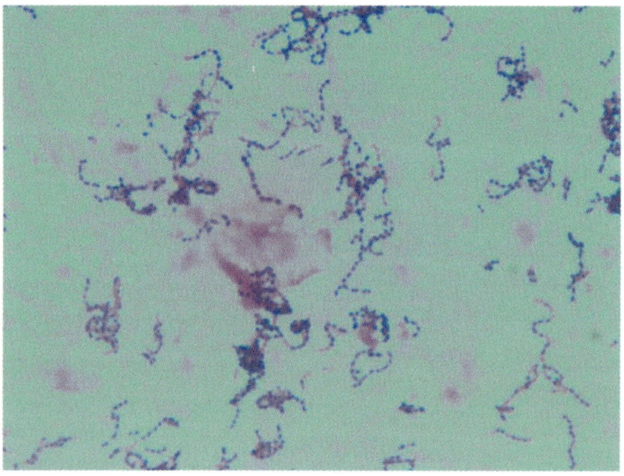

**Fig. 40.2** Gram-positive organisms on a smear

### Clinical Presentation

Common presenting symptoms include epiphora, swelling of the eyelid, pain, or redness (Fig. 40.1). Kaliki S et al. [3] in a very large series showed epiphora as the most common symptom (85 %) followed by swelling of the canalicular portion of the eyelid (32 %) and pain in 27 % of the cases. Rarely patient may even be asymptomatic [3].

On clinical examination, typical signs of canaliculitis include thickening of canalicular portion of the eyelid margin (72 %), expressible punctal discharge (36 %), and pouting erythematous punctum (34 %) (Fig. 40.1) or rarely a firm, non-tender nodule in the punctal and canalicular region [3].

## Diagnosis

Although canalicular imaging by dacryocystography and ultrasound biomicroscopy has been described for diagnosis and documentation of canaliculitis, a thorough clinical examination is sufficient for the diagnosis in most cases [26, 27].

The rarity of this disease may be attributed to the high rate of missed and delayed diagnosis. Furthermore, it may have atypical presentations, leading to additional difficulties in diagnosis [4, 28–30]. Canaliculitis can be misdiagnosed as chronic conjunctivitis, chalazion, hordeolum internum, or chronic dacryocystitis, causing a further delay in the initiation of effective treatment [3, 4, 31–33].

## Management

Various modalities of treatment have been described for canaliculitis [2–33]. Conservative measures include oral and topical antibiotics, punctal dilatation, and canalicular expression or canalicular irrigation with antibiotics [6–8]. Surgical measures include punctoplasty and canalicular curettage, canaliculotomy with canalicular curettage, or canaliculostomy [2, 3, 10–33].

However, with any of the modality of treatment, it is important to send the material for a meticulous microbiological examination.

### Conservative Medical Therapy

Initially, punctal dilatation with expression of canalicular discharge is performed under strict aseptic precautions under topical anesthesia. After instilling a drop of 0.5 % proparacaine hydrochloride in the conjunctival cul-de-sac, dilatation of the punctum is performed with Nettleship punctum dilator and manual expression of canalicular contents by a milking movement toward the punctum (Fig. 40.3). Mechanical expression is repeated until no further contents are expressed. The expressed contents are collected on a sterile cotton-tipped applicator and sent for microbiological workup. Broad-spectrum antibiotics can be started as dictated by regional isolates and their sensitivity, followed by specific antibiotics guided by patient-specific isolates. Conservative treatment in one of the largest series has shown to be effective in 59 % of the patients with a high rate or recurrence [3].

## Surgical Treatment

Surgical modalities include punctoplasty alone or in conjunction with canalicular curettage, performed under strict aseptic precautions, under local infiltrative anesthesia with 2 % lignocaine hydrochloride. A three-snip punctoplasty or the surgeon-preferred punctoplasty is performed with a small, straight Vannas scissors. To this a small canaliculotomy can be added (Fig. 40.4), and a 1-mm chalazion curette is used to curette out the granular material, concretions, or mucoid debris (Fig. 40.4). It is a good practice to evaluate walls of the ampulla, since concretions have a tendency to stack up and accumulate there. The curettage is repeated until there are no further contents. It is of utmost importance to avoid any damage to canalicular mucosa during this procedure. The curetted material is collected on a sterile surface or cotton-tipped applicator and sent for microbiological culture and sensitivity.

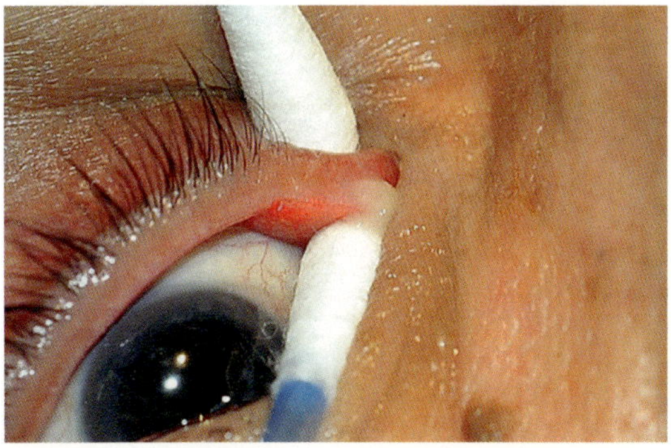

**Fig. 40.3** Late phase of canalicular milking

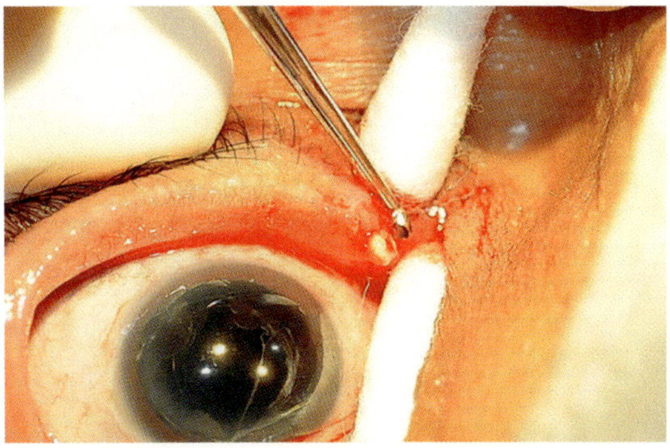

**Fig. 40.4** Pouting of concretions following canaliculotomy

Following any of the two interventions, the patient is prescribed a broad-spectrum antibiotic eye drop (e.g., 0.3 % ciprofloxacin four times per day) and is subsequently altered according to the results of the microbiology culture and sensitivity report.

Conservative treatment with topical antibiotics is associated with a high recurrence rate as high as 41 % [3, 4]. Canalicular curettage after canaliculotomy or punctoplasty carries a high-resolution rate and is the procedure of choice [2–4, 10, 31, 33]. Occasionally a repeat procedure may be required to manage recurrences. However, canaliculotomy can result in canalicular luminal narrowing or scarring, lacrimal pump dysfunction, and canalicular fistula formation [6, 31, 33]. In contrast, curettage through the punctum is a less-invasive procedure and preserves the lacrimal pump function [31, 33].

## Intracanalicular Foreign Bodies

Intracanalicular foreign bodies although rarely encountered can present as an ophthalmic emergency. Occasionally a broken cilia may enter the punctum and the canaliculus (Fig. 40.5). Careful removal under high magnification with a fine forceps is the usual management. The use of punctal plugs in the treatment of dry eye is well established [34, 35]. Collared silicone plugs of various sizes are available for managing dry eye on a semipermanent or permanent basis. Migrated punctal plugs into the canaliculus can cause

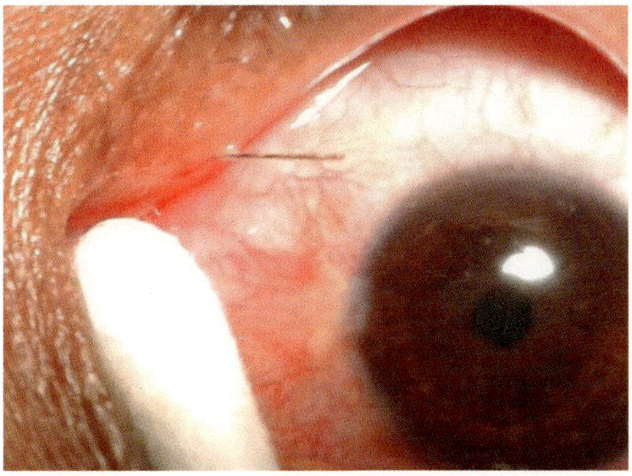

**Fig. 40.5** Eyelid cilia in lacrimal system. Note one end visible through the punctum

infection, granulomas, fibrosis, and canalicular obstructions [36]. Dacryoendoscopy has shown few typical features of migrated punctal plugs within a canaliculus [37]. If the plug is situated parallel to the canaliculus, the intracanalicular space is occluded along with granulomas and heavy debris. In contrast if the migrated plug is perpendicular to the intracanalicular space, it is not completely occluded and little granulation tissue and debris are found.

Such foreign-body reactions are more commonly encountered with long duration of intubation with a regular mono- or bicanalicular stents, which include canaliculitis (Fig. 40.6), canalicular traumatic tears (Fig. 40.7), and severe granulomatous response (Fig. 40.7). The treatment includes removal of the inciting agent like the stent and topical steroids.

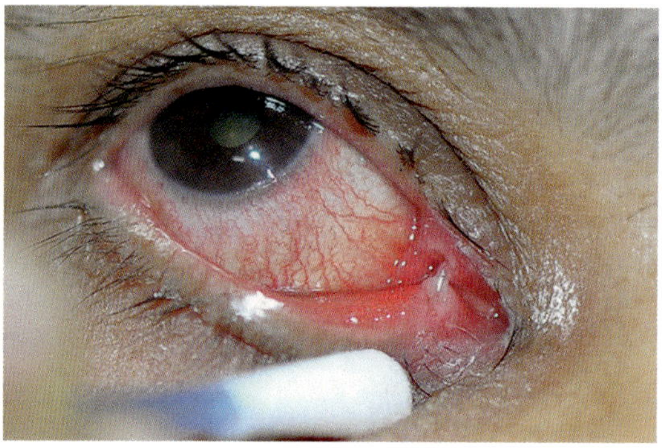

**Fig. 40.6** Lower canalicular trauma and upper canalicular granulomatous response to a tight bicanalicular silicone stents

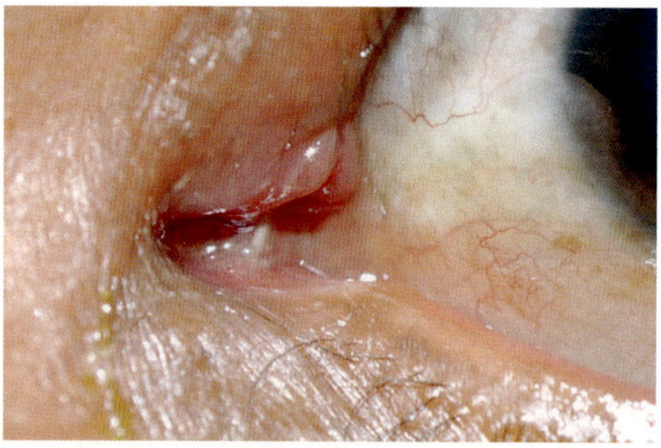

**Fig. 40.7** A severe canaliculitis and granuloma secondary to bicanalicular silicone stent

### Conclusion

In conclusion, a high index of suspicion is needed for the diagnosis of canaliculitis and intracanalicular foreign bodies. The microbiological profile of canaliculitis seems to be evolving with *Staphylococcus* emerging as the most common isolated species in South East Asia. Punctal dilatation with canalicular expression, though is effective in few patients, is more commonly associated with persistence of the disease. Punctoplasty with canalicular curettage is more efficacious with high success rates. In recurrent and persistent cases, conservative treatment is best avoided, and canalicular curettage should be done in all such cases to achieve a complete resolution.

## References


1. Anand S, Hollingworth K, Kumar V, et al. Canaliculitis: the incidence of long-term epiphora following canaliculotomy. Orbit. 2004;23:19–26.
2. Demant E, Hurwitz JJ. Canaliculitis: review of 12 cases. Can J Ophthalmol. 1980;15:73–5.
3. Kaliki S, Ali MJ, Honavar SG, Chandrasekhar G, Naik MN. Primary canaliculitis: clinical features, microbiological profile, and management outcome. Ophthal Plast Reconstr Surg. 2012;28:355–60.
4. Vécsei VP, Huber-Spitzy V, Arocker-Mettinger E, et al. Canaliculitis: difficulties in diagnosis, differential diagnosis and comparison between conservative and surgical treatment. Ophthalmologica. 1994;208: 314–7.
5. Brazier JS, Hall V. *Propionibacterium propionicum* and infections of the lacrimal apparatus. Clin Infect Dis. 1993;17:892–3.
6. McKellar MJ, Aburn NS. Cast-forming *Actinomyces israelii* canaliculitis. Aust N Z J Ophthalmol. 1997;25:301–3.
7. Sullivan TJ, Hakin KN, Sathananthan N, et al. Chronic canaliculitis. Aust N Z J Ophthalmol. 1993;21: 273–4.

8. Mohan ER, Kabra S, Udhay P, et al. Intracanalicular antibiotics may obviate the need for surgical management of chronic suppurative canaliculitis. Indian J Ophthalmol. 2008;56:338–40.
9. Briscoe D, Edelstein E, Zacharopoulos I, et al. *Actinomyces* canaliculitis: diagnosis of a masquerading disease. Graefes Arch Clin Exp Ophthalmol. 2004;242:682–6.
10. Hussain I, Bonshek RE, Loudon K, et al. Canalicular infection caused by *Actinomyces*. Eye. 1993;7:542–4.
11. Asghar S, Mahmood A, Khan MA. *Nocardia* canaliculitis presenting as pouted punctum. J Coll Phys Surg Pak. 2008;18:55–7.
12. Bharathi MJ, Ramakrishnan R, Meenakshi R, et al. *Nocardia asteroides* canaliculitis: a case report of uncommon aetiology. Indian J Med Microbiol. 2004;22:123–5.
13. Singh CN, Thakker M, Sires BS. Pyogenic granuloma associated with chronic *Actinomyces* canaliculitis. Ophthal Plast Reconstr Surg. 2006;22:224–5.
14. Eloy P, Brandt H, Nollevaux MC, et al. Solid cast-forming actinomycotic canaliculitis: case report. Rhinology. 2004;42:103–6.
15. Seal DV, McGill J, Flanagan D, et al. Lacrimal canaliculitis due *to Arachnia* (*Actinomyces*) *propionica*. Br J Ophthalmol. 1981;65:10–3.
16. Joseph TA, Paniker CK, Kumari S, et al. Actinomycotic lacrimal canaliculitis. Indian J Ophthalmol. 1980;28:157–9.
17. Fowler AM, Dutton JJ, Fowler WC, et al. *Mycobacterium chelonae* canaliculitis associated with SmartPlug use. Ophthal Plast Reconstr Surg. 2008;24:241–3.
18. Leung DY, Kwong YY, Ma CH, et al. Canaliculitis associated with a combined infection of *Lactococcus lactis cremoris* and *Eikenella corrodens*. Jpn J Ophthalmol. 2006;50:284–5.
19. de Koning EW, van Bijsterveld OP. *Herpes simplex virus* canaliculitis. Ophthalmologica. 1983;186:173–6.
20. Jordan DR, Agapitos PJ, McCunn PD. *Eikenella corrodens* canaliculitis. Am J Ophthalmol. 1993;115:823–4.
21. Chumbley LC. Canaliculitis caused by *Enterobacter cloacae*: report of a case. Br J Ophthalmol. 1984;68:364–6.
22. Romano A, Segal E, Blumenthal M. Canaliculitis with isolation of *Pityrosporum pachydermatis*. Br J Ophthalmol. 1978;62:732–4.
23. Newton JC, Tulevech CB. Lacrimal canaliculitis due to *Candida albicans*. Report of a case and a discussion of its significance. Am J Ophthalmol. 1962;53:933–6.
24. Weinberg RJ, Sartoris MJ, Buerger Jr GF, et al. *Fusobacterium* in presumed *Actinomyces* canaliculitis. Am J Ophthalmol. 1977;84:371–4.
25. Ali MJ, Pujari A, Motukupally S, et al. *Kocuria rosea* canaliculitis: a clinicomicrobiological correlation. Ophthal Plast Reconstr Surg. 2014;30(6):e139–40.
26. Sathananthan N, Sullivan TJ, Rose GE, et al. Intubation dacryocystography in patients with a clinical diagnosis of chronic canaliculitis ("*streptothrix*"). Br J Radiol. 1993;66:389–93.
27. Hurwitz JJ, Pavlin CJ. Proximal canalicular imaging utilizing ultrasound biomicroscopy B: canaliculitis. Orbit. 1998;17:31–6.
28. Moscato EE, Sires BS. Atypical canaliculitis. Ophthal Plast Reconstr Surg. 2008;24:54–5.
29. Charles NC, Lisman RD, Mittal KR. Carcinoma of the lacrimal canaliculus masquerading as canaliculitis. Arch Ophthalmol. 2006;124:414–6.
30. Fulmer NL, Neal JG, Bussard GM, et al. Lacrimal canaliculitis. Am J Emerg Med. 1999;17:385–6.
31. Pavilack MA, Frueh BR. Through curettage in the treatment of chronic canaliculitis. Arch Ophthalmol. 1992;110:200–2.
32. Lin SC, Kao SC, Tsai CC, et al. Clinical characteristics and factors associated the outcome of lacrimal canaliculitis. Acta Ophthalmol. 2011;89:759–63.
33. Lee MJ, Choung HK, Kim NJ, et al. One-snip punctoplasty and canalicular curettage through the punctum: a minimally invasive surgical procedure for primary canaliculitis. Ophthalmology. 2009;116:2027–30.e2.
34. Murube J, Murube E. Treatment of dry eye by blocking the lacrimal canaliculi. Surv Ophthalmol. 1996;40:463–80.
35. AltanYaycioglu R, Gencoglu EA, Akova YA, et al. Silicone versus collagen plugs for treating dry eye: results of a prospective randomized control trial including lacrimal scintigraphy. Am J Ophthalmol. 2005;140:88–93.
36. Soparkar CN, Patrinely JR, Hunts J, et al. The perils of permanent punctal plugs. Am J Ophthalmol. 1997;123:120–1.
37. Takahashi Y, Iwaki M, Nakamura Y, et al. Dacryoendoscopic findings of intracanalicular punctal plug migration with or without canaliculitis. Ophthal Plast Reconstr Surg. 2013;29:128–30.

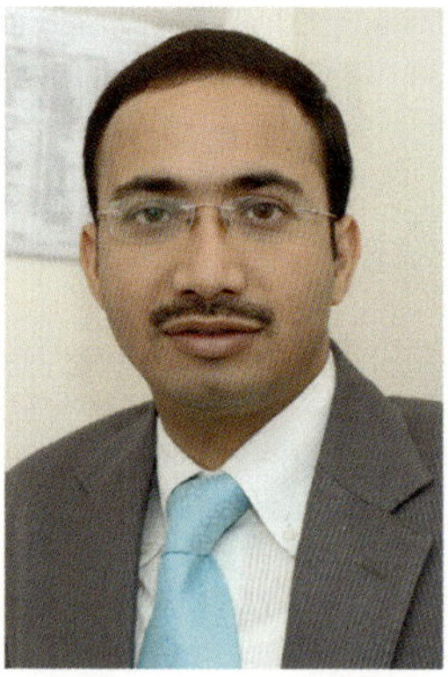

**Mohammad Javed Ali** Dr. Mohammad Javed Ali currently leads The Institute of Dacryology at the LV Prasad Eye Institute. Javed described two new diseases of the lacrimal system along with their classifications and clinicopathologic profiles. He is one among the rare recipients of The Experienced Researcher – Alexander Von Humbold Fellowship Award, one of the pinnacle awards in the research world. He was honored by the 2015 ASOPRS Merrill Reeh Award for his path-breaking work on etiopathogenesis of punctal stenosis. His textbook *Principles and Practice of Lacrimal Surgery* is considered to be the most comprehensive treatise on the subject. He is a section editor for 3 journals and reviewer for 16 major journals. He has to his credit a total of 203 publications, of which 141 are peer reviewed and 30 are non peer reviewed, 32 book chapters, 21 instruction courses, 3 keynote addresses, 214 conference presentations, 12 live surgical workshops, and 26 awards.

# 41 General Approach and Algorithm for Managing Emergent Neoplasms of the Orbit and Adnexa

Lora Rabin Dagi Glass, Seanna Grob, and Suzanne K. Freitag

Malignancies of the orbit can be classified into primary, secondary, or metastatic in nature. Primary orbital malignancies arise within the orbit, while secondary orbital malignancies are extensions of locally invasive tumors in adjacent structures. Metastatic orbital tumors are the result of hematogenous or lymphatic spread from primary tumors in remote sites.

Malignant neoplasm must be in the differential diagnosis of any patient presenting with proptosis or other globe displacement (Fig. 41.1), restriction of extraocular motility, globe compression, optic neuropathy, or other cranial neuropathies pertaining to the orbit or cavernous sinus. These orbital malignancies require different consideration than when they occur in other parts of the body because the orbit is a small confined space full of structures critical for vision. Prompt diagnosis is important to

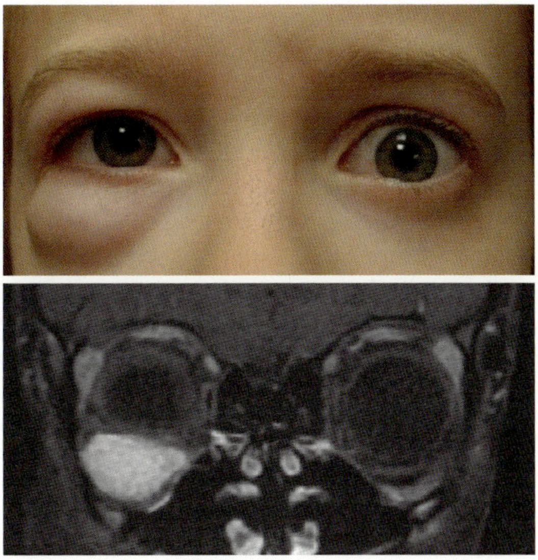

**Fig. 41.1** (**a**) An 8-year-old female presented with a rapidly progressive mass of the right orbit, causing globe displacement. (**b**) Coronal T1-weighted MRI with contrast showed a homogenously enhancing mass in the inferior orbit. Emergent biopsy showed embryonal rhabdomyosarcoma


L.R.D. Glass, MD
Ophthalmic Plastic and Reconstructive Surgery, Massachusetts Eye and Ear Infirmary, 243 Charles Street, 10th Floor, Boston, MA 02114, USA
e-mail: lora_dagiglass@meei.harvard.edu

S. Grob, MD, MAS
Ophthalmology, Massachusetts Eye and Ear Infirmary, Harvard Medical School, 243 Charles St, Boston, CA 02114, USA
e-mail: seanna_grob@meei.harvard.edu

S.K. Freitag, MD (✉)
Ophthalmic Plastic Surgery Service, Department of Oculoplastic and Reconstructive Surgery, Massachusetts Eye and Ear Infirmary, Harvard Medical School, 243 Charles Street, 10th Floor Oculoplastics Suite, Boston, MA 02114, USA
e-mail: suzanne_freitag@meei.harvard.edu



B. Mukherjee, H. Yuen (eds.), *Emergencies of the Orbit and Adnexa*,
DOI 10.1007/978-81-322-1807-4_41

prevent a rapidly enlarging lesion from causing permanent damage to orbital structures. If not carefully planned, treatments such as surgery or radiation therapy to the orbit may cause loss of vision or visual dysfunction such as diplopia. Certain pediatric neoplasms, such as rhabdomyosarcoma, neuroblastoma, and retinoblastoma, can be rapidly lethal. It is especially critical to recognize a potential neoplasm in this age group and address it immediately. Hence, it is crucial to identify the presence of an orbital lesion when a patient presents with symptoms, to suspect when it may be malignant, and to act carefully but expediently to save vision, eyes, and life.

## Examination

When an orbital neoplasm is suspected, a thorough examination is vital. The clinical history can elucidate helpful information regarding temporal onset of disease, rapidity of progression, and associated symptoms. These may serve as clues regarding tumor location and affected orbital structures. In addition to asking questions about onset, duration, severity, and progression, it is often useful to have the patient bring old photographs or request observations from close friends or family members to determine changes that may have occurred even earlier than the first reported symptoms. Sensory symptoms including pain, numbness, tingling, as well as severity and worsening of these symptoms with eye movements can provide additional information about the type or location of the tumor. For example, adenoid cystic carcinoma of the lacrimal gland is more commonly associated with pain due to its ability to infiltrate adjacent structures and invade orbital nerves. Symptoms suggesting disturbance of the optic nerve include changes in visual acuity or color vision, or awareness of a scotoma. Neoplasms affecting motor abilities of the eye can cause symptoms of diplopia, gaze or head positioning preference, pain with eye movements, and pulling or tugging sensations suggesting a restrictive component. Patients may notice changes in their appearance as a result of tumor growth, such as proptosis or enophthalmos, globe displacement in any direction, or swelling or fullness of eyelids (Fig. 41.2). If the tumor is affecting the orbital vascular system, the patient may notice conjunctival injection or eyelid erythema and edema.

A thorough discussion of past medical history and review of systems is also important, as neoplasms within the orbit are often associated with systemic abnormalities [1]. Review of systems may reveal symptoms of systemic illness such as fever or weight loss. Past medical, ocular, surgical, and family history can point to possible etiologies, particularly metastatic cancer or oncologic syndromes.

Physical examination is essential to collecting additional information that can be used to synthesize a plan for further clinical investigations and management. General observations such as facial contour and symmetry of facial, lid, orbital, and ocular structures are useful. The orbital structures should be palpated, as should the preauricular and cervical lymph nodes to check for enlargement, which would be concerning for nodal metastases. If tissues feel firm, nodular, nonmobile, or irregular, they should be investigated further. Resistance to retropulsion of the globe

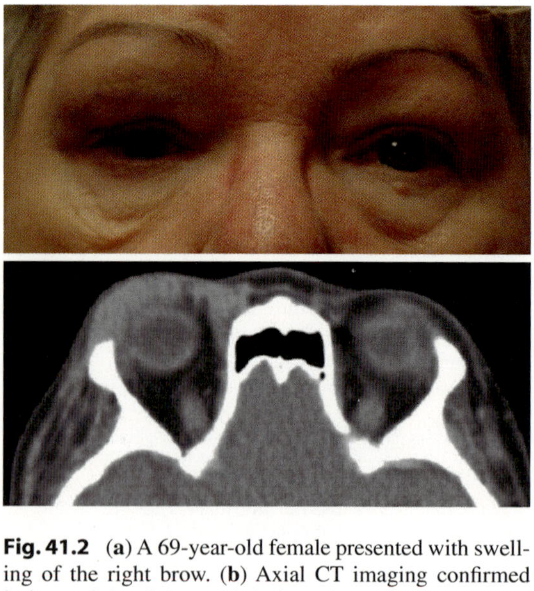

**Fig. 41.2** (**a**) A 69-year-old female presented with swelling of the right brow. (**b**) Axial CT imaging confirmed lesions of the right and left lids with extension into the right orbit, and biopsy confirmed a diagnosis of MALT lymphoma

should be assessed and compared to the contralateral orbit. Abnormal lid positioning or structural changes may be secondary to proptosis or other alterations in orbital anatomy. Measurements of interpalpebral fissure height, lid position lid crease position, lagophthalmos, and scleral show should all be documented. Slit lamp biomicroscopy may reveal the presence of tumor on the ocular surface (Fig. 41.3) or conjunctival injection, dilated episcleral vessels, or chemosis, especially when vascular congestion or malformations are present in the orbit.

Tests of vision and optic nerve function include best-corrected visual acuity, pupil evaluation for pupil asymmetry or afferent pupillary defect (Fig. 41.4), confrontational visual fields, Amsler grid testing of central vision, and color vision assessment. These measurements are helpful for evaluating compression of or the degree of damage to the optic nerve or other vital ocular structures, helping guide urgency of treatment.

The orbital exam should include exophthalmometry. Differences between the two eyes that are greater than 1–2 mm should be further investigated (Fig. 41.5) [2, 3]. Globe displacement horizontally or vertically should also be measured and documented. Ocular movements in all cardinal positions can be evaluated with ductions and versions. Hirschberg testing or prism measurements can provide information about the degree of ocular deviation. Additionally, a full eye examination including measurement of intraocular pressure and anterior segment and dilated funduscopic examination are important. Dilated examination can show optic nerve abnormalities, vascular congestion, or indentation of the globe from adjacent orbital masses.

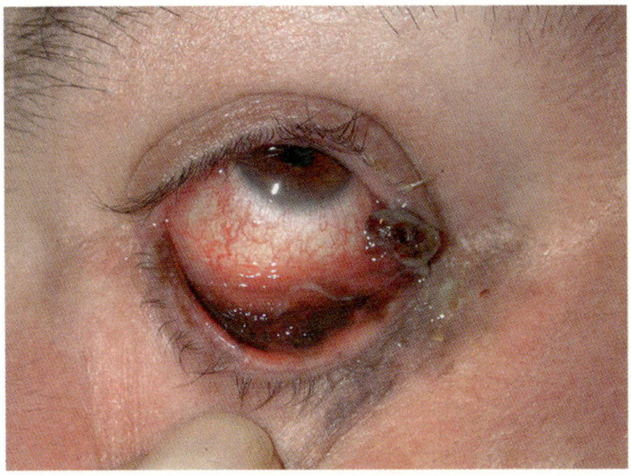

**Fig. 41.3** A 52-year-old male presented with a rapidly growing, melanotic mass of the right eye and was found to have both eyelid and caruncular melanomas. The neoplasm rapidly invaded the nasolacrimal system and metastasized to the lungs

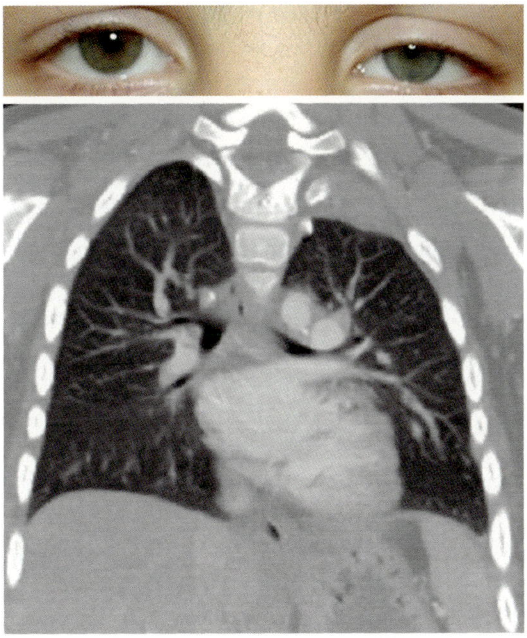

**Fig. 41.4** (**a**) A young boy presented with a history of congenital Horner syndrome; note ptosis of the left upper eyelid, ptosis of the left lower eyelid, miosis of the left pupil, and iris heterochromia with the affected pupil lighter than the unaffected pupil. (**b**) CT chest showed a left apical neuroblastoma (Figure courtesy of Gena Heidary, M.D)

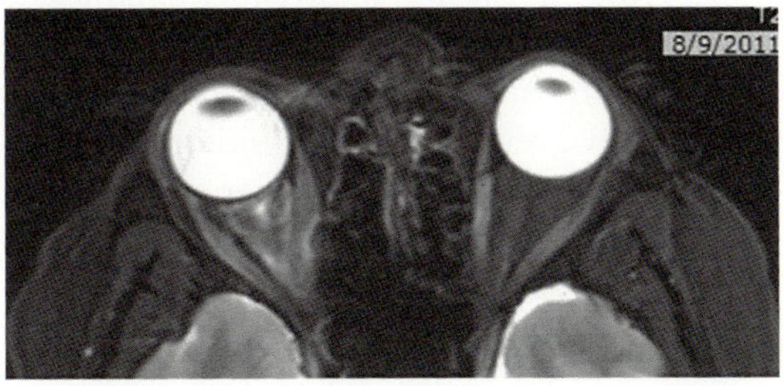

**Fig. 41.5** A 47-year-old female with a prior history of treated nonmetastatic breast cancer presented with amaurosis; clinical examination was notable for right-sided enophthalmos, and T2-weighted axial MRI showed an extensive right-sided intraconal mass. Orbital biopsy confirmed metastatic breast cancer

## Imaging and Clinical Investigations

The clinical examination can direct additional testing that may provide further information about the neoplasm and extent of disease.

Baseline visual field testing is recommended for all patients with orbital pathology. Although visual field defects are nonspecific for the type of neoplasm, they can provide information about the degree of optic nerve compression. Serial visual field tests can also provide information about disease progression and help guide management.

Orbital imaging is invaluable to the assessment of orbital malignancies. Imaging can provide information about the location of the tumor, relationship to adjacent structures, compression of orbital structures, involvement of the vascular system, and tissue characteristics such as cystic or solid, calcifications, and capsular definition. Orbital masses can be identified with both computed tomography (CT) and magnetic resonance imaging (MRI). Regardless of the imaging modality, thin axial, coronal and sagittal cuts through the orbit should be used. CT provides excellent detail of bony anatomy including details of bone tumors, bony infiltration, or calcification. CT can also provide soft tissue resolution because orbital fat is low density on CT imaging. CT with intravenous contrast is especially helpful in vascular lesions, lesions affecting the optic nerve, and for evaluating extra-orbital infiltration. MRI can provide soft tissue detail, allowing for further characterization of the neoplasm. Intravenous contrast is similarly helpful. Ultrasound is utilized for the evaluation of anterior orbital lesions in some centers; however, its utility is limited as it does not penetrate well into the deeper orbit and the image resolution is much poorer than that of CT or MRI.

Serologic laboratory testing may be indicated if there is suspicion for leukemia or lymphoma. Complete blood count with differential may show an elevated white blood cell count or other abnormalities. Serologic testing targeted for specific diseases such as IgG4, ANCA, and Lyme may be useful in distinguishing inflammatory or infectious conditions from malignancy.

## Multidisciplinary Approach

When an orbital mass is discovered and there is suspicion of malignancy, systemic evaluation by a medical oncologist may be helpful to screen for possible systemic findings, such a lymphadenopathy or a breast mass, which could help establish the diagnosis. When there is a known orbital malignancy, systemic evaluation is necessary for disease staging. Studies may include additional imaging of the brain, chest, abdomen, and pelvis or other laboratory serologic studies. Positron emission tomography (PET) may also be helpful in determining extent of disease.

## Biopsy and Histopathologic Analysis

Biopsy with histopathologic analysis provides a definitive diagnosis. Some orbital lesions are not easily accessible and may require the technical expertise of an experienced orbital surgeon to safely perform. Depending on the location, proximity to critical structures, size, evidence of infiltration, and presumed diagnosis, the decision may be made to perform either incisional biopsy or complete excision of the lesion. It is important to have a formulated plan for pathologic analysis prior to biopsy. For example, some lesions may need immediate evaluation with frozen section pathology to determine whether diagnostic tissue has been obtained at the time of biopsy. Additionally, special handling for flow cytometry is performed when lymphoma is suspected. Other possible areas of diagnostic analysis include cytology, immunohistochemistry, and electron microscopy. Good communication with a skilled ophthalmic pathologist can be invaluable in assistance with tissue handling and in making a proper diagnosis.

Some primary orbital malignancies involve the optic nerve or the dural sheath surrounding it. Biopsy of these lesions even in the case of a peripheral biopsy of a large lesion can lead to vision loss, the nerve or the vascular supply to the nerve can be disrupted leading to profound visual loss. However, if a malignant tumor is suspected based on tumor behavior or characteristics on imaging, biopsy may be required. In all cases, the risks of biopsy should be reviewed in detail with the patient, including the risk of visual loss, blindness, and double vision.

Fine needle aspiration biopsy (FNAB) is a minimally invasive technique to retrieve cytologic specimens and can at times be used to differentiate benign from malignant lesions. Cellular yields can be low, and interpretation of the specimen can be challenging, requiring additional biopsy. In addition, sticking a needle blindly into an orbit is not without risk. Critical structures can be damaged, and there is a risk of causing hemorrhage, which could lead to a compartment syndrome and visual loss.

Orbitotomy with direct visualization of tissue is safer and provides better tissue sampling for histopathologic analysis. The location of the tumor on imaging will direct the surgical approach for biopsy. A medial orbitotomy can be performed via a transcutaneous, transcaruncular, or transconjunctival approach and can provide access to medially located lesions as well as the optic nerve. A lateral orbitotomy, potentially with a bone window, allows for the best approach to laterally-based lesions [4–7]. Superiorly located lesions can also be approached via a lateral orbitotomy or transcutaneously along the upper lid crease. Inferiorly, orbital lesions can be approached through a lateral orbitotomy or transconjunctivally. A lateral canthotomy and cantholysis can provide additional exposure. Transnasal, transantral, and transethmoidal endoscopic approaches are being utilized more frequently to access orbital lesions and provide the benefit of less visible scarring. These are best for lesions located posteriorly in the orbit and medial to the optic nerve. Transcranial approaches may be utilized for posterior orbital lesions in conjunction with a neurosurgeon.

## Advances in Diagnosis and Treatment

Transnasal endoscopic surgery has proven to be a great advancement in access to the orbit. In conjunction with otolaryngologists, many new techniques have been developed by ophthalmologists to biopsy or remove orbital tumors, particularly in the medial and posterior orbit. The orbital apex and periorbital skull base have long been challenging to access. Murchison et al. reviewed 18 patients whereby an endoscopic approach was used to access a range of pathologies including cavernous hemangiomas, juvenile angiofibromas, and invasive cutaneous squamous cell carcinoma [8]. The majority of lesions were located in the medial orbit and/or optic canal [8].

The use of intraoperative stereotactic CT image guidance for anatomic localization in orbital and sinus surgery has become increasingly popular. Using a previously obtained CT scan, axial, coronal, and sagittal plane images are displayed simultaneously on a monitor in the operating room for real-time intraoperative localization of orbital and sinus structures using surgical instrument tips with tracking devices recognized by the image guidance system. A variety of these imaging guidance systems are available, and their use has been reported in numerous surgical approaches and orbital indications. There are reported cases of excision of an optic nerve glioma, recurrent pleomorphic adenoma of lacrimal gland, and secondary orbital meningioma [9]. Another case series, the image guidance system proved useful in localizing and obtaining a biopsy of three orbital apex tumors, two meningiomas and one osteoblastoma [10].

Advances in chemotherapeutic agents and use of multi-agent regimens have increased survival rates in patients with orbital malignancies. For example, the Intergroup Rhabdomyosarcoma Study Group suggests treatment with combined irradiation and chemotherapy, including vincristine and actinomycin with either cyclophosphamide, ifosfamide, or etoposide, with only 1 tumor-related death among 33 patients studied [11].

Recent data also suggests that neoadjuvant intra-arterial cytoreductive chemotherapy may allow for significantly higher survival rates in patients with adenoid cystic carcinoma who have intact lacrimal arteries, defined as not having undergone extensive debulking, and who follow with a course of orbital exenteration, with radiation and chemotherapy postoperatively [12, 13]. One center reported a 100 % 10-year disease-free survival with this regimen [12].

Proton beam therapy is a novel radiation treatment with fewer side effects than traditional external beam radiation. Its utilized has been increasing over the last decade. One significant benefit of proton beam radiation is its modulated, narrow radiation delivery zone that produces less collateral damage [14]. It can be especially helpful in the pediatric population, as there is less radiation dose delivery to vital structures such as the hypothalamic-pituitary system and decreased risk of development of secondary tumors [14]. This treatment is limited to several proton beam centers around the world.

**Conclusion**

Whether dealing with a primary, secondary, or metastatic malignancy of the orbit, careful examination of the patient is critical. Examination findings will help guide additional testing, which then leads to determination of a diagnosis, usually by means of a tissue biopsy. Having a high level of suspicion that an orbital lesion is malignant should lead to expeditious management and treatment in order to preserve vision, eye, and life.

## References


1. Rootman J. An approach to diagnosis of orbital disease. Can J Ophthalmol. 1983;18(3):102–7.
2. Rootman J. Diseases of the orbit: a multidisciplinary approach, vol. xxiv. Philadelphia: Lippincott; 1988. p. 628.
3. Fledelius HC, Stubgaard M. Changes in eye position during growth and adult life as based on exophthalmometry, interpupillary distance, and orbital distance measurements. Acta Ophthalmol. 1986;64(5):481–6.
4. McNab AA, Wright JE. Lateral orbitotomy – a review. Aust N Z J Ophthalmol. 1990;18(3):281–6.
5. Halli RC, Mishra S, Kini YK, Kharkar VR, Hebbale MA. Modified lateral orbitotomy approach: a novel technique in the management of lacrimal gland tumors. J Craniofac Surg. 2011;22(3):1035–8.
6. Berke RN. A modified Kronlein operation. AMA Arch Ophthalmol. 1954;51(5):609–32.
7. Harris GJ, Logani SC. Eyelid crease incision for lateral orbitotomy. Ophthal Plast Reconstr Surg. 1999;15(1):9–16; discussion 16–8.
8. Murchison AP, Rosen MR, Evans JJ, Bilyk JR. Endoscopic approach to the orbital apex and periorbital skull base. Laryngoscope. 2011;121(3):463–7.
9. Karcioglu ZA, Mascott CR. Computer-assisted image-guided orbit surgery. Eur J Ophthalmol. 2006;16(3):446–52.
10. Berger M, Char DH. Interactive image guidance for surgical localization of orbital apical tumors. Orbit. 2002;21(3):199–203.
11. Shields CL, Shields JA, Honavar SG, Demirci H. Primary ophthalmic rhabdomyosarcoma in 33 patients. Trans Am Ophthalmol Soc. 2001;99:133–42; discussion 142–3.
12. Tse DT, Kossler AL, Feuer WJ, Benedetto PW. Long-term outcomes of neoadjuvant intra-arterial cytoreductive chemotherapy for lacrimal gland adenoid cystic carcinoma. Ophthalmology. 2013;120(7):1313–23.
13. Tse DT, Benedetto P, Dubovy S, Schiffman JC, Feuer WJ. Clinical analysis of the effect of intraarterial cytoreductive chemotherapy in the treatment of lacrimal gland adenoid cystic carcinoma. Am J Ophthalmol. 2006;141(1):44–53.
14. Arvold ND, Niemierko A, Broussard GP, et al. Projected second tumor risk and dose to neurocognitive structures after proton versus photon radiotherapy for benign meningioma. Int J Radiat Oncol Biol Phys. 2012;83(4):e495–500.


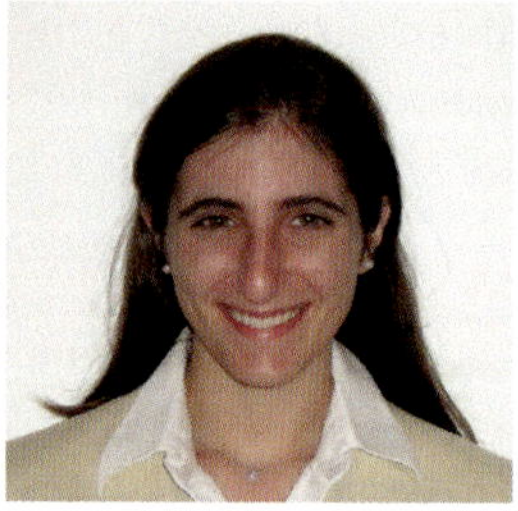

**Lora Rabin Dagi Glass** Lora Dagi Glass completed her ophthalmology residency at the Columbia University Medical Center, followed by a fellowship in oculoplastic surgery at the Massachusetts Eye and Ear Infirmary. Her research has focused on orbital processes ranging from thyroid eye disease to optic nerve glioma and orbital melanoma.

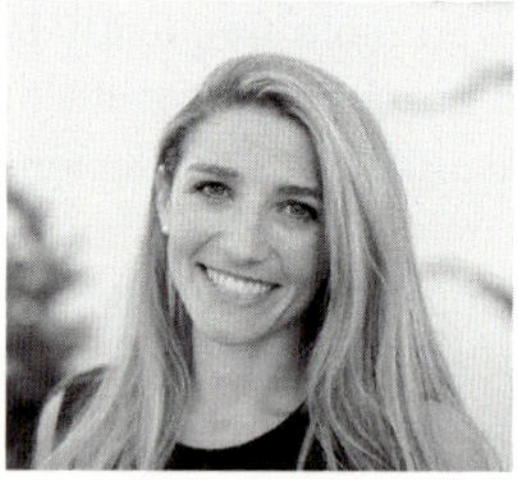

**Seanna Grob** MD, MAS received a BA in Molecular and Cellular Biology from the University of California, Berkeley and a MD and MAS from the University of California, San Diego. She completed her ophthalmology residency at Massachusetts Eye and Ear/Harvard Medical School. She is currently the Director of the Ocular Trauma Service at Massachusetts Eye and Ear and Brigham and Women's Hospital. She has been accepted into a 2-year American Society of Ophthalmic Plastic and Reconstructive Surgery-approved fellowship and will start in 2017.

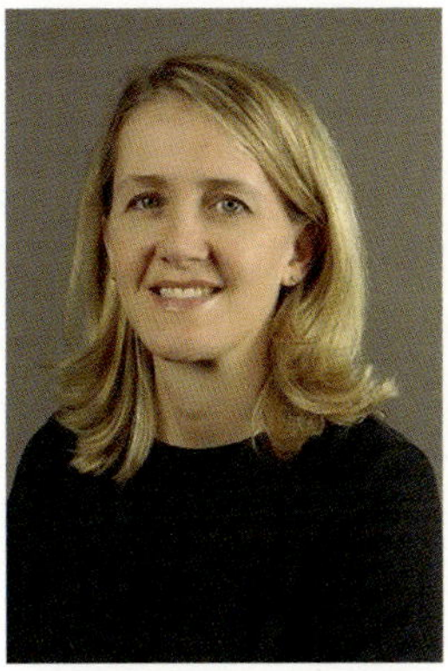

**Suzanne K. Freitag** Suzanne K Freitag, MD, received a BA from Duke University and MD from Jefferson Medical College in Philadelphia, PA. She completed ophthalmology residency at Wills Eye Hospital followed by a neuroophthalmology fellowship at the Wilmer Eye Institute at Johns Hopkins. She then completed a 2-year American Society of Ophthalmic Plastic and Reconstructive Surgery-approved fellowship in Boston. She is the Director of the Ophthalmic Plastic Surgery Service at Massachusetts Eye and Ear Infirmary and an Assistant Professor of Ophthalmology at Harvard Medical School.

# Primary Orbital Malignancies

# 42

Seanna R. Grob, Lora Rabin Dagi Glass,
and Suzanne K. Freitag

## Introduction

Malignancies of the orbit can be classified into primary, secondary, or metastatic. Primary orbital malignancies arise within the orbit, while secondary orbital malignancies are extensions of locally invasive tumors in adjacent structures, and metastatic tumors travel from remote sites in the body. This chapter will focus on malignancies that arise primarily in the orbit. Secondary and metastatic malignancies will be discussed in later chapters.

S.R. Grob, MD, MAS
Ophthalmology, Massachusetts Eye and Ear Infirmary, Harvard Medical School, Boston, CA, USA
e-mail: seanna_grob@meei.harvard.edu

L.R.D. Glass, MD
Ophthalmic Plastic Surgery Service, Department of Ophthalmology, Massachusetts Eye and Ear Infirmary, Harvard Medical School, Boston, MA, USA
e-mail: lora_dagiglass@meei.harvard.edu

S.K. Freitag, MD (✉)
Ophthalmic Plastic Surgery Service, Department of Oculoplastic and Reconstructive Surgery, Massachusetts Eye and Ear Infirmary, Harvard Medical School, 243 Charles Street, 10th Floor Oculoplastics Suite, Boston, MA 02114, USA
e-mail: suzanne_freitag@meei.harvard.edu

The incidence of primary orbital malignancies is low, with lymphoma being the most common in adults and rhabdomyosarcoma in children. Approximately 60 % of orbital tumors are benign, and 40 % are malignant [1]. Malignant lesions are more common in adults, with nearly 60 % of orbital tumors in adults over 60 being malignant [2]. The age-specific incidence of primary malignant orbital tumors is approximately two per million population until the sixth decade of life, increases to four per million population in those older than age 60 years, and further increases to ten per million population in those older than 80 years [3].

Rhabdomyosarcoma, a mesenchymal tumor, is the most common primary malignant orbital tumor in children. Six percent of childhood orbital tumors were rhabdomyosarcoma in a series by Rootman [1]. Other sarcomas make up a large majority of pediatric primary orbital malignancies. In adults, lymphoma is the most common orbital malignancy, accounting for approximately 24 % of all orbital malignancies in patients >59 years old [2, 4]. The next most common primary orbital malignancies in adults include other lymphoproliferative or hematopoietic malignancies and lacrimal gland malignancies. Although many patients present with similar symptoms, performing a detailed clinical history and examination as well as using other ancillary testing may reveal characteristics suggestive that an orbital lesion is malignant, hence requiring immediate management.


B. Mukherjee, H. Yuen (eds.), *Emergencies of the Orbit and Adnexa*,
DOI 10.1007/978-81-322-1807-4_42

## Clinical Presentation

Patients with orbital tumors can present with an array of different symptoms and chief complaints. If there is involvement or compression of the optic nerve, the patient may present with vision loss. Since the orbit is a relatively small, confined anatomical area, any space-occupying lesion within the orbit may result in proptosis or displacement of the globe. The patient then may notice a change in their appearance with fullness of their lids or protrusion or displacement of their eye in a particular direction. The patient may also note bruising or a change in the appearance of the periorbital skin. If there is displacement of the globe or a mass effect on the extraocular muscles, the patient may present with double vision. Pain is a common complaint and may be a sign of a more concerning lesion, as the neoplasm may be infiltrating surrounding structures and nerves. Pain can be described as pain with eye movements, pressure or pain behind the eyes, headaches, or even sinus pain or pressure. The patient's description of the rapidity of onset and progression is also vital to determining the level of concern that should be raised. In one series of 267 patients older than 60 years, the most common presenting clinical features of orbital malignancy were a palpable or visualized mass (26 %), proptosis (18 %), and pain (15 %) [2]. Of note, 6 % of the patients were asymptomatic [2]. Therefore, even routine ophthalmic examination may reveal findings concerning for orbital neoplasm.

## Classification

The list of primary orbital neoplasms is quite extensive. The number becomes much smaller when focusing on those that are malignant; however, these tumors are usually more aggressive and at risk of metastasizing. To simplify the process of listing orbital malignancies, it is helpful to think about basic orbital anatomy. Each structure within the orbit has its own list of associated neoplasms. However, not all primary malignant orbital tumors are derived from their respective tissue and may arise from undifferentiated tissues within the orbit. Table 42.1 lists primary orbital malignancies.

**Table 42.1** Primary orbital malignancies

| |
|---|
| 1. Malignant neurogenic tumors of the orbit |
| (a) Malignant optic nerve glioma of adulthood (glioblastoma) |
| (b) Malignant peripheral nerve sheath tumors |
| (c) Melanoma |
| 2. Malignant mesenchymal tumors of the orbit |
| (a) Malignant striated muscle tumors |
| (i) Rhabdomyosarcoma |
| (ii) Rhabdoid tumor |
| (iii) Endodermal sinus tumor |
| (b) Malignant smooth muscle tumors |
| (i) Leiomyosarcoma |
| (c) Malignant adipose tumors |
| (i) Liposarcoma |
| (d) Malignant fibrous tissue tumors |
| (i) Fibrosarcoma |
| (ii) Congenital and infantile fibrosarcoma |
| (iii) Epithelioid sarcoma |
| (iv) Malignant solitary fibrous tumor |
| (e) Malignant histiocytic tumors |
| (i) Malignant fibrous histiocytoma |
| 3. Malignant primary bone tumors of the orbit |
| (a) Osteosarcoma |
| (b) Chondrosarcoma |
| (c) Mesenchymal chondrosarcoma |
| (d) Ewing's sarcoma |
| (e) Giant cell tumor |
| (f) Hematopoietic and histiocytic lesions affecting the bone (e.g., myeloma) |
| 4. Lymphoproliferative, leukemic, and histiocytic lesions of the orbit |
| (a) Lymphocytic tumors |
| (i) Small B-cell lymphoma |
| (ii) Diffuse large B-cell lymphoma |
| (iii) Burkitt's lymphoma |
| (iv) T-cell lymphoma |
| (b) Leukemic tumors |
| (c) Plasma cell tumors |
| (d) Malignant histiocytosis |
| 5. Malignant lacrimal gland tumors |
| (a) Adenoid cystic carcinoma |
| (b) Carcinoma ex pleomorphic adenoma |
| (c) Mucoepidermoid carcinoma |
| (d) Adenocarcinoma |

## Acute Management for Primary Orbital Malignancies

Performing a careful history and clinical examination and ordering proper imaging are critical in the formulation of a differential diagnosis, which can aid in the rapid recognition of an orbital neoplasm. When this leads to a high index of suspicion for a malignant orbital process, rapid tissue diagnosis followed by thoughtful treatment decisions is critical. If there is concern for extension outside of the orbit, additional specialists such as head and neck surgeons, neurosurgeons, oncologists, and radiation oncologists should be consulted.

## Review of Some Primary Orbital Malignancies: Presentation and Management

This section will review some of the more common primary orbital malignancies in greater detail. Many orbital tumors present with signs and symptoms including proptosis, diplopia, globe displacement, pain, restriction of extraocular movements, and blurred vision. In addition to these nonspecific orbital findings, there are sometimes highly suggestive or pathognomonic findings leading to a specific diagnosis, which will be discussed below.

### Malignant Neurogenic Tumors of the Orbit

#### Malignant Optic Nerve Glioma (Glioblastoma)

Typical presentation and imaging:

- Age: middle age, more commonly males.
- Symptoms: rapid vision loss, monocular vision blurring, and retrobulbar pain.
- Signs: decreased visual acuity, afferent pupillary defect, visual field changes, enlarged blind spot or scotoma, strabismus, optic disk infarction, venous congestion and edema, hemiparesis, and hypothalamic abnormalities.
- Imaging: MRI orbits and brain with contrast is the preferred study.
  - CT scan: enlargement of optic nerve and/or chiasm.
  - MRI: similar to CT appearance but with more soft tissue detail. Useful to distinguish that the optic nerve itself and not the sheath is the source of the mass. The lesion is isointense or slightly hypointense on T1-weighted scans and variable on T2.

In 1973, Hoyt et al. described a malignant optic nerve glioma of adulthood [5]. It has a fulminant and relentless course that usually presents with monocular vision loss, retrobulbar pain, and edema that rapidly progresses to blindness, hemiparesis, and hypothalamic abnormalities. Pathologically, it is a glioblastoma that invades surrounding tissues. Ocular symptoms develop early as the tumor rapidly extends into the nervous system. Diagnosis is made by biopsy of the tumor, in contrast to pediatric optic nerve gliomas, which can often be diagnosed with imaging alone, grow very slowly, and can be observed until evidence of worsening symptoms or visual decline. Patients with malignant optic nerve glioma have a rapid downhill course that leads to death, and the lesion is usually unaffected by attempted therapeutic modalities [1].

### Malignant Mesenchymal Tumors of the Orbit

#### Rhabdomyosarcoma

Typical Presentation and Imaging

- Age: Young child (average age 7–8 years, with 70 % occurring in the first decade of life).
- Symptoms: Rapidly progressive proptosis or globe displacement, often minimal inflammation and pain.
- Signs: Acute and subacute proptosis, globe displacement (often down and out), eyelid edema, ptosis, and palpable mass.
- Imaging: MRI with contrast is the modality of choice in a young child to prevent radiation exposure. It may require sedation depending on the age of the child.

  - CT: homogenous, well-defined, soft tissue mass without bone destruction, isodense to normal muscle, and moderate to marked contrast enhancement (rarely may cause bony destruction with extension into other sites such as the sinuses, nasopharynx, oral cavity, intracranial space).
  - MRI: T1 is isointense to muscle, and T2 is hyperintense and appears hyperintense after contrast.

Rhabdomyosarcoma can be a devastating orbital malignancy. It is the most common primary orbital malignancy in children and the most common soft tissue sarcoma of childhood with approximately 10 % occurring primarily in the orbit [1]. The majority of rhabdomyosarcomas arise spontaneously, but other circumstances such as familial occurrences have been reported. Rhabdomyosarcoma can occur in primary sites throughout the body; of the 45 % occurring in the head and neck region, up to 35 % occur in the orbit [6]. Rhabdomyosarcoma is a primitive cancer that likely arises from undifferentiated mesenchymal cells [6]. While striated muscle is a histopathologic hallmark, the cancer most often arises independently of muscles in the orbit [6].

Most commonly, patients present in the first decade of life with acute or subacute proptosis with related globe displacement (often down and out from a superonasal lesion), ptosis, and swelling of the lids or conjunctiva [7] (see example Fig. 42.1). Pain is an uncommon presenting symptom. In many instances, parents may relate the exam findings to a recent trauma. Because of its often aggressive growth and potential mortality, any orbital mass in a child should be considered to be rhabdomyosarcoma until proven otherwise. Infants younger than 1 year have a worse prognosis [6].

Immediate imaging is indicated, demonstrating a well-defined, homogenous, enhancing orbital mass, which on occasion causes bony destruction with extension into other sites such as sinuses, nasopharynx, oral cavity, or intracranial space [6]. On MRI, the mass is isointense to muscle on T1 and hyperintense on T2 [6].

If rhabdomyosarcoma remains on the differential diagnosis after appropriate imaging studies are interpreted, there should be no delay in surgical biopsy, with many advocating for surgery on the same day as patient presentation. Current treatment regimens are based on whether or not the tumor has been debulked. Therefore, the tumor should be maximally debulked, but with care taken to preserve critical orbital structures.

Diagnosis is confirmed with histopathologic analysis. There are four main histopathologic subtypes depending on the morphologic pattern, which include embryonal, pleomorphic, alveolar, and botryoid. Embryonal is the most common and has the most favorable prognosis. Alveolar type tends to have a poorer prognosis [1, 7].

A diagnosis of rhabdomyosarcoma should be followed in short order with staging of disease and treatment. Uncontrolled disease can invade into the orbital bone and cranial cavity or rarely metastasize hematogenously to the bone, lung, and other sites. Therefore, the patient should be worked up for metastases at the time of diagnosis, which includes chest imaging, complete blood count, renal and liver function tests, bone marrow aspiration for cytology, and bone scan. The cerebral spinal fluid should be evaluated if there is concern for meningeal spread. An oncologist and radiation oncologist should be involved in the patient care and management.

Current management consists of a combination of systemic chemotherapy and targeted radiation therapy [4, 6, 8]. Exenteration is not thought to improve outcome, though it may be used for palliation in very advanced cases [6]. Survival rates are currently much improved over those reported in the past. Reports from the 1970s stated that only about 30 % of patients were alive at 5 years after diagnosis [9]. Survival rates now are greater than 95 % for orbital rhabdomyosarcoma [4, 6, 8], the embryonal subtype having a higher 5-year survival at 94 % and alveolar a 74 % 5-year survival [6].

## Leiomyosarcoma

Typical presentation and imaging:

- Age/gender: sixth decade/older individuals or as radiation induced in younger patients, slight female predilection
- Symptoms: rapidly progressive proptosis
- Signs: proptosis, palpable mass, generally located in extraconal space

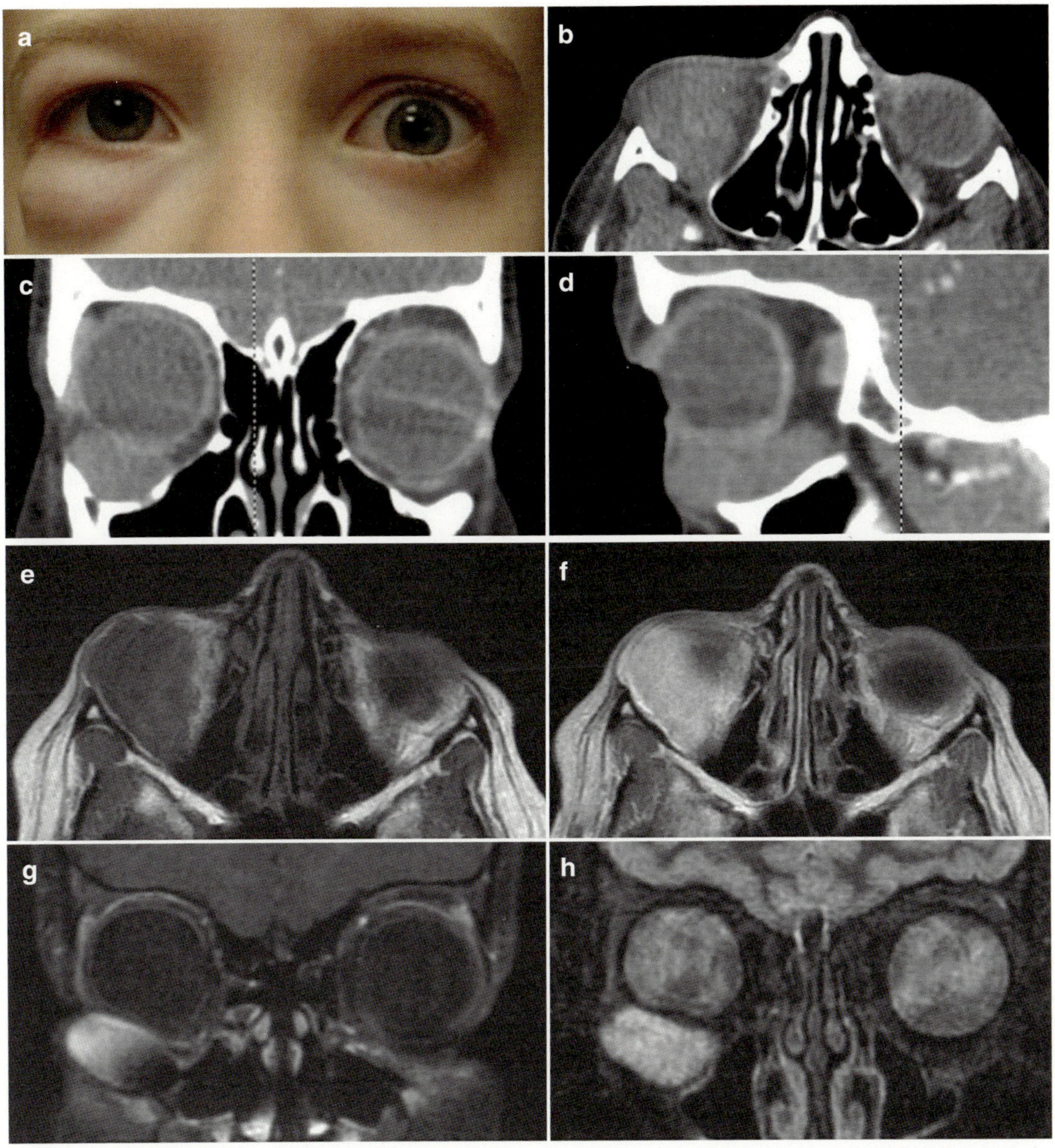


**Fig. 42.1** (**a**) Rhabdomyosarcoma; an 8-year-old female presented with swelling of her right lower eyelid for 1 month. (**b–d**) CT showed an extraconal soft tissue mass in the inferior aspect of the right orbit exerting a mass effect on the inferior portion of the globe. (**e**) In rhabdomyosarcoma, MRI showed multilobulated enhancing extraconal mass in the right inferior orbit. (**e–g**) The lesion has T1-intermediate signal and (**h**) T2 hyperintense signal. The patient underwent urgent biopsy and debulking of the tumor. Pathology was consistent with embryonal rhabdomyosarcoma. She subsequently underwent multi-agent systemic chemotherapy and proton beam therapy and is currently tumor-free

- Imaging: CT or MRI orbit and brain with contrast
  – Heterogeneous, lobulated, or cystic mass, which may infiltrate into surrounding structures

Leiomyosarcomas are rare tumors of the orbit with varying degrees of malignancy. Clinically, they are often rapidly progressive and on imaging show infiltration into surrounding tissues [10]. Due to their infiltrative nature, treatment recommendation is often extensive local surgical resection or exenteration, combined with chemotherapy or irradiation [4, 10]. Chemotherapy and radiation have been used in recurrent disease as well

[1, 11]. It is important for the patient to undergo a complete metastatic workup as these tumors more commonly arise from the uterus, gastrointestinal tract, or vascular tissue and the orbital lesion may represent a metastasis [11]. Primary orbital leiomyosarcomas are also commonly associated with distant metastases and local recurrence [10, 11]. The prognosis of patients with leiomyosarcoma has been reported to be quite poor due to hematogenous dissemination to the lungs, liver, brain, kidney, and skin [11]. However, with radical excision +/– adjuvant radiation therapy, more recent reports have shown no recurrence within 12 months [12] and 3 years [13].

### Liposarcoma

Typical presentation and imaging:

- Age: adulthood
- Extremely rare
- Symptoms: usually slowly progressive, proptosis, and globe displacement
- Signs: proptosis and other orbital signs
- Imaging: CT or MRI orbit and brain with contrast
  - CT: often appears cystic due to fat content
  - MRI: often appears cystic due to fat content, confirmed by hyperintensity on T1-weighted images

Liposarcomas are the most common soft tissue sarcoma of adults, but rarely occur in the orbit [14–17]. They are believed to arise from poorly differentiated mesenchymal cells rather than directly from fat. They are usually slowly progressive. Diagnosis requires imaging as well as biopsy with tissue analysis. There are four histologic subtypes: well-differentiated, myxoid, round cell, and pleomorphic [14]. Prognosis is dependent on size and tissue subtype with the pleomorphic and round cell types being more locally aggressive and likely to metastasize.

Treatment involves radical excision or exenteration. If the tumor is well circumscribed without infiltration and of one of the low-grade histopathological subtypes, it may be excised without exenteration [1]. Adjuvant radiation therapy is advocated. Since metastatic disease can occur, a thorough systemic evaluation should be completed. No recurrences were seen at mean 4-year follow-up of four cases of primary orbital liposarcoma treated with exenteration (and adjuvant radiation therapy in one patient) [18]. Other case reports have shown similar results, but the prediction of accurate prognosis is still difficult due to the rarity of the malignancy.

### Fibrosarcoma

Typical presentation and imaging:

- Age: Elderly
- Extremely rare
- Symptoms: proptosis over months and diplopia
- Signs: proptosis (can have massive proptosis at birth), usually in extraconal space, and other orbital signs
- Imaging: CT scan or MRI orbit and brain with contrast

Fibrosarcomas rarely occur in the head and neck region and the orbit [19, 20]. They are locally aggressive and infiltrative tumors and will engulf adjacent structures and expand posteriorly toward the orbital apex. It is important to ask about a history of irradiation, as these tumors can also arise as secondary tumors. Imaging and biopsy are recommended for diagnosis [21]. Wide local excision, including orbital exenteration when necessary, with pathologic control of margins is the recommended therapy. If the tumor is not completely excised, local recurrence, extension, and metastases are common. Radiotherapy, chemotherapy and other modalities are considered to be palliative [4]. One of the more comprehensive series of fibrosarcoma included 26 cases (none primary orbital) and found that survival was less than 70 % at 2 years and less than 50 % at 5 years [22].

## Malignant Primary Bone Tumors of the Orbit

### Osteosarcoma

Typical presentation and imaging:

- Age/Gender: second decade, slight male predilection
- Symptoms: rapid onset and progression of unilateral proptosis, averaging 4–6 months,

pain, diplopia, globe displacement, or decreased vision
- Signs: rapid progression, proptosis, facial asymmetry, and other orbital signs
- Imaging: CT best to delineate bone details
  - Mixed lytic and sclerotic mass with indistinct margins; can have soft tissue infiltration. MRI can better delineate soft tissue involvement if necessary.

Osteosarcoma is the most common primary neoplasm of the bone, but most commonly presents in long bones. Within the orbital bones, it can arise de novo most commonly in the maxillary bone, but can also be associated with previous radiation therapy, giant cell tumor, Paget's disease, fibrous dysplasia, or familial retinoblastoma [1, 23] (see example Fig. 42.2). Management of osteosarcoma involves preoperative chemotherapy, resection, and postoperative chemotherapy often modified by final pathology. Radiotherapy also has an adjuvant role in treatment. The prognosis for patients with osteosarcoma of the orbital bones is generally quite poor despite various treatment attempts [4].

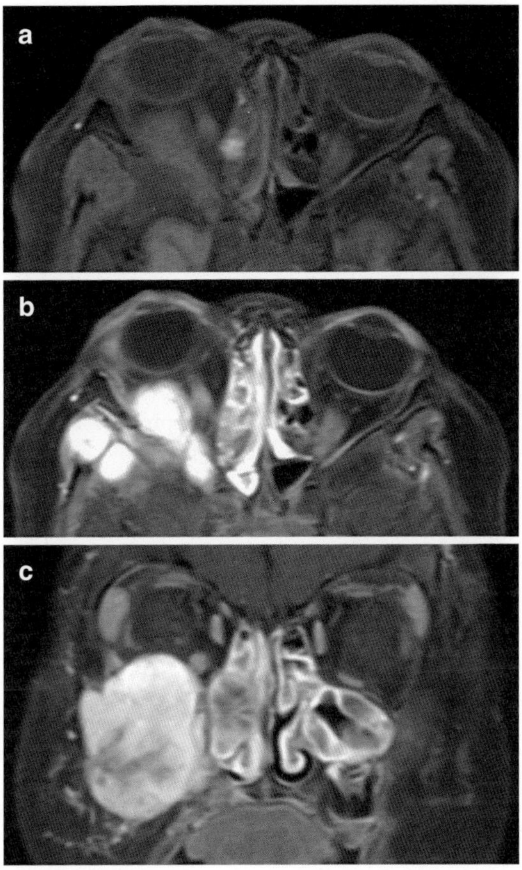


**Fig. 42.2** Osteosarcoma; a 5-year-old-female presented with facial asymmetry and a right maxillary lesion involving the inferior orbit. (**a**) Axial T1 pre-contrast MRI shows the mass involving the inferior orbit. (**b**) Axial T1 post-contrast MRI showing enhancement of the inferolateral intraconal lesion with extension into the temporal area. (**c**) Coronal T1 post-contrast MRI showing involvement of the inferior orbital wall and maxillary sinus. Biopsy was consistent with fibroblastic osteosarcoma. The patient subsequently underwent induction chemotherapy with debulking of the mass and proton beam radiotherapy

## Ewing's Sarcoma

Typical presentation and imaging:
- Age/gender: first two decades of life, slight predilection for males
- Symptoms: rapid progression, non-axial proptosis or globe displacement, diplopia, or decreased vision
- Signs: rapid progression, non-axial proptosis or globe displacement, restriction of eye movements, and other orbital signs
- Imaging: CT best to delineate bone details
  - Expansile or invasive mass with mottled bone destruction and possible soft tissue infiltration

Ewing's sarcoma is a small round cell tumor that usually arises in bone. The incidence in the head and neck region is approximately 4 % and most commonly presents in the maxilla and mandible [1]. Most orbital cases represent secondary extension or distant metastasis, so a rigorous systemic/metastatic workup for a primary source is recommended. Tissue biopsy and analysis will confirm the diagnosis showing sheets and clusters of small, round uniform cells. A tissue sample may be best accessed endoscopically. The patient should be immediately referred to an oncologist for systemic workup. Induction with multi-agent chemotherapy is often initiated, followed by radical local surgical excision or radiotherapy [1, 24, 25]. The development of multi-agent chemotherapy has increased the 5-year survival rate of Ewing's sarcoma patients from 5 to 10% more than 20 years ago, to greater than 70% now [25, 26].

## Malignant Lymphoproliferative Lesions of the Orbit

### Lymphoma

Typical presentation and imaging:

- Age: Elderly patients/sixth to seventh decade of life
- Symptoms: Painless, slowly progressive proptosis; may have a history of systemic lymphoma
- Signs: Mild to moderate proptosis, globe displacement, salmon patch if conjunctival involvement, possible lacrimal gland enlargement, possible bilateral findings, and other orbital signs
- Imaging: CT or MRI with contrast
  - CT: homogenous, mildly enhancing mass molding around the globe and orbital bones or other structures, typically with no bony destruction
  - MRI: similar to CT with T1 iso- to hypointense to muscle and T2 iso- to hyperintense

Orbital lymphoma is most commonly a low-grade malignancy and is found in older patients, with a slight female predilection. Orbital lymphoma has been associated with systemic lymphoma in 35–65% of cases, making it perhaps more strongly associated with systemic disease than conjunctival lymphoma, but definitively less so than eyelid lymphoma [27]. Twenty-five percent of patients with orbital disease alone at presentation will develop systemic lymphoma within 5 years [28]. Lymphoma is often multifocal in origin and can arise in multiple sites in the body. These other sites may be of a different histopathologic subtype than orbital lymphoma in the same patient.

The following risk factors likely portend a higher mortality rate: bilateral orbital lymphoma, older age, associated optic neuropathy, higher stage at presentation, histopathologic evidence of atypia, high proliferation index, p53 positivity, and more aggressive subtypes.

As with all lymphomas, orbital lymphoma is comprised of a clonal expansion of cells with features of lymphocytic lineage. The most commonly encountered primary orbital lymphoma subtype is low-grade extranodal marginal zone B-cell lymphoma of mucosa-associated lymphoid tissue (MALT) [27]. Other subtypes of orbital lymphoma include follicular lymphoma, diffuse large B-cell lymphoma, mantle cell lymphoma, and natural killer T-cell lymphoma [27].

Patients often present with a painless, slowly progressive orbital mass, proptosis, or diplopia. Clinical examination may demonstrate proptosis or globe displacement, restriction of extraocular motility, ptosis, or a firm palpable lacrimal gland or mass along the orbital rim. Bilateral orbital or adnexal findings may be noted. It is important to palpate for lymphadenopathy suggestive of extraorbital involvement.

On imaging, orbital lymphoma appears as a homogenous, moderately enhancing mass molding to but usually not displacing surrounding structures (Fig. 42.3). It may infiltrate the lacrimal gland or extraocular muscles [27]. Classically, lymphoma does not cause bony destruction, although this may be seen in diffuse large B-cell or natural killer T-cell subtypes [27]. On MRI, lymphoma is iso- to hypointense to muscle on T1 and iso- to hyperintense on T2 [27]. Because of the significant risk of systemic disease, neck and full body imaging should be performed, with consideration of positron emission tomography (PET) scanning because of its sensitivity for small foci of disease.

A tissue biopsy is necessary to confirm the diagnosis, and open biopsy is recommended because of the potential need for multiple modalities of tissue analysis. The specimen should be submitted in formalin for routine histopathology and immunohistochemistry, but in addition, consideration should be given to submission of fresh tissue in saline for flow cytometry.

Given the risk of concurrent undiagnosed or future systemic disease, all orbital lymphoma patients require a complete oncologic staging workup and periodic lifelong monitoring. While

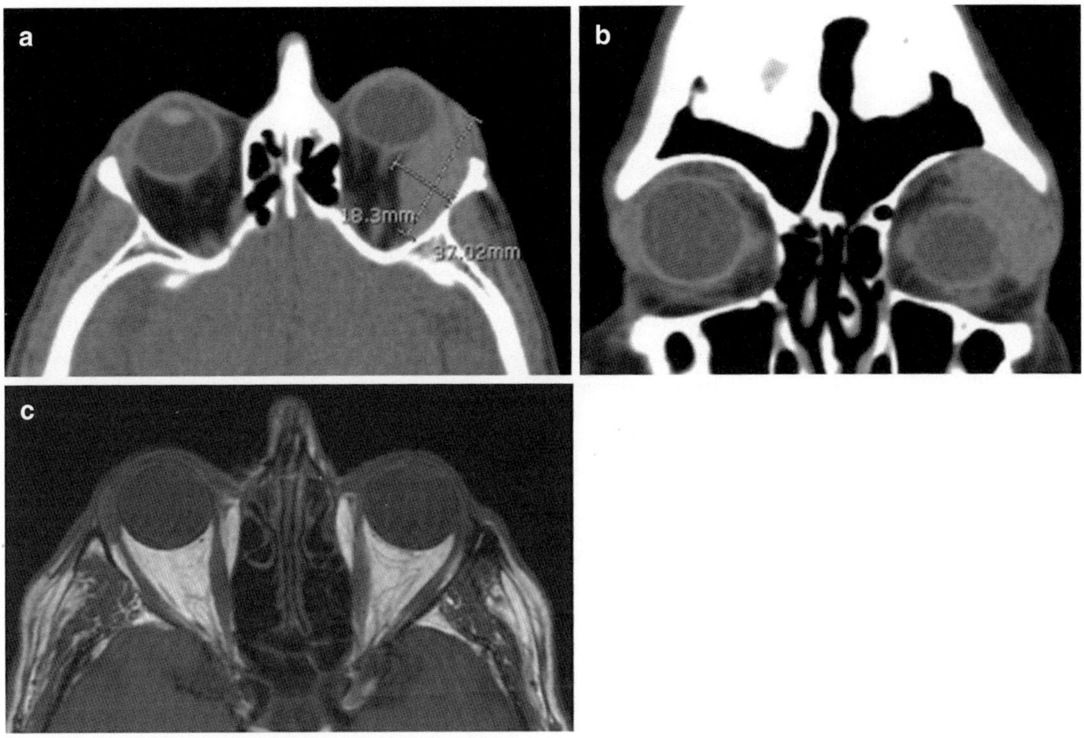


**Fig. 42.3** Orbital lymphoma; a 62-year-old male with a 7-year history of non-Hodgkin's lymphoma presented with 3 months of decreased vision and increasing proptosis of the left eye. Exam showed visual acuity of 20/400 on the left with decreased color vision, 8 mm of proptosis, and a palpable superotemporal mass. (**a**, **b**) CT scan demonstrated a large left orbital mass expanding the lateral orbital wall and lacrimal gland fossa with involvement of the lateral rectus and superior muscle complex. The patient underwent left orbitotomy with biopsy and received systemic chemotherapy. (**c**) Posttreatment MRI reveals interval resolution of the left orbital mass

low-grade systemic lymphomas often prove indolent in nature with excellent prognosis for long-term survival, high-grade lymphomas can be fatal within months.

If systemic disease is absent, some advocate for excision of any easily approached and well-circumscribed tumor. Radiation therapy is an often-utilized and effective treatment for orbital disease. Special consideration should be given to individuals with diabetes or other vasculopathic conditions, which would put them at higher risk for radiation-induced optic neuropathy or retinopathy. Chemotherapy and immunotherapy are generally considered for bilateral orbital disease or systemic disease. Rituximab, an immunotherapeutic agent, is approved with certain restrictions for low-grade, follicular, and diffuse large B-cell non-Hodgkin lymphomas [1, 29]. The number of treatment options for lymphoma continues to rapidly increase as new drugs and monoclonal antibody therapies enter the market. Fortunately, the prognosis for this most common orbital malignancy in adults is quite good. Local control rates were 100 % in a recent study of 81 patients with primary orbital lymphoma treated with primary radiotherapy [30]. Five percent of patients experienced disease relapse elsewhere and no patients died from lymphoma (median 4.4-year follow-up) [30].

## Malignant Lacrimal Gland Tumors

### Adenoid Cystic Carcinoma

Typical presentation and imaging:

- Age: younger patients, mean age of 40 years
- Symptoms: pain and sometimes numbness in the trigeminal region, subacute-chronic

progressive proptosis, inferonasal globe displacement, diplopia, and eyelid edema
- Signs: lacrimal gland with firm enlargement, ptosis, and strabismus
- Imaging: both CT and MRI with contrast recommended
  - CT: large, irregular lacrimal gland with bony erosion; may have calcification; potential intracranial spread
  - MRI: similar as for CT. T1 hypointense and T2 iso- or hypointense; important to evaluate for evidence of perineural spread

Adenoid cystic carcinoma (ACC) of the lacrimal gland is a rare, malignant, often painful epithelial neoplasm with risks of perineural invasion to the intracranial space, as well as distant metastasis (see example in Fig. 42.4). It accounts for over 60 % of malignant epithelial tumors of the lacrimal gland and 1 % of orbital lesions [4]. There is a biphasic age distribution, affecting those in their second or third decade of life as well as those in later middle age, with an average age at presentation of 40 years.

Urgent biopsy allows for histopathologic subtyping. ACC is a primary epithelial neoplasm. On histopathologic review, a cribriform "Swiss cheese" pattern is classically noted, consisting of lobules of tumor cells surrounding circular pools of mucin. Other histologic subtypes include sclerosing, basaloid, comedocarcinoma, and tubular. The basaloid variety has the poorest prognosis and portends a higher risk of metastatic disease.

Patients often present with complaints of orbital or periorbital pain or numbness and globe displacement and on examination may be found to have periorbital edema, proptosis, inferonasal globe displacement, or restriction of extraocular motility. A mass may be palpable along the orbital rim superotemporally. Given the risk of intracranial spread and distant metastases, a review of systems may suggest pathology at other sites.

Imaging shows a large, irregular lacrimal gland. CT may demonstrate calcification within the mass or erosion of the surrounding orbital bones [31]. Imaging likely greatly underestimates the presence of bony invasion [31]. On MRI, ACC is generally hypointense on T1 and iso- or hypointense on T2 and may be seen spreading along adjacent nerves and intracranially. Imaging may be helpful in distinguishing this tumor from pleomorphic adenoma of the lacrimal gland, which is important, as the surgical management differs greatly. On imaging, pleomorphic adenoma may be more well circumscribed than adenoid cystic carcinoma, can remodel but not erode bone, and calcifies in less than 5 % of cases. Pleomorphic adenoma should be removed in toto without incisional biopsy in order to preserve its pseudocapsule and prevent seeding of the surrounding area with tumor cells, which may then undergo malignant transformation.

Treatment of adenoid cystic carcinoma of the lacrimal gland is controversial, with different centers reporting varying rates of success with their specific treatment modalities. Exenteration is typically, though not always, performed, and may include concurrent adjacent bone removal. Chemotherapy is used in many cases, and postoperative radiation therapy is often employed, particularly in cases with perineural invasion [32, 33]. Though the AJCC grading system is lacking in detail, larger tumors (>T3) seem to have increased risk of recurrence if exenteration and postoperative radiation therapy are declined. These patients need to be urgently evaluated by a medical oncologist for metastatic workup and followed regularly after treatment of the primary lesion as metastatic lesions may arise many years later (see example Fig. 42.4).

The prognosis is generally thought to be poor. Only approximately one third of patients survive 10 years after diagnosis, and it is unusual for any to survive past 15 years. It has been suggested that children may have a more favorable prognosis [34]. However, recent data suggest that neoadjuvant intra-arterial cytoreductive chemotherapy may allow for significantly higher survival rates (reported 100 % 10-year disease-free survival at one center) in patients who have intact lacrimal arteries (i.e., have not undergone extensive debulking) and who follow a course of orbital exenteration, with radiation and chemotherapy postoperatively [35–37]. Future studies are required prior to making this protocol a standard of care.

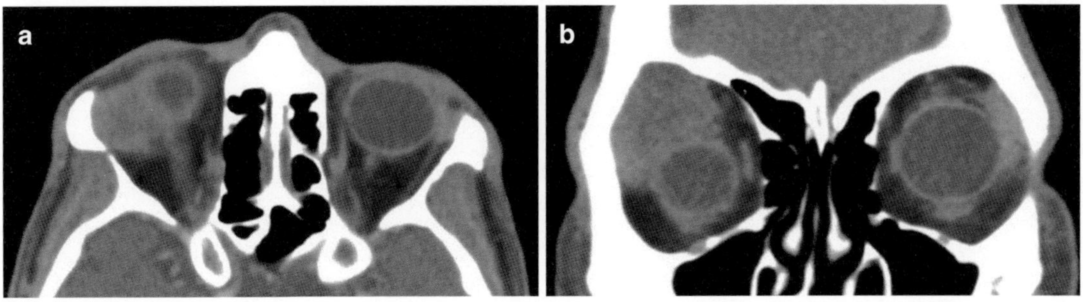

**Fig. 42.4** Adenoid cystic carcinoma; a 59-year-old male presented with upper eyelid ptosis, mild proptosis, and limitation of upgaze on the right. (**a**, **b**) CT shows a right lacrimal gland mass that appeared to depress the globe and erode adjacent bone. Fine-needle aspiration biopsy revealed small basaloid tumor cell clusters within entrapped stroma consistent with adenoid cystic carcinoma. Treatment included right orbitotomy and removal of the mass with adjuvant radiation therapy. Initial metastatic workup was negative, but 3 years later, the patient developed acute dyspnea and chest x-ray showed diffuse bilateral lung nodules. Fine-needle aspiration biopsy showed metastatic adenoid cystic carcinoma

## Summary

The list of primary malignant neoplasms of the orbit is extensive. Fortunately, many of them are exceedingly rare. Detailed ophthalmic and systemic evaluations both clinically and radiologically can narrow the differential diagnosis and further define the course of management. Tumors that are behaving aggressively require rapid biopsy and histopathological analysis. A multispecialty integrated team including ophthalmology, otolaryngology, neurosurgery, oncology, pediatrics, orbital surgery, radiology, ophthalmic pathology, and radiation oncology is beneficial to comprehensively care for these patients with complex, life-threatening orbital tumors.

## References

1. Rootman J. Diseases of the orbit: a multidisciplinary approach. Philadelphia: Lippincott; 1988. p. xxiv. 628 p.
2. Demirci H, Shields CL, Shields JA, Honavar SG, Mercado GJ, Tovilla JC. Orbital tumors in the older adult population. Ophthalmology. 2002;109(2): 243–8.
3. Margo CE, Mulla ZD. Malignant tumors of the orbit. Analysis of the Florida Cancer Registry. Ophthalmology. 1998;105(1):185–90.
4. Shields JA, Shields CL. Atlas of eyelid and conjunctival tumors. Philadelphia: Lippincott Williams & Wilkins; 1999. p. xvi. 350 p.
5. Hoyt WF, Meshel LG, Lessell S, Schatz NJ, Suckling RD. Malignant optic glioma of adulthood. Brain. 1973;96(1):121–32.
6. Shields JA, Shields CL. Rhabdomyosarcoma: review for the ophthalmologist. Surv Ophthalmol. 2003;48(1): 39–57.
7. Chess J, Ni C, Yin RQ, Wang WJ, Cassady JR, Weichselbaum RR, et al. Rhabdomyosarcoma. Int Ophthalmol Clin. 1982;22(1):163–82.
8. Shields CL, Shields JA, Honavar SG, Demirci H. Clinical spectrum of primary ophthalmic rhabdomyosarcoma. Ophthalmology. 2001;108(12):2284–92.
9. Abramson DH, Ellsworth RM, Tretter P, Wolff JA, Kitchin FD. The treatment of orbital rhabdomyosarcoma with irradiation and chemotherapy. Ophthalmology. 1979;86(7):1330–5.
10. Jakobiec FA, Howard GM, Rosen M, Wolff M. Leiomyoma and leiomyosarcoma of the orbit. Am J Ophthalmol. 1975;80(6):1028–42.
11. Meekins BB, Dutton JJ, Proia AD. Primary orbital leiomyosarcoma. A case report and review of the literature. Arch Ophthalmol. 1988;106(1):82–6.
12. Yeniad B, Tuncer S, Peksayar G, Mete O, Minareci O. Primary orbital leiomyosarcoma. Ophthal Plast Reconstr Surg. 2009;25(2):154–5.
13. Lin IC, Wu CT, Liao SL, Lin LL. Primary orbital leiomyosarcoma. Ophthal Plast Reconstr Surg. 2005; 21(6):451–3.
14. Jakobiec FA, Rini F, Char D, Orcutt J, Rootman J, Baylis H, et al. Primary liposarcoma of the orbit. Problems in the diagnosis and management of five cases. Ophthalmology. 1989;96(2):180–91.
15. Lane CM, Wright JE, Garner A. Primary myxoid liposarcoma of the orbit. Br J Ophthalmol. 1988;72(12): 912–7.
16. McNab AA, Moseley I. Primary orbital liposarcoma: clinical and computed tomographic features. Br J Ophthalmol. 1990;74(7):437–9.

17. Naeser P, Mostrom U. Liposarcoma of the orbit: a clinicopathological case report. Br J Ophthalmol. 1982;66(3):190–3.
18. Khurana S, Gupta AK, Sen S, Kashyap S. Primary liposarcoma of the orbit. Indian J Pathol Microbiol. 2014;57(4):617–9.
19. Eifrig DE, Foos RY. Fibrosarcoma of the orbit. Am J Ophthalmol. 1969;67(2):244–8.
20. Yanoff M, Scheie HG. Fibrosarcoma of orbit. Report of two patients. Cancer. 1966;19(11):1711–6.
21. Jakobiec FA, Tannenbaum M. The ultrastructure of orbital fibrosarcoma. Am J Ophthalmol. 1974;77(6):899–917.
22. Bahrami A, Folpe AL. Adult-type fibrosarcoma: a reevaluation of 163 putative cases diagnosed at a single institution over a 48-year period. Am J Surg Pathol. 2010;34(10):1504–13.
23. Dhir SP, Munjal VP, Jain IS, Banerjee AK, Sharma SK. Osteosarcoma of the orbit. J Pediatr Ophthalmol Strabismus. 1980;17(5):312–4.
24. Alio 2nd JL, Sales-Sanz M, Vaz MA, Barrancos C, Reguero ME, Diamantopoulus J, et al. Primary extraosseous Ewing sarcoma of the orbit. Ophthal Plast Reconstr Surg. 2013;29(3):e91–3.
25. Lam DS, Li CK, Cheng LL, Teo JG, Chik KW, Kwan WH, et al. Primary orbital Ewing's sarcoma: report of a case and review of the literature. Eye (Lond). 1999;13(Pt 1):38–42.
26. Vlasak R, Sim FH. Ewing's sarcoma. Orthop Clin N Am. 1996;27(3):591–603.
27. Demirci H, Shields CL, Karatza EC, Shields JA. Orbital lymphoproliferative tumors: analysis of clinical features and systemic involvement in 160 cases. Ophthalmology. 2008;115(9):1626–31. 31 e1-3.
28. Jenkins C, Rose GE, Bunce C, Cree I, Norton A, Plowman PN, et al. Clinical features associated with survival of patients with lymphoma of the ocular adnexa. Eye (Lond). 2003;17(7):809–20.
29. Piro LD, White CA, Grillo-Lopez AJ, Janakiraman N, Saven A, Beck TM, et al. Extended Rituximab (anti-CD20 monoclonal antibody) therapy for relapsed or refractory low-grade or follicular non-Hodgkin's lymphoma. Ann Oncol Off J Eur Soc Med Oncol/ESMO. 1999;10(6):655–61.
30. Woolf DK, Kuhan H, Shoffren O, Akinnawo EM, Sivagurunathan B, Boyce H, et al. Outcomes of primary lymphoma of the ocular adnexa (orbital lymphoma) treated with radiotherapy. Clin Oncol. 2014.
31. Williams MD, Al-Zubidi N, Debnam JM, Shinder R, DeMonte F, Esmaeli B. Bone invasion by adenoid cystic carcinoma of the lacrimal gland: preoperative imaging assessment and surgical considerations. Ophthal Plast Reconstr Surg. 2010;26(6):403–8.
32. Esmaeli B, Golio D, Kies M, DeMonte F. Surgical management of locally advanced adenoid cystic carcinoma of the lacrimal gland. Ophthal Plast Reconstr Surg. 2006;22(5):366–70.
33. Ahmad SM, Esmaeli B, Williams M, Nguyen J, Fay A, Woog J, et al. American Joint Committee on Cancer classification predicts outcome of patients with lacrimal gland adenoid cystic carcinoma. Ophthalmology. 2009;116(6):1210–5.
34. Tellado MV, McLean IW, Specht CS, Varga J. Adenoid cystic carcinomas of the lacrimal gland in childhood and adolescence. Ophthalmology. 1997;104(10):1622–5.
35. Tse DT, Benedetto P, Dubovy S, Schiffman JC, Feuer WJ. Clinical analysis of the effect of intraarterial cytoreductive chemotherapy in the treatment of lacrimal gland adenoid cystic carcinoma. Am J Ophthalmol. 2006;141(1):44–53.
36. Tse DT, Kossler AL, Feuer WJ, Benedetto PW. Long-term outcomes of neoadjuvant intra-arterial cytoreductive chemotherapy for lacrimal gland adenoid cystic carcinoma. Ophthalmology. 2013;120(7):1313–23.
37. Meldrum ML, Tse DT, Benedetto P. Neoadjuvant intracarotid chemotherapy for treatment of advanced adenocystic carcinoma of the lacrimal gland. Arch Ophthalmol. 1998;116(3):315–21.

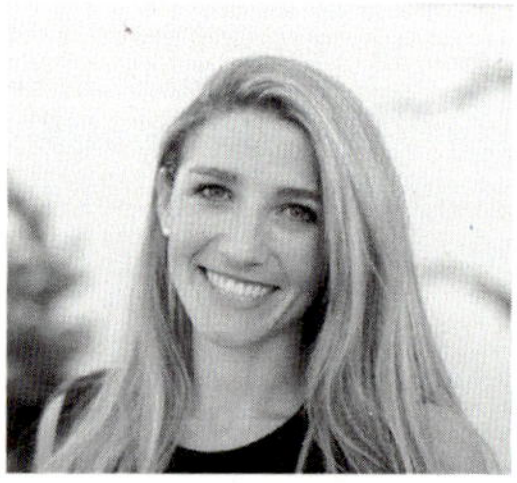

**Seanna Grob** Seanna Grob, MD, MAS received a BA in Molecular and Cellular Biology from the University of California, Berkeley and a MD and MAS from the University of California, San Diego. She completed her ophthalmology residency at Massachusetts Eye and Ear/Harvard Medical School. She is currently the Director of the Ocular Trauma Service at Massachusetts Eye and Ear and Brigham and Women's Hospital. She has been accepted into a 2-year American Society of Ophthalmic Plastic and Reconstructive Surgery-approved fellowship and will start in 2017.

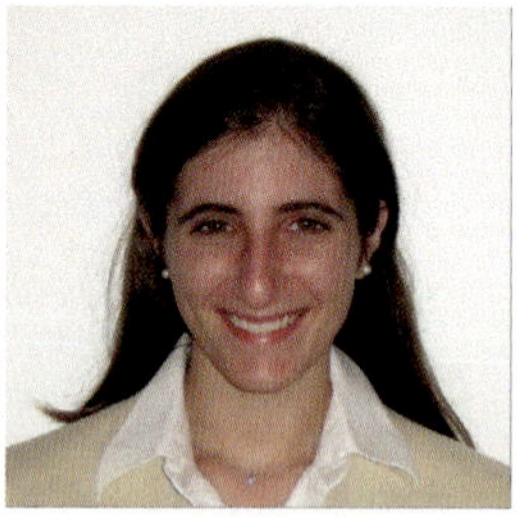

**Lora Rabin Dagi Glass** Lora Dagi Glass completed her ophthalmology residency at the Columbia University Medical Center, followed by a fellowship in oculoplastic surgery at the Massachusetts Eye and Ear Infirmary. Her research has focused on orbital processes ranging from thyroid eye disease to optic nerve glioma and orbital melanoma.

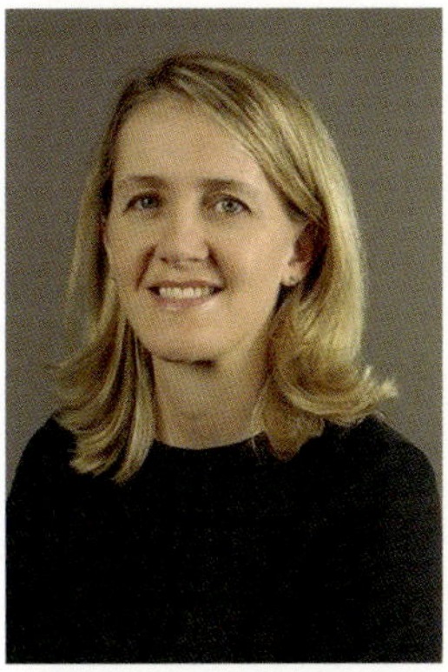

**Suzanne K. Freitag** Suzanne K Freitag, MD, received a BA from Duke University and MD from Jefferson Medical College in Philadelphia, PA. She completed ophthalmology residency at Wills Eye Hospital followed by a neuroophthalmology fellowship at the Wilmer Eye Institute at Johns Hopkins. She then completed a 2-year American Society of Ophthalmic Plastic and Reconstructive Surgery-approved fellowship in Boston. She is the Director of the Ophthalmic Plastic Surgery Service at Massachusetts Eye and Ear Infirmary and an Assistant Professor of Ophthalmology at Harvard Medical School.

# Secondary and Metastatic Tumors of the Orbit

# 43

Hunter Kwok-Lai Yuen, Lora Rabin Dagi Glass, and Suzanne K. Freitag

## Introduction

The orbit is surrounded by a number of significant structures, including the intracranial space and paranasal sinuses. A secondary orbital malignancy refers to a lesion arising from a surrounding structure which extends to the orbit by direct invasion. The primary tumor may arise in the paranasal sinuses, nasal cavity and nasopharynx, eyelid skin and face, eyeball, conjunctiva, lacrimal sac, or intracranial cavity [1]. Commonly encountered entities include epithelial tumors arising from the skin of the forehead, eyelid, and temple region, such as basal cell carcinoma and squamous cell carcinoma; carcinoma arising from glandular tissues of the eyelid such as sebaceous gland carcinoma (Fig. 43.1); carcinoma arising from the external surface of the eye such as conjunctival squamous cell carcinoma or melanoma; nasal cavity and paranasal sinus tumors (Fig. 43.2); and lacrimal sac malignancies (Fig. 43.3) [2].

In metastatic orbital disease, the primary malignancy originates at a remote site in the body and travels to the orbit via lymphatic or hematogenous spread. The most common sites of origin include the breast, lung, prostate, kidney, thyroid gland, and alimentary tract. Occasionally, metastasis from an unknown primary site may be encountered [3].

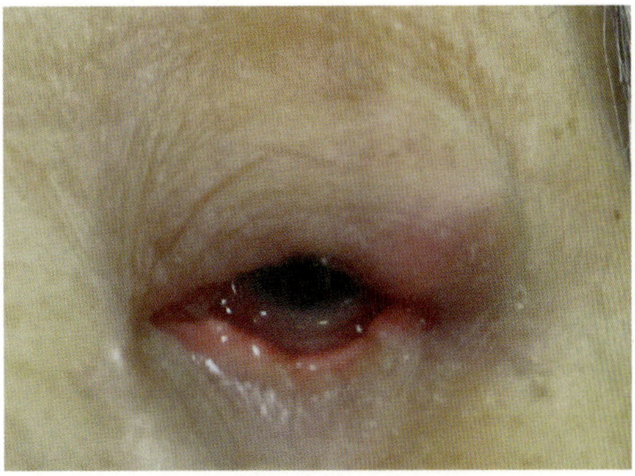

**Fig. 43.1** Left upper lid sebaceous gland carcinoma with orbital extension. There is a visible and palpable mass in the left upper eyelid and anterior orbit, with surrounding skin erythema and blepharoptosis. There is spread of tumor into the lower eyelid resulting in ectropion

H.K.-L. Yuen, FRCOphth, FRCSEd (✉)
Department of Ophthalmology and Visual Sciences, Hong Kong Eye Hospital, The Chinese University of Hong Kong, 147K, Argyle Street, Hong Kong, Hong Kong SAR, China
e-mail: hunterklyuen@gmail.com

L.R.D. Glass, MD
Ophthalmic Plastic Surgery Service, Department of Ophthalmology, Massachusetts Eye and Ear Infirmary, Harvard Medical School, Boston, MA, USA
e-mail: lora_dagiglass@meei.harvard.edu

S.K. Freitag, MD
Ophthalmic Plastic Surgery Service, Department of Ophthalmology, Massachusetts Eye and Ear Infirmary, Harvard Medical School, Boston, MA, USA
e-mail: suzanne_freitag@meei.harvard.edu


B. Mukherjee, H. Yuen (eds.), *Emergencies of the Orbit and Adnexa*,
DOI 10.1007/978-81-322-1807-4_43

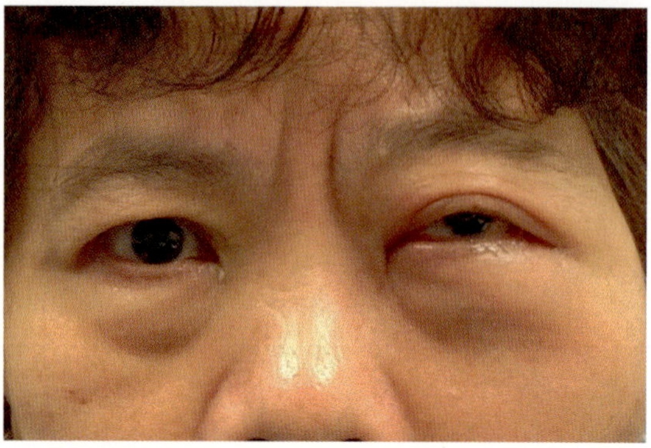

**Fig. 43.2** Left maxillary sinus carcinoma with orbital extension. The primary sinus mass is displacing the globe upward and causing visible fullness of the left lower eyelid

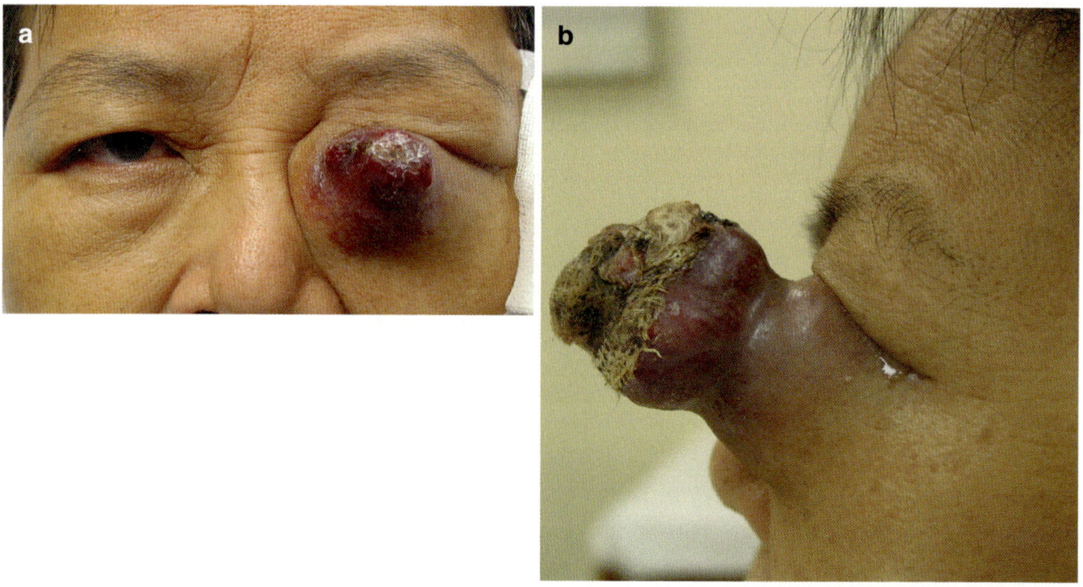


**Fig. 43.3** (**a**, **b**) Frontal and sagittal views of squamous cell carcinoma, presumably originating from the left lacrimal sac, with orbital extension. A large mass is seen projecting from the inferomedial orbital area. The tip of the lesion has a scaly, necrotic appearance, consistent with the histopathologic diagnosis

## Clinical Presentation

The clinical presentations of various secondary orbital malignancies differ depending on the primary pathology. For example, paranasal sinus and nasal tumors may have rhinologic symptoms, such as epistaxis, nasal obstruction, swelling or pain in the cheek basal cell carcinoma of the skin may be characterized by an ulcerated lesion with rolled edges; sebaceous gland carcinoma can cause a whitish-yellow lesion of the eyelid; lacrimal sac tumors may cause blood stained tears. Orbital extension of these tumors can result in non-axial proptosis, impaired ocular motility, and globe or optic nerve compression. As these secondary tumors originate from surrounding structures, they may develop over a longer period of time and can be quite extensive in size [4].

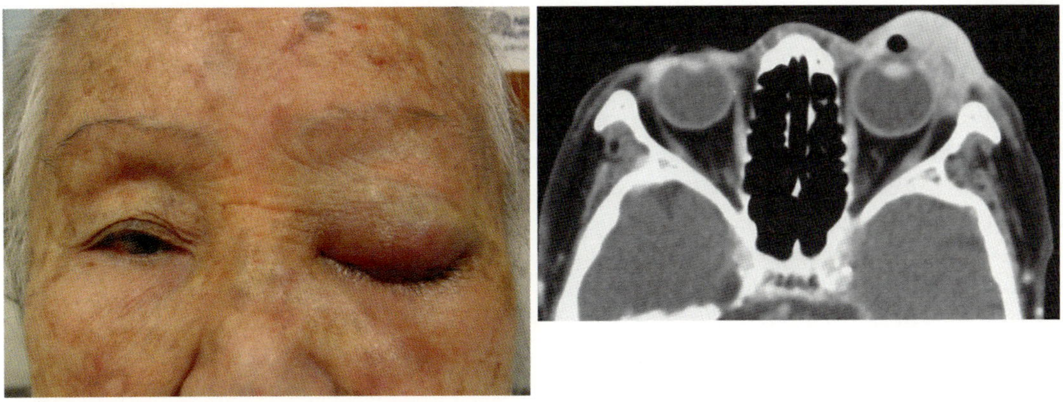

**Fig. 43.4** (**a**, **b**) Diffuse left upper lid swelling with erythema and secondary blepharoptosis. CT scan showed diffuse infiltrative left upper lid lesion. Subsequent biopsy confirmed eyelid T cell lymphoma

The clinical presentations of metastatic disease are more variable and include [5–7]:

1. Mass formation causing proptosis and globe or optic nerve compression
2. Infiltrative disease causing ocular motility disturbance, resistance to retropulsion, and enophthalmos (especially in metastatic carcinoma of the breast)
3. Cranial nerve palsies with functional symptoms such as diplopia
4. External eyelid erythema, edema, and pain simulating periorbital inflammatory diseases (Fig. 43.4)
5. Asymptomatic orbital disease detected incidentally by imaging for another reason

## Imaging and Investigations

**Imaging** Both MRI and CT are highly useful in the diagnosis of secondary and metastatic orbital tumors. CT is best for identifying tumor calcification and the location and extent of bone involvement, while MRI has better soft tissue definition [8]. T1 contrast-enhanced fat-suppressed MRI will show enhancement of the dura if early intracranial extension is present. PET imaging, based on metabolic activity of tissues, can be useful in the assessment of suspected metastatic disease, by identifying involved lymph nodes or sites of potential malignancy elsewhere in the body [9]. Chest x-ray is a simple and quick test to look for pulmonary primary and secondary malignancies. Ultrasonography of the abdomen may be useful to look for primary liver malignancy or liver metastases, as well as major lesions within the abdomen. Hematologic studies and gastrointestinal endoscopy may be helpful when certain diagnoses are suspected. For patients with orbital masses and known systemic metastatic disease, the diagnosis may be simpler, but these studies may be helpful for disease staging. Consultation of colleagues, including oncologists, otolaryngologists, and other specialists, is helpful, depending on the clinical indications.

**Role of Biopsy** In cases of secondary orbital tumors, surgical biopsy is usually required to determine the diagnosis [4]. Biopsy may be performed on the orbital portion of the tumor or on the portion of the mass in a surrounding structure, depending on the potential morbidities involved in operating on the various anatomic areas. For example, a sinonasal mass extending into the orbit may be best approached endoscopically via the nose for biopsy.

For orbital metastases with known primary disease or confirmed metastatic disease elsewhere, biopsy may not be needed. Nevertheless, when all investigations are noncontributory or no previous histopathologic diagnosis is available, an incisional biopsy is indicated; histopathologic studies may help identify the primary tumor site. Alternatively, fine-needle aspiration cytology can be considered [10].

## Management of Secondary and Metastatic Tumors of the Orbit

The first step for the management of secondary and metastatic orbital tumors should be confirmation of the diagnosis. Even though the patient may arrive with a previously established diagnosis, there are times when additional tissue sampling may be required to confirm the exact nature of the disease. It is important to have a trusted ophthalmic pathologist review the slides, especially in cases where the histopathologic diagnosis is one that is often confused, such as sebaceous gland carcinoma. Proper use of immunohistochemical staining is critical in establishing proper diagnoses.

Various factors should be considered when deciding on curative versus palliative management of the lesion in question, including the age and general status of the patient, co-morbidities, and the histopathologic subtype and stage of disease.

For localized secondary orbital tumors, surgical resection can be considered. Orbital exenteration with resection of the primary lesion may be required. Total exenteration was traditionally the most common type of exenteration, but recently more selective procedures have gained popularity, such as subtotal or skin-sparing exenteration (Fig. 43.5). For extensive cases, surgical resection can be challenging and may involve a craniofacial resection (Fig. 43.6) via a multidisciplinary approach, including oculoplastic surgeons, head and neck surgeons, neurosurgeons, and plastic surgeons. Surgical reconstruction with local or free flaps may be required [11–13]. Recently, preoperative or neoadjuvant chemoreduction has become a possibility [14, 15]. Advanced localized disease is difficult to eradicate and has a high rate of recurrence and a high mortality rate. Postoperative adjuvant chemotherapy and/or radiotherapy may be required [16]. For those tumors highly sensitive to chemotherapy or radiotherapy, such as lymphoma, surgery beyond diagnostic biopsy is generally not required.

The management of orbital metastases is largely dependent on the primary tumor. Even though the life expectancy and prognosis for these patients are poor in general, some may survive for years in light of advances in oncologic treatments and biologic medications. Management of orbital metastases may include supportive care, orbital irradiation, hormonal therapy, chemotherapy, surgical resection, and debulking [17]. For asymptomatic cases or advanced cases, observation and supportive care may be appropriate. For diffuse tumor or cases with bony involvement, orbital irradiation may be helpful in controlling the size of the tumor, thereby improving the orbital symptoms and perhaps vision in some cases. Hormonal therapy may be beneficial for hormone-sensitive tumors, such as carci-

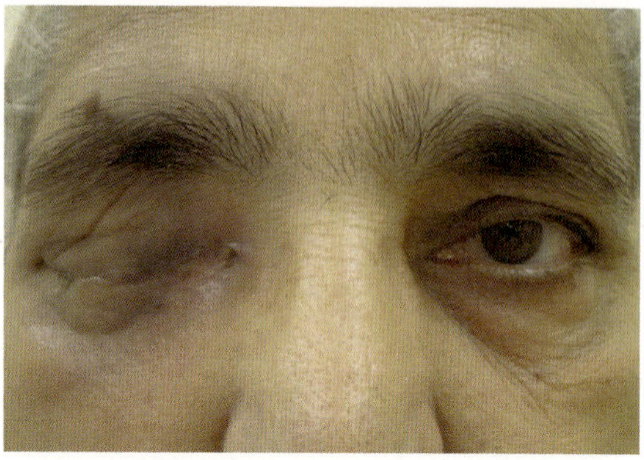

**Fig. 43.5** Right eyelid-sparing orbital exenteration performed for squamous cell carcinoma of the conjunctiva

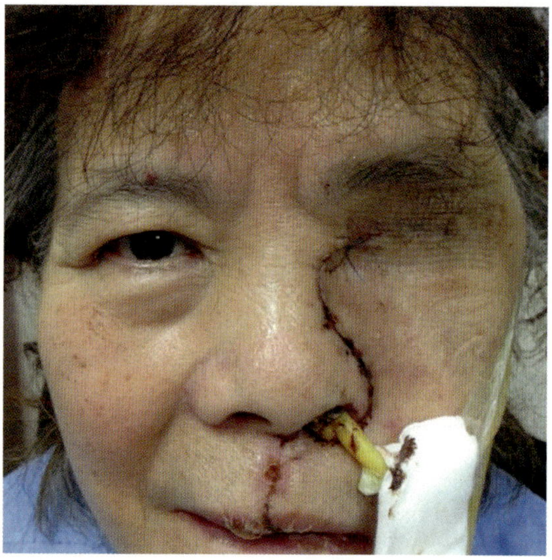

**Fig. 43.6** Left combined maxillectomy and eyelid-sparing orbital exenteration for the case in Fig. 43.2 with squamous cell carcinoma of the maxillary sinus, 1 week after surgery

noma of the breast and prostate. Carcinoma of the prostate may be responsive to orchiectomy as well. Chemotherapy is used in many patients with metastatic disease, with the choice of chemotherapeutic agents depending on the primary tumor and its biologic markers. In cases of solitary or circumscribed metastatic orbital tumors, surgical resection may provide symptomatic relief. For more extensive cases, surgical debulking may be helpful as well.

## Acute Management for Non-resectable Secondary Orbital Tumors or Orbital Metastases

In cases with poor patient prognosis, limited life expectancy, and the absence of definitive curative treatment regimens, palliative treatment may be performed to improve the quality of life and perhaps enhance the life expectancy. Acute bleeding from a tumor may be controlled with surgical intervention including coagulation or ligation. Secondary bacterial infection should be treated with systemic antibiotics. Other potential ophthalmic problems which may require management include elevated intraocular pressure, exposure keratopathy, neurotrophic ulcer, orbital compartment syndrome, and compressive optic neuropathy.

## Secondary Orbital Neoplasms in the Pediatric Population

Certain orbital neoplasms are particularly concerning and life threatening among the pediatric population; these include retinoblastoma, neuroblastoma, and leukemia. Although treatments for these disorders are variable, the primary focus is on patient survival. Given their importance, these three neoplasms have been highlighted in greater detail.

### Retinoblastoma with Orbital Extension

Retinoblastoma is the most common pediatric intraocular malignancy [18]. As intraocular retinoblastoma is becoming increasingly curable, orbital extension is rare, but when it occurs, it significantly increases the risk of metastatic disease and death. For this reason, the treatment of retinoblastoma should be both swift and multidepartmental, involving ophthalmology, oncology, genetics, and radiation oncology.

Orbital retinoblastoma extension can occur through the optic nerve or sclera. Patients with orbital involvement from retinoblastoma may present with a rapidly progressive orbital mass, causing proptosis, diplopia, or inflammatory signs that mimic cellulitis. They may have a known history of intraocular retinoblastoma and have undergone medical treatment or enucleation in the past. On examination, in addition to proptosis, globe displacement, and periorbital inflammation, a leukocoric reflex may be noted. Funduscopic examination will likely demonstrate intraocular tumor. In the case of previous enucleation for retinoblastoma, parents may complain of a change in the fit of the ocular prosthesis and examination may show proptosis of the orbital implant or a mass in the anophthalmic socket.

Imaging may demonstrate both intraocular and intraorbital neoplasms. Retinoblastoma shows homogenous enhancement, and areas of intralesional necrosis and resulting calcification maybe noted on CT. On MRI, the mass is hyperintense compared to vitreous on T1 and hypointense on T2. Optic nerve or choroidal involvement may be evident.

Should orbital disease be discovered, a biopsy is usually not necessary but may be performed if the diagnosis is not definite. Histopathology may demonstrate Flexner-Wintersteiner rosettes, Homer Wright rosettes, or fleurettes which are tumor cells with photoreceptor differentiation. Tissue necrosis and calcification are commonly seen. Systemic oncologic staging is required. For extraocular spread limited to the orbit, current therapeutic recommendations are for neoadjuvant chemotherapy to shrink the tumor, followed by surgical debulking, postoperative chemotherapy, and consideration of external beam radiation therapy [19]. Radiation should be used with caution in these patients as it may cause undesirable side effects, including other neoplasms in germline mutation patients [19]. Exenteration is rarely performed today for extraocular retinoblastoma but may still be beneficial in some cases as a palliative measure for extreme proptosis or pain.

Classically, orbital extension of retinoblastoma was considered a death sentence, with only anecdotal reports of survival. Over time, survival rates have improved, representing advances in detection and chemotherapeutic treatment of metastatic disease. Developing countries carry a heavy burden of orbital disease due to delayed diagnosis and treatment of intraocular retinoblastoma. While Western countries have 5-year survival rates of intraocular Rb up to 97 % and orbital disease in less than 10 % of patients, in developing countries, survival is only 10–50 %, and up to 50 % of patients have orbital disease [18–20].

## Neuroblastoma Metastatic to Orbit

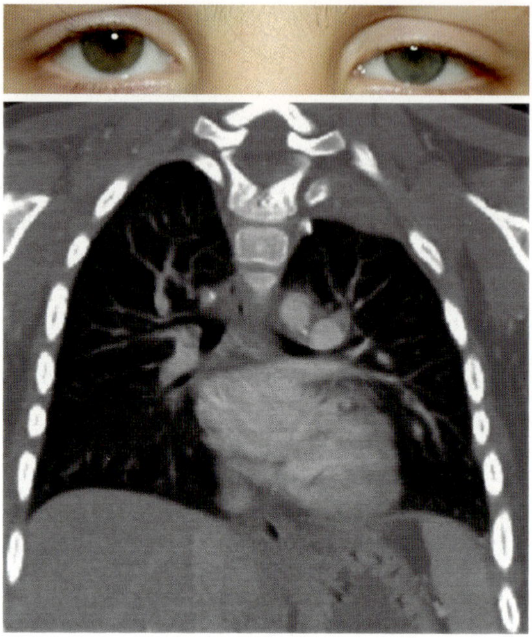

**Fig. 43.7** (**a**) A young boy presented with a history of congenital Horner syndrome; note ptosis of the left upper eyelid, ptosis of the left lower eyelid, miosis of the left pupil, and iris heterochromia with the affected iris lighter than the unaffected iris. (**b**) CT chest showed a left apical mass consistent with neuroblastoma (Figure courtesy of Gena Heidary, M.D.)

Neuroblastoma (Fig. 43.7) is generally found in the pediatric population, accounting for up to 10 % of childhood cancers, with 90 % occurring before the age of 10 [21, 22]. Ten to 43 % of neuroblastoma patients have metastatic orbital disease [21, 23].

Neuroblastoma arises from neural crest cells of the sympathetic nervous system and is usually a primary malignancy of the adrenal gland or paraspinal sympathetic chain. There are case reports of primary orbital neuroblastoma arising from the ciliary ganglion, but the vast majority are orbital metastases and can also involve the periorbital bones [22].

Patients may present with rapidly progressive unilateral or bilateral proptosis from retrobulbar tumors. "Raccoon eyes," or periorbital ecchymosis, is a common presenting finding and may be due to pancytopenia from bone marrow metastases. A miotic pupil, ptosis, and iris hypopigmentation are indicative of Horner syndrome from a sympathetic chain mass. Some patients with metastatic neuroblastoma present with paraneoplastic neurologic findings of opsoclonus-myoclonus syndrome or cerebellar ataxia [21].

Orbital imaging often shows a lateral, homogenously enhancing lesion, which is usually extraconal and may occasionally arise from the lateral wing of the sphenoid bone. The orbital lesion may be poorly or well circumscribed and may show areas of necrosis. On MRI, it is hypointense on T1. Imaging of the abdomen or chest may demonstrate the primary mass along the sympathetic chain or in the adrenal gland.

A biopsy of the orbital mass is diagnostic. Histopathology shows small blue cells which can demonstrate Homer Wright rosettes and intercellular neuropil. Urine or serum testing may be positive for elevated homovanillic acid, vanillylmandelic acid, or 3-methoxy-4-hydroxyphenylethyleneglycol.

The presence of orbital metastasis, which is sometimes the presenting sign of the disease, requires urgent oncologic care to preserve ocular function and life. Aggressive multi-agent chemotherapy is often initiated, with hopes of shrinking the primary tumor prior to resection [21]. Myeloablative chemotherapy is then administered; radiation therapy may be considered as well [21]. Finally, oral retinoic acid is given for 6 months [21].

Neuroblastoma has been shown to spontaneously regress in some cases in very young patients [22]. For patients with advanced disease, including orbital involvement, the prognosis is poor, with no survival beyond 1 year in one retrospective review [23]. The addition of stem cell transplant followed by immunotherapy has significantly improved survival [24].

## Leukemia

Whether acute, chronic, myeloid, or lymphocytic in nature, leukemia can rarely present with orbital involvement. Indeed, any extramedullary site can be involved, and such involvements are given a variety of names, including granulocytic sarcoma, myeloblastoma, myeloid sarcoma, and chloroma [25–27]. Orbital involvement most often presents prior to any known systemic leukemia diagnosis [25]. Once the orbit is involved, systemic disease is generally recognized within 1 year [27]. In fact, orbital leukemia is not actually considered a metastatic disease so much as part of a systemic process. Orbital leukemia is more common in Africa, Asia, Latin America, and the Middle East, and there may be a male preponderance [25].

Patients are generally pediatric and most present with proptosis and a palpable orbital mass. Examination may also demonstrate ptosis, eyelid edema, or restricted extraocular movements. Dilated funduscopic examination may show optic disc edema and retinal hemorrhages. It is of note that leukemia, like neuroblastoma, commonly presents bilaterally and shares the occasional finding of periorbital ecchymosis, also called "raccoon eyes" resulting from pancytopenia as a result of bone marrow infiltration.

Imaging shows a diffuse homogenous orbital lesion, often in the superomedial region, molding to the bone, rather than destroying it. Globe indentation may be noted. On MRI, leukemia is iso- to hypointense to muscle on T1 and iso- to hyperintense to muscle on T2 [26, 27].

Biopsy of the orbital lesion is recommended in these cases, and immunohistochemistry is critical in making the diagnosis. Histopathology demonstrates a clonal expansion of cells with features typical of immature hematopoietic stages. Controversy surrounds whether orbital biopsy can be avoided if a peripheral blood smear shows evidence of leukemic disease [27]. Whether diagnosis is confirmed on a peripheral blood smear or through orbital biopsy, an oncologist is needed to perform a complete workup for leukemia, including bone marrow biopsy.

Surgery is not considered therapeutic, and systemic chemotherapy is generally used to treat orbital leukemia [27]. Orbital radiation may be a necessary adjunct in certain cases [26]. Should systemic leukemia be uncovered, systemic chemotherapy is the mainstay of treatment, sometimes followed by bone marrow transplantation [26]. A negative systemic workup should not alleviate concerns; rather, frequent surveillance is necessary in order to detect the essentially inevitable occurrence of systemic disease.

## Summary

Secondary and metastatic tumors of the orbit are challenging to treat. Nevertheless, prompt diagnosis is required, and with appropriate treatment, patients can have significant symptomatic relief and possibly improved survival.

## References

1. Bonavolontà G, Strianese D, Grassi P, Comune C, Tranfa F, Uccello G, Iuliano A. An analysis of 2,480 space-occupying lesions of the orbit from 1976 to 2011. Ophthal Plast Reconstr Surg. 2013;29(2):79–86.
2. Shields JA, Shields CL, Scartozzi R. Survey of 1264 patients with orbital tumors and simulating lesions: the 2002 Montgomery lecture, part 1. Ophthalmology. 2004;111(5):997–1008.
3. Shields CL, Shields JA, Peggs M. Tumors metastatic to the orbit. Ophthal Plast Reconstr Surg. 1988;4(2):73–80.
4. Shields JA, Shields CL, Brotman HK, Carvalho C, Perez N, Eagle Jr RC. Cancer metastatic to the orbit: the 2000 Robert M. Curts lecture. Ophthal Plast Reconstr Surg. 2001;17(5):346–54.
5. Valenzuela AA, Archibald CW, Fleming B, Ong L, O'Donnell B, Crompton JJ, Selva D, McNab AA,

Sullivan TJ. Orbital metastasis: clinical features, management and outcome. Orbit. 2009;28(2-3):153–9.
6. Goldberg RA, Rootman J, Cline RA. Tumors metastatic to the orbit: a changing picture. Surv Ophthalmol. 1990;35(1):1–24. Review.
7. Goldberg RA, Rootman J. Clinical characteristics of metastatic orbital tumors. Ophthalmology. 1990; 97(5):620–4.
8. Peyster RG, Shapiro MD, Haik BG. Orbital metastasis: role of magnetic resonance imaging and computed tomography. Radiol Clin N Am. 1987;25(3): 647–62.
9. Hui KH, Pfeiffer ML, Esmaeli B. Value of positron emission tomography/computed tomography in diagnosis and staging of primary ocular and orbital tumors. Saudi J Ophthalmol. 2012;26(4):365–71.
10. Kennerdell JS, Slamovits TL, Dekker A, Johnson BL. Orbital fine-needle aspiration biopsy. Am J Ophthalmol. 1985;99(5):547–51.
11. Wong JC, Thampy R, Cook A. Life expectancy following orbital exenteration. Br J Ophthalmol. 2015;99(1):1–4.
12. Roche P, Timon C. Orbital exenteration in periorbital malignancies. Surgeon. 2012;10(4):189–93.
13. Kuo CH, Gao K, Clifford A, Shannon K, Clark J. Orbital exenterations: an 18-year experience from a single head and neck unit. ANZ J Surg. 2011;81(5):326–30.
14. Gill HS, Moscato EE, Chang AL, Soon S, Silkiss RZ. Vismodegib for periocular and orbital basal cell carcinoma. JAMA Ophthalmol. 2013;131(12):1591–4.
15. Murthy R, Honavar SG, Burman S, Vemuganti GK, Naik MN, Reddy VA. Neoadjuvant chemotherapy in the management of sebaceous gland carcinoma of the eyelid with regional lymph node metastasis. Ophthal Plast Reconstr Surg. 2005;21(4):307–9.
16. Garrity JA, Henderson JW. Henderson's orbital tumor. Philadelphia: JB Lippincott Co; 2007.
17. Karcioglu ZA. Orbital tumors diagnosis and treatment. New York: Springer; 2005.
18. Ali MJ, Reddy VAP, Honavar SG, Naik M. Orbital retinoblastoma: where do we go from here? J Cancer Res Ther. 2011;7(1):11–4.
19. Shields CL, Shields JA. Retinoblastoma management: advances in enucleation, intravenous chemoreduction, and intra-arterial chemotherapy. Curr Opin Ophthalmol. 2010;21(3):203–12.
20. Radhakrishnan V, Kashyap S, Pushker N, et al. Outcome, pathologic findings, and compliance in orbital retinoblastoma (International Retinoblastoma Staging System stage III) treated with neoadjuvant chemotherapy: a prospective study. Ophthalmology. 2012;119(7):1470–7.
21. Ahmed S, Goel S, Khandwala M, Agrawal A, Chang B, Simmons IG. Neuroblastoma with orbital metastasis: ophthalmic presentation and role of ophthalmologists. Eye (Lond). 2006;20(4):466–70.
22. Inazawa N, Hatakeyama N, Hori T, et al. Primary orbital neuroblastoma in a 1-month-old boy. Pediatr Int. 2014;56(1):122–5.
23. Smith SJ, Diehl NN, Smith BD, Mohney BG. Incidence, ocular manifestations, and survival in children with neuroblastoma: a population-based study. Am J Ophthalmol. 2010;149(4):677–682.e2.
24. Yu AL, Gilman AL, Ozkaynak MF, et al. Anti-GD2 antibody with GM-CSF, interleukin-2, and isotretinoin for neuroblastoma. N Engl J Med. 2010; 363(14):1324–34.
25. Shields JA, Stopyra GA, Marr BP, et al. Bilateral orbital myeloid sarcoma as initial sign of acute myeloid leukemia: case report and review of the literature. Arch Ophthalmol. 2003;121(1):138–43.
26. Bidar M, Wilson MW, Laquis SJ, et al. Clinical and imaging characteristics of orbital leukemic tumors. Ophthal Plast Reconstr Surg. 2007;23(2):87–93.
27. Murthy R, Vemuganti GK, Honavar SG, Naik M, Reddy V. Extramedullary leukemia in children presenting with proptosis. J Hematol Oncol. 2009;2:4.

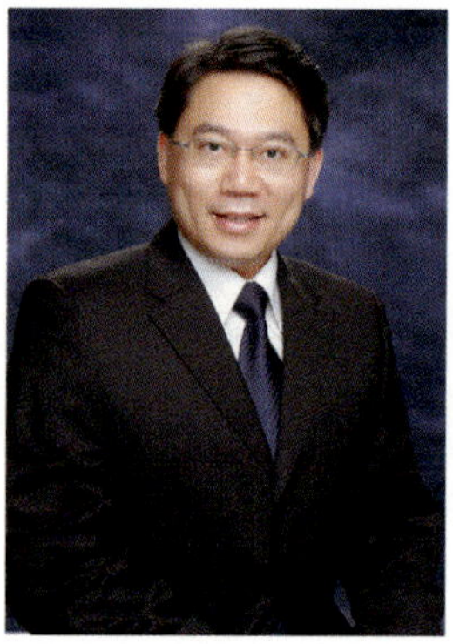

**Hunter Kwok-Lai Yuen** Dr. Hunter Kwok-Lai Yuen is the consultant ophthalmologist and head of the Oculoplastic & Orbital Surgery Service at Hong Kong Eye Hospital. Dr. Yuen was awarded as one of Ten Outstanding Youth Persons in 2007. Subsequently, he received The Fourth Hong Kong Volunteer Award in year 2011. He received Achievement Award and Distinguished Service Award from the Asian Pacific Academy of Ophthalmology in 2012. Moreover, he is the present first Vice President of Asia Pacific Society of Ophthalmic Plastic and Reconstructive Surgery (APSORPS), President of the Hong Kong Society of Ophthalmic Plastic and Reconstructive Surgery, Honorary Secretary of Asia-Pacific Society of Ocular Oncology and Pathology (APSOOP), and editorial member and reviewer of several journals.

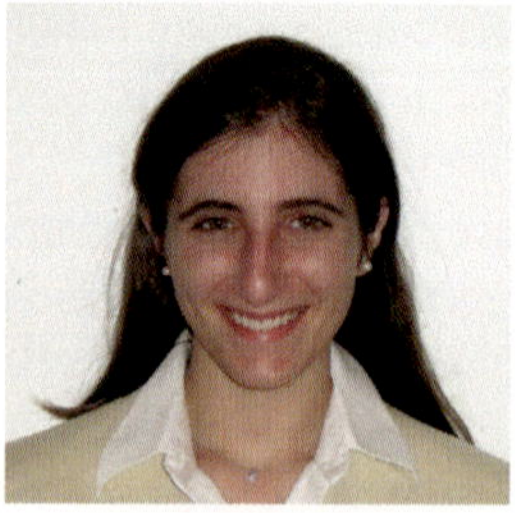

**Lora Rabin Dagi Glass** Lora Dagi Glass completed her ophthalmology residency at the Columbia University Medical Center, followed by a fellowship in oculoplastic surgery at the Massachusetts Eye and Ear Infirmary. Her research has focused on orbital processes ranging from thyroid eye disease to optic nerve glioma and orbital melanoma.

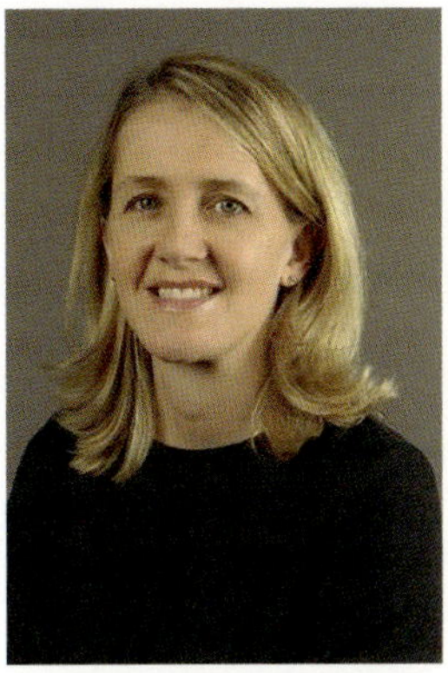

**Suzanne K. Freitag** Suzanne K Freitag, MD, received a BA from Duke University and MD from Jefferson Medical College in Philadelphia, PA. She completed ophthalmology residency at Wills Eye Hospital followed by a neuroophthalmology fellowship at the Wilmer Eye Institute at Johns Hopkins. She then completed a 2-year American Society of Ophthalmic Plastic and Reconstructive Surgery-approved fellowship in Boston. She is the Director of the Ophthalmic Plastic Surgery Service at Massachusetts Eye and Ear Infirmary and an Assistant Professor of Ophthalmology at Harvard Medical School.

# 44 Malignant Transformation in Benign Orbital Diseases

Bipasha Mukherjee

## Introduction

Malignant transformation of an existing benign tumor is a process by which the cells acquire properties of a cancerous phenotype and starts dividing uncontrollably.

The exact reason and process by which this transformation occurs is difficult to pinpoint. Certain types of benign tumor are known to undergo malignant transformation. One of the better-known examples of this phenomenon in the orbit is the progression of a benign pleomorphic adenoma of the lacrimal gland to a pleomorphic adenocarcinoma.

Initially, malignant transformation in a benign tumor may be detected only while pathologic examination of the lesion (carcinoma *in* pleomorphic adenoma). Later, the clinical signs and symptoms may signal malignant change. Unexplained, unremitting pain, sudden growth, change in texture (soft to hard), or neurological deficit in an area of a preexisting lesion should raise concern for malignant transformation.

B. Mukherjee, MS, DNB(Ophthalmology), FICO (✉)
Orbit, Oculoplasty, Reconstructive & Aesthetic Services, Sankara Nethralaya, Chennai, Tamil Nadu, India
e-mail: drbpm@snmail.org

## Predisposing Factors for Malignant Transformation

**Intrinsic factors:** defective genes or genetic mutations.

Two types of genes play a major role in malignant transformation: oncogenes and tumor suppressor genes.

*Oncogenes*: Healthy, unmutated oncogenes (also known as proto-oncogenes) take part in stimulating normal cell growth and division, whereas a mutated oncogene continuously commands the cell to proliferate, leading to unchecked, cancerous growth.

*Tumor suppressor genes*: In healthy cells, tumor suppressor genes keep the cell's growth in check. These genes stop working in a cancerous cell, allowing the cell to begin a malignant, destructive process.

Growth of normal tissues and organs is also controlled by a genetic phenomenon called programmed cell death, or *apoptosis*, in which a certain number of cells die and are eliminated after a finite number of divisions. Malignant transformation can impede programmed cell death, thus allowing the cells to grow uncontrollably and resulting in cancer [1].

**Extrinsic factors:** viruses, chemical carcinogens, or radiation damage by free radicals and ultraviolet radiation.


B. Mukherjee, H. Yuen (eds.), *Emergencies of the Orbit and Adnexa*,
DOI 10.1007/978-81-322-1807-4_44

Viruses of the family Polyomaviridae, a group of papovaviruses, are associated with malignancy in animals. Cancers caused by chemical or physical carcinogens in the environment probably often, if not invariably, are due to alterations in the sequences of proto-oncogenes that have converted them to oncogenes. Radiotherapy has emerged as a consistent and important risk factor for developing second malignancies due to their tumor suppressor gene defect [2, 3].

## Classification of Benign Orbital Lesions with Malignant Potential

Epithelial
Mesenchymal
Lymphoproliferative
Melanocytic
Neurogenic
Osseous and cartilaginous

## Epithelial Lesions

### Lacrimal Gland Tumors

The incidence of epithelial tumors of the lacrimal gland ranges from 5 to 8 % of orbital neoplasia [4]. The most common benign neoplasm of the lacrimal gland is the pleomorphic adenoma which usually presents as a unilateral painless, progressive, downward and inward displacement of the globe (Fig. 44.1).

CT and MRI are invaluable in assessing lacrimal gland lesions. Radiologically benign lesions are round or oval, smooth in outline, displacing the globe and deforming the lacrimal gland fossa, but not causing any bony erosion (Fig. 44.2). Calcifications are not seen. On the contrary, malignant lacrimal gland lesions are irregular in outline, cause bony erosions and may demonstrate calcifications (Fig. 44.3).

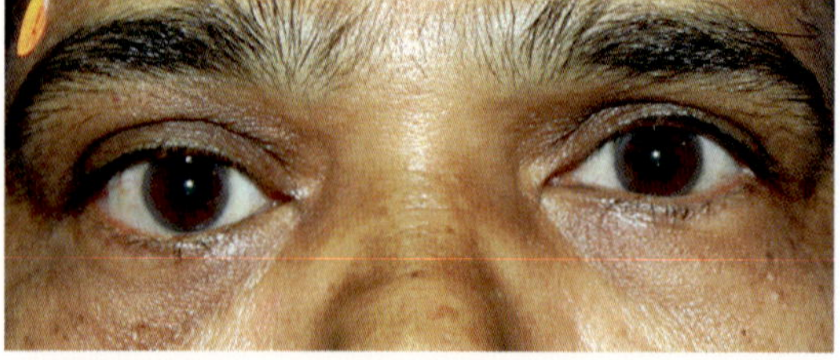

**Fig. 44.1** Clinical photograph of patient with lacrimal gland pleomorphic adenoma of the right orbit

Malignant mixed tumor, also called carcinoma ex pleomorphic adenoma, pleomorphic carcinoma or carcinoma in pleomorphic adenoma, represents a pleomorphic adenoma that has undergone malignant degeneration [5]. These tumors can be seen in a patient who had undergone an incomplete resection of a benign mixed tumor and can present with a recurrence decades later [6]. Malignant transformation of a long-standing, indolent lacrimal gland tumor can be heralded by sudden acute expansion of the mass with pain and swelling of the upper eyelid [7].

Font and Gamel reported a 10 % incidence of malignant transformation of recurrent adenomas by 20 years after treatment and 20 % by 30 years [8].

A high index of suspicion and knowledge of the radiologic findings and clinical behavior of the different lesions is imperative when dealing with lacrimal tumors (Table 44.1).

Histologically, benign and malignant components of the lesion need to be identified. A malignant mixed tumor shows features of a benign mixed tumor with areas of malignant transformation [9]. In most cases, these elements are poorly differentiated adenocarcinomas, but squamous cell carcinoma, adenoid cystic carcinoma, or even a sarcoma can be found [10, 11].

**Management:** All lacrimal gland pleomorphic adenomas should be excised completely, along with its intact pseudo-capsule, as untreated or partially excised tumors carry a significant long-term risk of recurrence and malignant transformation. Incisional biopsy of a suspected benign lesion also should be avoided as it carries the risk of cellular seeding beyond the pseudo-capsule, which forms an effective physical barrier around the intact tumor [12].

Management of malignant lacrimal gland tumors is still unsatisfactory and requires an aggressive approach including exenteration, en bloc craniofacial orbitectomy, lymph node

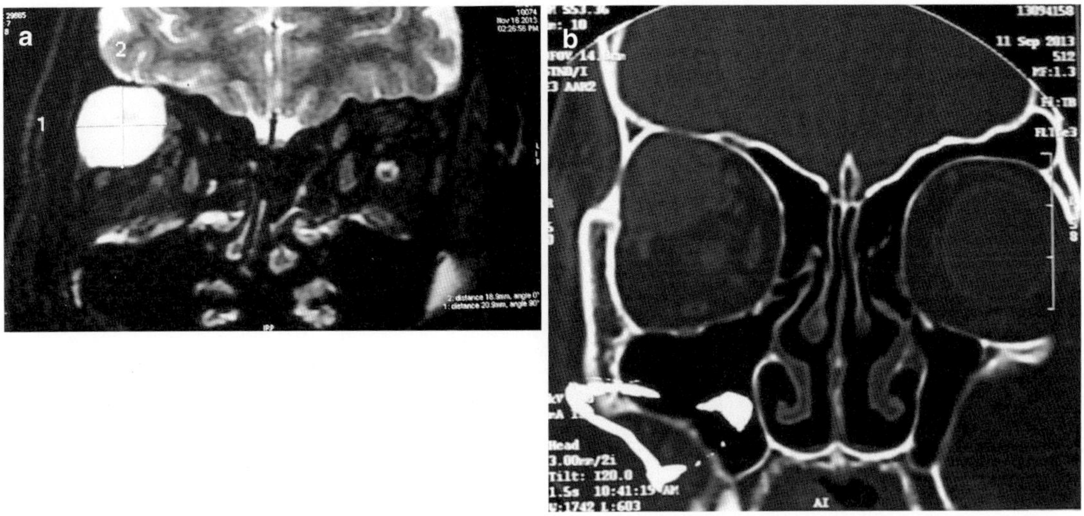


**Fig. 44.2** T2-weighted coronal MRI scan showing a well-circumscribed round soft tissue lesion in the right lacrimal gland fossa (**a**); CT scan of the same patient showing fossa formation without bony erosion or calcification (**b**)

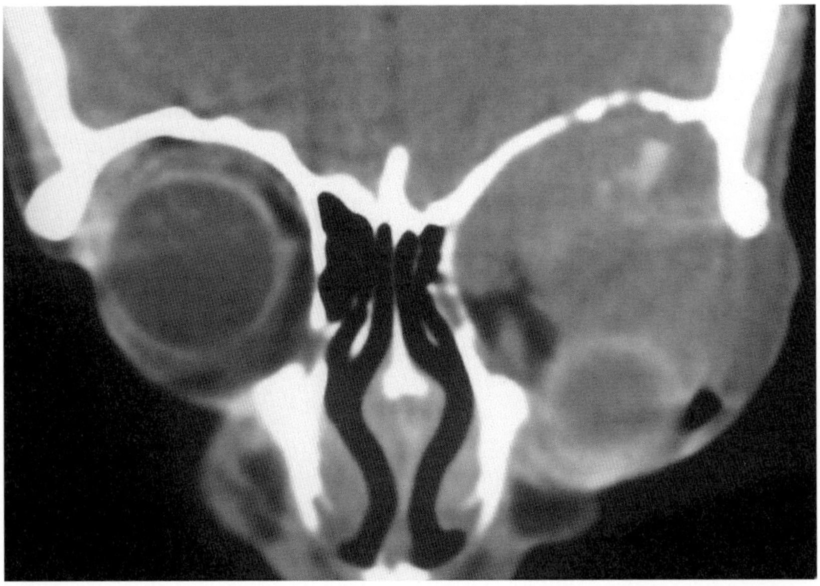

**Fig. 44.3** CT scan of patient with malignant lacrimal gland tumor showing bone erosion

dissection, and subsequent radiotherapy. A potentially promising option is intra-arterial administration of neo-adjuvant chemotherapy [13].

## Mesenchymal Tumors

Prior to the use of immunohistochemical techniques, the diagnosis of orbital spindle cell neoplasms like solitary fibrous tumor (SFT) used to be confused with fibrous histiocytoma, giant cell angiofibroma and hemangiopericytoma. Microscopically, they all show considerable similarity, varying in degree of cellularity, stromal collagen, and the presence of giant cells. However, immunohistochemistry reveals positivity for CD34 in all cases (100 %), and these lesions are nowadays designated as solitary fibrous tumor [14].

Local recurrences of SFT are possible and usually follow an incomplete initial excision.

**Table 44.1** Clinicopathological features of benign and malignant lacrimal gland tumors

| | Benign | Malignant | Malignant transformation |
|---|---|---|---|
| Commonest | Pleomorphic adenoma | Adenoid cystic carcinoma | Malignant mixed tumor |
| Duration | >1 year | <1 year | Sudden recurrence in an incompletely removed lacrimal gland mass or sudden expansion in a long-standing benign neoplasm |
| Clinical features | 4th–5th decade of life; painless | Younger age group (ave. age: 40 years); painful; rarely numbness | Older patients; painful sudden proptosis |
| Imaging findings | Well-circumscribed mass lesion; expansion/remodeling of the lacrimal gland fossa; without bone invasion; no calcification | Bone invasion; calcification | May or may not show bony changes |
| Histopathology | Mixture of epithelial and mesenchymal elements (benign mixed tumor) | Five histological patterns: cribriform; solid (basaloid); sclerosing; comedocarcinomatous; tubular (ductal) | Features of benign mixed tumor with areas of malignant change |

Recurrent orbital SFT has the potential for malignant transformation even several years after surgery [15].

**Management** The treatment of choice of orbital SFT is complete surgical excision and careful follow-up [16].

## Lymphoproliferative Lesions

Ocular and adnexal lymphomas (OAL) constitute 8 % of extranodal lymphomas and are the most common malignant tumors of the orbit [17]. Lymphoid hyperplasia (LH) is a term used to describe benign lymphoproliferative lesions of the orbit. It has been hypothesized that it represents a temporary benign precursor lesion with the potential to progress to lymphoma [18].

The term 'reactive' LH (RLH) has been used for lesions with a benign morphology and immunophenotype, whereas 'atypical' LH (ALH) applies to borderline lesions [19]. The association between LH and autoimmune diseases like Sjogren's syndrome, Grave's disease, lupus erythematosus etc suggests chronic stimulation by autoimmune antigens may play a role in the developement of polyclonal BRLH which can progress to monoclonality and lymphoma [20]. Recent studies suggest that the risk of progression to malignant lymphoma is about 10 % [21].

It is at times difficult to distinguish LH from malignant lymphoma on the basis of histomorphology alone. Ancillary techniques like immunohistochemistry (IHC), flow cytometry and molecular genetic analyses based on clonality are necessary to distinguish benign from malignant lymphoproliferative processes.

RLH accounts for 10–20 % of all OALs [22]. The majority of OAL are B-cell non-Hodgkin's lymphoma (NHL), predominantly extranodal marginal zone lymphoma (ENMZL) of mucosa –associated lymphoid tissue (MALT). The clinical manifestations of these lesions depend on the site of involvement. Anatomic sites usually affected by BRLH and OAL are the lacrimal glands, extra ocular muscles, lacrimal sac, conjunctiva, eyelids and the entire orbit. Orbital LH is predominately extraconal and found above the horizontal midline, being most commonly centered in the lacrimal gland. Patients with conjunctival lesions may present with complaints of foreign body sensation and redness [19]. Both LH and malignant lymphomas can present as a visible mass beneath the conjunctiva, described as a "salmon patch" (Fig. 44.4). Lymphoproliferative lesions involving the orbits and eyelids present

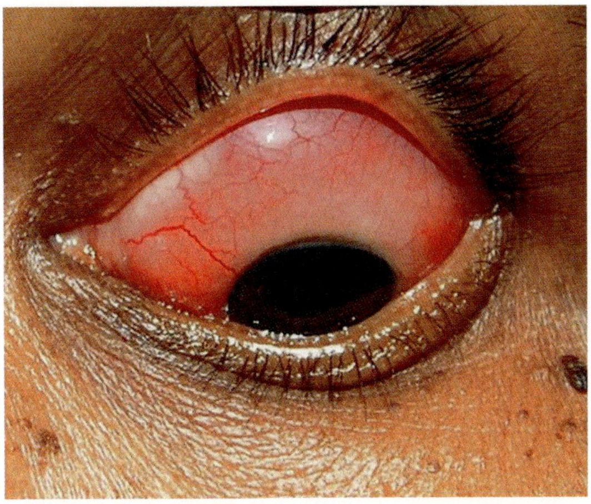

**Fig. 44.4** Salmon patch: Pink hyperemic infiltrative mass over bulbar conjunctiva extending from medial to lateral canthus and up to superior fornix

with swelling or with painless proptosis. Imaging will demonstrate an infiltrative contrast enhancing mass lesion with molding of the globe and the adjacent structures without invasion (Fig. 44.5).

Reactive LH and low-grade OAL are clinically and radiologically indistinguishable from each other, requiring tissue biopsy in all cases followed by IHC and systemic workup to classify the nature of the lesion under the Revised European and American Lymphoma (REAL) classification [23].

Benign lesions show polymorphous array of small round lymphocytes and plasma cells whereas malignant lymphomas show anaplastic cells with nuclear pleomorphism and prominent nucleoli. Lesions beginning as polyclonal reactive processes can succumb to malignant transformation with light chain restriction. The clonality of lymphoid proliferations is assessed using immunophenotyping (immunohistochemistry or flow cytometry) to detect immunoglobulin light chain restriction and molecular genetic techniques–polymerase chain reaction (PCR) [19].

**Castleman's Disease (CD):** Castleman disease is a non-neoplastic abnormal follicular proliferation of uncertain pathogenesis. They can present with lacrimal gland enlargement, peri-optic swelling, or orbital mass lesions. The rare plasma cell variant of CD has an increased association with lymphoma [24, 25].

**IgG4-related Disease:** A subtype of Idiopathic orbital Inflammatory Disease (IOID) caused by raised tissue and serum immunoglobulin G4 (IgG4) has been recently described. There are reports suggesting that B-cell lymphoma can arise on a background of IgG4-related chronic inflammation [26, 27]. Using diagnostic thresholds of >10 IgG4+cells/high power field (HPF) and IgG4+/IgG+ cell ratio >40 %, several centers have found IgG4-related disease to account for 50 % of benign lymphoid hyperplasia and 23 % of orbital lymphoproliferative disease [28].

**Management:** Currently there are no definitive guidelines for treatment of LH. The most important aspect of management is careful monitoring for both signs of recurrence and/or malignant transformation to systemic lymphoma. Histological and cytological evaluation is mandatory by IHC and flow cytometry in the diagnosis of suspected orbital and adnexal lymphoproliferative masses. Management of LH depends on the clinical features, co-morbidities, and location of the disease.

Specific therapy of LH includes systemic and /or intraorbital steroids, local radiotherapy (15–20Gy), biologoical response modifiers like rituximab and intralesional bevacizumab, and chemotherapy [29]. Radiotherapy is a particularly useful modality in unilateral cases, when corticosteroids are contra-indicated, or for recurrences. Radiotherapy may also confer some protection against recurrence and malignant transformation. Radioimmunotherapy is another interesting modality since these lesions.

## Neurogenic Tumors

Irradiation and neurofibromatosis type 1(NF1) may, in combination, pose a significant risk for the development of malignancies. There is a significantly increased risk of new glioma and malignant peripheral nerve sheath tumors

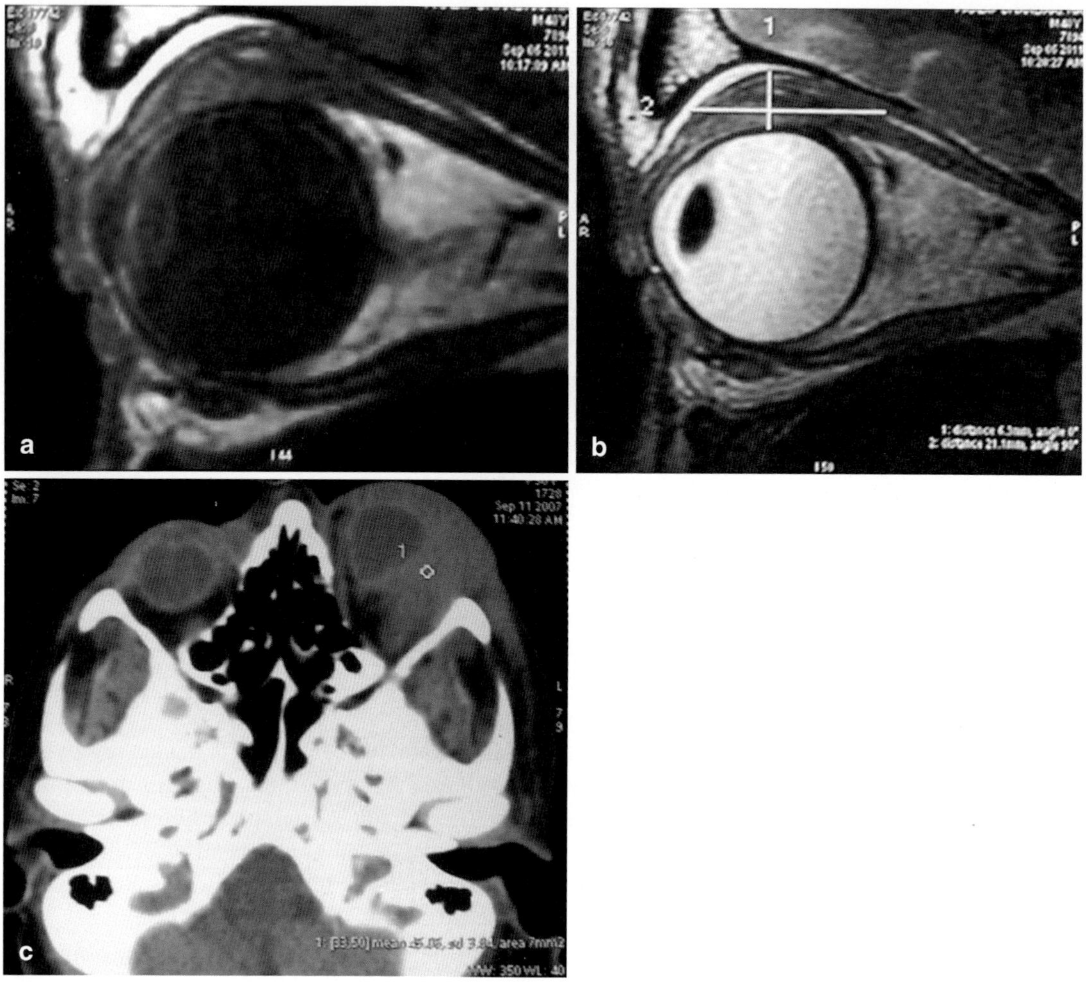


**Fig. 44.5** BRLH: well-defined homogenous soft tissue lesion extending from superior limbus to superior rectus insertion, moderately thickened SR and LPS muscle isointense on T1 W (**a**) and T2W (**b**). CT scan showing lymphoproliferative lesion involving left orbit molding the globe (**c**)

(MPNST) in NF1 patients who are irradiated for optic nerve glioma [30, 31]. MPNSTs typically arise from preexisting plexiform neurofibroma in an individual with NF1 in their third to fourth decade of life. In one study, a tenfold increased significant risk of a malignant tumor in the radiation field was seen compared to NF2 patients who had not undergone radiotherapy [32]. Malignant transformation can occur after radiation probably because insufficient cells are killed in the tumor, and some of the surviving cells acquire mutations in genes, such as TP53, that can transform a benign tumor into a malignant one. These malignant lesions are highly aggressive, almost universally fatal and frequently metastasize [33].

Neurilemomas (benign schwannomas) are found in 1.5–18 % of patients with von Recklinghausen's neurofibromatosis. However, malignant transformation of this by and large benign tumor also has been reported to occur in this condition [34].

A benign medulloepithelioma in the orbit has been reported which underwent malignant transformation 10 months after removal. The authors suggested that a medulloepithelioma of the optic nerve should be considered malignant despite morphology with tendency to spread to the CNS [35].

**Management:** Overall, these studies indicate that the risk of radiation-induced tumors after radiotherapy for benign disease is 0.5–3 % after 30 years. While MRI can detect volumetric changes and may predict malignant change, positron emission tomography (PET) is the most sensitive and specific test to diagnose NF1-associated MPNSTs [36]. However, the significant dose of radiation involved in PET precludes its use in routine screening in a cancer prone syndrome [37].

The mainstay of treatment of MPNSTs is wide surgical resection followed by local radiotherapy, but the prognosis is poor [38].

The relatively small risk of malignant transformation and new primary tumors, when compared to the benefits of radiation treatment for certain benign tumors, justifies the use of radiation in specific circumstances, for example, when surgery is refused or in an elderly patient. Nonetheless, people who have such treatment should be made aware of the potential risks [3]. We recommend that if irradiation is necessary in persons with neurofibromatosis, regular follow-up is imperative.

## Melanocytic

Nevi by definition are benign proliferations of melanocytes. However, 50 % of malignant melanomas arise from preexisting nevi [39]. Melanomas can develop due to DNA damage to cells (most often caused by ultraviolet radiation from chronic sun exposure or tanning beds) triggering genetic mutations. Primary orbital melanomas are usually associated with periorbital pigmentary disorders, such as oculodermal melanocytosis, blue nevus, and ocular melanocytosis [40]. Malignant melanoma associated with nevus of Ota has been reported to occur in the uveal tract, optic nerve head, brain, and orbit. The incidence of malignant change in nevus of Ota (oculodermal melanocytosis) is 0.5 % for East Asians and about 25 % for Caucasians [41].

**Management:** Systemic metastasis should be ruled out by PET scan. Exenteration is the treatment of choice of most ophthalmologists for orbital malignant melanoma. It should be kept in mind that even such an extensive surgery offers no assurance of cure and lifelong follow-up is of utmost importance.

## Osseous and Cartilaginous Lesions

Excessive exposure to radiation, especially at a young age, and combinations of radiation and chemotherapy for treating prior cancer may increase risk of bone cancer at a later age. Individuals treated with certain kinds of anticancer drugs (alkylating agents) may be at increased risk for malignant bone tumors. Certain genetic risk factors may be associated with a propensity for the development of sarcomas. Individuals who have had multiple benign tumors (osteochondromas), who have been diagnosed with Paget's disease, or who have a long-term bone infection (osteomyelitis) may also be more likely to develop primary sarcomas [42]. Chondrosarcomas may also arise from benign lesions (e.g., enchondromas and osteochondromas) or in individuals with hereditary multiple exostosis or enchondromatosis; the risk of malignant transformation in these individuals may be as high as 25 % [43]. Patients of familial retinoblastoma can develop second malignant tumors like osteosarcoma even without radiation therapy [44].

## Premalignant Conditions

### Paget's Disease

Both benign and malignant neoplasms arise in the setting of Paget's disease. The incidence of sarcoma has been estimated at approximately 1 %. Osteosarcoma is by far the most common, and fibrosarcoma and chondrosarcoma are rarely observed. The prognosis of sarcoma in a patient with Paget's disease is considerably worse than for similar primary tumors, with the 5-year survival as low as 8 %.

## Chronic Osteomyelitis

The interval to the development of malignancy in a patient of chronic osteomyelitis is highly variable, from as little as 1 year to decades. The clinical clues that suggest malignant transformation include a growing mass, increased pain, bleeding, or a purulent discharge in a long-standing sinus. Radiographically, acceleration in the destructive nature of the lesion and a soft tissue mass are the rule. Histologically, most cases are well-differentiated squamous cell carcinoma, although osteosarcoma, fibrosarcoma, and undifferentiated sarcoma have also been reported.

## Osteochondroma

The incidence of chondrosarcoma arising in patients with multiple osteochondromas has been estimated at 5–35 % [43].

## Fibrous Dysplasia

Malignant transformation in fibrous dysplasia, most commonly to osteosarcoma, has been documented at a rate of 0.4–2.0 %.

## Postradiation Sarcoma

Sarcoma is now a well-documented detrimental effect of ionizing radiation. To use the term postradiation sarcoma, the bone must have been included in the radiation field. Most cases present at least 4 years after irradiation, and the most common postradiation sarcoma is osteosarcoma [45].

**Management:** Management of malignant osseous and cartilaginous lesions of the orbit comprises of a combination of chemotherapy, total resection, and adjuvant radiotherapy. In spite of aggressive treatment, the prognosis remains poor.

In summary, ophthalmologists should be aware of the fact that many benign orbital lesions have the potential to undergo malignant transformation. Benign lesions which are known to become cancerous over time, like pleomorphic adenoma of the lacrimal gland, should be completely excised as early as possible and the patients followed up for signs of recurrence. Incisional biopsy should be avoided as seeding during biopsy can cause recurrence of the tumor. Radiation exposure should be curtailed and avoided altogether, if possible, in young children. The role of external carcinogens specially nicotine is a well-known fact and should remain a public concern. Follow-up of all patients with orbital lesions, even if benign, even after complete excision, is mandatory.

## References


1. Birch JM. Genes and cancer. Arch Dis Child. 1999;80(1):1–3.
2. Klein G, Michaelis J, Spix C, Wibbing R, Eggers G, Ritter J, Kaatsch P. Second malignant neoplasms after treatment of childhood cancer. Eur J Cancer. 2003; 39:808–17.
3. Evans DGR, Birch JM, Ramsden RT, Sharif S, Baser ME. Malignant transformation and new primary tumours after therapeutic radiation for benign disease: substantial risks in certain tumour prone syndromes. J Med Genet. 2006;43:289–94.
4. Rootman JA. Diseases of the orbit: a multidisciplinary approach. Philadelphia: JB Lippincott; 1988. p. 384–405.
5. Weis E, Rootman J, Joly J. Epithelial lacrimal gland tumors. Pathologic classification and current understanding. Arch Ophthalmol. 2009;127:1016–28.
6. Shields JA, Shields C. Malignant transformation of presumed pleomorphic adenoma of lacrimal gland after 60 years. Arch Ophthalmol. 1987;105(10): 1403–5.
7. Duck Kim Y. Lacrimal gland tumors. In: Karcioglu ZA, editor. Orbital tumors, diagnosis and treatment. New York: Springer; 2005. p. 204–20.
8. Font RL, Gamel JW. Epithelial tumors of the lacrimal gland: an analysis of 265 cases. In: Jacobiec FA, editor. Ocular and adnexal tumors. Birmingham: Aesculapius Publishing; 1978. p. 787–805.
9. Font RL, Smith SL, Bryan RG. Malignant epithelial tumors of the lacrimal gland. A clinicopathologic study of 21 cases. Arch Ophthalmol. 1998;116:613–6.
10. Ishida M, Hotta M, Kushima R, Tsuruoka S, Ohji M, Okabe H. Case of ductal adenocarcinoma ex pleomorphic adenoma of the lacrimal gland. Rinsho Byori. 2009;57:746–51.
11. Takahira M, Minato H, Takahashi M, et al. Cystic carcinoma ex pleomorphic adenoma of the lacrimal gland. Ophthal Plast Reconstr Surg. 2007;23:407–9.

12. Rose GE. To crash or not to crash? Probability in the management of benign lacrimal gland tumours. Eye. 2009;23:1625–8.
13. Tse DT, Benedetto P, Dubovy S, et al. Clinical analysis of the effect on intraarterial cytoreductive chemotherapy in the treatment of lacrimal gland adenoid cystic carcinoma. Am J Ophthalmol. 2006;141:44–53.
14. Furusato E, Valenzuela IA, Fanburg-Smith JC, Auerbach A, Furusato B, Cameron JD, Rushing EJ. Orbital solitary fibrous tumor: encompassing terminology for hemangiopericytoma, giant cell angiofibroma, and fibrous histiocytoma of the orbit: reappraisal of 41 cases. Hum Pathol. 2011;42:120–8.
15. Carrera M, Prat J, Quintana M. Malignant solitary fibrous tumor of the orbit: report of a case with 8 years follow-up. Eye. 2001;15:102–4.
16. Bernardini FP, de Conciliis C, Schneider S, Kersten RC, Kulwin DR. Solitary fibrous tumor of the orbit: is it rare? Report of a case series and review of the literature. Ophthalmology. 2003;110:1442–8.
17. Freeman C, Berg JW, Cutler SJ. Occurence and prognosis of extranodal lymphomas. Cancer. 1972;29:252–60.
18. Jakobiec FA. Ocular adnexal lymphoid tumors: progress in need of clarification. Am J Ophthalmol. 2008;86:948–66.
19. Andrew NH, Coupland SE, Pirbhai A, Selva D. Lymphoid hyperplasia of the orbit and ocular adnexa: A clinical pathologic review. Surv Ophthalmol. 2016 Apr 26. pii: S0039-6257(16)30060-1. doi: 10.1016/j.survophthal.2016.04.004. [Epub ahead of print].
20. Kubota T, Moritani S. High incidence of autoimmune disease in Japanese patients with ocular adnexal reactive lymphoid hyperplasia. Am J Ophthalmol. 2007;144:148–9.
21. Mannami T, Yoshino K, et al. Clinical, histopathological, and immunogenetic analysis of ocular adnexal lymphoproliferative disorders: characterization of malt lymphoma and reactive lymphopid hyperplasia. Mod Pathol. 2001;14:641–9.
22. Shinder R, Al-Zubaidi N, Esmaeli B. Survey of orbital tumors at a comprehensive cancer center in the United States. Head Neck. 2010;33:610–4.
23. Coupland SE, Hummel M, Stein H. Ocular adnexal lymphomas: five case presentations and a review of the literature. Surv Ophthalmol. 2002;47:470–90.
24. Mukherjee B, Alam MS, Krishnakumar S. A rare case of bilateral orbital castleman disease. Orbit. 2014;15:1–4.
25. Venizelos I, Papathomas TG, Papathanasiou M, Cheva A, Garypidou V, Coupland S. Orbital involvement in Castleman disease. Surv Ophthalmol. 2010;55:247–55.
26. Sato Y, Takata K, Ichimura K, Tanaka K, Morito T, Tamura M, et al. IgG4-producing marginal zone B-cell lymphomas. Int J Hematol. 2008;88:428–33.
27. Kubota T, Moritani S, Yoshino T, Nagai H, Terasaki H. Ocular adnexal marginal zone B cell lymphoma infiltrated by IgG4-positive plasma cells. J Clin Pathol. 2010;63:1059–65.
28. Andrew NH, Sladden N, Kearney DJ, Selva D. An analysis of IgG4-related disease (IgG4-RD) among idiopathic orbital inflammations and benign lymphoid hyperplasias using two consensus-based diagnostic criteria for IgG4-RD. Br J Ophthalmol. 2015;99(3):376–81. doi: 10.1136/bjophthalmol-2014-305545. PubMed PMID: 25185258.
29. Singh AD, editor. Ocular and adnexal lymphoma, essentials in ophthalmology. Berlin: Springer; 2014.
30. Sharif S, Ferner R, Birch J, et al. Second primary tumours in NF1 patients treated for optic glioma: substantial risks post radiotherapy. J Clin Oncol. 2006;16:2570–5.
31. Ducatman B, Scheithauer B, Piepgras D, Reiman H, Istrup D. Malignant peripheral nerve sheath tumors: a clinicopathological study of 120 patients. Cancer. 1986;57:2006–21.
32. Baser ME, Evans DGR, Jackler RK, Sujansky E, Rubinstein A. Malignant peripheral nerve sheath tumours, radiotherapy and neurofibromatosis 2. Br J Cancer. 2000;82:998.
33. Lyons CJ, McNab AA, Garner A, et al. Orbital MPNSTs. BJO. 1989;73:731–8.
34. Schatz H. Benign orbital neurilemoma. Sarcomatous transformation in von Recklinghausen's disease. Arch Ophthalmol. 1971;86(3):268–73.
35. Lindegaard J, Heegaard S, Toft PB, Nysom K, Prause JU. Malignant transformation of a medulloepithelioma of the optic nerve. Orbit. 2010;29:161–4.
36. Ferner RE, Golding JF, Smith M, Calonje E, Jan W, Sanjayanathan V, O'Doherty M. [18F]2-fluoro-2-deoxy-D-glucose positron emission tomography (FDG PET) as a diagnostic tool for neurofibromatosis 1 (NF1) associated malignant peripheral nerve sheath tumours (MPNSTs): a long-term clinical study. Ann Oncol. 2008;19(2):390–4.
37. Evans DGR, Huson SM, Birch JM. Malignant peripheral nerve sheath tumours in inherited disease. Clin Sarcoma Res. 2012;2:17.
38. Dutton JJ, Tawfik HA, DeBacker CM, Lipham WJ, Gayre GS, Klintworth GK. Multiple recurrences in malignant peripheral nerve sheath tumor of the orbit: a case report and a review of the literature. Ophthal Plast Reconstr Surg. 2001;17:293–9.
39. Taloni A, Alemi AA, Ciusani E, Sethna JP, Zapperi S, et al. Mechanical properties of growing melanocytic nevi and the progression to melanoma. PLoS One. 2014;9(4):e94229.
40. Rice CD, Brown HH. Primary orbital melanoma associated with orbital melanocytosis. Arch Ophthalmol. 1990;108:1130–4.
41. Nitta K, Kashima T, Mayuzumi H, et al. Animal-type malignant melanoma associated with nevus of Ota in the orbit of a Japanese woman: a case report. Melanoma Res. 2014;24:286–9.
42. Horvai A, Krishnan KU. Premalignant conditions of bone. J Orthop Sci. 2006;11:412–23.
43. Baker LH. Bone tumors: primary and metastatic bone lesions. In: Goldman L et al., editors. Cecil medicine. 23rd ed. Saunders Elsevier; 2007. MD Consult. Elsevier. 9 Sep 2009.
44. Abramson DH, Ronner HJ, Ellsworth RM. Second tumors in non-irradiated bilateral retinoblastoma. Am J Ophthalmol. 1979;87:624–7.
45. Cahan WG. Radiation-induced sarcoma – 50 years later. Cancer. 1998;82:6–7.

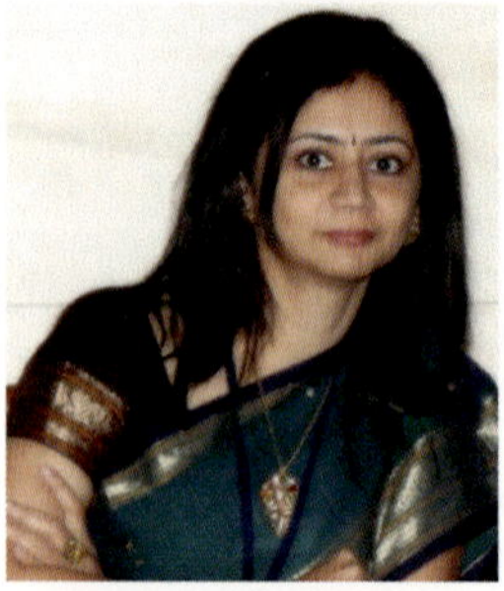

**Bipasha Mukherjee** Dr. Bipasha Mukherjee is a fellow in Orbit & Oculoplasty from Aravind Eye Hospitals, India, and ICO fellow from University Hospital of Limoges, France, under Prof. Jean-Paul Adenis. She has undergone clinical observerships with stalwarts like Jack Rootman, Richard Collins, Geoff Rose, Mark Duffy, and Robert Goldberg.

She currently heads the department of Orbit, Oculoplasty, Aesthetic & Reconstructive services in Medical Research Foundation, Chennai. She has numerous presentations in national and international conferences and publications in peer-reviewed journals and text books. Her areas of interest include diseases of the orbit and adnexa including tumors, lacrimal surgery, socket reconstruction, traumatic lid and adnexal injuries, training residents and fellows, and photography.

# Sebaceous Gland Carcinoma

# 45

Md. Shahid Alam, Akshay Gopinathan Nair, and Bipasha Mukherjee

## Introduction

Sebaceous gland carcinoma (SGC), sebaceous cell carcinoma, and meibomian gland carcinoma are all terms used in the literature to describe a malignant neoplasm of sebaceous origin, commonly found in the eyelids and adnexa [1]. It was first described as a malignant ocular entity of the ocular adnexa as early as the nineteenth century [2]. Straatsma presented the first series of 16 patients with sebaceous carcinoma in 1956 [3]. The tumor is notorious, for mimicking various benign and malignant clinical entities and for its aggressive local behavior and the potential to metastasize regionally to lymph nodes and to distant organs.

M.S. Alam, MS (✉)
Orbit Oculoplasty Reconstructive and Aesthetic Services, Sankara Nethralaya, 18 College Road, Chennai, Tamil Nadu 600006, India
e-mail: mshahidalam@gmail.com

A.G. Nair, MBBS, DNB
Ophthalmic Plastic Surgery, L V Prasad Eye Institute, Hyderabad, Telangana, India
e-mail: akshaygn@gmail.com

B. Mukherjee, MS, DNB (Ophthalmology), FICO
Orbit Oculoplasty Reconstructive and Aesthetic Services, Sankara Nethralaya, 18 College Road, Chennai, Tamil Nadu 600006, India

Medical Research Foundation, Chennai, Tamil Nadu, India
e-mail: drbpm@snmail.org

## Origin

The most common location for SGC is within the meibomian glands of the upper eyelids followed by the lower eyelids [2]. The upper eyelid is involved more frequently because of more number of meibomian glands. It can also arise from the gland of Zeis and the sebaceous glands associated with the caruncle.

## Incidence and Demographics

Sebaceous gland carcinoma accounts for almost 5 % of all eyelid malignancies in the United States [1]. A higher incidence has been reported in Asian and Indian population [1, 4]. Ni and associates reported that sebaceous carcinoma accounted for 33 % of all malignant eyelid tumors in China [5].

Sebaceous carcinoma occurs more commonly in females than males, and the average age of detection is between 60 and 69 years. There is a second younger age of incidence in children who develop sebaceous carcinoma as a secondary cancer after radiation for bilateral inherited retinoblastoma [6].

**Risk factors:** the following are some of the risk factors for the development of sebaceous gland carcinoma of the ocular adnexa:

(a) Irradiation: There are reports of cases of sebaceous gland carcinoma occurring in patients who received radiotherapy for retinoblastoma


B. Mukherjee, H. Yuen (eds.), *Emergencies of the Orbit and Adnexa*,
DOI 10.1007/978-81-322-1807-4_45

in the past. A review of nine such cases revealed that all cases were hereditary, and sebaceous carcinoma occurred after a mean duration of 11 years of exposure [7].

(b) Human papillomavirus (HPV) infection: HPV infection and integration of DNA have been implicated in many cancers including sebaceous gland carcinoma. Hayashi et al. found HPV infection in 61.9 % of sebaceous carcinoma specimens [8].

(c) Immunosuppression: Like many other malignancies, immunosuppression is a risk factor for development of sebaceous gland carcinoma too. In patients infected with HIV, the tumor occurs at a younger age and is more aggressive. There is a report of sebaceous carcinoma occurring in two patients infected with HIV. Both the patients were in their 30s and developed aggressive tumor over 6–9 months of duration, requiring exenteration in one of them [9]. Autoimmune diseases also represent a suppressed immune system. There is a report of a case of multiple scalp sebaceous adenomas and solitary sebaceous carcinoma occurring in a patient of multiple sclerosis [10].

(d) Muir-Torre syndrome: There are occasional reports of patients with Muir-Torre syndrome developing periocular sebaceous carcinoma [11].

(e) Diuretics: A relationship between the use of thiazide diuretics and sebaceous carcinoma has been postulated in a report of 20 cases [12]. However, there is no firm evidence of relationship between the two.

## Clinical Features

Sebaceous gland carcinoma most commonly presents as a solitary painless nodule, arising from the meibomian glands of the upper eyelid followed by that of the lower eyelid [1, 13] (Fig. 45.1). Since the epidermis of the eyelid skin is not involved in the initial stages, there are chances of misdiagnosing as a chalazion. As the tumor starts invading the epidermis, it gives a yellow cast because of the lipid deposition. It also begins to disrupt the lid architecture and leads to loss of eyelashes which can be seen even in the earlier stages in a mass arising from the glands of Zeis [14]. Other suspicious signs include telangiectasia, ulceration, and bleeding (Fig. 45.2).

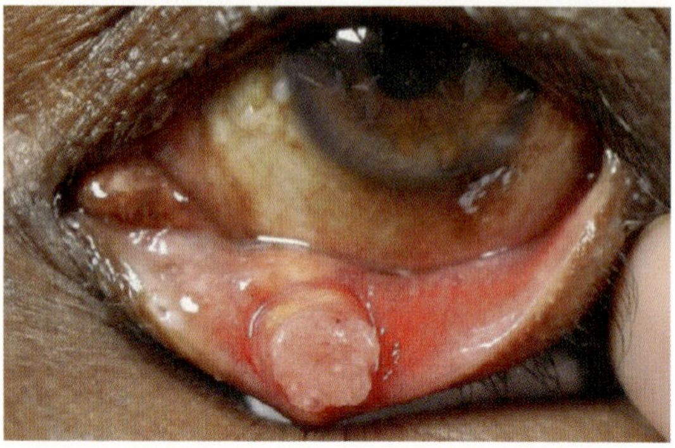

**Fig. 45.1** Sebaceous gland carcinoma (SGC) of the lower lid presenting as a lid nodule, which on eversion showed an irregular, elevated mass

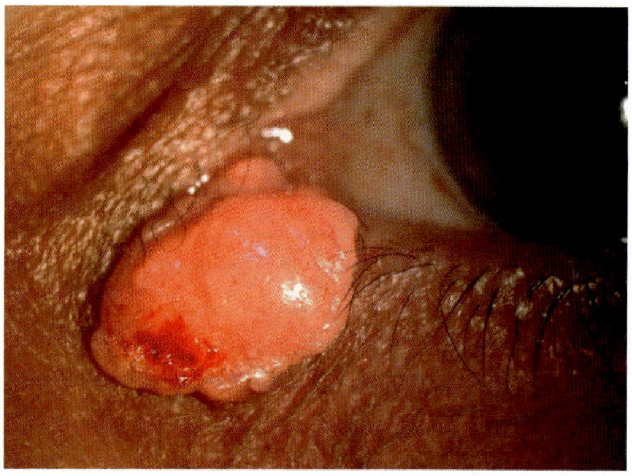

**Fig. 45.2** SGC presenting as a yellowish, nodular mass arising from the lower eyelid with surface ulceration

The second most frequent presentation is a diffuse unilateral thickening of the eyelid [1]. This variant can spread intraepithelially (pagetoid spread) into the fornices and the bulbar conjunctiva. It is often misdiagnosed as blepharitis or blepharoconjunctivitis. Any middle-aged or elderly patient presenting with long-standing unilateral blepharitis or blepharoconjunctivitis not responding to standard treatment is a candidate for lid biopsy. This intraepithelial (pagetoid) invasion of the overlying conjunctival epithelium has been reported in up to 40–80 % of cases of SGC [15] (Fig. 45.3).

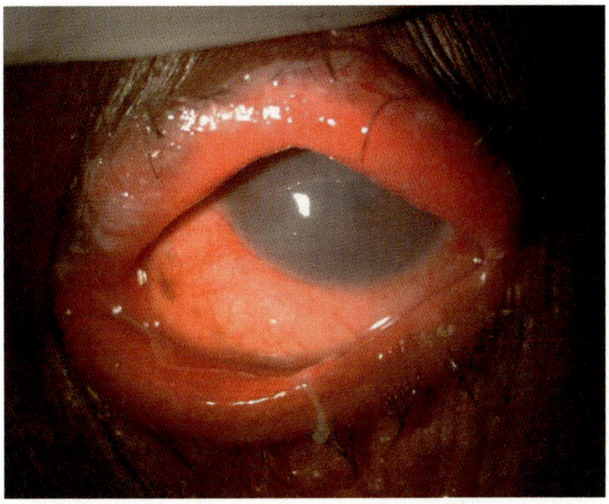

**Fig. 45.3** SGC with pagetoid spread: note the diffuse epithelial involvement over the ocular surface

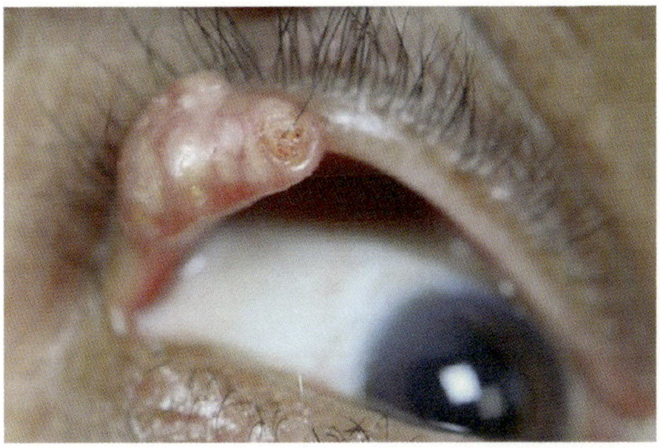

**Fig. 45.4** SGC of the upper lid presenting as a cutaneous horn with ulceration at the tip

Rarely, SGC can present as a pedunculated lesion, just like a cutaneous horn [16] (Fig. 45.4). In neglected cases, sebaceous gland carcinoma can involve the orbital structures, eyelids, and conjunctiva and rarely can also mimic a lacrimal gland mass (Fig. 45.5).

## Differential Diagnosis [1]

1. Basal cell carcinoma, squamous cell carcinoma, sweat gland tumors, and pilomatrixoma
2. Eyelid lymphomas
3. Chalazion
4. Blepharitis

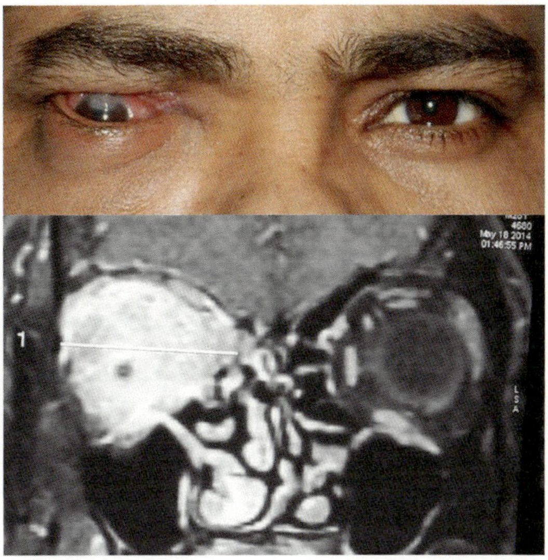

**Fig. 45.5** SGC of the right eyelid with orbital invasion presented with proptosis and restricted ocular motility. An MRI (*below*) shows the orbital component of the tumor as a hyperintense mass lesion

5. Keratoconjunctivitis
6. Inflammatory conditions like allergic conjunctivitis and cicatricial pemphigoid

## Diagnostic Modalities

The diagnosis of adnexal sebaceous gland carcinoma starts with a high degree of clinical suspicion. An incisional biopsy is then carried out which should be a full-thickness eyelid biopsy containing the skin, tarsus, and bulbar conjunctiva [1]. Orbital imaging is necessary in cases of diffuse eyelid and conjunctival involvement, to rule out orbital involvement. Map biopsy as described by Putterman is imperative in determining the extent of disease, in cases where pagetoid spread is suspected [17].

Fine-needle aspiration biopsy (FNAB) is not of much diagnostic importance as the amount of tissue aspirated is inadequate. However FNAB can be utilized in cases with established diagnosis and with lymph node involvement for the purpose of staging.

## Histopathological Features

Sebaceous gland carcinoma is a well-encapsulated infiltrating mass with cells showing mitotic activity and having vacuolated cytoplasm [13] (Fig. 45.6a, b). The lipid content of the tumor can be demonstrated with Oil Red O stain on frozen section. Histopathologically, SGC can be classified into four distinct variants: lobular, comedocarcinoma, papillary, and mixed [13, 18]. Immunohistochemical techniques should be utilized to differentiate sebaceous carcinoma from

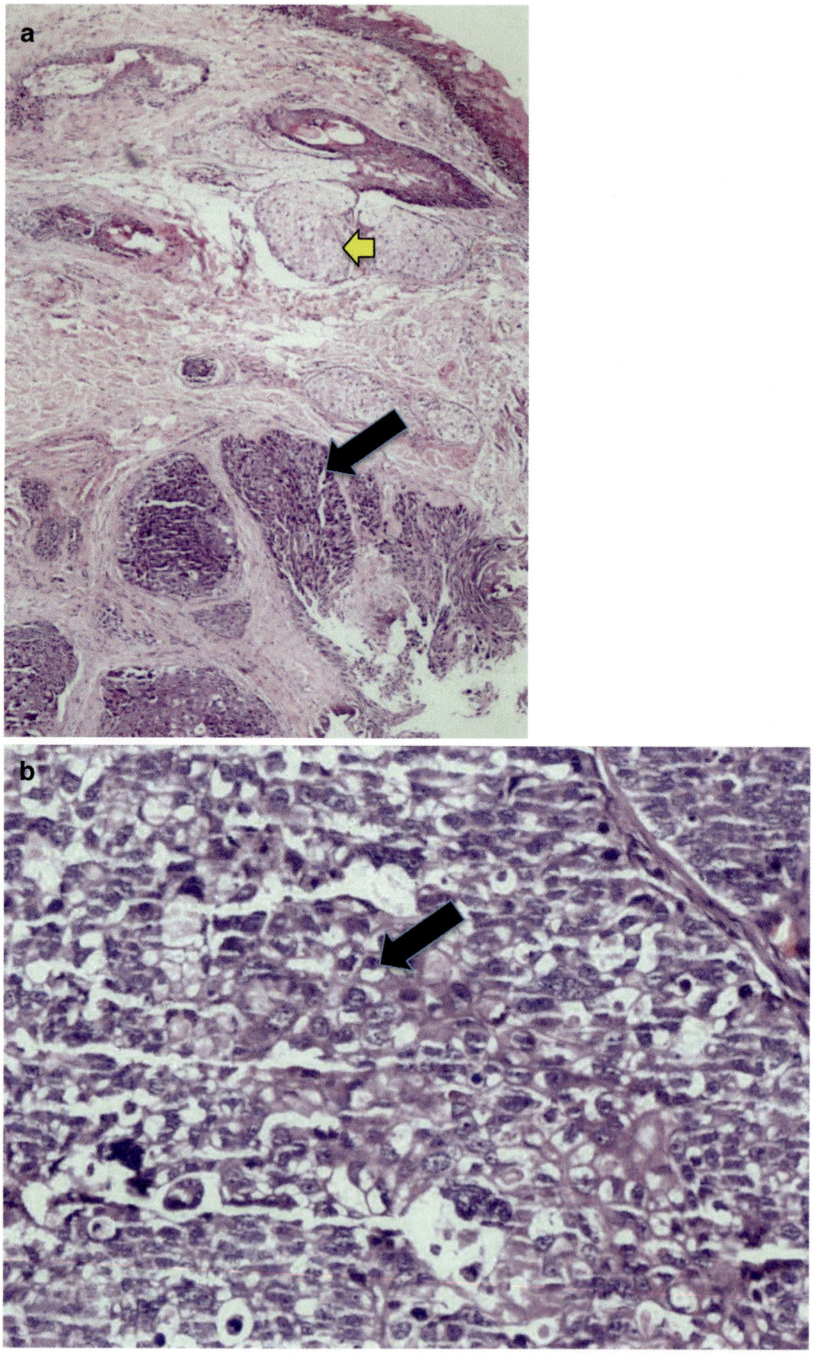


**Fig. 45.6** (**a**) This hematoxylin and eosin-stained section shows sebaceous cell carcinoma in the lower field of this photomicrograph with atypical, dark, pleomorphic sebaceous cells (*black arrows*). These are in contrast to the normal foamy sebaceous glands (*yellow arrowhead*) seen in the upper part of this photomicrograph (10×) (From Dr. Saurabh Kamal, MS, FAICO (New Delhi, India) and Dr. Indumati Gopinathan, MD (Mumbai, India)). (**b**) High-magnification view of the section shows irregularly arranged sebaceous and undifferentiated tumor cells. These cells show nuclear pleomorphism. The undifferentiated cells show eosinophilic cytoplasm with fine lipid globules. Lipid-laden foamy cells with vacuolated cytoplasm (*black arrow*) are characteristic of sebaceous gland carcinoma. (Hematoxylin and eosin, 40×) (From Dr. Saurabh Kamal, MS, FAICO (New Delhi, India) and Dr. Indumati Gopinathan, MD (Mumbai, India))

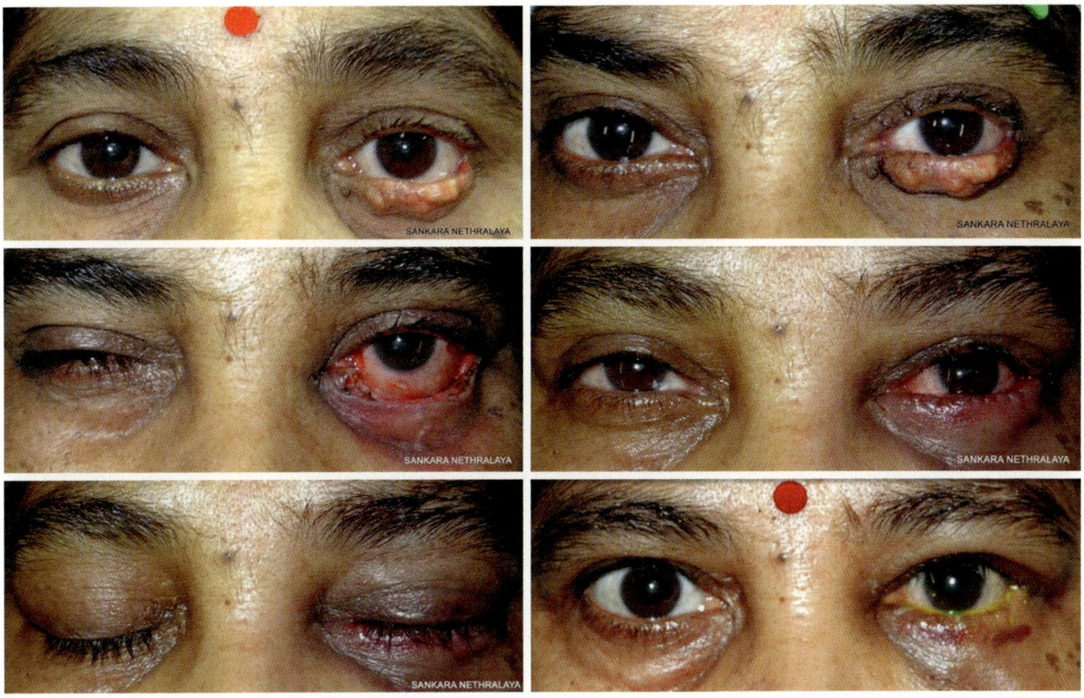


**Fig. 45.7** Left lowed lid, multifocal SGC occupying almost the entire lid (*left upper*). The tumor was resected with margin control (*right upper*), following which the patient underwent lid reconstruction by Hughes procedure (*left middle*). Subsequently, the flap was divided as a secondary procedure with good cosmetic outcome (*right* and *left lower* photos)

squamous cell carcinoma and basal cell carcinoma in cases where there is a resemblance in microscopic features. Epithelial membrane antigen (EMA), Cam 5.2, and BRST-1 are three such immunohistochemical markers [19]. In a cohort of patients reported by Shields et al., 50 % of the patients of SGC who were biopsied prior to referral were misdiagnosed [20]. This probably reflects the pressing need for ophthalmologists and pathologists to be more sensitive regarding the prevalence and diagnosis of SGC. This is of much more relevance in countries like India and China, where the incidence of SGC is much higher.

## Management

A thorough preoperative evaluation is essential before deciding the line of management. The preauricular, submandibular, and anterior cervical lymph nodes, in particular, should be clinically evaluated to rule out lymph node metastasis. If found suspicious, FNAB of the lymph node is performed under ultrasound guidance before primary tumor management. It has been reported that the size of the tumor may provide vital clues to the possibility of regional lymph node and systemic metastatic spread [21, 22].

1. Non-pagetoid local disease: Complete excision with margin clearance under frozen section is the management of choice for tumors localized to lids and presenting as solitary nodule (Fig. 45.7). In a group of 14 patients analyzed by Dogru, there were five recurrences in the group with surgical margins 1–3 mm, while no recurrence was seen in patients with 5 mm surgical margin [23]. There are reports of good results with low recurrence rates with Mohs micrographic surgery [24]. However, it has got its own limitations, keeping in view the pagetoid nature of spread.
2. Pagetoid local disease: Intraepithelial involvement of the conjunctiva poses a difficult

problem. Excision of tumor with application of cryotherapy to the conjunctiva was presented as a method to control conjunctival disease by Lisman and Jakobiec [25]. Shields presented a series of four patients treated successfully with Mitomycin-C (MMC). Patients in this series were treated with topical 0.4 % MMC four times daily for 1 week, followed by a 1 week drug-free period. The cycle was repeated until the resolution of the malignancy [26].

3. Extensive disease with orbital extension: extensive orbital spread often requires exenteration (total or lid sparing). Recently there are reports of cases where neoadjuvant chemotherapy in the form of systemic 5-fluorouracil and cisplatin has been tried to chemoreduce the tumor and later excising it or attempting a lid-sparing exenteration [27]. Sebaceous gland carcinoma is not radiosensitive, and radiotherapy is used either as a palliative measure or after orbital extension.

## Prognostic Factors

According to Rao et al., the following are the poor prognosis factors for sebaceous gland carcinoma [18]:

(a) Vascular invasion
(b) Lymphatic invasion
(c) Upper and lower lid involvement
(d) Orbital invasion
(e) Poor differentiation
(f) Pagetoid invasion
(g) Tumors larger than 10 mm
(h) Highly infiltrative pattern
(i) Multicentric origin

### Conclusion

Sebaceous carcinoma of the eyelids is a malignant neoplasm notorious for local extension and distant metastasis. The tumor can masquerade as benign conditions like chalazion and blepharoconjunctivitis. Greater awareness among clinicians in the recent years and resection of tumor with margin control, along with modalities like topical Mitomycin-C and neoadjuvant chemotherapy, have resulted in better treatment outcomes.

## References


1. Shields JA, Demirci H, Marr BP, Eagle RC, Shields CL. Sebaceous carcinoma of the ocular region: a review. Surv Ophthalmol. 2005;50:103–22.
2. Kass LG, Hornblass A. Sebaceous carcinoma of the ocular adnexa. Surv Ophthalmol. 1989;33:477–90.
3. Straatsma BR. Meibomian gland tumors. Arch Ophthalmol. 1956;56:71–93.
4. Chee SP, Goh SH. Sebaceous carcinoma of the eyelids: a review of six cases. Ann Acad Med Singapore. 1996;25:273–8.
5. Ni C, Searl SS, Kuo PK, et al. Sebaceous cell carcinoma of the ocular adnexa. Int Ophthalmol Clin. 1982;22:23–61.
6. Boniuk M, Zimmerman LE. Sebaceous carcinoma of the eyelid, eyebrow, caruncle, and orbit. Trans Am Acad Opthalmol Otolaryngol. 1968;72:619–41.
7. Kivela T, Asko-Seljavaara S, Pihkala U, et al. Sebaceous carcinoma of the eyelid associated with retinoblastoma. Ophthalmology. 2001;108:1124–8.
8. Hayashi N, Furihata M, Ohtsuki Y, Ueno H. Search for accumulation of p53 protein and detection of human papilloma virus genomes in sebaceous gland carcinoma of the eyelid. Virchows Arch. 1994;424:503–9.
9. Yen MT, Tse DT. Sebaceous cell carcinoma of the eyelid and the human immunodeficiency virus. Ophthal Plast Reconstr Surg. 2000;16:206–10.
10. Akhtar SS, Oza KK, Roulier RG. Multiple sebaceous adenomas and extraocular sebaceous carcinoma in a patient with multiple sclerosis: case report and review of literature. J Cutan Med Surg. 2001;5:490–6.
11. Stockl FA, Dolmetsch AM, Codere F, et al. Sebaceous carcinoma of the eyelid in an immunocompromised patient with Muir-Torre syndrome. Can J Ophthalmol. 1995;30:324–6.
12. Khan JA, Grove AS, Joseph MP, et al. Sebaceous carcinoma. Diuretic use, lacrimal system spread, and surgical margins. Ophthal Plast Reconstr Surg. 1989;5:227–34.
13. Bernardino CR, Bernardino VB. Sebaceous gland neoplasms. In: Albert DM, Jakobiec FA, editors. Principles and practice of ophthalmology, vol. 3. 3rd ed. Philadelphia: Saunders Elsevier; 2008. p. 3309–21.
14. Kato N, Sotodate A, Tomita Y. Zeis gland carcinoma. J Dermatol. 1997;24:595–600.
15. Margo CE, Lessner A, Stern GA. Intraepithelial sebaceous carcinoma of the conjunctiva and skin of the eyelid. Ophthalmology. 1992;99:227–31.
16. Baumuller S, Herwig MC, Mangold E, Holz FG, Loeffler KU. Sebaceous gland carcinoma of the eyelid masquerading as a cutaneous horn in Li-Fraumani syndrome. Br J Ophthalmol. 2011;95:1470–8.
17. Putterman AM. Conjunctival map biopsy to determine pagetoid spread. Am J Ophthalmol. 1986;102:87–90.
18. Rao NA, Hidayat AA, Mc Lean JW, et al. Sebaceous carcinoma of the ocular adnexa: a clinicopathologic study of 104 cases, with five- year follow-up data. Hum Pathol. 1982;13:113–22.

19. Sinard JH. Immunohistochemical distinction of ocular sebaceous carcinoma from basal cell and squamous cell carcinoma. Arch Ophthalmol. 1999;117:776–83.
20. Shields JA, Demirci H, Marr BP, et al. Sebaceous carcinoma of the eyelids: personal experience with 60 cases. Ophthalmology. 2004;111:2151–7.
21. Esmaeli B, Nasser QJ, Cruz H, Fellman M, Warneke CL, Ivan D. American joint committee on cancer T category for eyelid sebaceous carcinoma correlates with nodal metastasis and survival. Ophthalmology. 2012;119(5):1078–82.
22. Nair AG, Kaliki S, Ali MJ, Honavar SG, Naik MN. Sebaceous gland carcinoma: clinical profile, management, and outcomes in 147 patients. Paper presented at the American Society of Ophthalmic Plastic and Reconstructive surgery 44th annual fall scientific symposium, New Orleans. Nov 2013.
23. Dogru M, Matsui H, Inoue M, et al. Management of eyelid sebaceous carcinoma. Ophthalmologica. 1997;211:40–3.
24. Spencer JM, Nossa R, Tse DT, Sequeira M. Sebaceous carcinoma of the eyelid treated with Mohs micrographic surgery. J Am Acad Dermatol. 2001;44:1004–9.
25. Lisman RD, Jakobiec FA, Small P. Sebaceous carcinoma of the eyelids. The role of adjunctive cryotherapy in the management of conjunctival pagetoid spread. Ophthalmology. 1989;96:1021–6.
26. Shields CL, Naseripour M, Shields JA, Eagle Jr RC. Topical mitomycin-C for pagetoid invasion of the conjunctiva by eyelid sebaceous gland carcinoma. Ophthalmology. 2002;109:2129–33.
27. Murthy R, Honavar SG, Burman S, et al. Neoadjuvant chemotherapy in the management of sebaceous gland carcinoma of the eyelid with regional lymph node metastasis. Ophthal Plast Reconstr Surg. 2005;21:307–9.

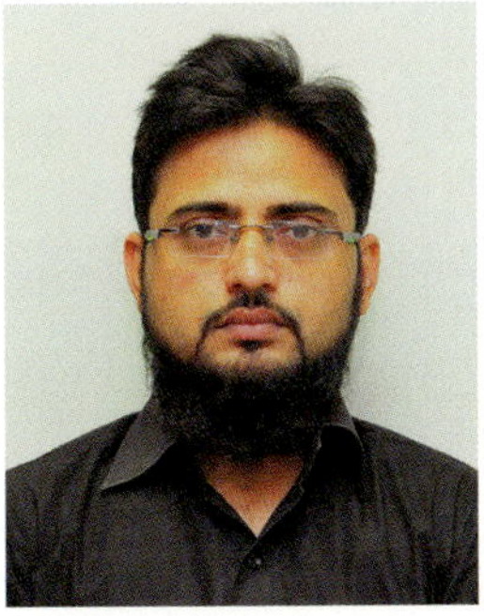

**Md. Shahid Alam** Dr. Md. Shahid Alam did his masters in Ophthalmology from the prestigious Aligarh Muslim University. He completed his long term fellowship training in Orbit and oculoplastics from Sankara Nethralaya. Presently he is working as an associate consultant in the department of orbit oculoplasty reconstructive and aesthetic services, Sankara Nethralaya, Chennai. His area of interest is orbital and adnexal oncology and ocular trauma.

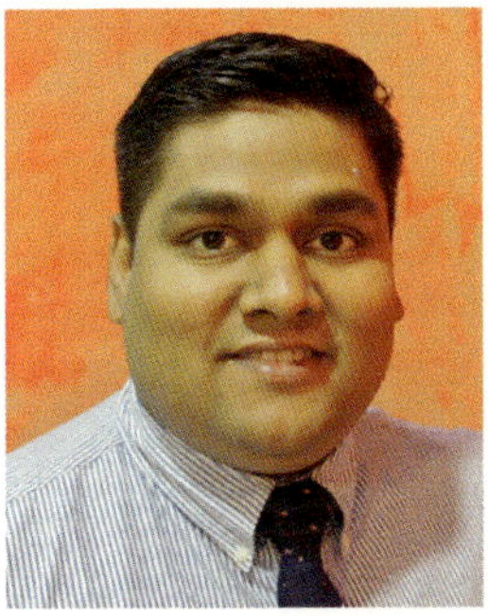

**Akshay Gopinathan Nair** Akshay Gopinathan Nair received his medical degree from Maharashtra University of Health Sciences, India and completed his residency training in ophthalmology from Sankara Nethralaya in Chennai, India. Following this, he underwent fellowship training in ophthalmic plastic surgery, ocular oncology and facial aesthetics at L V Prasad Eye Institute, Hyderabad, India and New York Eye & Ear Infirmary of Mount Sinai, USA. Dr. Nair has over 50 peer-reviewed publications, 8 book chapters in ophthalmology. His areas of special interest are ocular surface and eyelid tumours, ophthalmic imaging and neuroimaging. Dr. Nair is a faculty member at Lokmanya Tilak Municipal Medical College, Mumbai, India and is also affiliated with Advanced Eye Hospital & Institute and Aditya Jyot Eye Hospital in Mumbai.

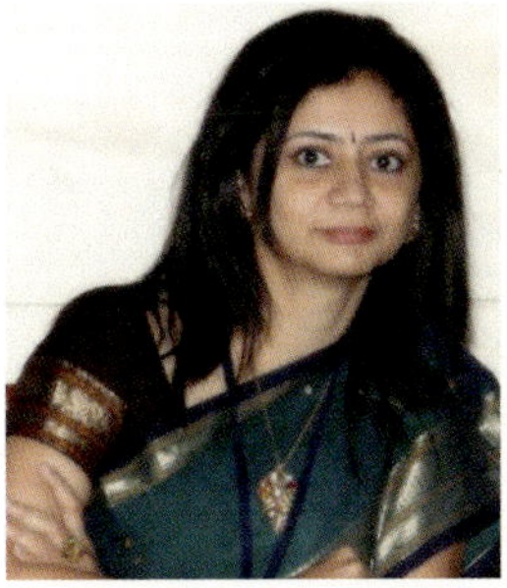

**Bipasha Mukherjee** Dr. Bipasha Mukherjee is a fellow in Orbit & Oculoplasty from Aravind Eye Hospitals, India, and ICO fellow from University Hospital of Limoges, France, under Prof. Jean-Paul Adenis. She has undergone clinical observerships with stalwarts like Jack Rootman, Richard Collins, Geoff Rose, Mark Duffy, and Robert Goldberg.

She currently heads the department of Orbit, Oculoplasty, Aesthetic & Reconstructive services in Medical Research Foundation, Chennai. She has numerous presentations in national and international conferences and publications in peer-reviewed journals and text books. Her areas of interest include diseases of the orbit and adnexa including tumors, lacrimal surgery, socket reconstruction, traumatic lid and adnexal injuries, training residents and fellows, and photography.

# 46 Squamous Cell Carcinoma

Md. Shahid Alam and Bipasha Mukherjee

## Introduction

Squamous cell carcinoma (SCC) is the second most common malignancy of the eyelid in Caucasians [1]. It is an invasive epithelial malignancy of keratinocytic differentiation and comprises 5–10 % of all eyelid malignancies [2]. Clinically it is liable to be misdiagnosed as basal cell carcinoma (BCC), owing to its relatively rare incidence as compared to BCC and diverse clinical presentations. Unlike BCC, it shows aggressive clinical behavior and is capable of metastasizing to lymph nodes and distant organs, causing significant morbidity and even mortality.

M.S. Alam, MS (✉)
Orbit Oculoplasty Reconstructive and Aesthetic Services, Sankara Nethralaya, 18 College Road, Chennai, Tamil Nadu, India
e-mail: mshahidalam@gmail.com

B. Mukherjee, MS, DNB (Ophthalmology), FICO
Orbit Oculoplasty Reconstructive and Aesthetic Services, Sankara Nethralaya, 18 College Road, Chennai, Tamil Nadu, India

Medical Research Foundation, 18 College Road, Chennai, Tamil Nadu, India
e-mail: drbpm@snmail.org

## Incidence and Demographics

The incidence of eyelid SCC is reported to be between 0.09 and 2.42 cases per 100,000 population [3]. The highest incidence in the world is found in areas of significant ultraviolet radiation exposure, with the incidence of SCC doubling with each 10° reduction in latitude [4]. Queensland has got the highest incidence of cutaneous SCC (2,400 per 100,000) [5]. It generally affects people over 60 years of age and there is slight male preponderance [2, 6].

## Precursors

SCC can arise de novo from an otherwise normal skin. It can also arise from one of the following preexisting skin lesions:

(a) Actinic keratosis: It is a partial-thickness infiltration of the epidermis by atypical keratinocytes without any violation of the basement membrane.
(b) Intraepidermal carcinoma or SCC in situ: Intraepidermal carcinoma (IEC) or SCC in situ is a full-thickness infiltration of the epidermis by atypical keratinocytes without any violation of the basement membrane.
(c) Bowen's disease: It is a variant of IEC with well-defined clinical margins.


B. Mukherjee, H. Yuen (eds.), *Emergencies of the Orbit and Adnexa*,
DOI 10.1007/978-81-322-1807-4_46

(d) Keratoacanthoma: A variant of pseudocarcinomatous hyperplasia characterized by a well-defined elevated lesion with central keratin-filled crater. It has been classified by some authors as low-grade SCC or a precursor of SCC [7].

## Risk Factors

1. Chronic sun exposure and acute sunburns: Chronic sun exposure is a known risk factor for the development of SCC. There is an increased incidence of SCC in the sun-exposed skin, and the incidence increases with the decrease in latitude [4]. UVB radiation (wavelength between 290 and 320 nm) induces reactive oxygen species formation and plays an important role in the formation of SCC [8].
2. Carcinogens: Exposure to various carcinogens like arsenic and coal tar and industrial chemicals like vinyl chloride and polycyclic aromatic hydrocarbons has been linked to the development of SCC [9–11].
3. Human papillomavirus infection [12]
4. Immunosuppression and organ transplant: Immunosuppression in any form is a risk factor for the development of SCC [13]. The risk of developing SCC in organ transplant recipients is 18 times higher when compared to the general population, and the tumor tends to be multiple and presents two decades earlier [14].
5. Intrinsic risk factors: Intrinsic risk factors for the development of SCC include albinism, preexisting chronic skin lesions, and genetic skin disorders such as xeroderma pigmentosum and epidermodysplasia verruciformis [2].

## Clinical Features

SCC most commonly involves the lower lid, followed by the medial canthus, upper lid, and lateral canthus in decreasing order of frequency [3]. Usually it presents as a sessile or pedunculated plaque with telangiectasia and ulceration (Fig. 46.1a). Patients generally have other signs of skin damage in the form of actinic keratosis and chronic dermatitis [1]. SCC has got variable presentation and can be confused with other lid tumors, most commonly basal cell carcinoma [2].

## Presenting as Emergency

Perineural spread is a characteristic feature of SCC. An orbital invasion of SCC can involve the orbital nerves and can present with ptosis and complete ophthalmoplegia, without proptosis [1]. It can give the impression of a cavernous sinus lesion. It can also present in emergency with bleeding, infection, or ocular and adnexal myiasis [15]. Ophthalmomyiasis can lead to destruction of globe and the surrounding structures.

## Tumor Spread

Locally the tumor can spread to the orbit if left neglected, making the prognosis even worse with high chances of mortality due to perineural spread into the brain.

Regional lymph nodes are the first site of metastasis, with parotid and preauricular nodes being the most commonly affected followed by submandibular, submental, and lower cervical nodes [16].

Reported rate of metastasis for SCC varies from 1 % to 21 % [17].

## Histopathological Features

Histopathologically, the tumor demonstrates nests, sheets, and strands of malignant epithelial cells, showing mitotic figures that arise from the keratinocytes of stratum spinosum [4]. Keratinization is evident from the formation of keratin cysts and keratin pearls (Fig. 46.1b). Depending upon differentiation, the tumor can be graded as "well," "moderately," and "poorly" differentiated.

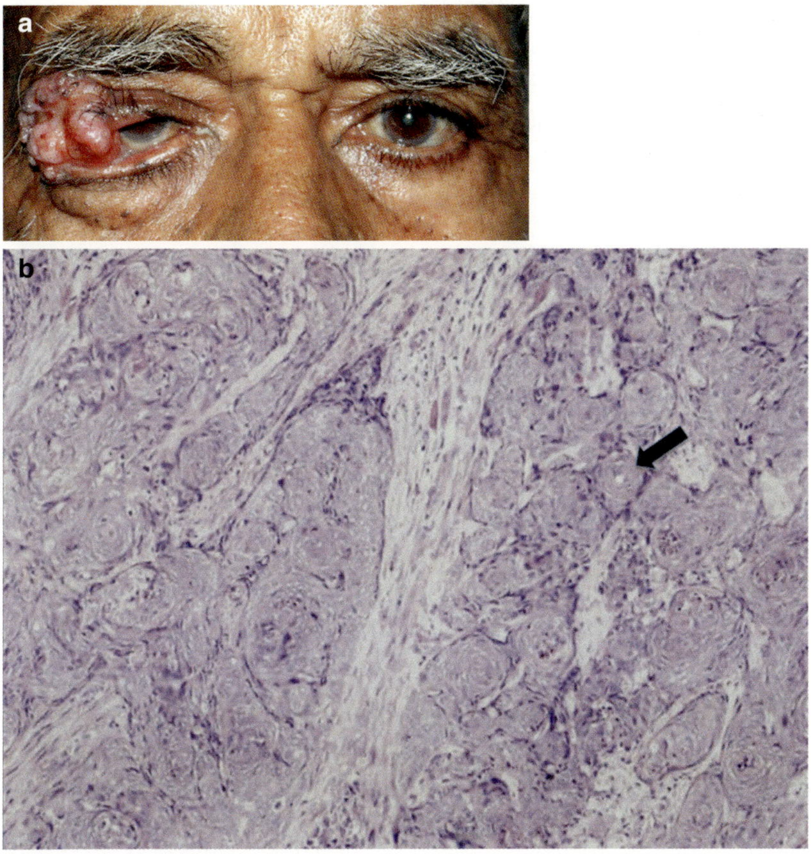


**Fig. 46.1** Cutaneous squamous cell carcinoma. (**a**) Colored photograph showing an ill-defined sessile ulcerated mass lesion involving the lateral half of the upper lid, lateral canthus, and lateral-most portion of the lower lid. Mass can be seen involving the bulbar and inferior palpebral conjunctiva (acknowledgement: Dr Saurabh Kamal, MS, FAICO and Dr Indumati Gopinathan, MD). (**b**) The section shows irregular tumor cells with keratin differentiation and formation of keratin pearls. Proliferation of anastomosing nests, sheets, and strands of atypical keratinocytes is also seen. They are originating in the epidermis and infiltrating into the dermis to form "eddy" or keratin pearls (*black arrow*) (hematoxylin and eosin stain, 20×) (Acknowledgement: Dr Saurabh Kamal, MS, FAICO and Dr Indumati Gopinathan, MD)

## Management

Incisional biopsy is usually done to confirm the diagnosis before planning any definite management. Taking a punch biopsy is an outpatient procedure, and the patient can then be sent home with a small dressing. It is always good to include a margin of healthy tissue for comparison. Another option is to do the biopsy under frozen section and plan for complete excision and reconstruction in the same setting. However, squamous cell carcinomas are liable to be misdiagnosed on frozen section, and it is always better to rely upon the permanent section diagnosis [18].

Magnetic resonance imaging (MRI) is frequently required in cases with suspected orbital extension. SCC has got the potential to metastasize, and occult lymph node involvement cannot be ruled out clinically. To assess lymph node involvement, lymphatic mapping with sentinel lymph node biopsy (SLNB) is being investigated [19]. At the same time, the use of SLNB for cutaneous SCC may be limited due to less metastatic spread as compared to melanoma [20]. Further study of

SLNB is necessary before its implementation in the management of high-risk cutaneous SCC [21].

Positron emission tomography (PET) scan is required in cases where distant metastasis is suspected.

## The American Joint Committee on Cancer (AJCC) Staging System for Eyelid Carcinoma: Seventh Edition [22]

All eyelid malignancies should be staged according to the revised AJCC staging system for eyelid carcinoma (Tables 46.1 and 46.2). It not only aids in the management but also helps in predicting the prognosis.

For a better understanding, the management can be divided as follows depending upon its extent and involvement:

(a) Tumors localized to the lid: Complete surgical excision with margin controls under frozen section is the treatment of choice for SCC primarily localized to the lids. Mohs reported a recurrence rate of 1.9% in 161 cases of periocular SCC who underwent Mohs' micrographic surgery [23].

The National Comprehensive Cancer Network (NCCN) guidelines classify eyelid squamous cell carcinoma as high-risk tumor [24]. The NCCN guidelines recommend a surgical margin of 4–6 mm for low-risk cutaneous SCC [24]. Larger margins (up to 6 mm) or complete circumferential peripheral and deep margin assessment with frozen section analysis is needed for high-risk tumors, like eyelid SCC [24].

(b) Perineural spread: Postoperative radiotherapy is indicated for all cases having clinical or pathological perineural invasion [2].

(c) Infiltrative and metastatic tumors: Tumors infiltrating the orbit require extended enucleation or exenteration depending upon the extent of involvement. Adjuvant radiotherapy should be considered in patients with positive surgical margins or aggressive histology. Chemotherapy is reserved for patients having extensive and infiltrative disease with local or distant metastasis. Cisplatin alone or in combination with doxorubicin is the chemotherapeutic agent of choice [25].

(d) Chemoimmune therapy and targeted therapy:

Fluoropyrimidines such as 5-fluorouracil (5-FU) have been used successfully in the treatment of cutaneous SCC [26]. A combination of capecitabine, an oral fluoropyrimidine

**Table 46.1** Primary tumor definition for carcinoma of the eyelid

| | |
|---|---|
| TX | Primary tumor cannot be assessed |
| T0 | No evidence of primary tumor |
| Tis | Carcinoma in situ |
| T1 | Tumor ≤5 mm in greatest dimension; no invasion of the tarsal plate or eyelid margin |
| T2a | Any tumor >5 mm but <10 mm in greatest dimension; any tumor that invades the tarsal plate or eyelid margin |
| T2b | Any tumor >10 mm but <20 mm in greatest dimension; any tumor that invades the full thickness of the eyelid |
| T3a | Any tumor >20 mm in greatest dimension, any tumor that invades adjacent ocular or orbital structures, any tumor with perineural tumor invasion |
| T3b | Complete resection of tumor requires enucleation, exenteration, or bone resection |
| T4 | Tumor is not resectable because of extensive invasion of ocular, orbital, or craniofacial structures or of the brain |

**Table 46.2** Stage grouping for carcinoma of the eyelid

| Stage | T | N | M |
|---|---|---|---|
| 0 | Tis | N0 | M0 |
| 1A | T1 | N0 | M0 |
| 1B | T2a | N0 | M0 |
| 1C | T2b | N0 | M0 |
| 2 | T3a | N0 | M0 |
| 3A | T3b | N0 | M0 |
| 3B | Any T | N1 | M0 |
| 3C | T4 | Any N | M0 |
| 4 | Any T | Any N | M1 |

which gets converted into 5-FU into tumor cells, and interferon alpha subcutaneously has shown promising results in a small series [27].

Cetuximab is a mouse-human chimeric monoclonal antibody which prevents the binding of epithelial growth factor (EGF) to epithelial growth factor receptors (EGFR). A phase 2 clinical trial of cetuximab for metastatic or unresectable cutaneous SCC, used as a single agent, showed a disease control of 69 % on the basis of intention-to-treat analysis and 81 % based on the actual treatment received [28].

Gefitinib is a tyrosine kinase inhibitor. In a study of 22 patients with recurrent aggressive disease, defined as lesions that were 2 cm or larger in greatest diameter, invaded deep tissues, or were associated with perineural invasion and/or metastasis to the lymph nodes, neoadjuvant therapy with gefitinib 250 mg daily produced an overall response rate of 46.5 % [29].

Erlotinib is a tyrosine kinase inhibitor through competitive inhibition of ATP. Clinical trials of erlotinib for cutaneous SCC have not yet been completed; however, case reports have indicated favorable results in locally advanced adnexal [30] and metastatic cutaneous SCC [31].

## Ocular Surface Squamous Neoplasia (OSSN)

The term "ocular surface squamous neoplasia" (OSSN) was coined by Lee and Hirst to incorporate three broad categories of lesions including benign dysplasia, conjunctival and corneal carcinoma in situ, and invasive squamous cell carcinoma [32]. OSSN primarily occurs in elderly males. The age of presentation is earlier in cases of xeroderma pigmentosum and HIV. A number of risk factors such as genetic predisposition, ultraviolet light exposure, immunosuppression, and HPV infection have been implicated in the development of OSSN [33].

OSSN typically occurs in the interpalpebral region arising from the limbal stem cells and involving the bulbar conjunctiva, cornea, or both [34]. Clinically OSSN can either present as a well-circumscribed gelatinous lesion or leukoplakic, papillary growth. Circumscribed gelatinous lesion is the most common variant. Feeder vessels can be seen in many cases (Fig. 46.2a).

The typical appearance of the lesion is enough to make a clinical diagnosis. Definitive diagnosis is made by incisional or excisional biopsy. Impression cytology, exfoliative cytology, and fine-needle aspiration biopsy are other less-invasive methods to make a definitive diagnosis.

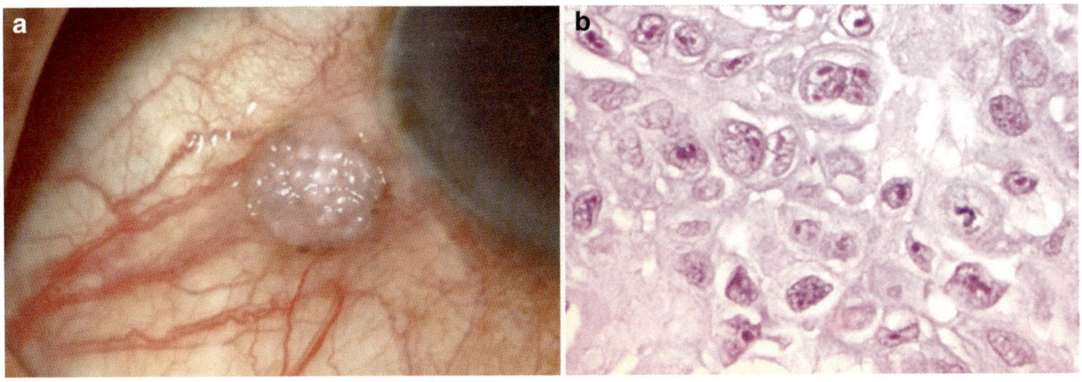


**Fig. 46.2** OSSN. (**a**) Slit lamp photograph demonstrating a typical ocular surface neoplasm with an elevated nodular limbal mass showing feeder vessels, intrinsic vascularity, and keratin debris over it. (**b**) High-magnification photomicrograph showing cells with abundant cytoplasm, large nuclei with prominent nucleoli and bizarre giant tumor cells (hematoxylin and eosin stain, 40×) (Acknowledgement: Dr. Saurabh Kamal, MS, FAICO and Dr Indumati Gopinathan, MD)

Confocal microscopy has shown good results in the evaluation of OSSN [35]. Ultrahigh-resolution optical coherence tomography is a newer modality which provides a cross-sectional evaluation of the mass and is quite useful in equivocal cases and treatment monitoring [36].

Histopathologically, carcinoma in situ shows partial- or full-thickness epithelial dysplasia. Invasive OSSN shows nests of infiltrating tumor cells that have breached the epithelial basement membrane and reached the conjunctival or corneal stroma (Fig. 46.2b).

Complete surgical excision with margin control under frozen section is the treatment of choice for OSSN. In an attempt to prevent recurrence, it is recommended to excise the tumor tissue with wide surgical margin of 2–3 mm [37]. Cryotherapy can be applied to the tumor bed. When the deep cornea or sclera is involved, deep lamellar keratectomy or sclerectomy is applied [38].

Postoperative chemotherapy in the form of topical Mitomycin C (0.02–0.04 %) has shown reduced recurrence rates in both positive and negative surgical margins [39, 40]. A 1-week-on and 1-week-off regime is followed. The chemotherapy-free period allows the slow-growing normal epithelial and limbal cells to regenerate.

Most eyes with intraocular invasion of OSSN require enucleation [41]; in cases of orbital extension, exenteration is needed [42].

Topical 1 % 5-fluorouracil applied four times daily for a 14–21-day cycle has shown promising results in preinvasive lesions [43, 44]. Interferon alpha-2b has shown promising results in primary and recurrent cases. However it takes longer duration for complete resolution and is more toxic than Mitomycin C. It is used either as drops (1 million IU/ml) or as subconjunctival injection [45].

**Conclusion**

SCC is the most frequent cause of death from an eyelid cancer, with mortality rate being as high as 15 % in some series [1]. Complete surgical excision with margin control offers high cure rate for the patients. Topical chemotherapeutic agents like Mitomycin C, 5-fluorouracil, and interferon alpha-2b have opened new options in the nonsurgical management of OSSN.

Since sun exposure is an important proven risk factor, protection in the form of sunglasses, sunscreens and protective clothing should be emphasized upon patients with outdoor activities.

## References

1. Reifler DM, Hornblass A. Squamous cell carcinoma of the eyelid. Surv Ophthalmol. 1986;30:349–65.
2. Donaldson MJ, Sullivan TJ, Whitehead KJ, Williamson RM. Squamous cell carcinoma of the eye lids. Br J Ophthalmol. 2002;86:1161–5.
3. Cook BE, Bartley GB. Epidemiologic characteristics and clinical course of patients with malignant eye lid tumors in an incidence cohort in Olmsted County, Minnesota. Ophthalmology. 1999;106:746–50.
4. Valenzuela AA, Sullivan TJ. Squamous cell carcinoma in the eyelids. In: Albert DM, Jakobiec FA, editors. Principles and practice of ophthalmology, vol. 3. 3rd ed. Philadelphia: Saunders Elsevier; 2008. p. 3293–307.
5. Green A. Changing patterns in incidence of non-melanoma skin cancer. Epithelial Cell Biol. 1992;1:47–51.
6. Vitaliano PP, Urbach F. The relative importance of risk factors in nonmelanoma carcinoma. Arch Dermatol. 1980;116:454–6.
7. Requena L, Romero E, Sanchez M, et al. Aggressive keratoacanthoma of the eyelid: malignant keratoacanthoma or squamous cell carcinoma? J Dermatol Surg Oncol. 1990;16:564–8.
8. Kubo Y, Murao K, Matsumoto K, Arase S. Molecular carcinogenesis of squamous cell carcinomas of the skin. J Med Invest. 2002;49:111–7.
9. Simeonova PP, Luster MI. Mechanisms of arsenic carcinogenicity: genetic or epigenetic mechanisms? J Environ Pathol Toxicol Oncol. 2000;19:281–6.
10. Langard S, Rosenberg J, Anderson A, Heldaas SS. Incidence of cancer among workers exposed to vinyl chloride in polyvinyl chloride manufacture. Occup Environ Med. 2000;57:65–8.
11. Hussain M, Rae J, Gilman A, Kauss P. Lifetime health risk assessment from exposure of recreational users to polycyclic aromatic hydrocarbons. Arch Environ Contam Toxicol. 1998;35:527–31.
12. Nguyen M, Song S, Liem A, et al. A mutant of human papillomavirus type 16 E6 deficient in binding alpha-helix partners displays reduced oncogenic potential in vivo. J Virol. 2002;76:13039–48.
13. Maclean H, Dhilon B, Ironside J. Squamous cell carcinoma of the eyelid and the acquired immunodeficiency syndrome. Am J Ophthalmol. 1996;121:219–21.
14. Lindelof B, Sigurgeirsson B, Gabel H, Stern RS. Incidence of skin cancer in 5356 patients following organ transplantation. Br J Dermatol. 2000;143:513–9.

15. Khurana S, Biswal M, Bhatti HS, Pandav SS, Gupta A, Chatterjee SS, et al. Ophthalmomyiasis: three cases from North India. Indian J Med Microbiol. 2010;28:257–61.
16. Faustina M, Diba R, Ahmadi MA, Esmaeli B. Patterns of regional and distant metastasis in patients with eye lid and periocular squamous cell carcinoma. Ophthalmology. 2004;111:1930–2.
17. Loeffler M, Hornblass A. Characteristics and behavior of eye lid carcinoma. Ophthalmic Surg. 1990;21:513–8.
18. Turner RJ, Leonard N, Malcolm AJ, Lawrence CM, Dahl MGC. A retrospective study of outcome of Mohs' micrographic surgery for cutaneous squamous cell carcinoma using formalin fixed sections. Br J Dermatol. 2000;142:752–7.
19. Mich C, Starz H, Bachter D, Balda BR. Sentinel lymphonodectomy in nonmelanoma skin malignancies. Br J Dermatol. 2003;149:763–9.
20. Vauterin TJ, Veness MJ, Morgan GJ, Poulsen MG, O'Brien CJ. Patterns of lymph node spread of cutaneous squamous cell carcinoma of the head and neck. Head Neck. 2006;28:785–91.
21. Weisberg NK, Bertagnolli MM, Becker DS. Combined sentinel lymphadenectomy and Mohs' micrographic surgery for high risk cutaneous squamous cell carcinoma. J Am Acad Dermatol. 2000;43:483–8.
22. Ainbinder DJ, Esmaeli B, Groo SC, Finger PT, Brooks JP. Introduction of the 7th edition eye lid carcinoma classification system from the American joint committee on cancer- international union against cancer staging manual. Arch Pathol Lab Med. 2009;133:1256–61.
23. Mohs FE. Micrographic surgery for the microscopically controlled excision of eye lid cancers. Arch Ophthalmol. 1986;104:901–9.
24. National Comprehensive Cancer Network. Practice guidelines in oncology: basal and squamous cell skin cancer. http://www.nccn.org/. 2010.
25. Motley R, Kersey P, Lawrence C. Multiprofessional guidelines for the management of the patient with primary cutaneous squamous cell carcinoma. Br J Dermatol. 2002;146:18–25.
26. Czarnecki D, Meehan CJ, Bruce F, Culjak G. The majority of cutaneous squamous cell carcinomas arise in actinic keratoses. J Cutan Med Surg. 2002;6:207–9.
27. Wollina U, Hansel G, Koch A, Kostler E. Oral capecitabine plus subcutaneous interferon alpha in advanced squamous cell carcinoma of the skin. J Cancer Res Clin Oncol. 2005;131:300–4.
28. Maubec E, Petrow P, Scheer-Senyarich I, et al. Phase II study of cetuximab as first-line single-drug therapy in patients with unresectable squamous cell carcinoma of the skin. J Clin Oncol. 2011;29:3419–26.
29. Lewis CM, Glisson BS, Feng L, et al. A phase II study of gefitinib for aggressive cutaneous squamous cell carcinoma of the head and neck. Clin Cancer Res. 2012;18:1435–46.
30. Yin VT, Pfeiffer ML, Esmaeli B. Targeted therapy for orbital and periocular basal cell carcinoma and squamous cell carcinoma. Ophthalmol Plast Reconstr Surg. 2013;29:87–92.
31. Engelhardt C, Curiel-Lewandrowski C, Warneke J, Cranmer L. Metastatic cutaneous squamous cell carcinoma responding to erlotinib therapy. J Am Acad Dermatol. 2011;65:237–8.
32. Lee GA, Hirst LW. Ocular surface squamous neoplasia. Surv Ophthalmol. 1995;39:429–50.
33. Pe'er J, Frucht-Pery J. Ocular surface squamous neoplasia. In: Singh AD, Pe'er J, Murphree AL, editors. Clinical ophthalmic oncology. Philadelphia: Elsevier; 2007. p. 136.
34. Kiire CA, Srinivasan S, Karp CL. Ocular surface squamous neoplasia. Int Ophthalmol Clin. 2010;50: 35–46.
35. Xu Y, Zhou Z, Xu Y, et al. The clinical value of in vivo confocal microscopy for diagnosis of ocular surface squamous neoplasia. Eye. 2012;26:781–7.
36. Kieval JZ, Karp CL, AbouShousha M, et al. Ultrahigh resolution optical coherence tomography for differentiation of ocular surface squamous neoplasia and pterygia. Ophthalmology. 2012;119:481–6.
37. Iliff WJ, Marback R, Green WR. Invasive squamous cell carcinoma of the conjunctiva. Arch Ophthalmol. 1975;93:119–22.
38. Freedman J, Rohm G. Surgical management and histopathology of invasive tumors of the cornea. Br J Ophthalmol. 1979;63:632–5.
39. Ballalai PL, Erwenne CM, Martins MC, et al. Long-term results of topical mitomycin C 0.02% for primary and recurrent conjunctival corneal intraepithelial neoplasia. Ophthalmol Plast Reconstr Surg. 2009;25: 296–9.
40. Chen C, Louis D, Dodd T, Muecke J. Mitomycin C as an adjunct in the treatment of localized ocular surface squamous neoplasia. Br J Ophthalmol. 2004;88: 17–8.
41. Schlote T, Mielke J, Rohrback JM. Massive intraocular invasion of conjunctiva by squamous cell carcinoma: a case report. Klin Monatsbl Augenheilkd. 2001;218:518–21.
42. Shields JA, Shields CL, Suvaramani C, Tantisina M, Shah P. Orbital exenteration with eyelid sparing: indications, technique, and results. Ophthalmic Surg. 1991;22:292–7.
43. Kim JW, Abramson DH. Topical treatment options for conjunctival neoplasms. Clin Ophthalmol. 2008;2: 503–15.
44. Midena E, Angeli CD, Valenti M, et al. Treatment of conjunctival squamous cell carcinoma with topical 5-fluorouracil. Br J Ophthalmol. 2000;84:268–72.
45. Holocombe DJ, Lee GA. Topical interferon alfa-2b for the treatment of recalcitrant ocular surface squamous neoplasia. Am J Ophthalmol. 2006;142:568–71.

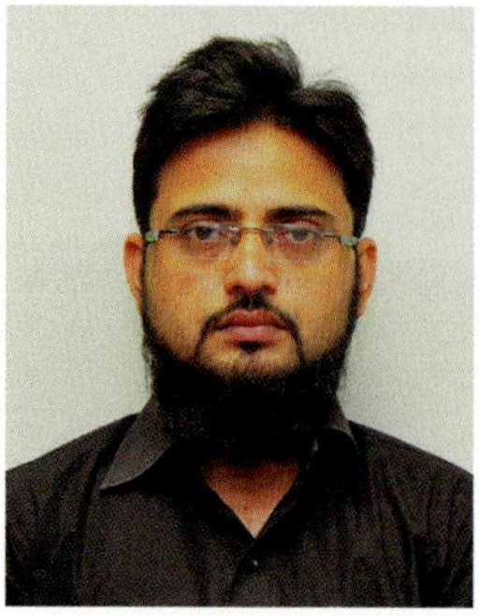

**Md. Shahid Alam** Dr. Md. Shahid Alam did his masters in Ophthalmology from the prestigious Aligarh Muslim University. He completed his long term fellowship training in Orbit and oculoplastics from Sankara Nethralaya. Presently he is working as an associate consultant in the department of orbit oculoplasty reconstructive and aesthetic services, Sankara Nethralaya, Chennai. His area of interest is orbital and adnexal oncology and ocular trauma.

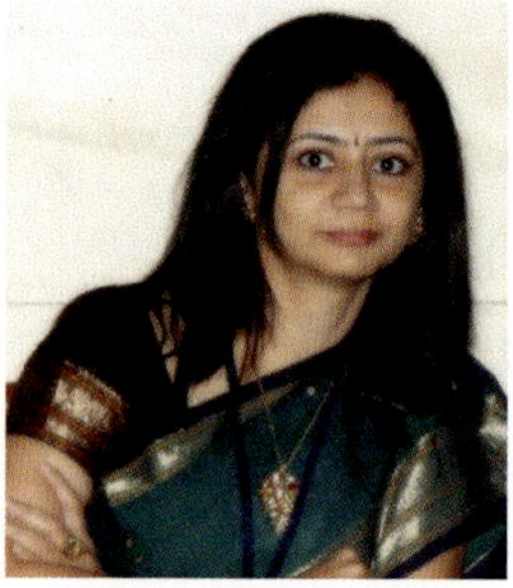

**Bipasha Mukherjee** Dr. Bipasha Mukherjee is a fellow in Orbit & Oculoplasty from Aravind Eye Hospitals, India, and ICO fellow from University Hospital of Limoges, France, under Prof. Jean-Paul Adenis. She has undergone clinical observerships with stalwarts like Jack Rootman, Richard Collins, Geoff Rose, Mark Duffy, and Robert Goldberg.

She currently heads the department of Orbit, Oculoplasty, Aesthetic & Reconstructive services in Medical Research Foundation, Chennai. She has numerous presentations in national and international conferences and publications in peer-reviewed journals and text books. Her areas of interest include diseases of the orbit and adnexa including tumors, lacrimal surgery, socket reconstruction, traumatic lid and adnexal injuries, training residents and fellows, and photography.

# 47 Melanoma

Meghana Anika Varde

## Melanoma

Malignant melanoma (MM) is a potentially life-threatening tumour. Cutaneous melanomas account for about 7 % of skin malignancies but are responsible for 90 % of skin cancer-related deaths according to the National Cancer Institute in the USA [1]. The prognosis is mainly dependent on the size of the tumour at presentation, so that timely diagnosis is of utmost importance. The growth rate of melanomas is variable, but about a third of cutaneous melanomas can exhibit a fairly fast growth of 0.5 mm per month or more [2]. These tumours have to be treated on an emergent basis (Fig. 47.1).

Malignant melanomas of the eyelid may involve the skin as well as the conjunctiva and in many cases a combination of the two. When examining a case of eyelid melanoma, it is essential to evert the lids and rule out any involvement of the palpebral or bulbar conjunctiva.

M.A. Varde, MS, FEBO, FMRF (Oculoplasty)
Department of Ophthalmology,
Klinikum Region Hannover, Haltenhoffstr. 41,
Hannover 30167, Germany
e-mail: thelivingcompass@gmail.com

## Cutaneous Eyelid Melanoma

### Introduction and Epidemiology

Cutaneous melanoma of the eyelid is a rare tumour representing less than 1 % of all eyelid malignancies [3, 4]. The incidence is significantly lower in darker-skinned individuals with persons of African origin rarely affected. Eyelid melanoma is a disease of the older population and shows a peak incidence in the sixth and seventh decades of life.

Eyelid skin melanoma can occur as primary lesion, as metastasis from cutaneous melanoma at another site or by extension of a conjunctival melanoma. The clinical features, histopathology, treatment and prognosis are comparable to that of cutaneous malignant melanoma elsewhere [5].

### Aetiology and Pathogenesis

Cutaneous melanoma may arise de novo most likely to ultraviolet (UV) radiation-induced skin damage or appear as malignant transformation of a precursor lesion.

There are four major types of cutaneous melanomas in the periocular region:

- *Lentigo maligna melanoma* (LMM)
- *Nodular melanoma* (NM)
- *Superficial spreading melanoma* (SSM)
- *Desmoplastic melanoma* (DM)

*Lentigo maligna* (LM, Hutchinson's freckle) represents a *melanoma in situ*. It presents as a flat,


B. Mukherjee, H. Yuen (eds.), *Emergencies of the Orbit and Adnexa*,
DOI 10.1007/978-81-322-1807-4_47

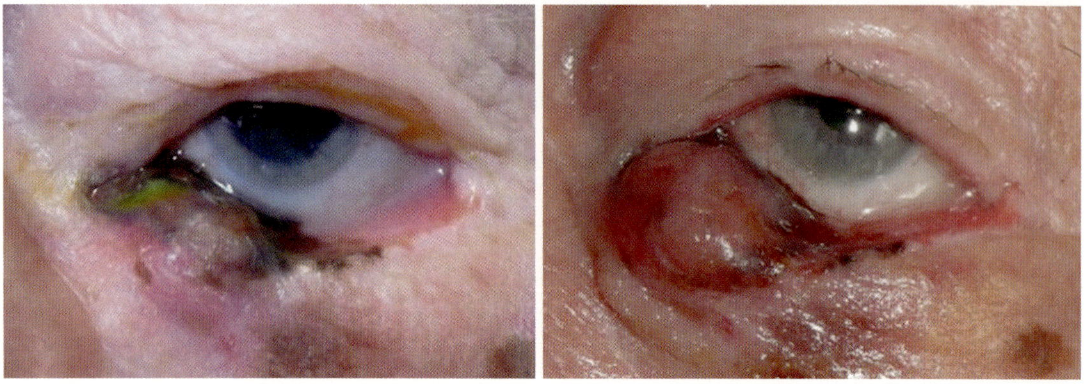

**Fig. 47.1** Growth of a lid melanoma in 6 weeks

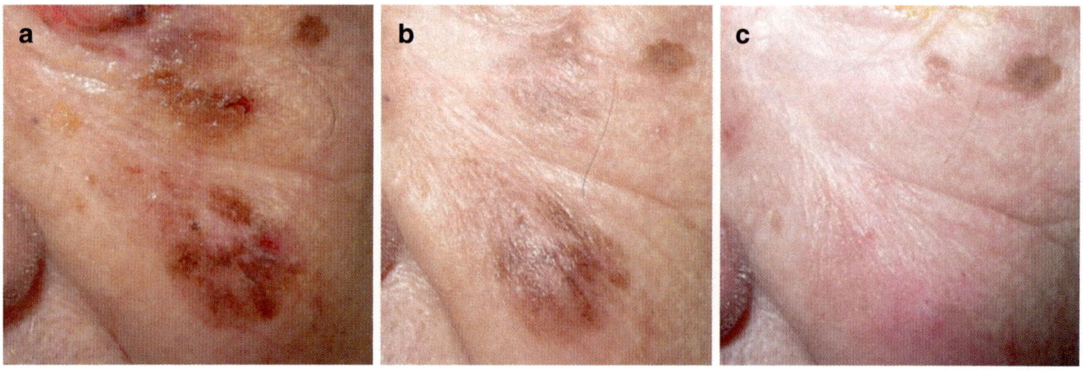


**Fig. 47.2** Spontaneous regression of lentigo maligna over the course of 2.5 years. (**a**) 09/2011, (**b**) 03/2012, (**c**) 03/2014

non-palpable pigmented macule, which is found mostly in elderly white-skinned individuals on sun-exposed skin. The lesions exhibit irregular pigmentation and margins. Some areas may show spontaneous involution (Fig. 47.2). An invasive melanoma commonly presents as a firm nodule of variable pigmentation within the lesion (Fig. 47.3).

About 61 % of eyelid cutaneous melanomas arise from LM [3].

*Nodular melanomas* represent about 15–30 % of eyelid melanomas. They tend to show early vertical growth with little horizontal spread and arise de novo without a precursor lesion.

*Superficial spreading melanomas* often arise from pre-existing *dysplastic naevi*. In the eyelid, this type of melanoma is the least common [3].

*Desmoplastic melanomas* are rare. They present as firm, indurated, nonpigmented mass with ill-defined borders, can resemble a scar and any benign or malignant lesion [6] and are associated with perineural invasion.

## Clinical Presentation

Eyelid melanomas occur most frequently in the lower lid [7]. The pigmentation can vary from dark black to amelanotic. Melanomas of the lid often involve the lid margin. If associated with a conjunctival component, it may be difficult to distinguish the origin of the melanoma. These tumours seem to have a worse prognosis because of possible late detection of the conjunctival growth [8].

The rare desmoplastic variant of melanoma is often a tumour of the deeper structures and can thus appear as subcutaneous nodule or even as a chalazion.

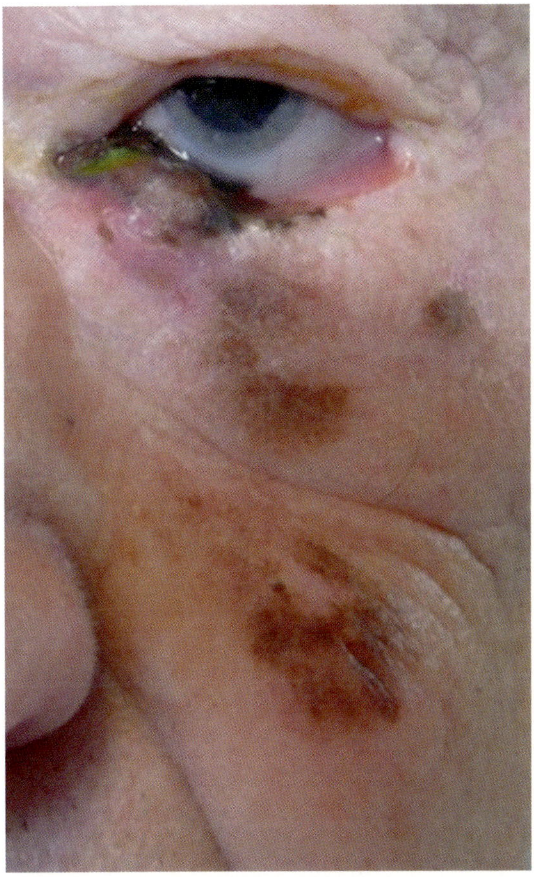

**Fig. 47.3** Lentigo maligna melanoma with conjunctival involvement in a 98-year-old patient

## Differential Diagnosis

*Naevocellular naevi* can involve the skin as well as the lid margin. Another entity found in the eyelid is the *Spitz naevus*. It arises before the fourth decade of life and can exhibit morphological features similar to melanoma although it is commonly perceived as a benign lesion. It might be considered as potential precursor for a melanoma, similar to dysplastic naevi [9].

Another important differential diagnosis is *seborrhoeic keratosis* (SK). *Basal cell carcinoma* (BCC) may be pigmented, especially in individuals with increased skin pigmentation (Fig. 47.4) and can be mistaken for nodular melanoma.

## Histopathology

Cutaneous melanomas normally arise from the junctional area between the dermis and epidermis.

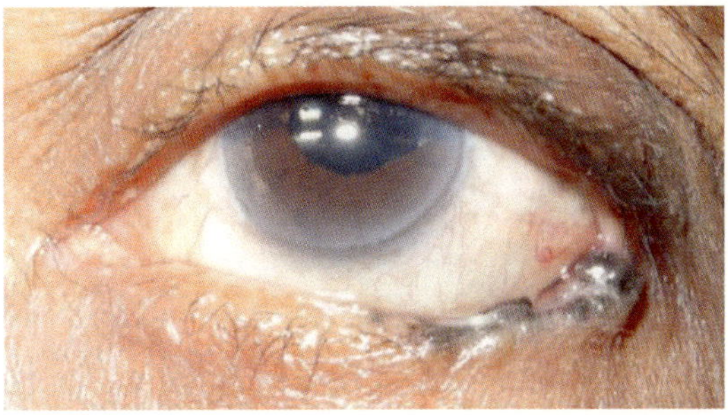

**Fig. 47.4** Pigmented BCC of the left lower lid in an Indian patient

Cell pleomorphism and a high mitosis rate might help in the differential diagnosis to a compound naevus [10]. The tumour may sometimes show ulceration. Melanoma cells are mainly of two morphologic types: epithelioid and spindle cells. Epithelioid cells are round and large with prominent nuclei, large nucleoli and a broad rim of eosinophilic cytoplasm. Spindle cells on the other hand are narrow, spindle-shaped with less cytoplasm (Fig. 47.5). Desmoplastic melanomas present a challenge also on histologic and immunohistochemical analysis.

Three histologic characteristics correlate strongly with the outcome of the disease and thus should be reported for adequate staging [11]:

- *Breslow*'s depth of invasion: In the histological slide, the maximum vertical extent of the tumour is measured in millimetres.
- Presence or absence of *histological ulceration* (tumour-induced full-thickness loss of the epidermis) [12].
- *Mitotic rate*: measured as number of dermal mitoses per square millimetre [13].

Special immunohistochemical (IHC) staining is done for confirmation of diagnosis. Among the antibodies most commonly used are:

- *S100* with a very high sensitivity (97–100 %) for the detection of cells from melanocytic origin but with a low specificity (75–87 %), staining nucleus and cytoplasm [14].
- *HMB45*, *MART-1*/*Melan-A* or *Tyrosinase* with lower sensitivities (69–93 %, 75–92 %,

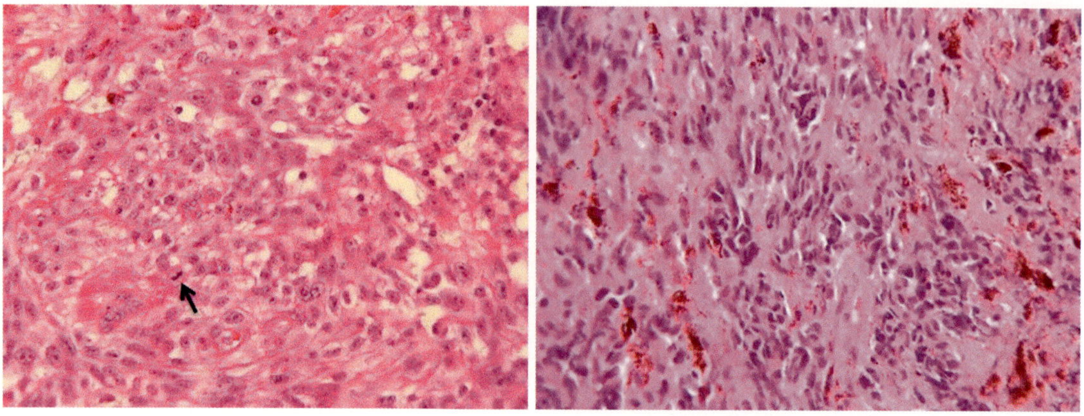

**Fig. 47.5** Haematoxylin and eosin staining of lid melanoma with areas of epithelioid cells (large cells with abundant nuclei and pleomorphism, arrow pointing to a mitosis) and spindle cells (elongated cells with scarce cytoplasm). The tumour exhibits few areas of pigmentation

84–94 %, respectively) but very high specificities for melanocytes (near 100 %, 95–100 %, 97–100 %, respectively) [14].

- *Ki-67* as marker of tumour cell proliferation. In naevi, less than 5 % of cell nuclei are stained; in Spitz and dysplastic naevi, it can be up to 15 %. In general, the stained cells will be seen mainly in the apical regions of the tumour, whereas in melanoma, about 13–30 % stain positive, and they may be located also in the deeper parts of the lesion. This marker can be used to distinguish melanoma from benign lesions of melanocytic origin, such as naevi [14, 15].

## Classification and Staging

The TNM (tumour, node, metastasis) staging system is used for cutaneous melanomas (Tables 47.1, 47.2, and 47.3).

According to the American Joined Committee on Cancer (AJCC), the tumours are grouped by their TNM status into groups that define the treatment or enrolment into clinical studies (Table 47.4).

*Staging procedures* for cutaneous melanoma are designed to help detect treatable locoregional or distant metastasis. Staging procedures should be tailored to the stage of the disease and the possibility of correct identification of prognostically relevant systemic involvement.

The staging procedures in tumours clinically not suspicious for metastatic disease up to *Stage IIB* involve:

**Table 47.1** Primary tumour (pT) staging of cutaneous melanoma [31, 89–91]

| pT | Meaning |
|---|---|
| pTX | Primary tumour cannot be assessed |
| pT0 | No evidence of primary tumour |
| pTis | Melanoma in situ |
| pT1 | ≤1.0 mm thickness (*a* without ulceration, mitotic rate <1/mm$^2$; *b* with ulceration or mitotic rate ≥1/mm$^2$) |
| pT2 | 1.01–2.0 mm thickness (a or b) |
| pT3 | 2.01–4.0 mm thickness (a or b) |
| pT4 | >4.0 mm thickness (a or b) |

Mitotic rate as seen in haematoxylin and eosin-stained tissue

**Table 47.2** Regional lymph node status (N) of cutaneous melanoma [31, 90, 91]

| N | Meaning |
|---|---|
| NX | Regional lymph nodes cannot be assessed |
| N0 | No regional lymph node metastasis |
| N1 | 1 node involved (*a* microscopic metastasis, *b* macroscopic metastasis, *c* in-transit metastasis without lymph node involvement) |
| N2 | 2–3 nodes involved |
| N3 | ≥4 nodes involved *or* matted LN *or* satellites or in-transit metastasis with LN involvement |

*LN* lymph node

- *Detailed local examination* (e.g. involvement of the lid margin, bulbar or palpebral conjunctiva, motility, globe integrity, dilated fundus examination, any other skin lesion such as lentigo maligna, in-transit lesions (subcutaneous nodules in the path between primary tumour and regional lymph nodes), seborrhoeic keratosis, and BCC)

- *Palpation of regional lymph nodes* (i.e. preauricular, parotid, submandibular, cervical) as well as drainage channels to rule out in-transit metastasis
- *General skin examination* to rule out metastatic disease to the lids
- *Sonography of the regional lymphatic basins* from Stage IB onwards
- *Serum S100* as tumour marker
- *Wide local excision* with histopathological confirmation of diagnosis (type of melanoma, Breslow's depth, presence of ulceration and mitotic level)

**Table 47.3** Distant metastasis (M) of cutaneous melanoma [90, 91]

| M | Meaning |
|---|---|
| MX | Distant metastasis cannot be assessed |
| M0 | No distant metastasis |
| M1 | Distant metastasis present |
| M1a | Skin, subcutaneous tissue, distant lymph nodes |
| M1b | Lung |
| M1c | Other or any M1 with elevated serum LDH |

*LDH* lactate dehydrogenase

- *Sentinel lymph node biopsy* (SLNB) for tumours thicker than 1 mm or thicker than 0.75 mm in patients with higher risk of metastatic disease (age <40, ulceration, high mitotic rate)

In *Stage IIC and III* melanomas, *additional* staging procedures are recommended:

- *Cranial MRI*
- *Cross-sectional imaging* (PET/CT, CT or MRI of the whole body, wherein PET/CT has superior diagnostic accuracy)
- *Serum lactate dehydrogenase (LDH)* as tumour marker

In *Stage IV* melanomas, recommendations for staging are as follows:

- *Cranial MRI*
- *Cross-sectional imaging* (PET/CT, CT or MRI of the whole body)
- *Serum LDH* as tumour marker
- *Abdominal sonography*
- *Lymph node sonography*
- *Skeletal scintigraphy*
- *Serum S100* and *serum LDH* as tumour markers

**Table 47.4** AJCC treatment groups of cutaneous melanoma [31, 91, 92]

| Group | pT | N | M |
|---|---|---|---|
| 0 | In situ | 0 | 0 |
| IA | ≤1 mm, no ulceration | 0 | 0 |
| IB | ≤1 mm with ulceration or MR ≥1/mm$^2$<br>1.01–2 mm, no ulceration | 0 | 0 |
| IIA | 1.01–2 mm with ulceration<br>2.01–4 mm, no ulceration | 0 | 0 |
| IIB | 2.01–4 mm with ulceration<br>>4 mm, no ulceration | 0 | 0 |
| IIC | >4 mm with ulceration | 0 | 0 |
| IIIA | Any Ta (without ulceration) | Microscopic mets≤ 3 LN | 0 |
| IIIB | Any Tb (with ulceration)<br>Any Ta<br>Any Ta | Microscopic mets≤ 3 LN<br>Macroscopic mets≤ 3 LN<br>No LN involvement, but satellites or in-transit mets | 0 |
| IIIC | Any Tb<br>Any T a *or* b | Macroscopic mets≤ 3 LN *or* satellites or in-transit mets without LN involvement<br>Macroscopic mets≥ 4 LN *or* matted LN *or* satellites or in-transit mets with LN involvement | 0 |
| IV | | | 1 |

## Treatment

### Surgical Treatment

#### Primary Excision

*Stage 0, I and II* melanomas are local tumours without lymphatic spread and thus considered primarily resectable.

In periocular tumours, wide local excision as recommended for cutaneous melanomas elsewhere is associated with significant morbidity and the necessity to excise structurally important tissue. According to recent studies analysing the target excision margin for periocular skin melanomas, a 3 mm surgical margin (2 mm histologic margin) for the excision of melanomas less than 1 mm Breslow thickness and 5 mm in thicker melanomas is recommended. The excision should include the full thickness of the lid in tumours thicker than 1 mm [16, 17].

The current AJCC guidelines suggest *micrographically controlled surgery* for lesions in these regions. In lentigo maligna melanoma, there is marked subclinical extension, so modified Mohs procedure (*mapped serial excision*) was able to show unpredictability of margin clearance of the disease requiring multiple excisions. A 3 % recurrence rate [18] as compared to previously published recurrence rates of 9–10 % [19, 20] was reported.

*Exenteration* for cutaneous melanoma of the lid is very rare. Most of the exenterations associated with melanomas are conjunctival or orbital in origin [21].

If the initial tumour resection yields R1 (microscopic) or R2 (macroscopic remnants) status on permanent histological sections, re-excision is recommended if possible until histological clearance is achieved.

#### Lymph Node Dissection

*Stage III* disease displays lymph node involvement but no distant metastases. The theory of metastasis development in melanoma is that primary metastasis occurs into the sentinel lymph node (SLN), from there into the regional lymphatic basin and only after a delay via further lymphatic and haematogenous spread to the rest of the body. Thus, in early stages of melanoma without distant micrometastasis, cure could possibly be achieved by targeting the SLN or regional lymph nodes before further spread occurs. If anatomically possible, complete excision should be done for satellite lesions, in-transit and lymph node metastases.

In cases of positive sentinel lymph node biopsy, completion regional lymph node dissection (CLND) is recommended to achieve R0 state. Elective therapeutic lymph node dissection (TLND) is not recommended.

#### Excision of Distant Metastases

Patients with *Stage IV* disease (distant metastasis) need to be individually assessed by an interdisciplinary team regarding the indication for surgical intervention. Excision of distant metastases can be considered if R0 excision is possible and morbidity associated with surgery is acceptable, the number of metastases limited, disease-free interval long and other therapeutic modalities have been unsuccessful or less promising [22].

### Medical Treatment

#### Primary Medical Treatment

The primary treatment of cutaneous melanomas is surgical excision.

The lifetime risk for the development of LMM in a 45-year-old patient diagnosed with LM is approximated to 5 % [23]. LM in the periocular region can be of considerable size thus causing significant morbidity if excised. In biopsy-proven LM when surgical treatment is not feasible or refused by the patient, immune response therapy with *imiquimod* 5 % cream can be started. Application is once or twice daily for 6 weeks to 3 months. The response rate is excellent with complete remission reported in 93 [24] – 100 % [25]. Because of the inflammatory response, periocular use may be limited by ocular irritation and chemical conjunctivitis [26]. Imiquimod can also be used as adjunctive treatment prior to micrographically controlled excision [27]. Development of amelanotic melanomas within the lesion has to be kept in mind when using conservative treatment in these patients, and they have to be closely followed. *Radiotherapy* is another option for the treatment of LM [28].

### Adjuvant and Palliative Medical Treatment

Adjuvant or palliative medical treatment is recommended for *Stage III* and *Stage IV* melanomas.

*Radiotherapy* is administered to the lymphatic basin after lymph node dissection in certain conditions [29–31].

Adjuvant radiotherapy may be an option to enhance local control of resected desmoplastic melanoma in the head and neck region [32].

Radiotherapy can be administered to non-resectable metastases of the bone and brain especially for palliation [33, 34].

*Interferon α-2b* is an immunomodulatory as well as antiproliferative agent used mainly in viral hepatitis. Trials show a small but significant benefit for overall disease-free survival. Interferon can be given as high-dose, low-dose or pegylated therapy. The main limiting factors are the side effects causing discontinuation of treatment [35, 36]. Adjuvant interferon therapy is recommended for melanomas at high risk of metastasis, ulcerated melanomas as well as those with micrometastases.

*Interleukin-2* is an immunomodulatory agent targeting natural killer cells. High-dose therapy has been shown to benefit some patients with Stage IV melanoma. Overall response rates vary from 8 % to 16 %. Toxicity is high.

*Dacarbazine* is the standard chemotherapeutic agent for non-resectable and metastasized melanomas. It acts via DNA alkylation. Polychemotherapy is also available and can be used in progressive disease [22].

Certain mutations in activating oncogenes of melanomas can be targeted with new medications. These are mainly the *BRAF mutation* (36–57 % of cutaneous melanomas [37, 38]), the *NRAS mutation* in 11–15 % [37, 38] and the *c-KIT mutation* mainly in acral and mucosal melanomas [39].

In cutaneous melanomas of the lid, mainly BRAF and NRAS mutations can be targeted with specific medications. BRAF and KIT mutations have been found in some conjunctival melanomas [40].

*Vemurafenib* is a specific inhibitor of BRAF (V600E) kinase, and treatment in conjunction with clinical trials is recommended in case the molecular testing is positive for the mutation [31, 41]. The response rate in melanomas showing the respective mutation is almost complete. Main side effects include the development of secondary neoplasms. The main problem encountered is resistance to the drug after several months [42].

There is no specific inhibitor for NRAS-mutated oncogenes. MEK inhibitors (MAP kinase pathway inhibitors), specifically *trametinib*, show effects on affected cells and can be used to treat metastatic melanoma positive for NRAS mutations [43].

*Imatinib* mesylate, an orally available c-KIT inhibitor, has shown some effect in treating metastatic melanoma with the respective mutation with good tumour regression rates of 42 % [40, 44].

*Ipilimumab* is a novel immunomodulator targeting cytotoxic T-lymphocyte-associated antigen 4 (CTLA-4), a suppressor for T lymphocyte activity. Treatment with this agent has been promising for some patients with Stage III or IV melanoma. The response rate is relatively limited (10–15 %), but responders treated over a short period of time were able to exhibit significant survival of up to 10 years [45].

Recent advances in the development of drugs targeting melanoma cells give hope in the treatment of Stage III and IV melanomas. Adjuvant treatment with radiotherapy in Stage III and recurrent melanoma is recommended. Adjuvant treatment with targeted immunotherapy is recommended in BRAF-positive Stage III and IV disease. Ipilimumab is promising in BRAF-negative tumours, especially as combination therapy with radiation or with targeted immunotherapy.

Therapy in these advanced stages has to be done in a dermato-oncological setting especially in regard to the option of enrolling the patient into current trials.

## Prognosis and Follow-Up

The prognosis for cutaneous melanoma is generally dependent on the stage of the disease.

In *localised disease* (Stages I and II), the prognosis is generally favourable. Small T1a tumours as in Stage I show 10-year survival rates of 93 %. T4b tumours as in Stage II disease, although localised, have less favourable 5-year/10-year survival rates of 53/39 %, respectively [46]. Tumours located in the lower lid had a higher risk of recurrence in one study [16]. Negative prognostic factors regarding the lid are lid margin and conjunctival involvement [47]. Desmoplastic melanoma seems to have lower risk for developing metastatic disease, albeit a higher risk for local recurrence [48, 49].

In *Stage III* disease, 5-year survival rates were 70 % for N1a nodal involvement and 39 % for N3 nodal involvement, putting emphasis on the prognostic importance of micrometastastatic disease, low tumour burden, and absence of in-transit metastases [46].

*Stage IV* melanoma has a generally poor prognosis with 5-year survival rates reported less than 10 % and mean survival of 6 months [50].

Risk-adapted follow-up of the patients has been recommended for 10 years from diagnosis [31].

Newer adjuvant treatment are promising in terms of prolonging life, but metastatic cutaneous melanoma remains an incurable cancer nevertheless, and the goal has to be early recognition and complete micrographically controlled excision with adequate reconstruction in the periocular area wherever possible.

## Eyelid Conjunctival Melanoma

### Introduction and Epidemiology

Conjunctival melanomas comprise about 5 % of all periocular and ocular melanomas. They are predominantly seen in Whites older than 60 years and rarely in Blacks, although the White-to-Black (WBR) ratio of conjunctival melanoma seems to be less pronounced (2:1) than that of cutaneous (about 16:1) or uveal (18:1) melanoma [51].

Conjunctival melanoma can occur as primary lesion, as metastasis from cutaneous melanoma or by extension from a cutaneous melanoma of the lid. Uveal melanomas, which are by far more common, can appear as pigmented subconjunctival mass if extrascleral extension is present.

### Aetiology and Pathogenesis

Conjunctival melanomas can arise from precursor lesions such as primary acquired melanosis (PAM) with atypia also termed conjunctival melanocytic intraepithelial neoplasia (C-MIN), from preexisting naevi or de novo. The role of possible UV-induced damage underlying this disease has not been established. They are mostly unilateral and can occasionally be multifocal.

About 75 % of conjunctival melanomas arise from *PAM with atypia* [52]. The incidence of PAM itself is not known; it is estimated to be present in about 36 % of Caucasians [53]. Clinically, PAM is an acquired flat pigmented lesion on mostly the bulbar conjunctiva. The risk of developing melanoma from PAM with severe atypia is about 13 %, dependent on the extent of PAM [54].

Roughly 12–17 % of melanomas arise from preexisting naevi. The risk of malignant conversion of a conjunctival naevus is less than 1 % [55].

The remaining 12 % of conjunctival melanomas arise de novo without any precursor lesion [56].

### Clinical Presentation

Conjunctival melanomas are irregular, prominent lesions that can present with variable pigmentation, are unilateral in most cases and can be multifocal or involve the lid margin in case of underlying PAM. In any pigmented lesion occurring in adulthood, especially if there is evidence of colour change, growth or location in the forniceal or palpebral conjunctiva, melanoma should be suspected. Melanomas can exhibit "feeder vessels", dilated conjunctival vessels leading to the lesion (Fig. 47.6).

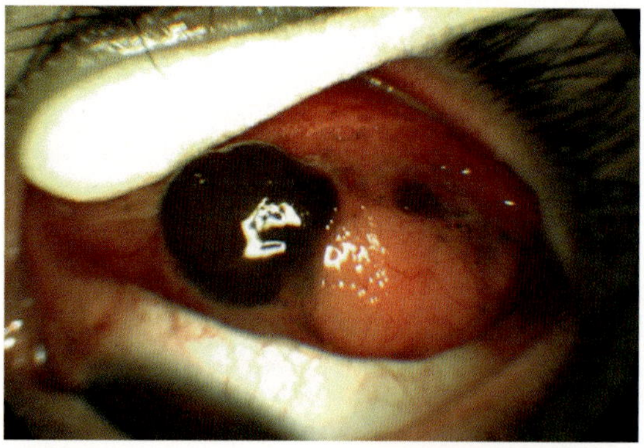

**Fig. 47.6** Conjunctival melanoma of the upper lid with a pigmented and an unpigmented mass in the palpebral conjunctiva with seedings

Clinical examination should involve slit lamp biomicroscopy, dilated fundus examination, if indicated gonioscopy and ultrasound biomicroscopy to detect deep invasion.

## Differential Diagnosis

Differential diagnoses for PAM include *racial melanosis* [47] and *congenital ocular melanocytosis*. Ocular and oculodermal melanocytosis can be associated with uveal melanomas and can give rise to cutaneous melanomas [57]. *Naevi* are the most common melanocytic tumours of the conjunctiva. Congenital naevi are present at birth or can appear up to 6 months thereafter. Acquired naevi normally appear during the first two decades of life. Naevi exhibit variable pigmentation and frequently show intralesional cysts on slit lamp biomicroscopy [10]. Conjunctival *Spitz naevus* shows rapid growth despite its benign nature and is mostly amelanotic. Conjunctival *blue naevus* presents as very dark pigmented lesion in the deep substantia propria of the conjunctiva. Other differential diagnoses for amelanotic melanomas include *papillomas*, *squamous cell carcinomas* and *metastases* [58].

## Histopathology

In primary acquired melanosis without atypia, the number as well as the melanin deposition increases with the cells, retaining their normal morphology. In PAM with atypia, the cells show enlargement of the nucleus, prominent nucleolus, and they may form nests and invade the more superficial structures of the epithelial layer. Some authors have suggested naming the lesion *conjunctival melanocytic intraepithelial neoplasia* (C-MIN), parallel to the conjunctival intraepithelial neoplasia (CIN) as precursor lesion of squamous cell carcinomas of the ocular surface [59, 60]. Atypias can progress to melanoma in situ.

*Conjunctival naevi* are either compound (involving the epidermal/dermal junction as well as the substantia propria) or subepithelial when excised in adulthood. Junctional naevi (only involving the epidermal/dermal junction) are found very early in life. C-MIN with atypia should be suspected if found in an adult.

The cell types as well as the immunohistochemical staining of conjunctival melanoma are essentially the same as in cutaneous melanoma. Histologic characteristics that should be reported for accurate staging are [61]:

- Jakobiec modification of the *Breslow* thickness in millimetres
- *Invasion* of adjacent structures (globe, orbit, lacrimal system)
- Evidence of the tumour arising from a *precursor lesion* or de novo

## Classification and Staging

The TNM staging system is also used for conjunctival melanomas. There is a separate clinical and histopathological staging for the tumour (Tables 47.5, 47.6, 47.7, and 47.8).

Unlike cutaneous melanoma, there are no treatment groups defined for conjunctival melanoma.

Workup recommendations for conjunctival melanoma have not been as extensively evaluated as those for their cutaneous counterparts. Initial workup of a patient *without clinical suspicion for metastatic disease* would include:

- *Detailed local examination* (e.g. localisation, size, involvement of the lid margin, mobility

**Table 47.5** Clinical tumour (cT) staging of conjunctival melanoma [92]

| cT | Meaning |
|---|---|
| cTX | Primary tumour cannot be assessed |
| cT0 | No evidence of primary tumour |
| cTis | Melanoma in situ confined to conjunctival epithelium |
| cT1 | Invasive melanoma of the *bulbar* conjunctiva: *a* ≤ 1 quadrant; *b* >1, ≤2 quadrants; *c* >2, ≤3 quadrants; *d* >3 quadrants |
| cT2 | Invasive melanoma of the *palpebral*, *forniceal* or *caruncular* conjunctiva: *a* no caruncular involvement, ≤ 1 quadrant; *b* no caruncular involvement, >1 quadrant; *c* caruncular involvement, ≤ 1 quadrant; *d* caruncular involvement, >1 quadrant |
| cT3 | Any melanoma with *local invasion*: *a* globe, *b* eyelid, *c* orbit, *d* sinus |
| cT4 | Invasion of the central nervous system |

Quadrants are defined by clock hour extending from the centre of the cornea

**Table 47.6** Pathologic primary tumour (pT) staging of conjunctival melanoma [92]

| pT | Meaning |
|---|---|
| pTX | Primary tumour cannot be assessed |
| pT0 | No evidence of primary tumour |
| pTis | Melanoma in situ confined to conjunctival epithelium (including PAM with atypia replacing >75 % of epithelium) |
| pT1 | Invasive melanoma of the *bulbar* conjunctiva: $a \leq 0.5$ mm; $b > 0.5$ mm, $\leq 1.5$ mm; $c > 1.5$ mm |
| pT2 | Invasive melanoma of the *palpebral, forniceal* or *caruncular* conjunctiva: $a \leq 0.5$ mm; $b > 0.5$ mm, $\leq 1.5$ mm; $c > 1.5$ mm |
| pT3 | Any melanoma with *local invasion* |
| pT4 | Invasion of the central nervous system |

**Table 47.7** Regional lymph node status (N) of conjunctival melanoma [92]

| N | Meaning |
|---|---|
| NX | Regional lymph nodes cannot be assessed |
| N0 | No regional lymph node metastasis |
| N1 | Regional lymph node metastasis present |

**Table 47.8** Distant metastasis (M) of conjunctival melanoma [92]

| M | Meaning |
|---|---|
| MX | Distant metastasis cannot be assessed |
| M0 | No distant metastasis |
| M1 | Distant metastasis present |

of the conjunctiva over the globe, evidence of precursor lesion, multifocal disease, motility, globe integrity, dilated fundus examination, evidence of spread into lacrimal drainage pathway or sinuses)

- *Palpation of regional lymph nodes* (i.e. preauricular, parotid, submandibular, cervical) as well as drainage channels to rule out in-transit metastasis
- *General skin examination* to rule out metastatic disease to the lids
- *Sonography of the regional lymphatic basins* [62]
- *Imaging* of the orbit and brain [62]
- *Imaging* (CT) of the chest, abdomen and pelvis for melanomas thicker than 2 mm, local recurrences or diameter more than 10 mm [62] or *liver ultrasound* and *chest x-ray* [63]
- *Liver function tests* [63]
- *Excision* with histopathological confirmation of diagnosis and staging
- *Sentinel lymph node biopsy* (SLNB) for tumours thicker than 2 mm, lid involvement or local recurrences

Unlike cutaneous melanoma, distant metastasis may be found without evidence of regional lymphatic involvement in 26–60 % of cases [64–66]. This may be the reason for more extensive initial screening for metastasis. The role of sentinel lymph node biopsy (SLNB) in conjunctival melanoma has not been established as clearly as in cutaneous melanoma. There is evidence for at least prognostic use of SLNB in tumours with higher risk for metastasis, i.e. depth >2 mm, unfavourable location (including involvement of the lid) and multiple local recurrences as are often seen in melanoma arising from C-MIN with atypia [67].

## Treatment

### Surgical Treatment

#### Primary Excision

The treatment of *C-MIN with atypia* has not reached consensus statement as yet. It is justifiable to observe small lesions in the bulbar conjunctiva of less than 1 clock hour in extent every 6–12 months. In case of larger lesions or involvement of unfavourable locations (e.g. palpebral conjunctiva, fornix, lid margin) excisional biopsy is recommended with adjuvant cryotherapy or chemotherapy (as discussed below), depending on histopathological grading. For diffuse disease, map biopsies of the conjunctiva are recommended followed by either cryotherapy [54] or chemotherapy with Mitomycin C (MMC). Generally, C-MIN associated with invasive melanoma is treated more aggressively, and follow-up is more frequent [60].

Local control of the tumour is very important in the management of *conjunctival melanomas*, since local recurrence is a negative predictor for systemic spread. Concentrating on conjunctival melanomas involving the lid margin, fornix and bulbar conjunctiva, wide, micrographically controlled *excision* is recommended. Some authors advocate a

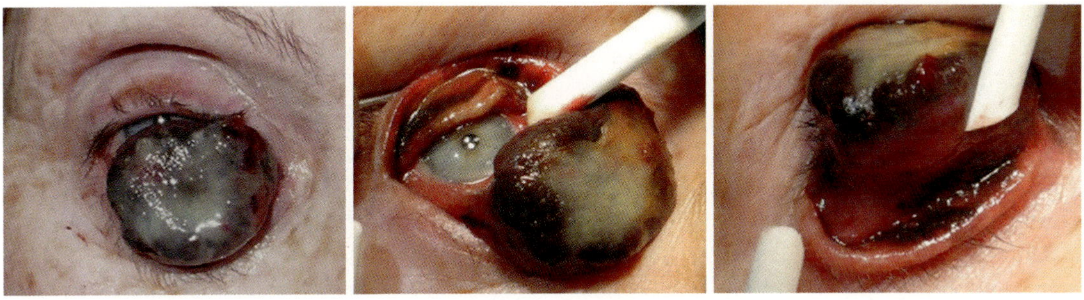

**Fig. 47.7** Large conjunctival melanoma of the inferior fornix with extensive C-MIN

margin of 4 mm [68]. Micrographic R0 excision is difficult to achieve, especially in cases of C-MIN and pagetoid spread. Even with good margin control, recurrences from C-MIN can occur in 26 % of patients by 5 years and 68 % of patients by 15 years [69]. Conjunctival melanomas involving the lid will be staged at T2 or T3 by definition. It is recommended to completely excise smaller tumours with the "*no-touch*" *technique* as described by Shields et al. [68]. Herein it is mandatory to not touch the tumour with the instruments, keep the surgical field dry, not to use irrigation until the tumour has been excised and change of instruments for reconstructive procedures. The specimen has to be handled very gently in order to prevent crush artefacts.

Larger tumours might warrant an incisional biopsy before planning surgery, although for melanomas incisional biopsy is not advised because of the risk of tumour spread [70].

Tumours involving the lid margin have to be excised in full thickness.

Many studies in the last years have shown the significant benefit in local tumour control from adjuvant procedures [60, 66, 71].

*Exenteration* of the orbit may be required in cases of orbital invasion and/or extensive involvement of the conjunctival circumference for local tumour control. Exenteration for conjunctival melanoma as such does not improve the overall prognosis [21] (Fig. 47.7).

#### Lymph Node Dissection

Prophylactic radical neck dissection is controversial.

If *SLNB* turns out positive, a *regional dissection* of lymph nodes is recommended, followed by *radiation* of the lymph node basin if additional nodes turn out positive or if extracapsular extension is noted.

#### Excision of Distant Metastases

Patients with distant metastases need to be individually assessed by an interdisciplinary team regarding the indication for surgical intervention. As in cutaneous melanoma, excision of distant metastases can be considered if R0 excision is possible and morbidity associated with surgery is acceptable.

### Medical Treatment

#### Adjuvant Medical Treatment

Conventional intraoperative adjuvant treatments for excised C-MIN with atypia or melanoma include *cryotherapy* of the surrounding bulbar conjunctiva, lifting it from the sclera during the double freeze-thaw cycle and treatment of bare sclera with absolute *alcohol* [68]. Cryotherapy should not be applied to the sclera for possibility of necrosis.

Chemotherapy with Mitomycin C as 0.04 or 0.02 % drops can be used as an adjuvant therapy after excision of C-MIN or melanoma, especially if there is evidence of R1 resection [72]. Primary treatment of conjunctival melanoma is not recommended since the penetration is not sufficient and recurrence rates near 100 % [73]. Side effects of topical MMC therapy are commonly conjunctival redness, chemosis and irritation, superficial punctate keratitis, punctal and canalicular stenosis and most seriously limbal stem cell insufficiency [74]. Different treatment regimens have been described, ranging from 0.04 % MMC four times a day for 2 weeks, followed by a 2 week treatment gap, followed by a second cycle of chemotherapy 0.02 % MMC four times a day for 2 weeks [75] to 0.02 % drops in four 7-day cycles each separated by a week [76]. Punctal occlusion may be considered before starting treatment. There are a few case series supporting the use of MMC as primary treatment for C-MIN with atypia and as adjuvant treatment for conjunctival melanoma [73, 77]. One study examined the effect on topical MMC as primary treatment for conjunctival melanoma and found good response to treatment but for the tumours involving the lid [78].

In summary, chemotherapy with MMC should be considered as adjuvant treatment after micrographically controlled excision of conjunctival melanomas involving high-risk areas like the lid, especially if it arises from C-MIN. MMC can be considered as primary treatment of disseminated C-MIN with atypia following map biopsies. Nevertheless, recurrence rates are considerable and close follow-up is recommended.

*Radiation therapy* can be administered as brachytherapy, proton or external beam therapy. External beam radiotherapy is mainly administered to the regional lymph node basin after lymph node dissection.

Brachytherapy has been shown beneficial as adjuvant therapy after excision of conjunctival melanomas, and many authors advocate its use as standard procedure [64, 76]. Nevertheless, brachytherapy applicators suitable for the palpebral conjunctiva are not yet available.

For primary treatment and local control of lid-involving conjunctival melanomas not accessible to excision, *brachytherapy with Iodine-125* has been successfully used in 14 patients with incomplete excision or recurrence of conjunctival melanoma involving the lid [79].

P*roton beam* irradiation was used for extensive disease involving the lid in 11 cases as alternative to exenteration [80].

Radiotherapy as primary or adjuvant therapy seems to be beneficial in terms of local tumour control and also in high-risk cases of conjunctival melanoma involving the lid.

*Interferon α-2b* (*IFN α-2b*) might be a good alternative to MMC in the treatment of C-MIN with atypia and as adjuvant treatment after excision of conjunctival melanoma, especially if there is intolerance to MMC [81, 82].

*BRAF* (mainly V600E) mutations were found in conjunctival melanomas in 22–29 % of cases [37, 83, 84], *NRAS* mutations in 0–18 % [37, 40, 83] and *c-KIT* mutations in 0–8 % [37, 40].

There is one case report of a multiple recurrent BRAF mutation-positive conjunctival melanoma involving the lids, which was successfully treated with systemic *Vemurafenib* [85].

Treatment options for metastatic conjunctival melanoma follow the guidelines of those for cutaneous melanoma.

## Prognosis and Follow-Up

The prognosis for conjunctival melanoma is dependent mainly on the location and size of the tumour. Eyelid conjunctival melanomas have a significantly worse prognosis than do those involving the bulbar conjunctiva.

Depending on patient selection and treatment, local recurrence is reported in 30–60 % of cases [65, 71, 86, 87].

There is no standardised follow-up protocol as there is for cutaneous melanoma. The authors of a recent review suggest six monthly clinical evaluations of the local and regional lymph basin status, liver function tests and in high-risk patients as stated above, sonography of the abdomen and chest x-ray for 5 years after initial treatment [63]. Distant metastases appear in roughly 30 % of patients after 10 years [66, 88]. Frequent site of metastasis are the lungs, liver, skin and brain. Generally, prognosis of metastasized conjunctival melanoma is poor.

Five-year survival rate has been reported at 83–86 % and 10-year survival 69–71 % [21, 64].

## References

1. Black EHN, FA, Calvano CJ, Gladstone GJ, Levine MR. Smith and Nesi's ophthalmic plastic and reconstructive surgery. 3rd ed. New York: Springer; 2012.
2. Liu W, Dowling JP, Murray WK, McArthur GA, Thompson JF, Wolfe R, et al. Rate of growth in

melanomas: characteristics and associations of rapidly growing melanomas. Arch Dermatol. 2006; 142(12):1551–8.
3. Kostopoulos E, Champsas G, Konofaos P, Kostaki M, Papadopoulos O. Eyelid melanoma: our experience a propos of 23 cases. Ann Chir Plast Esthet. 2012; 57(2):158–63.
4. Cook Jr BE, Bartley GB. Treatment options and future prospects for the management of eyelid malignancies: an evidence-based update. Ophthalmology. 2001;108(11):2088–98; quiz 99–100, 121.
5. Char DH. Ocular melanoma. Surg Clin North Am. 2003;83(2):253–74, vii.
6. Busam KJ. Desmoplastic melanoma. Clin Lab Med. 2011;31(2):321–30.
7. Vaziri M, Buffam FV, Martinka M, Oryschak A, Dhaliwal H, White VA. Clinicopathologic features and behavior of cutaneous eyelid melanoma. Ophthalmology. 2002;109(5):901–8.
8. Tahery DP, Goldberg R, Moy RL. Malignant melanoma of the eyelid. A report of eight cases and a review of the literature. J Am Acad Dermatol. 1992;27(1):17–21.
9. Sepehr A, Chao E, Trefrey B, Blackford A, Duncan LM, Flotte TJ, et al. Long-term outcome of Spitz-type melanocytic tumors. Arch Dermatol. 2011;147(10):1173–9.
10. Rohrbach JM, Lieb WE. Tumoren des Auges und seiner Adnexe. Stuttgart: Schattauer; 1998.
11. Bichakjian CK, Halpern AC, Johnson TM, Foote Hood A, Grichnik JM, Swetter SM, et al. Guidelines of care for the management of primary cutaneous melanoma. American Academy of Dermatology. J Am Acad Dermatol. 2011;65(5):1032–47.
12. Eigentler TK, Buettner PG, Leiter U, Garbe C, Central Malignant Melanoma Registry of the German Dermatological S. Impact of ulceration in stages I to III cutaneous melanoma as staged by the American Joint Committee on Cancer Staging System: an analysis of the German Central Malignant Melanoma Registry. J Clin Oncol Off J Am Soc Clin Oncol. 2004;22(21):4376–83.
13. Azzola MF, Shaw HM, Thompson JF, Soong SJ, Scolyer RA, Watson GF, et al. Tumor mitotic rate is a more powerful prognostic indicator than ulceration in patients with primary cutaneous melanoma: an analysis of 3661 patients from a single center. Cancer. 2003;97(6):1488–98.
14. Ohsie SJ, Sarantopoulos GP, Cochran AJ, Binder SW. Immunohistochemical characteristics of melanoma. J Cutan Pathol. 2008;35(5):433–44.
15. Prieto VG, Shea CR. Immunohistochemistry of melanocytic proliferations. Arch Pathol Lab Med. 2011;135(7):853–9.
16. Harish V, Bond JS, Scolyer RA, Haydu LE, Saw RP, Quinn MJ, et al. Margins of excision and prognostic factors for cutaneous eyelid melanomas. J Plast Reconstr Aesthet Surg JPRAS. 2013;66(8):1066–73.
17. Esmaeli B, Youssef A, Naderi A, Ahmadi MA, Meyer DR, McNab A, et al. Margins of excision for cutaneous melanoma of the eyelid skin: the Collaborative Eyelid Skin Melanoma Group Report. Ophthal Plast Reconstr Surg. 2003;19(2):96–101.
18. Malhotra R, Chen C, Huilgol SC, Hill DC, Selva D. Mapped serial excision for periocular lentigo maligna and lentigo maligna melanoma. Ophthalmology. 2003;110(10):2011–8.
19. Coleman 3rd WP, Davis RS, Reed RJ, Krementz ET. Treatment of lentigo maligna and lentigo maligna melanoma. J Dermatol Surg Oncol. 1980;6(6):476–9.
20. Pitman GH, Kopf AW, Bart RS, Casson PR. Treatment of lentigo maligna and lentigo maligna melanoma. J Dermatol Surg Oncol. 1979;5(9):727–37.
21. Paridaens AD, McCartney AC, Minassian DC, Hungerford JL. Orbital exenteration in 95 cases of primary conjunctival malignant melanoma. Br J Ophthalmol. 1994;78(7):520–8.
22. Pflugfelder A, Kochs C, Blum A, Capellaro M, Czeschik C, Dettenborn T, et al. S3-guideline "diagnosis, therapy and follow-up of melanoma" – short version. J Dtsch Dermatol Ges J Ger Soc Dermatol JDDG. 2013;11(6):563–602.
23. Weinstock MA, Sober AJ. The risk of progression of lentigo maligna to lentigo maligna melanoma. Br J Dermatol. 1987;116(3):303–10.
24. Naylor MF, Crowson N, Kuwahara R, Teague K, Garcia C, Mackinnis C, et al. Treatment of lentigo maligna with topical imiquimod. Br J Dermatol. 2003;149 Suppl 66:66–70.
25. Buettiker UV, Yawalkar NY, Braathen LR, Hunger RE. Imiquimod treatment of lentigo maligna: an open-label study of 34 primary lesions in 32 patients. Arch Dermatol. 2008;144(7):943–5.
26. Cannon PS, O'Donnell B, Huilgol SC, Selva D. The ophthalmic side-effects of imiquimod therapy in the management of periocular skin lesions. Br J Ophthalmol. 2011;95(12):1682–5.
27. Cotter MA, McKenna JK, Bowen GM. Treatment of lentigo maligna with imiquimod before staged excision. Dermatol Surg: Off Publ Am Soc Dermatol Surg [et al]. 2008;34(2):147–51.
28. Hedblad MA, Mallbris L. Grenz ray treatment of lentigo maligna and early lentigo maligna melanoma. J Am Acad Dermatol. 2012;67(1):60–8.
29. Bibault JE, Dewas S, Mirabel X, Mortier L, Penel N, Vanseymortier L, et al. Adjuvant radiation therapy in metastatic lymph nodes from melanoma. Radiat Oncol. 2011;6:12.
30. Burmeister BH, Henderson MA, Ainslie J, Fisher R, Di Iulio J, Smithers BM, et al. Adjuvant radiotherapy versus observation alone for patients at risk of lymph-node field relapse after therapeutic lymphadenectomy for melanoma: a randomised trial. Lancet Oncol. 2012;13(6):589–97.
31. Pflugfelder A, Kochs C, Blum A, Capellaro M, Czeschik C, Dettenborn T, et al. Malignant melanoma S3-guideline "diagnosis, therapy and follow-up of melanoma". J Dtsch Dermatol Ges J Ger Soc Dermatol: JDDG. 2013;11 Suppl 6:1–116, 1–26.
32. Guadagnolo BA, Prieto V, Weber R, Ross MI, Zagars GK. The role of adjuvant radiotherapy in the local

management of desmoplastic melanoma. Cancer. 2014;120(9):1361–8.
33. Fogarty GB, Hong A. Radiation therapy for advanced and metastatic melanoma. J Surg Oncol. 2014; 109(4):370–5.
34. Silk AW, Bassetti MF, West BT, Tsien CI, Lao CD. Ipilimumab and radiation therapy for melanoma brain metastases. Cancer Med. 2013;2(6):899–906.
35. Eggermont AM, Suciu S, Santinami M, Testori A, Kruit WH, Marsden J, et al. Adjuvant therapy with pegylated interferon alfa-2b versus observation alone in resected stage III melanoma: final results of EORTC 18991, a randomised phase III trial. Lancet. 2008;372(9633):117–26.
36. Hancock BW, Wheatley K, Harris S, Ives N, Harrison G, Horsman JM, et al. Adjuvant interferon in high-risk melanoma: the AIM HIGH Study – United Kingdom Coordinating Committee on Cancer Research randomized study of adjuvant low-dose extended-duration interferon Alfa-2a in high-risk resected malignant melanoma. J Clin Oncol: Off J Am Soc Clin Oncol. 2004;22(1):53–61.
37. Beadling C, Jacobson-Dunlop E, Hodi FS, Le C, Warrick A, Patterson J, et al. KIT gene mutations and copy number in melanoma subtypes. Clin Cancer Res: Off J Am Assoc Cancer Res. 2008;14(21):6821–8.
38. Goel VK, Lazar AJ, Warneke CL, Redston MS, Haluska FG. Examination of mutations in BRAF, NRAS, and PTEN in primary cutaneous melanoma. J Invest Dermatol. 2006;126(1):154–60.
39. Torres-Cabala CA, Wang WL, Trent J, Yang D, Chen S, Galbincea J, et al. Correlation between KIT expression and KIT mutation in melanoma: a study of 173 cases with emphasis on the acral-lentiginous/mucosal type. Mod Pathol: Off J US Can Acad Pathol. 2009;22(11):1446–56.
40. Wallander ML, Layfield LJ, Emerson LL, Mamalis N, Davis D, Tripp SR, et al. KIT mutations in ocular melanoma: frequency and anatomic distribution. Mod Pathol: Off J US Can Acad Pathol. 2011;24(8): 1031–5.
41. Institute NC. Melanoma treatment 2014. Available from: http://www.cancer.gov/cancertopics/pdq/treatment/melanoma/healthprofessional. Accessed 20.04.2014.
42. Garbe C, Abusaif S, Eigentler TK. Recent results in cancer research Fortschritte der Krebsforschung Progres dans les recherches sur le cancer. Vemurafenib. 2014;201:215–25.
43. Lawrence L. MEK inhibitor active in NRAS-mutated melanoma 2013. Available from: http://www.cancernetwork.com/melanoma/mek-inhibitor-active-nras-mutated-melanoma. Accessed 30.04.2014.
44. Guo J, Si L, Kong Y, Flaherty KT, Xu X, Zhu Y, et al. Phase II, open-label, single-arm trial of imatinib mesylate in patients with metastatic melanoma harboring c-Kit mutation or amplification. J Clin Oncol: Off J Am Soc Clin Oncol. 2011;29(21):2904–9.
45. Hodi FS, O'Day SJ, McDermott DF, Weber RW, Sosman JA, Haanen JB, et al. Improved survival with ipilimumab in patients with metastatic melanoma. N Engl J Med. 2010;363(8):711–23.
46. Balch CM, Gershenwald JE, Soong SJ, Thompson JF, Atkins MB, Byrd DR, et al. Final version of 2009 AJCC melanoma staging and classification. J Clin Oncol: Off J Am Soc Clin Oncol. 2009;27(36):6199–206.
47. Singh BE, Pe'er J, Murphree AL, Perry JD. Clinical ophthalmic oncology. Philadelphia: Saunders Elsevier; 2007.
48. Hawkins WG, Busam KJ, Ben-Porat L, Panageas KS, Coit DG, Gyorki DE, et al. Desmoplastic melanoma: a pathologically and clinically distinct form of cutaneous melanoma. Ann Surg Oncol. 2005;12(3):207–13.
49. Pawlik TM, Ross MI, Prieto VG, Ballo MT, Johnson MM, Mansfield PF, et al. Assessment of the role of sentinel lymph node biopsy for primary cutaneous desmoplastic melanoma. Cancer. 2006;106(4):900–6.
50. Manola J, Atkins M, Ibrahim J, Kirkwood J. Prognostic factors in metastatic melanoma: a pooled analysis of Eastern Cooperative Oncology Group trials. J Clin Oncol: Off J Am Soc Clin Oncol. 2000;18(22):3782–93.
51. Hu DN, Yu G, McCormick SA, Finger PT. Population-based incidence of conjunctival melanoma in various races and ethnic groups and comparison with other melanomas. Am J Ophthalmol. 2008;145(3):418–23.
52. Jakobiec FA, Folberg R, Iwamoto T. Clinicopathologic characteristics of premalignant and malignant melanocytic lesions of the conjunctiva. Ophthalmology. 1989;96(2):147–66.
53. Gloor P, Alexandrakis G. Clinical characterization of primary acquired melanosis. Invest Ophthalmol Vis Sci. 1995;36(8):1721–9.
54. Shields JA, Shields CL, Mashayekhi A, Marr BP, Benavides R, Thangappan A, et al. Primary acquired melanosis of the conjunctiva: risks for progression to melanoma in 311 eyes. The 2006 Lorenz E. Zimmerman lecture. Ophthalmology. 2008;115(3):511–9 e2.
55. Shields CL, Fasiuddin AF, Mashayekhi A, Shields JA. Conjunctival nevi: clinical features and natural course in 410 consecutive patients. Arch Ophthalmol. 2004;122(2):167–75.
56. Network AC. Clinical practice guidelines for the management of melanoma in Australia and New Zealand; Ocular and periocular melanoma: Supplementary document 2008. Available from: http://www.cancer.org.au/content/pdf/HealthProfessionals/ClinicalGuidelines/ManagementofOcularmelanomasupplementarydocument2008.pdf. Accessed 30.04.2014.
57. Sinha S, Cohen PJ, Schwartz RA. Nevus of Ota in children. Cutis. 2008;82(1):25–9.
58. Kiratli H, Shields CL, Shields JA, DePotter P. Metastatic tumours to the conjunctiva: report of 10 cases. Br J Ophthalmol. 1996;80(1):5–8.
59. Varde MA, Biswas J. Ocular surface tumors. Oman J Ophthalmol. 2009;2(1):1–2.
60. Damato B, Coupland SE. Management of conjunctival melanoma. Expert Rev Anticancer Ther. 2009; 9(9):1227–39.

61. Pathologists TRCo. Dataset for the histopathological reporting of conjunctival melanoma and melanosis 2007. Available from: http://www.rcpath.org/Resources/RCPath/MigratedResources/Documents/G/g054datasetconjunctivalmelanoma-finaloct07.pdf.. Accessed 01.05.2014.
62. Esmaeli B. Ophthamic oncology. Pollok RE, editor. Springer Science and Business Media, LLC 2011.
63. Missotten GS, de Wolff-Rouendaal D, de Keizer RJ. Screening for conjunctival melanoma metastasis: literature review. Bull Soc Belge Ophtalmol. 2007; 306:23–30.
64. Missotten GS, Keijser S, De Keizer RJ, De Wolff-Rouendaal D. Conjunctival melanoma in the Netherlands: a nationwide study. Invest Ophthalmol Vis Sci. 2005;46(1):75–82.
65. Esmaeli B, Wang X, Youssef A, Gershenwald JE. Patterns of regional and distant metastasis in patients with conjunctival melanoma: experience at a cancer center over four decades. Ophthalmology. 2001;108(11):2101–5.
66. De Potter P, Shields CL, Shields JA, Menduke H. Clinical predictive factors for development of recurrence and metastasis in conjunctival melanoma: a review of 68 cases. Br J Ophthalmol. 1993;77(10):624–30.
67. Pfeiffer ML, Savar A, Esmaeli B. Sentinel lymph node biopsy for eyelid and conjunctival tumors: what have we learned in the past decade? Ophthal Plast Reconstr Surg. 2013;29(1):57–62.
68. Shields CL, Shields JA. Tumors of the conjunctiva and cornea. Surv Ophthalmol. 2004;49(1):3–24.
69. Shields CL, Shields JA, Gunduz K, Cater J, Mercado GV, Gross N, et al. Conjunctival melanoma: risk factors for recurrence, exenteration, metastasis, and death in 150 consecutive patients. Arch Ophthalmol. 2000;118(11):1497–507.
70. Shields CL, Markowitz JS, Belinsky I, Schwartzstein H, George NS, Lally SE, et al. Conjunctival melanoma: outcomes based on tumor origin in 382 consecutive cases. Ophthalmology. 2011;118(2):389–95 e1–2.
71. Werschnik C, Lommatzsch PK. Long-term follow-up of patients with conjunctival melanoma. Am J Clin Oncol. 2002;25(3):248–55.
72. Hirst LW. Randomized controlled trial of topical mitomycin C for ocular surface squamous neoplasia: early resolution. Ophthalmology. 2007;114(5):976–82.
73. Kurli M, Finger PT. Topical mitomycin chemotherapy for conjunctival malignant melanoma and primary acquired melanosis with atypia: 12 years' experience. Graefe's Arch Clin Exp Ophthalmol Albrecht Graefes Arch Klin Exp Ophthalmol. 2005;243(11):1108–14.
74. Lichtinger A, Pe'er J, Frucht-Pery J, Solomon A. Limbal stem cell deficiency after topical mitomycin C therapy for primary acquired melanosis with atypia. Ophthalmology. 2010;117(3):431–7.
75. Schallenberg M, Niederdraing N, Steuhl KP, Meller D. Topical Mitomycin C as a therapy of conjunctival tumours. Der Ophthalmol: Z Dtsch Ophthalmol Ges. 2008;105(8):777–84.
76. Damato B, Coupland SE. An audit of conjunctival melanoma treatment in Liverpool. Eye. 2009;23(4):801–9.
77. Pe'er J, Frucht-Pery J. The treatment of primary acquired melanosis (PAM) with atypia by topical Mitomycin C. Am J Ophthalmol. 2005;139(2): 229–34.
78. Groh MJ, Holbach LM, Kuhnel B, Conway RM, Naumann GO. Management of conjunctival malignant melanoma associated with primary acquired melanosis (PAM) using 0.02% mitomycin C eye-drops. Der Ophthalmol: Z Dtsch Ophthalmol Ges. 2003;100(9):708–12.
79. Stannard CE, Sealy GR, Hering ER, Pereira SB, Knowles R, Hill JC. Malignant melanoma of the eyelid and palpebral conjunctiva treated with iodine-125 brachytherapy. Ophthalmology. 2000; 107(5):951–8.
80. Wuestemeyer H, Sauerwein W, Meller D, Chauvel P, Schueler A, Steuhl KP, et al. Proton radiotherapy as an alternative to exenteration in the management of extended conjunctival melanoma. Graefe's Arch Clin Exp Ophthalmol Albrecht Graefes Arch Klin Exp Ophthalmol. 2006;244(4):438–46.
81. Finger PT, Sedeek RW, Chin KJ. Topical interferon alfa in the treatment of conjunctival melanoma and primary acquired melanosis complex. Am J Ophthalmol. 2008;145(1):124–9.
82. Herold TR, Hintschich C. Interferon alpha for the treatment of melanocytic conjunctival lesions. Graefe's Arch Clin Exp Ophthalmol Albrecht Graefes Arch Klin Exp Ophthalmol. 2010;248(1):111–5.
83. Griewank KG, Westekemper H, Murali R, Mach M, Schilling B, Wiesner T, et al. Conjunctival melanomas harbor BRAF and NRAS mutations and copy number changes similar to cutaneous and mucosal melanomas. Clin Cancer Res: Off J Am Assoc Cancer Res. 2013;19(12):3143–52.
84. Gear H, Williams H, Kemp EG, Roberts F. BRAF mutations in conjunctival melanoma. Invest Ophthalmol Vis Sci. 2004;45(8):2484–8.
85. Pahlitzsch M, Bertelmann E, Mai C. Conjunctival melanoma and BRAF inhibitor therapy. J Clin Exp Ophthalmol. 2014;5(1):322. doi: 10.4172/2155-9570.1000322.
86. Paridaens AD, Minassian DC, McCartney AC, Hungerford JL. Prognostic factors in primary malignant melanoma of the conjunctiva: a clinicopathological study of 256 cases. Br J Ophthalmol. 1994;78(4):252–9.
87. Lommatzsch PK, Lommatzsch RE, Kirsch I, Fuhrmann P. Therapeutic outcome of patients suffering from malignant melanomas of the conjunctiva. Br J Ophthalmol. 1990;74(10):615–9.
88. Tuomaala S, Eskelin S, Tarkkanen A, Kivela T. Population-based assessment of clinical characteristics predicting outcome of conjunctival melanoma in whites. Invest Ophthalmol Vis Sci. 2002;43(11): 3399–408.
89. Breslow A. Thickness, cross-sectional areas and depth of invasion in the prognosis of cutaneous melanoma. Ann Surg. 1970;172(5):902–8.

90. Gershenwald JE, Soong SJ, Balch CM, American Joint Committee on Cancer Melanoma Staging C. 2010 TNM staging system for cutaneous melanoma… and beyond. Ann Surg Oncol. 2010;17(6):1475–7.
91. Edge SB. American Joint Committee on Cancer. AJCC cancer staging manual. 7th ed. New York: Springer; 2010. xiv, 648 p.
92. AJCC. American Joint Committee Cancer Staging Manual. 7th ed. New York: Springer; 2010.

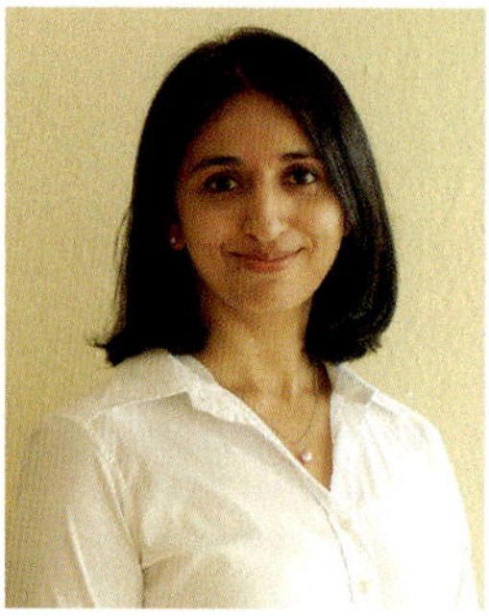

**Meghana Anika Varde** Meghana Anika Varde received her medical degree from the University of Frankfurt am Main, Germany, and did her residency in ophthalmology at the Universities of Tübingen, Erlangen and Kiel. She completed a fellowship in Oculoplastics and Trauma at SankaraNethralaya Eye Hospital in Chennai, India.

Dr. Varde has been working as a consultant at the KlinikumNordstadt in Hannover, Germany, for the past 6 years. Her main interests are Oculoplastics as well as Traumatology and globe reconstruction.

She is a full member of the European Society of Ophthalmic Plastic and Reconstructive Surgery and teaches Oculoplastic Surgery at Acha Eye Hospital in Cameroon. She is also examiner for the European Board of Ophthalmology.

# 48 Merkel Cell Carcinoma (Cutaneous Neuroendocrine Carcinoma)

Meghana Anika Varde

## Introduction and Epidemiology

Merkel cell carcinoma (MCC) is a rare, highly aggressive malignant tumour of the skin. The tumour is fast growing and tends to metastasize regionally and systemically. It usually presents in the white, elderly population, especially in immunosuppressed individuals. More than half of the MCCs are found in light-exposed areas of the head and neck.

The face is involved in about 27 % and the eyelids in 2.5–10 % of all cases [1, 2]. The upper eyelid seems to be more often affected than the lower lid [3]. MCC represents an uncommon tumour in the eyelid. In a population-based study from Florida, it represented only 2.9 % of all non-basal cell and non-squamous cell carcinomas of the lid (both accounting for about 90 % of eyelid malignancies) [4].

Incidence of MCC is stated at 0.1–0.3 per 100,000 per year [5] although in the last years, an increase in incidence to 0.44/100,000 has been recorded in the USA [6]. Ninety-three percent of the tumours arise in white-skinned patients and only 1.2 % in blacks. Male preponderance for MCC in general has been reported, although in the periocular region, females seem to be affected more often [7]. The tumour is mainly found in patients above 65 years of age [8].

## Aetiology and Pathogenesis

MCC is thought to be derived from Merkel cells, which are touch-sensitivity-associated cells located in the dermo-epidermal junction of the skin. In the eyelid, these cells are mainly found near the lashes, associated with touch receptors [7]. The origin of the cells has been unclear until recently, since they exhibit neuroendocrine and epidermal properties. However, a recent study suggests the development of Merkel cells from epidermal stem cells rather than neural crest progenitors [9]. Interestingly, MCC is located almost exclusively in the dermis and subcutis, although Merkel cells are epithelial cells. This might suggest the cellular origin of this tumour being in dermal progenitor cells rather than in the cell itself [10].

Recent research suggests a DNA virus named Merkel cell polyomavirus (MCV) to be a causative factor for the development of MCC. Integration of a part of the viral genome has been found in 80 % of MCC [11].

MCC is found mainly in whites on UV-exposed skin and incidence is higher in Australia. Moreover, patients receiving PUVA therapy (psoralen + UVA) for psoriasis have been found

M.A. Varde, MS, FEBO, FMRF (Oculoplasty)
Department of Ophthalmology, Klinikum Region Hannover, Haltenhoffstr. 41, Hannover 30167, Germany
e-mail: thelivingcompass@gmail.com


B. Mukherjee, H. Yuen (eds.), *Emergencies of the Orbit and Adnexa*,
DOI 10.1007/978-81-322-1807-4_48

to present with a higher incidence of MCC [12]. MCC incidence is also higher, and age of onset is lower in immunocompromised individuals following organ transplants, HIV infection or haematolymphoid diseases [13]. Complete regression of metastatic Merkel cell carcinoma has been described [14]. MCC is a dermal tumour and might not be directly related to UV skin damage, but rather to UV-induced downregulation of immune responses [15].

## Clinical Presentation and Macroscopic Differential Diagnosis

Merkel cell carcinoma presents commonly as red or violaceous firm, painless nodule that can grow rapidly within weeks to months (Fig. 48.1). The surface is often smooth and shiny and ulceration is uncommon [15]. Necrosis can occur in very fast-growing tumours. If the eyelid is involved, the margin is predisposed for the development of these tumours corresponding to the distribution of Merkel cells in the lid in the outer root layer of the cilia [16]. Growth is usually as a nodule, inducing a variable amount of cilia loss and exhibiting telangiectasia. Satellite lesions can occur.

Macroscopic differential diagnoses include chalazion, basal cell carcinoma, sebaceous gland carcinoma, cavernous haemagioma, pyogenic granuloma and metastasis [17, 18].

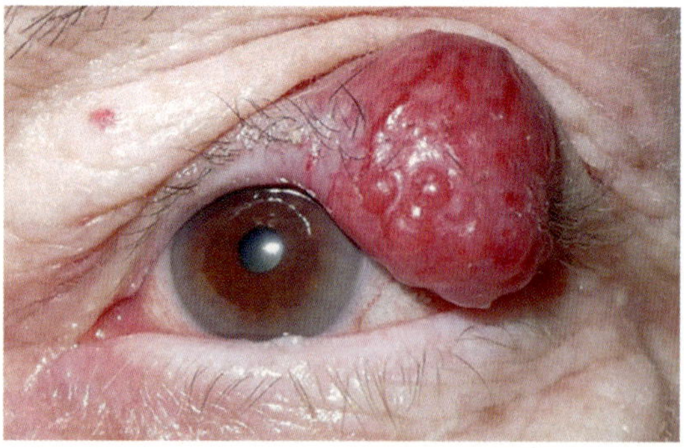

**Fig. 48.1** Merkel cell carcinoma of the *left upper* lid in an 87-year-old patient. Nodular appearance, shiny, red surface and dilated vessels

## Histopathology and Microscopic Differential Diagnosis

Histopathology shows a solid, sometimes septate tumour in the dermis with uniform, small, monomorphous cells with basophilic cytoplasm and large, round, clear nuclei with prominent nucleoli. Many mitoses can be seen throughout. The tumour is characteristically separated from the overlying epidermis by a free zone of uninvolved dermis [10]. Sometimes there are pseudorosettes and signs of high cell turnover such as necrosis and apoptosis. Lymphocytic and plasmacellular infiltrates commonly surround the lesion [18] (Fig. 48.2).

Microscopic differential diagnoses are mainly lymphoma, metastasis of small cell (neuroendocrine) carcinoma of the lung and amelanotic melanoma. As discussed above, the tumour cells exhibit epithelial and neuroendocrine histologic properties, which are represented in the positive immunohistochemical (IHC) staining which is usually positive for low-molecular-weight cytokeratin (cytokeratin 20), neuroendocrine markers (neuron-specific enolase, synaptophysin) and neurofilament protein. Differentiation from amelanotic melanoma is with S100 and HMB-45 stains and from metastatic small cell carcinoma is with thyroid transcription factor-1 for which MCC is usually negative [3]. Differentiation from cutaneous non-Hodgkin lymphoma can be made through the positive staining for cytokeratin and negative CD45 staining [19].

## Classification and Staging

Staging and grouping of MCCs in general are done according to the ninth edition of the American Joint Committee on Cancer (AJCC) on the basis of Lemos et al. [20] wherein the eyelid is not included. Eyelid carcinomas are staged by the system designed by AJCC [21].

Tumours are grouped by their Tumour-node-metastasis (TNM) status into groups that define the treatment or enrolment into clinical studies as in cutaneous melanoma.

The staging of MCC in the eyelid and general skin differs to a significant extent because the

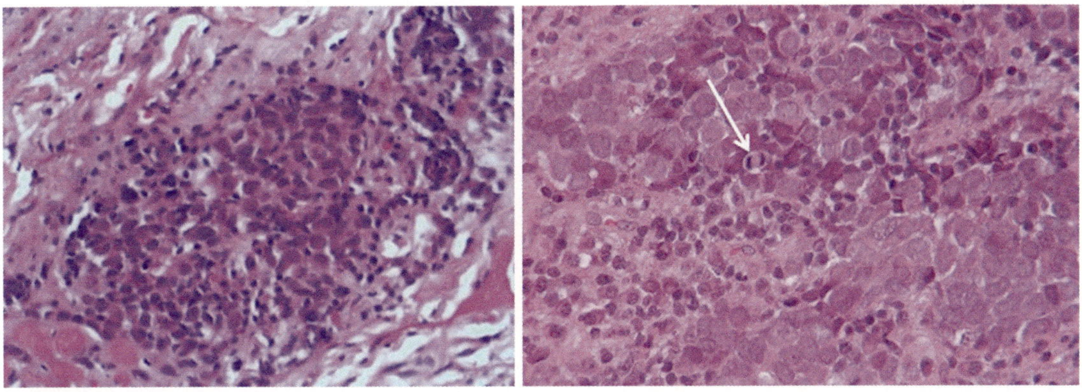

**Fig. 48.2** Merkel cell carcinoma H&E staining. Large monomorphous cells with basophilic cytoplasm and lymphocytic infiltrate. *Arrow* showing mitosis

proximity of the eyelid skin to other crucial structures (muscle, tarsal plate) renders it special treatment, and smaller tumours have greater impact on prognosis.

Although *SLNB* is generally recommended for skin MCCs, the use of it in eyelid Merkel cell carcinomas is still under debate. Histopathological evaluation of the lymph nodes (via SLNB or elective lymph node resection such as neck dissection or parotid gland dissection in case of eyelid tumours) has been shown to significantly improve prognostic accuracy in MCC [20] and that around one third of patients undergoing only clinical nodal evaluation are understaged because occult microscopic nodal involvement is overlooked [22]. Currently, some authors recommend SLNB for Merkel cell carcinoma of any size, mainly for prognostic purposes [23, 24]. Distant metastases of MCCs have been found in node-negative patients, so that treatment of occult nodal disease might not necessarily mean a better prognosis in eyelid MCC.

Because of the rare occurrence, there is no consensus statement as to the preoperative metastatic workup of patients with MCC. In general, careful clinical examination and palpation of the regional lymph nodes (i.e. preauricular and parotid, cervical and submandibular) are recommended and as per clinical judgement ultrasonography of the lymph node basins and CT or MRI of the chest and abdomen. CT of the chest may be required to rule out neuroendocrine small cell carcinoma of the lung as differential diagnosis might be difficult even with IHC. Abdominal sonography and chest X-ray may be performed, although with limited sensitivity and specificity as discussed in the chapter for cutaneous melanoma. SLNB as stated above is currently controversial. PET/CT can accurately detect Merkel cell carcinoma and might be an adjunct in preoperative assessment [25]. It is to be noted that in large prospective studies of MCC, 27–31 % of patients presented with nodal disease [1, 20]; hence primary nodal involvement has to be taken into account when evaluating this aggressive tumour.

There are no serum markers specific for MCC as of now.

## Treatment

### Surgical Treatment

Surgical excision is the standard treatment in Merkel cell carcinomas. In locations other than the face, surgical margins of 2–3 cm are recommended [26–28]. In the eyelid, margins are not specified, and some surgeons advocate micrographically controlled surgery, although this might miss some of the satellite lesions for which this tumour is known. Since MCC is radiosensitive, adjuvant treatment with radiotherapy might be advocated in cases that have undergone micrographic excision [29]. Currently, most eyelid MCCs are treated without irradiation [15].

Local recurrences should be excised with the same curative concepts.

In case of lymph node involvement, resection of regional lymphatics is recommended [30], combined with adjuvant radiotherapy.

The excision of distant metastases can be considered if associated morbidity is acceptable, in combination with radiotherapy and chemotherapy and for palliative purposes.

## Radiotherapy

Radiotherapy can be administered as adjuvant treatment for excised primary or recurrent tumours of the eyelid. The dose should be ≥50 Gy [31]. A significant decrease in local recurrence following adjuvant radiotherapy has been demonstrated; unfortunately it does not seem to have an effect on overall survival [32–34].

Radiotherapy is recommended as adjuvant treatment following regional lymphadenectomy with a dose of 50 Gy.

In cases of macroscopic (residual) tumour or metastasis, the recommended radiation dose is ≥55 Gy [28].

### Medical Treatment

Medical treatment has so far been limited to the treatment of systemic disease, adjuvant treatment in locally advanced disease and in palliative situations. The treatment is based on the *chemotherapy* used for small cell lung cancer, but a standardised chemotherapeutic regimen does not exist. Remission occurs partially in about 70–75 % of cases, and complete remission is seen in 40 %, although this does not seem to have an influence on survival [15, 35]. The significant toxicity of these substances has to be weighed against the expected benefit and the patient's quality of life.

Future treatment strategies are targeted towards MCV-positive Merkel cell tumours. Immune response alteration might have a benefit in localised tumours. In one case report of an MCC treated with intralesional *Interferon* $\alpha_{-2b}$, the tumour responded well [36], but in another report of two cases with MCV-positive disseminated disease, systemic treatment with interferon did not alter the course of the disease and had severe side effects [37]. Nevertheless, further research regarding the role of MCV in the treatment of MCC is currently under way. Intralesional *tumour necrosis factor alpha* (TNF-α) showed regression of a tumour in one case report [38].

## Prognosis and Follow-Up

Merkel cell carcinoma is an aggressive, potentially fatal tumour with a high propensity for local recurrence as well as regional and distant spread. Relative 10-year survival rates were dependent on age, sex and tumour stage in a large, population-based study. Localised disease had a rate of 71 %, regional spread disease of 48 % and distant metastatic disease of 20 %, respectively [1]. Another study showed relative tumour-related survival in 5 years to be 54 % [20].

Unfavourable prognostic markers in MCC are male sex, larger tumour size and disseminated disease. Another negative prognostic marker seems to be high proliferation rate indexed by more than 50 % of Ki67-positive cells in histopathology [39].

Interestingly, spontaneous regression of Merkel cell carcinomas in the skin and in the eyelid have been reported [40]. These may occur following reinstatement of immunocompetence or, in the case of the lid tumours, following incisional or incomplete excisional biopsy [3]. Even metastatic disease has been shown to exhibit rapid, spontaneous regression [41]. In 15–20 % of metastatic MCC, no primary tumour could be diagnosed in one series, underlining the possibility that spontaneous regression of these tumours is more frequent than expected [42].

There is no consensus regarding the follow-up frequency of Merkel cell carcinoma patients. German guidelines recommend 3-month metastatic screening in the first, thereafter every 6 months for 5 years in the absence of clinical evidence for metastasis. This comprises clinical and ultrasonographic evaluation of the regional lymph node basins as well as screening for lung or liver metastases once a year [43].

Merkel cell carcinoma of the eyelid is a rare and potentially lethal tumour, which shows rapid progression. The prognosis is mainly dependent on the tumour size and stage. Early diagnosis and treatment are therefore mandatory in the management of these tumours. MCCs are mainly found in the white, elderly population, especially in immunocompromised individuals. Treatment involves micrographically controlled surgical excision and adjuvant radiotherapeutic treatment. Sentinel lymph node biopsy is advised if possible in all cases. The discovery of Merkel cell polyomavirus associated with MCC development is providing hope for the development of newer treatment tactics.

## References


1. Albores-Saavedra J, Batich K, Chable-Montero F, Sagy N, Schwartz AM, Henson DE. Merkel cell carcinoma demographics, morphology, and survival based on 3870 cases: a population based study. J Cutan Pathol. 2010;37(1):20–7.
2. Rice Jr RD, Chonkich GD, Thompson KS, Chase DR. Merkel cell tumor of the head and neck. Five new cases with literature review. Arch Otolaryngol Head Neck Surg. 1993;119(7):782–6.
3. Missotten GS, de Wolff-Rouendaal D, de Keizer RJ. Merkel cell carcinoma of the eyelid review of the literature and report of patients with Merkel cell carcinoma showing spontaneous regression. Ophthalmology. 2008;115(1):195–201.
4. Margo CE, Mulla ZD. Malignant tumors of the eyelid: a population-based study of non-basal cell and non-squamous cell malignant neoplasms. Arch Ophthalmol. 1998;116(2):195–8.
5. Goessling W, McKee PH, Mayer RJ. Merkel cell carcinoma. J Clin Oncol Off J Am Soc Clin Oncol. 2002;20(2):588–98.
6. Hodgson NC. Merkel cell carcinoma: changing incidence trends. J Surg Oncol. 2005;89(1):1–4.
7. Kivela T, Tarkkanen A. The Merkel cell and associated neoplasms in the eyelids and periocular region. Surv Ophthalmol. 1990;35(3):171–87.
8. Agelli M, Clegg LX. Epidemiology of primary Merkel cell carcinoma in the United States. J Am Acad Dermatol. 2003;49(5):832–41.
9. Van Keymeulen A, Mascre G, Youseff KK, Harel I, Michaux C, De Geest N, et al. Epidermal progenitors give rise to Merkel cells during embryonic development and adult homeostasis. J Cell Biol. 2009;187(1): 91–100.
10. Proenca R, Santos MF, Cunha-Vaz JG. Primary neuroendocrine carcinoma of the eyelid, immunohistochemical and ultrastructural study. Int Ophthalmol. 1990;14(4):251–8.
11. Feng H, Shuda M, Chang Y, Moore PS. Clonal integration of a polyomavirus in human Merkel cell carcinoma. Science. 2008;319(5866):1096–100.
12. Lunder EJ, Stern RS. Merkel-cell carcinomas in patients treated with methoxsalen and ultraviolet A radiation. N Engl J Med. 1998;339(17):1247–8.
13. Zwald FO, Brown M. Skin cancer in solid organ transplant recipients: advances in therapy and management: part II. Management of skin cancer in solid organ transplant recipients. J Am Acad Dermatol. 2011;65(2):263–79; quiz 80.
14. Wooff JC, Trites JR, Walsh NM, Bullock MJ. Complete spontaneous regression of metastatic merkel cell carcinoma: a case report and review of the literature. Am J Dermatopathol. 2010;32(6):614–7.
15. Schrama D, Ugurel S, Becker JC. Merkel cell carcinoma: recent insights and new treatment options. Curr Opin Oncol. 2012;24(2):141–9.
16. May CA, Osterland I. Merkel cell distribution in the human eyelid. Eur J Histochem EJH. 2013;57(4), e33.
17. Heath M, Jaimes N, Lemos B, Mostaghimi A, Wang LC, Penas PF, et al. Clinical characteristics of Merkel cell carcinoma at diagnosis in 195 patients: the AEIOU features. J Am Acad Dermatol. 2008;58(3):375–81.
18. Rohrbach JM, Lieb WE. Tumoren des Auges und seiner Adnexe. Stuttgart: Schattauer; 1998.
19. Chu PG, Weiss LM. Modern immunohistochemistry. 2nd ed. Cambridge: Cambridge University Press; 2014.
20. Lemos BD, Storer BE, Iyer JG, Phillips JL, Bichakjian CK, Fang LC, et al. Pathologic nodal evaluation improves prognostic accuracy in Merkel cell carcinoma: analysis of 5823 cases as the basis of the first consensus staging system. J Am Acad Dermatol. 2010;63(5):751–61.
21. Edge SB, American Joint Committee on Cancer. AJCC cancer staging manual. 7th ed. New York: Springer; 2010. xiv, 648 p.
22. Gupta SG, Wang LC, Penas PF, Gellenthin M, Lee SJ, Nghiem P. Sentinel lymph node biopsy for evaluation and treatment of patients with Merkel cell carcinoma: the Dana-Farber experience and meta-analysis of the literature. Arch Dermatol. 2006;142(6):685–90.
23. Pfeiffer ML, Savar A, Esmaeli B. Sentinel lymph node biopsy for eyelid and conjunctival tumors: what have we learned in the past decade? Ophthal Plast Reconstr Surg. 2013;29(1):57–62.
24. Herbert HM, Sun MT, Selva D, Fernando B, Saleh GM, Beaconsfield M, et al. Merkel cell carcinoma of the eyelid: management and prognosis. JAMA Ophthalmol. 2014;132(2):197–204.
25. Hui KH, Pfeiffer ML, Esmaeli B. Value of positron emission tomography/computed tomography in diagnosis and staging of primary ocular and orbital tumors. Saudi J Ophthalmol Off J Saudi Ophthalmol Soc. 2012;26(4):365–71.
26. Kukko H, Bohling T, Koljonen V, Tukiainen E, Haglund C, Pokhrel A, et al. Merkel cell carcinoma – a population-based epidemiological study in Finland

with a clinical series of 181 cases. Eur J Cancer. 2012;48(5):737–42.
27. Kokoska ER, Kokoska MS, Collins BT, Stapleton DR, Wade TP. Early aggressive treatment for Merkel cell carcinoma improves outcome. Am J Surg. 1997; 174(6):688–93.
28. Becker JC, Assaf C, Vordermark D, Reske SN, Hense J, Dettenborn T, Seitz O, Grabbe SJ. Brief S2k guidelines-Merkel cell carcinoma Dtsch Dermatol Ges. 2013;11 Suppl 3:29–36, 31–8. doi: 10.1111/ddg.12015_6.
29. Levy RM, Hanke CW. Mohs micrographic surgery: facts and controversies. Clin Dermatol. 2010;28(3): 269–74.
30. Fields RC, Busam KJ, Chou JF, Panageas KS, Pulitzer MP, Kraus DH, et al. Recurrence and survival in patients undergoing sentinel lymph node biopsy for merkel cell carcinoma: analysis of 153 patients from a single institution. Ann Surg Oncol. 2011;18(9): 2529–37.
31. Plunkett TA, Subrumanian R, Leslie MD, Harper PG. Management of Merkel cell carcinoma. Expert Rev Anticancer Ther. 2001;1(3):441–5.
32. Meeuwissen JA, Bourne RG, Kearsley JH. The importance of postoperative radiation therapy in the treatment of Merkel cell carcinoma. Int J Radiat Oncol Biol Phys. 1995;31(2):325–31.
33. Gillenwater AM, Hessel AC, Morrison WH, Burgess M, Silva EG, Roberts D, et al. Merkel cell carcinoma of the head and neck: effect of surgical excision and radiation on recurrence and survival. Arch Otolaryngol Head Neck Surg. 2001;127(2): 149–54.
34. Lewis KG, Weinstock MA, Weaver AL, Otley CC. Adjuvant local irradiation for Merkel cell carcinoma. Arch Dermatol. 2006;142(6):693–700.
35. Tai PT, Yu E, Winquist E, Hammond A, Stitt L, Tonita J, et al. Chemotherapy in neuroendocrine/Merkel cell carcinoma of the skin: case series and review of 204 cases. J Clin Oncol Off J Am Soc Clin Oncol. 2000;18(12):2493–9.
36. Durand JM, Weiller C, Richard MA, Portal I, Mongin M. Treatment of Merkel cell tumor with interferon-alpha-2b. Br J Dermatol. 1991;124(5):509.
37. Biver-Dalle C, Nguyen T, Touze A, Saccomani C, Penz S, Cunat-Peultier S, et al. Use of interferon-alpha in two patients with Merkel cell carcinoma positive for Merkel cell polyomavirus. Acta Oncol. 2011;50(3):479–80.
38. Ito Y, Kawamura K, Miura T, Ueda K, Onodera H, Takahashi H, et al. Merkel cell carcinoma. A successful treatment with tumor necrosis factor. Arch Dermatol. 1989;125(8):1093–5.
39. Llombart B, Monteagudo C, Lopez-Guerrero JA, Carda C, Jorda E, Sanmartin O, et al. Clinicopathological and immunohistochemical analysis of 20 cases of Merkel cell carcinoma in search of prognostic markers. Histopathology. 2005;46(6):622–34.
40. Connelly TJ, Cribier B, Brown TJ, Yanguas I. Complete spontaneous regression of Merkel cell carcinoma: a review of the 10 reported cases. Dermatol Surg Off Publ Am Soc Dermatol Surg [et al]. 2000;26(9):853–6.
41. Connelly TJ, Kowalcyk AP. Another case of spontaneous regression of Merkel cell (neuroendocrine) carcinoma. Dermatol Surg Off Publ Am Soc Dermatol Surg [et al]. 1997;23(7):588–90.
42. Boyle F, Pendlebury S, Bell D. Further insights into the natural history and management of primary cutaneous neuroendocrine (Merkel cell) carcinoma. Int J Radiat Oncol Biol Phys. 1995;31(2):315–23.
43. Hauschild A, Garbe C. Cutaneous neuroendocrine carcinoma (Merkel cell carcinoma). Quality Assurance Committee of the German Society of Dermatology and the Professional Organization of German Dermatologists e. V. Der Hautarzt; Zeitschrift fur Dermatologie, Venerologie, und verwandte Gebiete. 1998;48 Suppl 1:S27–9.

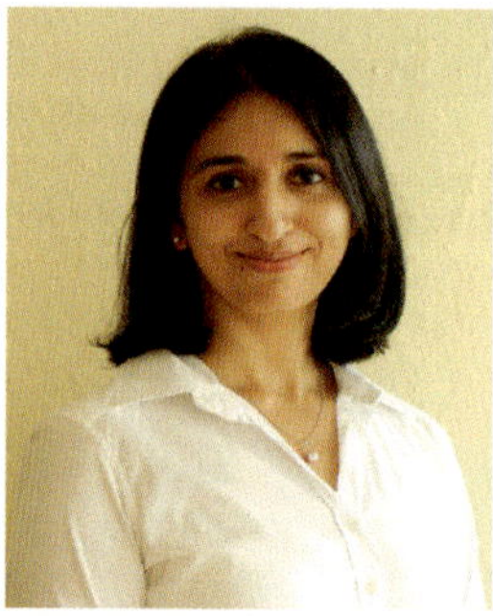

**Meghana Anika Varde** Meghana Anika Varde received her medical degree from the University of Frankfurt am Main, Germany, and did her residency in ophthalmology at the Universities of Tübingen, Erlangen and Kiel. She completed a fellowship in Oculoplastics and Trauma at Sankara Nethralaya Eye Hospital in Chennai, India.

Dr. Varde has been working as a consultant at the KlinikumNordstadt in Hannover, Germany, for the past 6 years. Her main interests are Oculoplastics as well as Traumatology and globe reconstruction.

She is a full member of the European Society of Ophthalmic Plastic and Reconstructive Surgery and teaches Oculoplastic Surgery at Acha Eye Hospital in Cameroon. She is also examiner for the European Board of Ophthalmology.

# 49 Acute Presentation of Vascular Lesions in the Orbit

David H. Verity, Usha R. Kim, and Geoffrey E. Rose

## Introduction

Orbital vascular disease can present with acute symptoms and, if untreated, can lead to loss of visual functions. In general, such a presentation is due to orbital haemorrhage, acute arteriovenous shunting or subacute thrombosis with resultant local changes in orbital perfusion. On occasion, the clinical presentation heralds the presence of previously unrecognised disease, whereas in others, it occurs against a background of a known diagnosis of vascular disorder.

## Pathogenesis

Visual loss occurs when the elevation of orbital pressure causes decrease in central retinal artery perfusion or compression of the long and short posterior ciliary arteries resulting in retina and optic nerve ischaemia, respectively. Increased orbital pressure can also cause vision loss secondary to central retinal vein occlusion or compressive optic neuropathy [1].

D.H. Verity, MD, MA, FRCOphth (✉)
Adnexal Service, Moorfields Eye Hospital, 162 City Road, London EC1V 2PD, UK
e-mail: david.verity@moorfields.nhs.uk

U.R. Kim, DO, DNB
Orbit, Oculoplasty & Ocular Oncology, Aravind Eye Hospital, 1, Anna Nagar, Madurai 625 020, Tamil Nadu, India
e-mail: usha@aravind.org

G.E. Rose, MS, DSc, MRCP, FRCS, FRCOphth
Orbital, Lacrimal and Oculoplastic Service, Moorfields Eye Hospital NHS Trust, London, UK
e-mail: geoff.rose@moorfields.nhs.uk

## Clinical Features

Typical symptoms and signs of an acute vascular event within the orbit include sudden onset of proptosis, usually occurring overnight (Fig. 49.1), painful periorbital oedema, decreased or double vision and nausea or vomiting. Any pathology at the orbital apex leads to impairment of the venous drainage manifesting as episcleral venous congestion and a secondary rise in intraocular

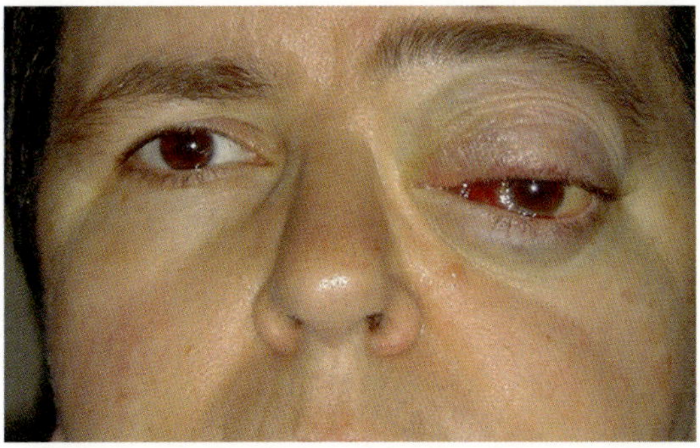

**Fig. 49.1** Sudden onset of proptosis and partial visual loss due to acute haemorrhage in a patient with a mixed orbital venous-lymphatic malformation


B. Mukherjee, H. Yuen (eds.), *Emergencies of the Orbit and Adnexa*,
DOI 10.1007/978-81-322-1807-4_49

pressure. If acute extravascular haemorrhage or intravascular pathology occurs at the orbital apex, embarrassment of the posteriorly directed venous drainage occurs and manifests as a episcleral venous congestion and a secondary rise in intraocular pressure. Periocular bruising appears after a delay, which depends on the depth of the haemorrhage within the orbit. The rapid expansion of the intraorbital volume and sudden stretching of the extraocular muscles can lead to severe pain, nausea and vomiting; nausea and vomiting are mediated through the oculo-cardiac vagal reflex and are particularly troublesome in children, in whom the symptoms can be incorrectly attributed to presumed intracranial injury (a scenario that can also occur following blowout fractures in children; see Chap. 14). In cases of significant arteriovenous shunting, the intraocular pressure will often also show an abnormally high variation during the cardiac cycle (as high as 10 mmHg), and, when suspected, this sign should actively be elicited on applanation tonometry. A secondary effect of such vascular congestion and fluid leakage is an increased intercellular fluid volume, resulting in oedematous extraocular muscles (manifest as a global reduction in eye movements) and caruncular or subconjunctival oedema. Very rarely, frank bleeding can occur from the orbit and on occasion patients can be aware of a sudden onset of a 'pulsation' or 'rushing sound' within their head in high-flow carotid-cavernous fistula.

## Vascular Lesions of the Orbit

### Acute Orbital Haemorrhage [2–6]

Spontaneous haemorrhage from a normal orbital vessel is exceptionally rare. It may occur during an acute increase in the orbital venous pressure during a significant Valsalva manoeuvre (e.g. during delivery, exertional sports, such as weightlifting, severe vomiting or strangulation). Bleeding can also occur following an orbital fracture if the small vessels which perforate the orbital walls are sheared; in some cases, the site of blow can be outside the orbit (particularly with frontal fractures), and this should be considered where there is loss of vision in the absence of direct injury to the globe.

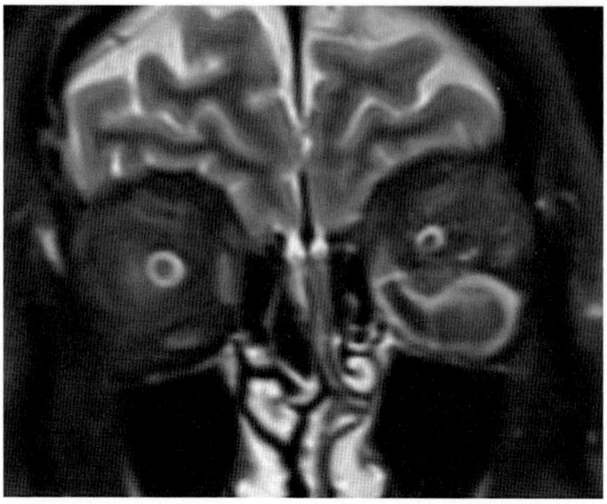

**Fig. 49.2** T2-weighted MR showing typical appearance of an acute haemorrhage, biassed inferolaterally within the left orbit, it having a hyperintense 'capsule' surrounding the lower signal blood products

In contrast to the rarity of orbital haemorrhage from healthy vessels, bleeding from fragile vessels in the elderly patient is relatively common (and the most common cause of all orbital haemorrhages). Associated risk factors are the concurrent use of anti-platelet agents (aspirin and other nonsteroidal anti-inflammatory agents, warfarin and clopidogrel), long-standing (or uncontrolled) hypertension and chronic diabetes in younger patients. In these patients, a precipitating event, such as a severe bout of coughing, can result in a rapid onset of unilateral proptosis, usually with minimal reduction of vision or ocular ductions. Imaging with CT typically identifies such spontaneous haemorrhages in the posterior half of the infero-temporal quadrant of the orbit, these sometimes described as having a 'beached whale' configuration (Fig. 49.2).

In both congenital and acquired orbital vascular lesions, haemorrhage usually occurs with low-pressure venous or venous-lymphatic ('lymphangioma') anomalies and not, as might be expected, with high-pressure (or high-flow) arteriovenous malformations or fistulas. In patients with orbital lymphangiomas, spontaneous haemorrhages tend to occur in the first decade

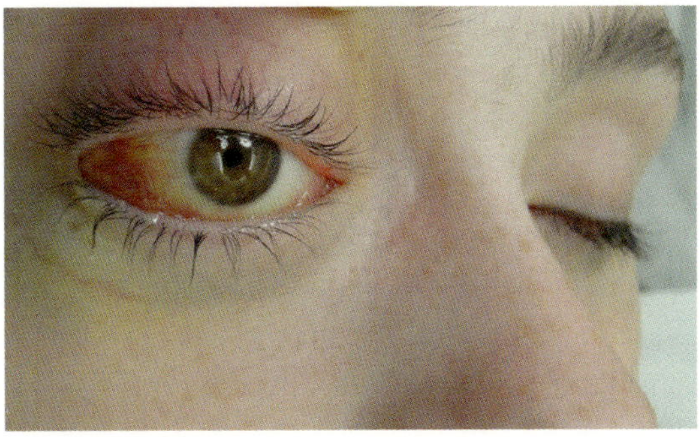

**Fig. 49.3** Preoperative image showing a 12-year-old patient with a known deep orbital venous-lymphatic malformation, presenting with sudden onset of proptosis and partial visual loss due to acute orbital haemorrhage

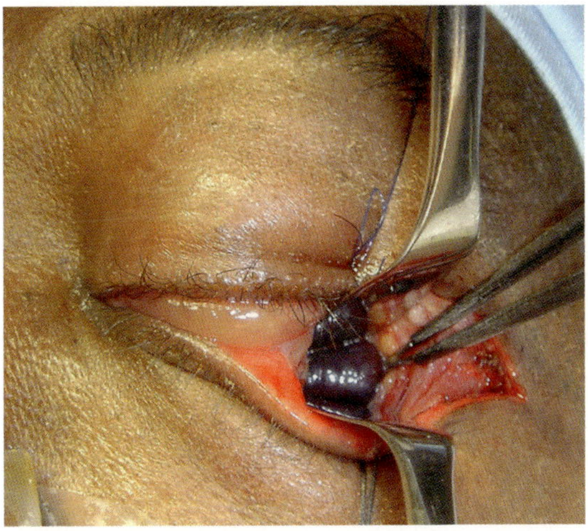

**Fig. 49.4** Acute orbital haemorrhage in a young male presenting with proptosis and early optic neuropathy; haemorrhage related to a bi-lobed varix was identified at surgery and the haemorrhage drained and venous anomaly excised

of life (Fig. 49.3) and seem to become less frequent with advancing years – this possibly occurring as a result of perivascular fibrosis in regions of prior haemorrhage. Infrequently, haemorrhage in adults can arise from a previously unrecognised venous anomaly (Fig. 49.4) and can also occur in orbital tumours undergoing necrosis.

Finally, spontaneous haemorrhage can also occur into the fibrous sheath around long-standing silicone implants (such as floor implants); again, such patients present with acute proptosis – and often with hyperglobus – but the appearance of periocular bruising can be delayed for up to a week.

Orbital haemorrhage following trauma [7] can be accidental or iatrogenic. Haemorrhage within the orbit may occur as a postoperative complication of orbital or periorbital surgeries, certain oculoplastic and lacrimal procedures, most commonly orbitotomies, fracture repairs, blepharoplasties and dacryocystorhinostomies [8, 9]. Retrobulbar haemorrhage occurs in less than 2 % of retrobulbar and peribulbar anaesthetic injections and may result in devastating visual loss if not promptly managed [10] (See Chap. 11).

Diagnosis is clinical and should be suspected in patients presenting with acute proptosis, rapid vision loss, ophthalmoplegia and relative afferent pupillary defect [11]. Evaluation and treatment must be prompt to ensure the best possible outcome. Determining the location of the haemorrhage and the etiologic mechanism is essential for providing the most appropriate intervention and requires a thorough understanding of the orbital and periorbital anatomy.

## Treatment of Spontaneous Orbital Haemorrhage [12–14]

Irrespective of the cause, the hydrostatic pressure generated by an arterial haemorrhage can be sufficient to arrest vascular perfusion at the orbital apex or in the peripapillary area, both carrying a dire visual prognosis. In the presence of dramatic proptosis, marked loss of eye movements and increased resistance to retropulsion, immediate treatment is imperative if visual function is to be saved. Treatment should be directed to drainage of the haemorrhage or creation of more space for the orbital contents by disrupting the orbital septum. Once a rupture of the globe has been excluded, intermittent firm pressure should be applied to tamponade the orbit until the bleeding subsides (due to vasospasm, platelet action and coagulation) and whilst secondary treatment is being organised. The firm tamponade should be released at regular intervals to permit optic nerve perfusion, and urgent arrangements made to drain the haemorrhage or reduce the intraorbital pressure by disrupting the orbital septum. In the case of acute postoperative haemorrhage, the incision should be widely reopened, and, with blunt dissection, the tissues are spread to permit release of the haematoma; the clinician should not be concerned if orbital fat prolapses from the incision, as this will result in further lowering of the orbital pressure.

One of two methods can generally be used to reduce the hydrostatic pressure in a tense orbit with progressive visual loss. Where the site of haemorrhage is known or suspected on clinical grounds – for example, in a patient with hypoglobus due to haemorrhage alongside an orbital roof fracture – direct drainage of the collection can readily be achieved. A long horizontal incision is placed in the corresponding upper or lower lid skin crease, and, using a pair of blunt-ended scissors, the deeper tissues and orbital fat pads are gently spread apart to release blood and tissue fluid. A pair of malleable retractors is placed in the cavity, and care should be taken to ensure that the majority of blood is aspirated, any actively bleeding vessels cauterised and consideration given to placing a surgical drain.

Where the focus of haemorrhage is not readily apparent, the intraorbital pressure can be released by performing a lateral canthotomy and wide lateral cantholysis, this releasing the orbital septum and thus lowering the intraorbital pressure. It is imperative to recognise that horizontal canthotomy alone leaves the septum intact and thus will have no effect on intraorbital pressure; in order to be effective, the orbital septum must be divided by at least 1–2 cm both upwards and downwards around the rim. An alternative approach is to perform a full-thickness perpendicular incision, about 1 cm in height, through the far lateral ends of both the upper and lower eyelids. In neither case should the incision be closed, since natural drainage is required in the event of further haemorrhage and both approaches typically heal with minimal visible scarring.

Acute intervention is seldom required with a spontaneous vasculopathic haemorrhage and most will reabsorb over many months. In the absence of failing vision due to a new-onset optic neuropathy, these patients can safely be monitored, although consideration should be given to repeat imaging and orbital drainage in the event of a deterioration of clinical signs. However, it should be noted that, despite arrest of the haemorrhage, it is common for proptosis to increase slightly over the first few weeks due to the hyperosmotic effect of blood breakdown products. Stopping all anti-platelet agents and anticoagulants will have no effect on the original haemorrhage, but may reduce the small risk of further haemorrhage.

Orbital haemorrhages from venous-lymphatic malformations tend to absorb gradually over a period of several months. However, where a large hematoma is causing severe proptosis, cosmetic disfigurement, diplopia and persistent optic neuropathy, surgical debulking of the lesion and/or sclerotherapy may be attempted.

Although blood cysts are readily exposed and drained, the risk of further bleeding can be reduced by excising the ochre membrane around the haemorrhage. In the case of persistent lymphatic malformations, occlusive sclerotherapy provides a useful alternative treatment: Large cysts are drained under radiographic control, and alcohol and another surface-active agent are sequentially injected to destroy the endothelial lining; firm occlusive pressure is then applied to allow the inflamed tissues to seal closed, and, in some techniques, a vacuum drain is placed. Although sclerotherapy will not eliminate large mixed venous-lymphatic malformations, residual lesions can be often removed intact.

## Acute Periorbital and Orbital Vascular Shunts [15–22]

Vascular shunts between arterial and venous circulations are usually of acute onset, with the presenting features in the orbit including episcleral vascular engorgement, typically with a 'corkscrew' configuration (Fig. 49.5), chemosis, a moderately raised intraocular pressure, diplopia due to lateral rectus paresis, and, on occasion, marked pulsation of the mires on applanation tonometry.

Carotico-cavernous fistulas (CCFs) are abnormal communications between the carotid arterial

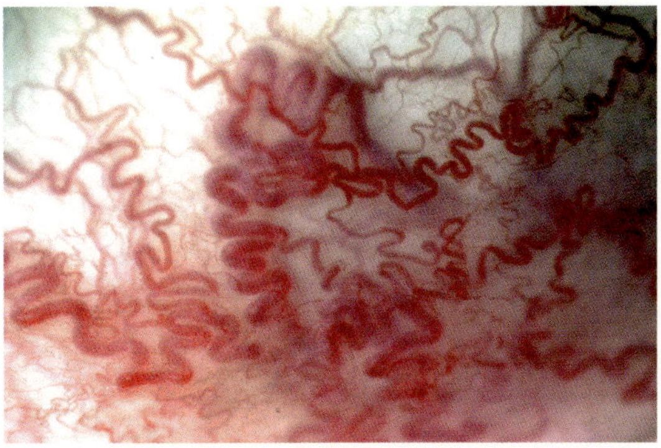

**Fig. 49.5** Dilated episcleral vessels – with a 'corkscrew configuration' – in a patient with a high-flow carotid-cavernous sinus fistula

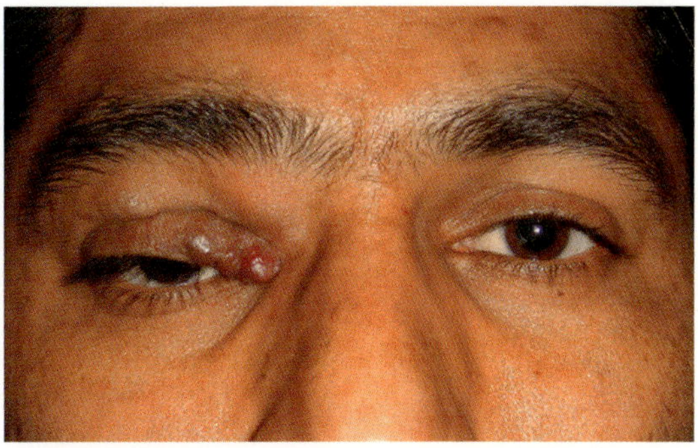

**Fig. 49.6** High-flow carotid-cavernous sinus fistula presenting with marked proptosis and chemosis with gross conjunctival prolapse

system and the venous cavernous sinus and are classified as *direct type A* and *dural type B*, *C* and *D*. Direct CCFs are usually seen in major cranial injury and in patients with systemic vascular disease. Due to their high flow, type A CCFs have an acute presentation with complications that can include compressive optic neuropathy, central retinal vein occlusion, proliferative retinopathy and glaucoma. They typically present with acute onset of marked proptosis, chemosis, global reduction of eye movements and, in many patients, an awareness of a pulsatile sensation in the head (Fig. 49.6).

The most common orbital arteriovenous abnormality is the so-called 'low-flow' dural shunt, resulting from an intracranial communication between a meningeal arteriole and the venous circulation in the region of the cavernous sinus, having a gradual onset, with generally milder presentations. Such low-flow shunts occur in the context of systemic vascular disease, and the majority will close spontaneously after several months to a year or so. In view of the natural history of these vascular communications, patients are managed conservatively – with topical medications to reduce intraocular pressure if necessary – and intervention is reserved for those in whom vision is threatened or where there is likely risk of cerebral venous thrombosis.

Colour Doppler ultrasonography is diagnostic, identifying reversal of flow (from posterior to anterior) within a dilated superior ophthalmic vein; this occurs during cardiac systole, although it can rarely occur throughout the cardiac cycle (Fig. 49.7). CT imaging typically identifies an enlarged superior ophthalmic vein, with a mild degree of proptosis and engorgement of the extraocular muscles (Fig. 49.8). Magnetic resonance angiogram (MRA) and digital subtraction angiography (DSA) are helpful and confirmatory tests for CCF. Between 25 % and 50 of dural CCFs resolve spontaneously. The accepted practice is to treat ocular symptoms conservatively with medical management or manual carotid compression. Unresponsive CCFs are treated by endovascular embolisation with a combination of detachable balloons, coils, stents or liquid embolic agents [21].

Intraorbital arteriovenous fistulas (AVFs) are rare vascular malformations which can mimic carotid-cavernous fistulas (CCFs) or present with a localised pulsatile mass (Fig. 49.9). These involve a fistula from the ophthalmic artery to one of the draining ophthalmic veins (Figs. 49.10 and 49.11) and can occur either spontaneously or following injury. These vascular lesions can be treated by direct surgical ligation but are best approached by prior transarterial or transvenous embolisation with coils or glue and subsequent surgical excision (Fig. 49.12).

## Orbital Vascular Occlusion

Acute occlusion of the orbital venous or arterial vasculature is exceptionally rare and usually seen

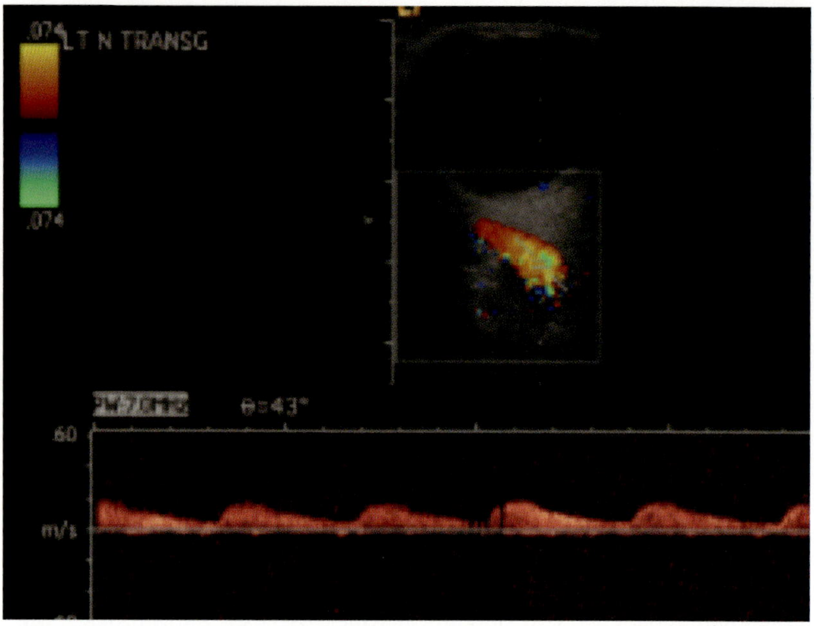


**Fig. 49.7** Slow-flow dural sinus fistula: diagnostic colour-coded Doppler ultrasonography showing reversal of flow (shown as *red*), from posterior to anterior within the dilated superior ophthalmic vein and also an arterial waveform with a flow rate of over 20 cm/s

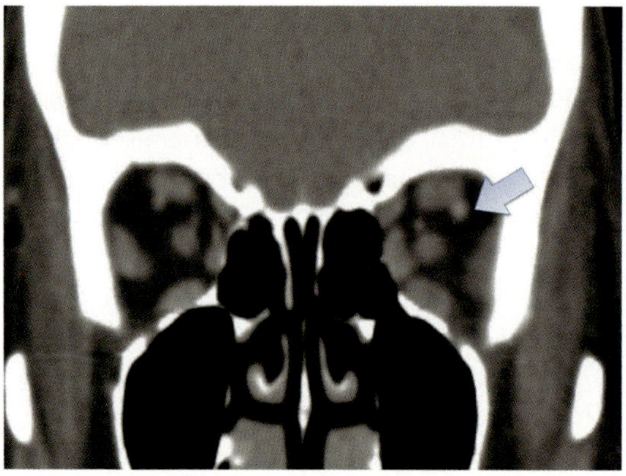

**Fig. 49.8** Dural fistula with CT imaging identifying an enlarged left superior ophthalmic vein (*arrow*) and engorgement of the ipsilateral extraocular muscles

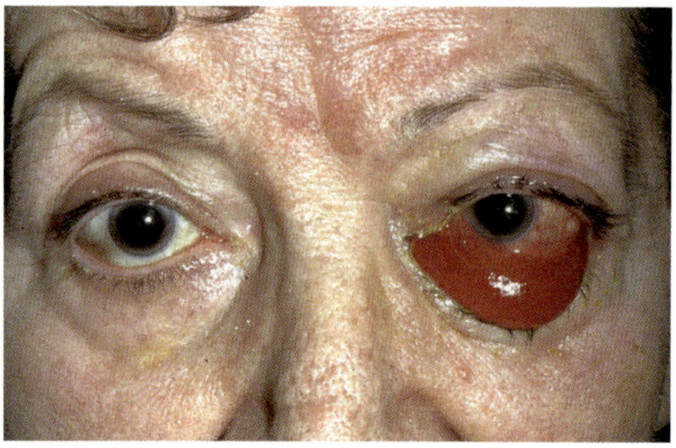

**Fig. 49.9** Anterior orbital arteriovenous fistula (AVF) presenting with orbital ache and a progressively enlarging, pulsatile, multilobed anterior orbital vascular lesion

in the background of vascular anomaly, injury or infection.

Patients with known orbital venous malformations can occasionally experience a dramatic worsening of symptoms, which may either be due to haemorrhage from the fragile abnormal vessels or due to thrombosis within the lesion. The ensuing secondary orbital congestion can threaten vision. The potential benefits of surgery, if contemplated, should always be weighed against significant risks. With recanalisation, the signs and symptoms abate spontaneously [23].

Severe periorbital infections, particularly those arising in the sinuses, can lead to thrombosis of the superior ophthalmic vein or the cavernous sinus and can also cause an occlusive arteritis with secondary orbital necrosis; the latter scenario is a particular risk with aggressive fungal sinusitis, including mucormycosis. This life-threatening infection (with a risk of cerebral

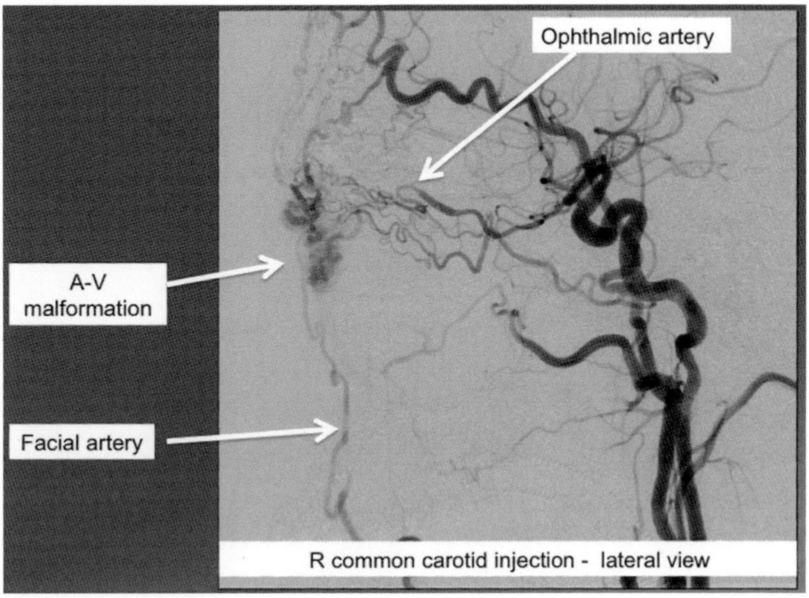


**Fig. 49.10** Arterial phase of the digital subtraction angiogram of patient shown in Fig. 49.9, identifying arterial feeder vessels (Figure courtesy of Fergus Robertson, FRCR, Consultant Neuroradiologist, NHNN, Queen Square, London)

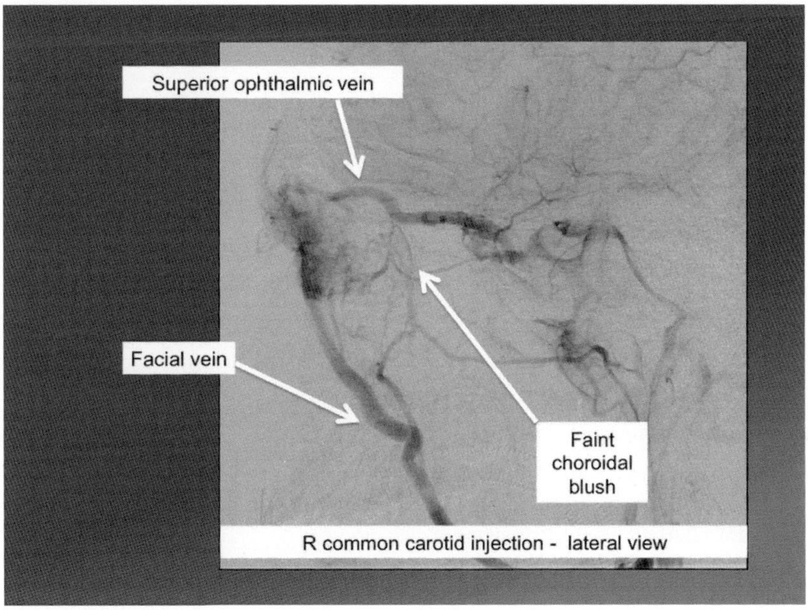


**Fig. 49.11** Venous phase of the angiogram showing drainage of the AVF through the facial and superior ophthalmic veins (Figure courtesy of Fergus Robertson, FRCR, Consultant Neuroradiologist, NHNN, Queen Square, London)

vasculitis and infection) requires urgent treatment with the advice and support of infectious disease and intensive care physicians and also head-and-neck surgeons. Management typically involves surgical excision of infected or necrotic tissues, high-dose systemic antibacterial or antifungal agents and can also include anticoagulation (See Chap. 35).

Occlusion of the orbital arterial circulation per se is a rare event and usually occurs after external orbital pressure – as can occur during prolonged neurosurgical procedures in which the patient is placed in the prone position or in an unconscious individual after a prolonged period of inadvertent pressure on the globe and orbit (See Chap. 21).

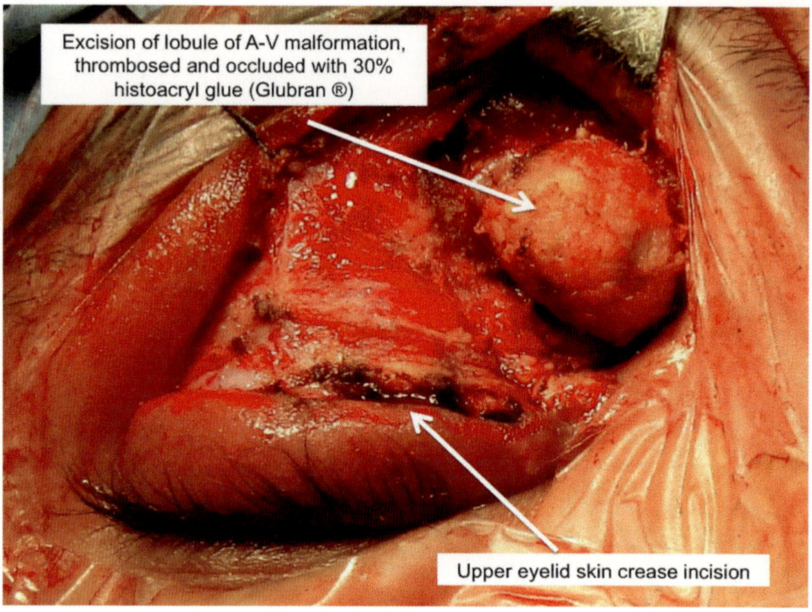


**Fig. 49.12** Surgical excision of the AVF identified in Figs. 49.9, 49.10, and 49.11, 1 week after endo-arterial occlusion with histoacryl glue

## Summary

Sudden orbital vascular events are usually due to acute haemorrhage; arteriovenous shunts occurring either spontaneously or following injury are uncommon, and intraorbital vascular occlusion is exceptionally rare. As with all orbital disease, the most likely diagnosis is reached through careful history taking, examination and appropriate imaging. The majority of patients can safely be observed, but where excessive pressure at the orbital apex threatens perfusion of the optic nerve, urgent intervention should be considered.

Prompt diagnosis and management can prevent devastating visual impairment.

## References


1. Lima V, Burt B, Leibovitch I, Prabhakaran V, Goldberg RA, Selva D. Orbital compartment syndrome: the ophthalmic surgical emergency. Surv Ophthalmol. 2009;54:441–9.
2. Wright JE, Sullivan TJ, Garner A, Wulc AE, Moseley IF. Orbital venous anomalies. Ophthalmology. 1997;104:905–13.
3. Sullivan TJ, Wright JE. Non-traumatic orbital haemorrhage. Clin Experiment Ophthalmol. 2000;28: 26–31.
4. Atalla ML, McNab AA, Sullivan TJ, Sloan B. Nontraumatic subperiosteal orbital hemorrhage. Ophthalmology. 2001;108:183–9.
5. Moin M, Kersten RC, Bernardini F, Kulwin D, Biddinger PW, Ernst RJ, Khouri LM. Spontaneous hemorrhage in an intraorbital arteriovenous malformation. Ophthalmology. 2000;107:2215–9.
6. Gilhotra JS, McNab AA, McKelvie P, O'Donnell BA. Late orbital haemorrhage around alloplastic orbital floor implants: a case series and review. Clin Experiment Ophthalmol. 2002;30:352–5.
7. Wood GD. Blindness following fracture of the zygomatic bone. Br J Oral Maxillofac Surg. 1992;24:12–6.
8. Nicholson DH, Guzak SW. Visual loss complicating repair of orbital floor fractures. Arch Ophthalmol. 1971;86:369–75.
9. Lederman IR. Loss of vision associated with surgical treatment of zygomatic-orbital floor fractures. Plast Reconstr Surg. 1981;68:94–9.
10. Puustjarvi T, Purhonen S. Permanent blindness following retrobulbar hemorrhage after peribulbar anesthesia for cataract surgery. Ophthalmic Surg. 1992;23: 450–2.
11. Kloss BT, Patel R. Orbital compartment syndrome from retrobulbar hemorrhage. Int J Emerg Med. 2010;3:521–2.
12. Winterton JV, Patel K, Mizen KD. Review of management options for a retrobulbar hemorrhage. J Oral Maxillofac Surg. 2007;65:296–9.
13. Zimmerer R, Schattmann K, Essig H, Jehn P, Metzger M, Kokemüller H, Gellrich NC, Tavassol F. Efficacy of transcutaneous transseptal orbital decompression in treating acute retrobulbar hemorrhage and a literature review. Craniomaxillofac Trauma Reconstr. 2014;7:17–26.

14. Burkat CN, Lemke BN. Retrobulbar hemorrhage: inferolateral anterior orbitotomy for emergent management. Arch Ophthalmol. 2005;123:1260–2.
15. Tan B, Rootman J, Seah LL. Combined radiological intervention and surgical excision of a periorbital arteriovenous fistula. Orbit. 2013;32:181–3.
16. Naqvi J, Laitt R, Leatherbarrow B, Herwadkar A. A case of a spontaneous intraorbital arteriovenous fistula: clinico-radiological findings and treatment by transvenous embolisation via the superior ophthalmic vein. Orbit. 2013;32:124–6.
17. de Keizer R. Carotid-cavernous and orbital arteriovenous fistulas: ocular features, diagnostic and hemodynamic considerations in relation to visual impairment and morbidity. Orbit. 2003;22:121–42.
18. Miller NR. Dural carotid-cavernous fistulas: epidemiology, clinical presentation, and management. Neurosurg Clin N Am. 2012;23:179–92.
19. Gemmete JJ, Ansari SA, Gandhi DM. Endovascular techniques for treatment of carotid-cavernous fistula. J Neuroophthalmol. 2009;29:62–71.
20. Tjoumakaris SI, Jabbour PM, Rosenwasser RH. Neuroendovascular management of carotid cavernous fistulae. Neurosurg Clin N Am. 2009;20:447–52.
21. Gemmete JJ, Chaudhary N, Pandey A, Ansari S. Treatment of carotid cavernous fistulas. Curr Treat Options Neurol. 2010;12:43–53.
22. Williamson RW, Ducruet AF, Crowley RW, McDougall CG, Albuquerque FC. Transvenous coil embolization of an intraorbital arteriovenous fistula: case report and review of the literature. Neurosurgery. 2013;72:E130–4.
23. Rose GE, Verity DH. Acute presentation of vascular disease within the orbit—a descriptive synopsis of mechanisms. Eye. 2013;27:299–307.

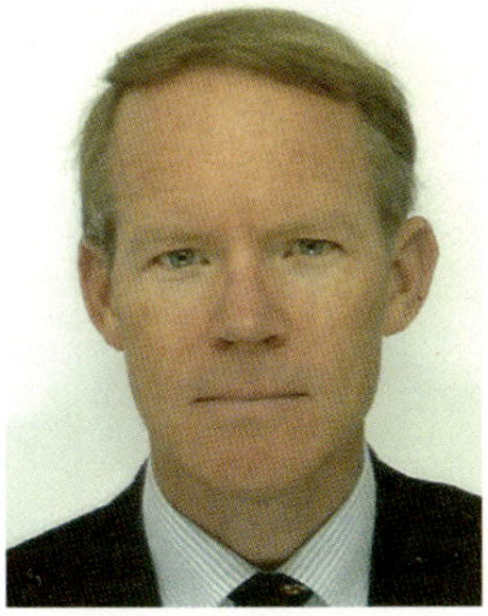

**David H. Verity** Dr. Verity is a Consultant Ophthalmic Surgeon, and Adnexal Service Director, Moorfields Eye Hospital, London.

He is a Honorary Senior Clinical Lecturer, University College London.

Trained in ophthalmology in the UK, Dr. Verity undertook two Fellowships in ophthalmic adnexal disease before joining the Consultant staff at Moorfields Eye Hospital in 2004.

He is a Full Member of the British Oculoplastic Surgery Society (current Treasurer), Treasurer Elect for the European Society of Ophthalmic Plastic and Reconstructive Surgery, and Full Member of the International Society of Ocular Oncology.

In 2009, he was elected to the Orbital Society, in 2010 became Editor-in Chief of the journal ORBIT, and in 2016 became Oculoplastic Section Editor for the Journal of Ophthalmic and Vision Research.

His medical publications in peer-reviewed journals and books include 90(+) publications, and with a wide range of research interests, he is an active national and international teacher and surgical trainer.

Dr. Verity also has a life-long interest in the charitable work of the St John Eye Hospital Group. In 2014, he was invested in the Order of St John, and in 2016 he joined the Board as Trustee of the Hospital Group.

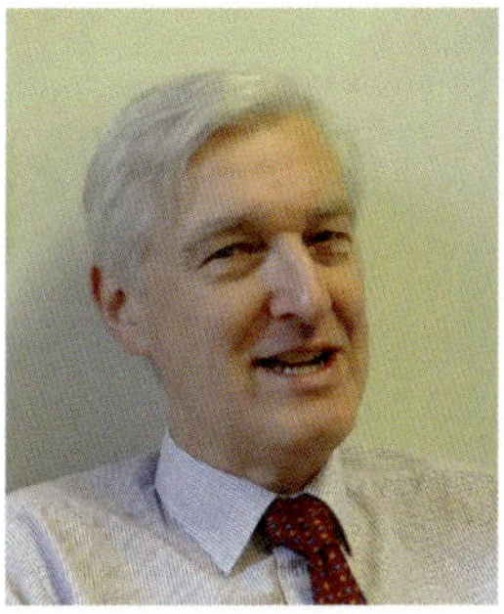

**Geoffrey E. Rose** Geoffrey Rose graduated BSc Pharmacology, MBBS, and MRCP. His postgraduate ophthalmic training culminated in award of FRCS in 1985 and FRCOphth at its foundation in 1988. In 1990, the University of London granted an MS doctorate for corneal research and, in 2004, a Doctor of Science in Ophthalmology and Ophthalmic Surgery.

Professor Rose was appointed consultant to Moorfields Eye Hospital, London, in 1990 and is also a Senior Research Fellow of the NIHR Biomedical Research Centre of the Institute of Ophthalmology. He served as the British Council member of the European Society of Ophthalmic Plastic and Reconstructive, is a Past-President of the British Oculoplastic Surgical Society, and is President of the European Society of Oculoplastic and Reconstructive Surgeons.

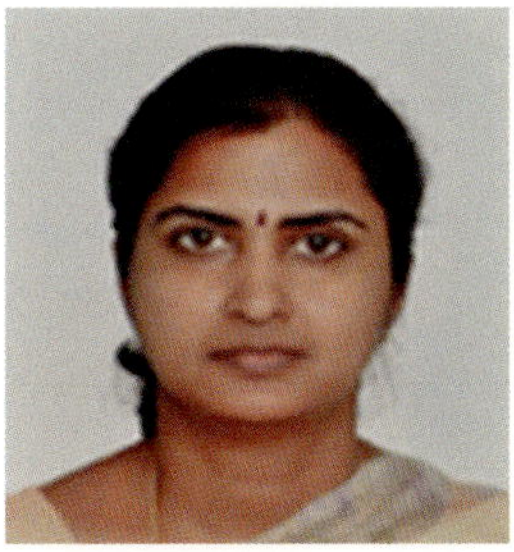

**Usha R. Kim** ***Current Position*** Head of the Department of Orbit, Oculoplasty and Ocular Oncology Services, Professor in Ophthalmology, Director of Mid-Level Ophthalmic Personnel, Head of Telemedicine-Supported Vision Centers Network at Aravind Eye Care System, Madurai.

***Qualification*** Dr. Usha Kim received her MBBS from Bharathiar University, Coimbatore, in 1991, Diploma in Ophthalmology and MNAMS (Oph), from Aravind Eye Hospital, Madurai, in the year 1994 and 1995 respectively. She completed her specialty training under the guidance of Dr. William B. Stewart at University of California, San Francisco, and at Salt Lake City, Utah, in the United States of America.

Dr. Usha Kim is heading the Department of Orbit, Oculoplasty and Ocular Oncology at Aravind Eye Hospital since 1998. Under her efficient leadership, the clinic has seen several innovations such as the addition of Ocular Oncology Services and an Ocular Prosthesis Center. She is actively involved in various teaching programs at Aravind Eye Hospital and Lions Institute of Community Ophthalmology (LAICO). She has trained nearly 55 national and 16 international candidates as fellows in the field of Orbit, Oculoplasty, and Ocular Oncology. She has also trained 41 ocularists both at the national and international level.

She has been a member of Aravind Research Committee since March 1998 and is a principal investigator for many studies conducted at Aravind Eye Care System. She is actively involved in various research activities and currently focuses on genetics of retinoblastoma.

She has presented papers, delivered lectures, and chaired various international, national, and state-level ophthalmic conferences.

**She has 43 publications to her credit – 23 international and 18 national.** She has also written chapters in many books and co-authored a book on Imaging in Orbit and Neuro-ophthalmology.

She established 'The Ring of Hope' in 2004, a program that provides free service to patients, children, and adults who have life-threatening cancers in the eye like retinoblastoma. The Ring of Hope Fund, since its inception, has supported 1600 ocular cancer patients, who would otherwise not have been able to receive treatment.

***Awards***

- **CP Gupta Award** for '**Best Paper**' from TNOA in 2002
- '**Best Orbital Photography**' **award** in Joint Meeting of the Oculoplastics Association of India & Asia Pacific Society of Ophthalmic Plastic and Reconstructive Surgery in 2007
- **'Best Poster' award for Prospective Evaluation of Contracted Anophthalmic Sockets** in the Indo Israel Meeting held in Chennai in 2005
- '**Vocational excellence Award**' from Rotary Club of Madurai in 2010 for her work in the community
- **International Women's day Excellence award** by the Lions Club of Madurai District 324-B3 March 8, 2015, for her work in the field of Ocular Oncology
- **PSG & Sons' Charities, Coimbatore Scroll of Honour awarded** for her an eminent expert in diagnosis, treatment, rehabilitation, and research in ophthalmology holding a key leadership position in a reputed Eye Care system, for having conducted a large number of cataract surgeries in addition to her widely acclaimed expertise in orbit oculoplasty, ocular prosthetic services, ocular oncology, and her personal involvement in the Ring of Hope initiative

# 50 Exposure Keratopathy Due to Facial Palsy

Darmayanti Siswoyo

## Introduction

Facial nerve palsy causes paralysis of the orbicularis oculi which results in atony of the muscle, elongation of the tarsal plate, medial and lateral canthal ligaments, and laxity of the upper and lower lid, resulting in lagophthalmos and corneal exposure and culminating in exposure keratopathy (Figs. 50.1 and 50.2).

Paralytic lagophthalmos denotes incomplete closure of the eyelid as a result of paralysis of the seventh cranial nerve, usually from lesions affecting the nuclear or peripheral portion of the nerve.

Facial nerve paralysis with resultant lagophthalmos and ectropion can occur from many causes, including Bell's palsy, tumors, trauma, injury, or vascular accidents affecting the facial nerve. Whatever the cause, the ocular complications of inadequately or improperly managed facial paralysis range in severity from corneal irritation and punctate keratopathy to corneal ulceration, perforation, and blindness (Fig. 50.3).

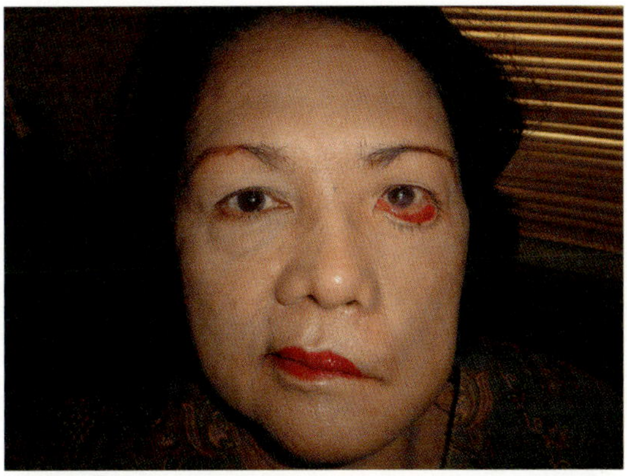

**Fig. 50.1** Left eye facial nerve palsy with severe ectropion and corneal exposure

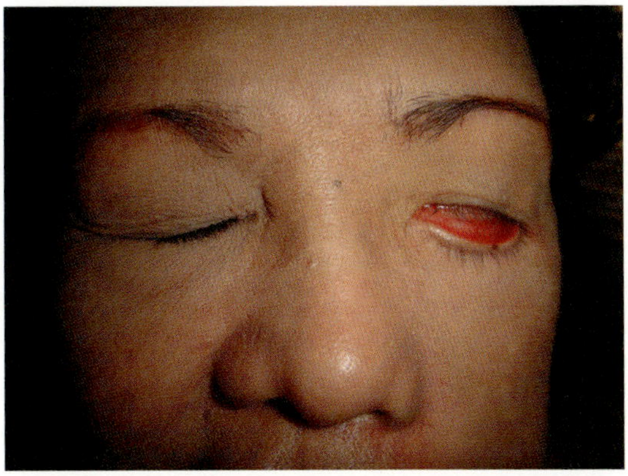

**Fig. 50.2** Left eye facial nerve palsy with severe ectropion and corneal exposure

D. Siswoyo
Oculoplastic & Eye Reconstructive Surgery, Jakarta-Eye-Center, CIK Ditiro no. 46 Menteng, Jakarta 10310, Indonesia
e-mail: darmayanti_spm@yahoo.com; yanti@jec.co.id


B. Mukherjee, H. Yuen (eds.), *Emergencies of the Orbit and Adnexa*, DOI 10.1007/978-81-322-1807-4_50

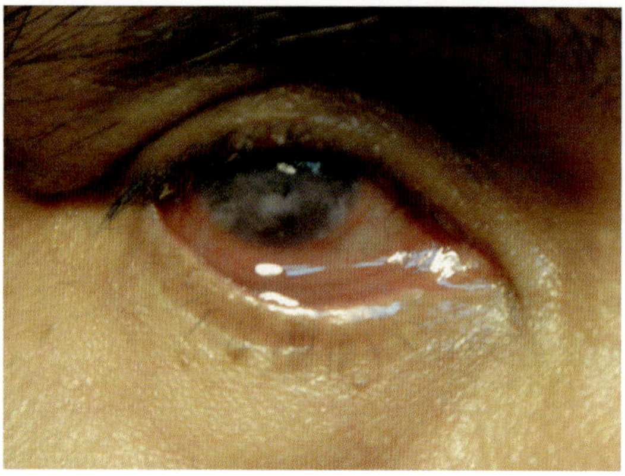

**Fig. 50.3** Corneal perforation

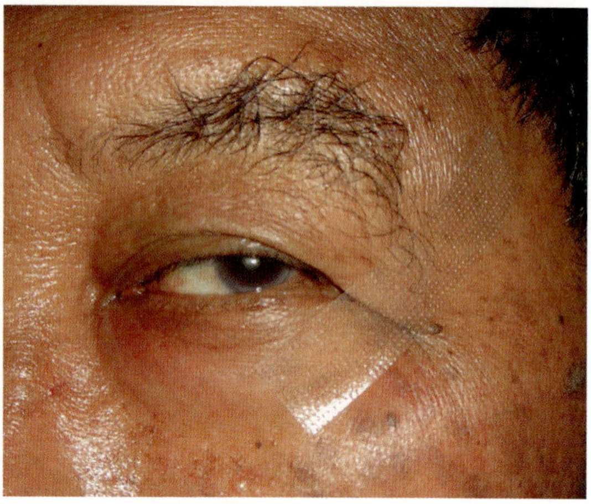

**Fig. 50.4** Taping the lower eyelid

The facial nerve innervates both the frontalis muscle, which raises the eyebrow, and the orbicularis oculi muscle, which closes the eyelids [1, 4, 7]. Loss of function of the facial nerve inhibits eyelid closure as well as the blink reflex and the lacrimal pumping mechanism. In addition, the facial nerve innervates the muscles of facial expression including the zygomaticus muscles, which elevate the cheeks as well as the corrugator supercilii and procerus muscles, which depress the eyebrow. These muscles play an important role in maintaining facial symmetry.

## Etiology

Facial nerve palsy may result from a broad spectrum of causes largely due to its topographic complexity [7, 8].

Trauma: The facial nerve is susceptible to blunt trauma or laceration along its bony course. Fractures to the skull base or mandible can damage the nerve or one of its branches.

Cerebrovascular accidents: The facial nerve receives its blood supply from the anterior inferior cerebellar artery. It is most susceptible to ischemic damage just proximal to the geniculate ganglion.

Bell's palsy: This is an idiopathic facial nerve palsy that is thought to be associated with an acute viral infection or reactivation of Herpes simplex virus.

Tumors: Acoustic neuromas in the cerebellopontine angle and metastatic lesions are most commonly associated with lagophthalmos.

Iatrogenic trauma after the removal of tumors.

Infectious, immune-mediated causes: Less common causes of lagophthalmos include Lyme diseases, chickenpox, mumps, polio, Guillain–Barre syndrome, leprosy, diphtheria, and botulism.

Moebius' syndrome: This rare, congenital condition is characterized by cranial nerve palsies (especially sixth and seventh cranial palsies), motility disturbances, limb anomalies, and orofacial defects.

## Medical Therapy

Medical therapy includes emollient eyedrops [3, 8], as well as taping. The tape should be passed from lateral one-third of the lower eyelid and then pulled up to the temple (Fig. 50.4) to reduce exposure of the cornea. Do not use gauze for dressing, as it will stick to the cornea and cause more severe corneal damage. Botox injection to the levator muscle can be done to induce ptosis of the upper lid [6], as well as tarsorrhaphy [2, 8] as a temporary measure for corneal protection, but sometimes this is cosmetically unacceptable to the patient. The majority of patients require definitive surgical treatment to correct this chronic impairment.

## **Surgical Management** (Table 50.1)

Surgical intervention is primarily considered in cases in which medical management has failed or the condition is unlikely to improve over time.

In facial nerve palsy, laxity occurs in all parts of the lower lid.

When there is laxity and poor lateral canthal fixation to the lateral orbital wall, refixation of the eyelid to the lateral orbital tubercle with tarsal strip procedure corrects the laxity and restores the contour of the lateral canthal angle [9].

When the lateral canthal tendon is stable and there is marked redundancy to lower lid skin, the Byron Smith modification of the Kuhnt–Szymanowski procedure combines horizontal full-thickness eyelid shortening with a blepharoplasty – type skin incision is desirable [9].

In the author's experience, if only the lower lid margin is shortened, without enhancement with ear cartilage graft or synthetic material, the laxity will recur again usually 6 months after surgery due to the absence of orbicularis muscle contraction.

### Shortening Lower Lid Margin by Lateral Tarsal Strip Procedure Enhanced with Ear Cartilage Graft with a Blepharoplasty: Type Skin Incision

Subciliaris skin incision and then orbicularis muscle dissection to expose the inferior orbital rim, lateral canthotomy is done, and inferior cantholysis is completed to mobilize the lateral aspect of the eyelid for its advancement superiorly and laterally. The tarsal strip is made by excising the mucosa, cilia, and orbicularis at the lateral edge of the eyelid. The length of the tarsal strip to be excised is determined depending on the laxity of the eyelid. At least 4–5 mm of bare tarsal strip is left intact for attachment to the lateral orbital rim. Residual mucosa on the posterior surface of the tarsus is deepithelized (Fig. 50.30). Then harvest the graft from ear

**Table 50.1** System for facial nerve palsy

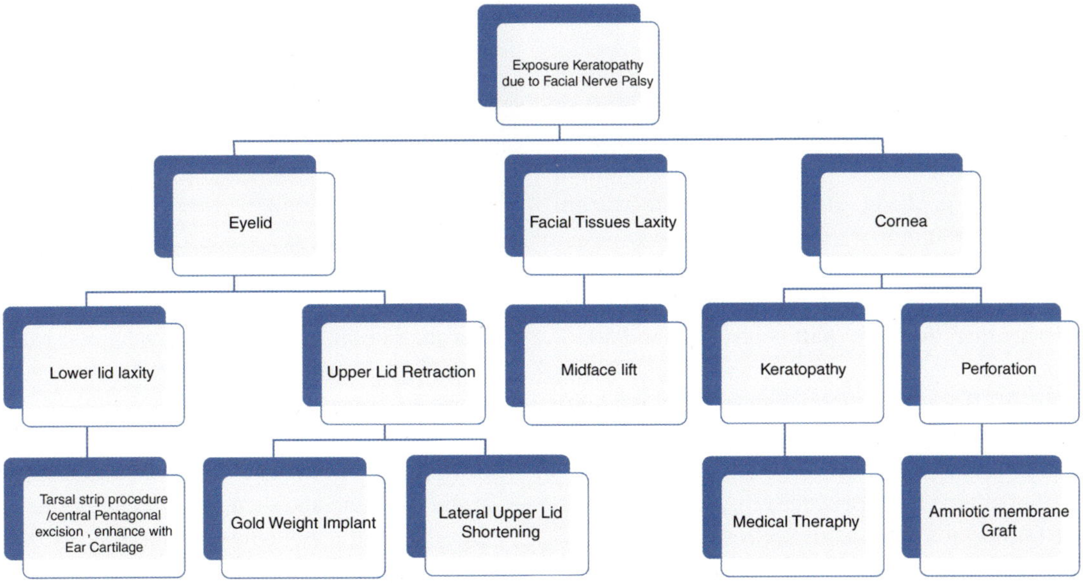

cartilage as mentioned below in (Figs. 50.22, 50.23a–d, and 50.24). Suture the graft as the same as mentioned in Fig. 50.25a and 50.25b then continue suturing the lateral tarsal strip. A 5.0 suture is passed into the periorbita 2–4 mm within the lateral orbital rim above the level of the lateral commissure; the suture is then passed through the stump of the tarsus, and then it is brought back through the tarsus. The needle is again passed into the periorbita, just above the initial periorbital bite, and then the suture is tightened. Reinforce the lateral lower eyelid tarsus and orbicularis to the periorbital with two or three additional sutures to tighten the lower lid tissues (Fig. 50.31). Redefine the lateral commissure.

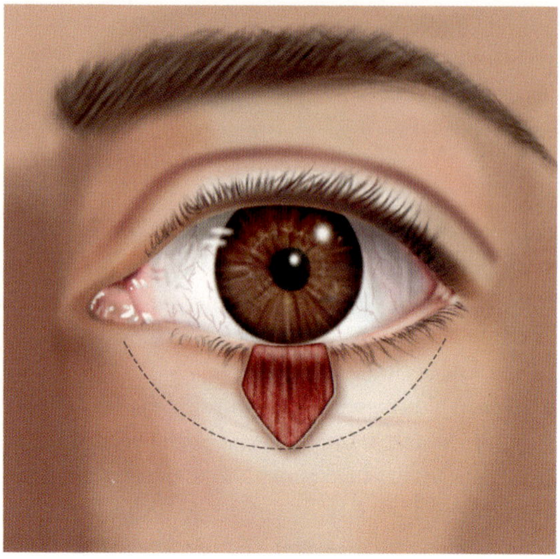

**Fig. 50.5** Central pentagonal excision

## Shortening Lower Lid Margin by Khunt–Szymanowski Combines Central Full: Thickness Eyelid Excision Enhanced with Ear Cartilage Graft with a Blepharoplasty-Type Skin Incision

In the author's experience, tightening the central part of the lower lid by excision of the central lower lid tissues, and then suturing layer by layer, makes the entire lower lid structure stronger (Fig. 50.5), compared to excision of the lateral part of the lower lid tissue (Fig. 50.6).

A central part lower lid shortening procedure enhanced with ear cartilage graft or synthetic material fixed at the inferior tarsal plate and at the lower orbital rim will maintain a normal position of the lower lid margin (Figs. 50.7 and 50.8).

How to prevent lid margin notching:

The superior part of the excision should be shorter than the lower part (Figs. 50.5 and 50.9). To create slight eversion of the wound edges (Fig. 50.10), prevent late depression or notching of the resulting scar (Fig. 50.11).

1. Subciliaris skin incision (Fig. 50.12).
2. Orbicularis muscle dissection to expose the inferior orbital rim (Fig. 50.13a, b).
3. Cut the nasal lower lid for pentagonal excision (Fig. 50.14).
4. Fold the tarsal plate over and estimate excess lower lid margin (Fig. 50.15).

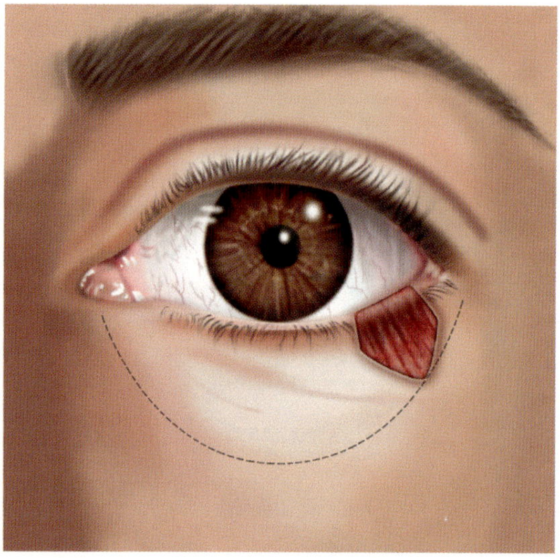

**Fig. 50.6** Lateral pentagonal excision

5. Cut the lateral lower lid for pentagonal excision (Fig. 50.16).
6. Complete pentagonal excision (Fig. 50.17).
7. The first suture should be at the gray line, from inside the wound (Fig. 50.18a).Emerge at the gray line and then pinch the gray line at the other side at the same position (Fig. 50.18b) to get a good approximation of the lid margin. Tighten the suture (Fig. 50.18c). Cut the suture (Fig. 50.18d).
8. Suture the lid margin at the skin border (Fig. 50.19).

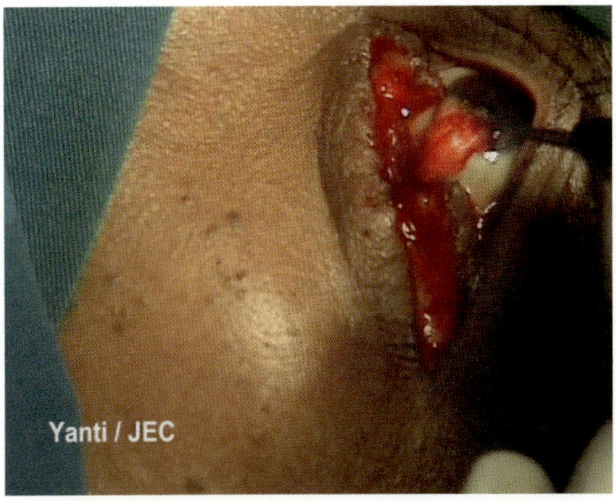


**Fig. 50.7** Central pentagonal excision

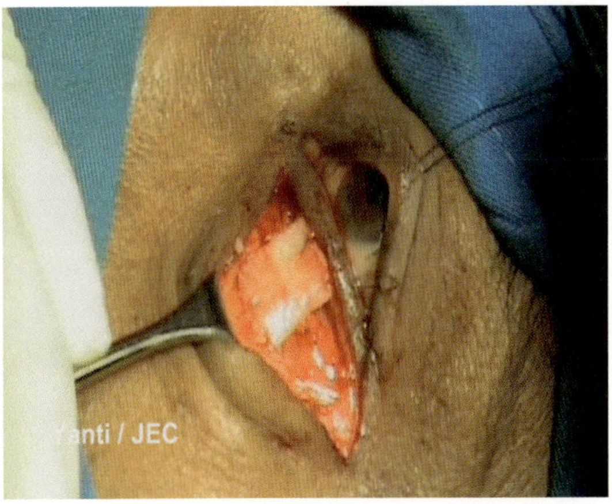


**Fig. 50.8** Ear cartilage graft

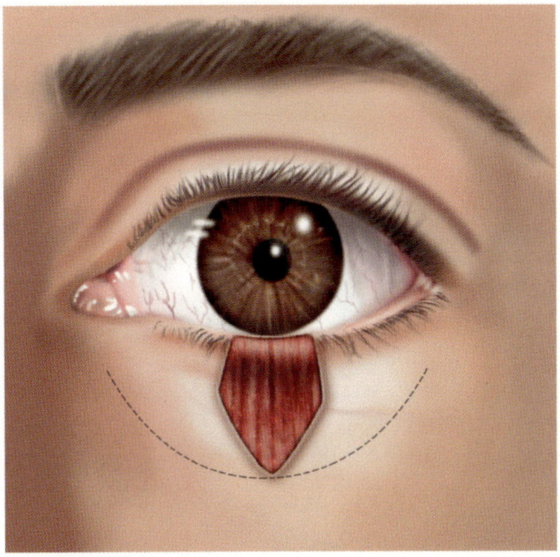

**Fig. 50.9** To prevent lid margin notching, the superior part of the excision should be shorter than the lower part

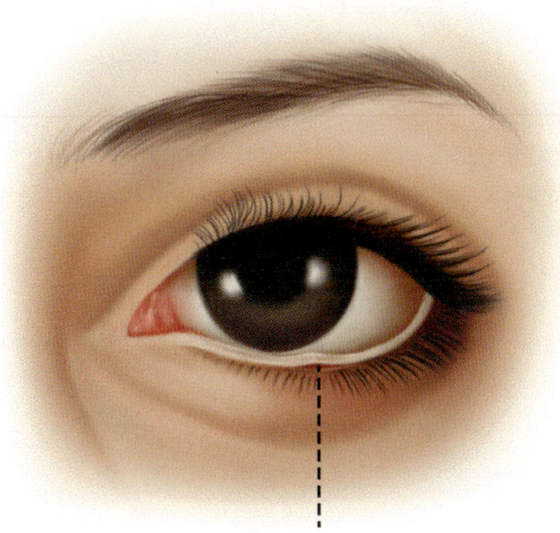

**Fig. 50.10** Slight eversion of the wound edges

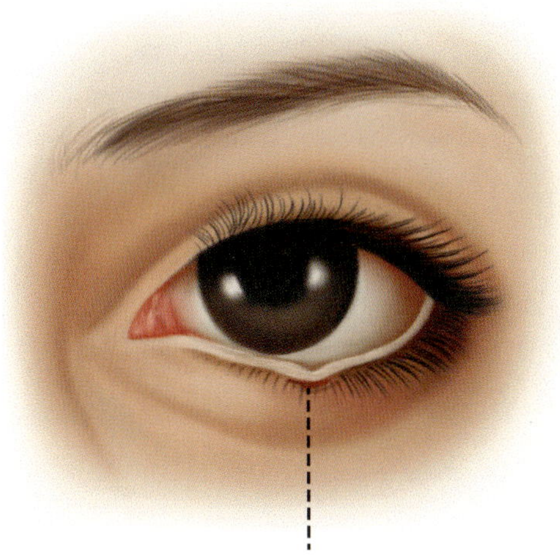

**Fig. 50.11** Notching of the wound edges

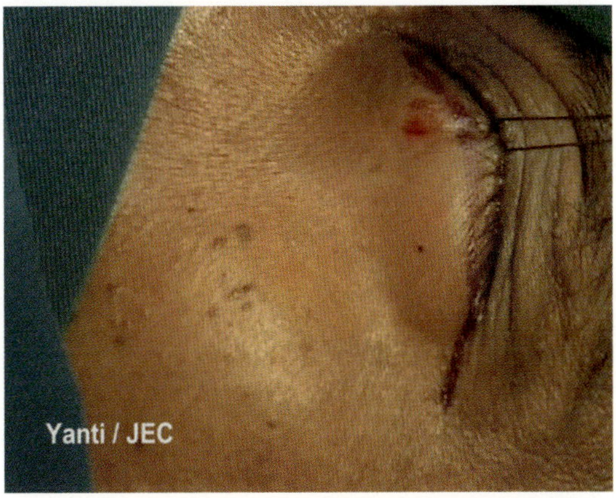


**Fig. 50.12** Subciliaris skin incision

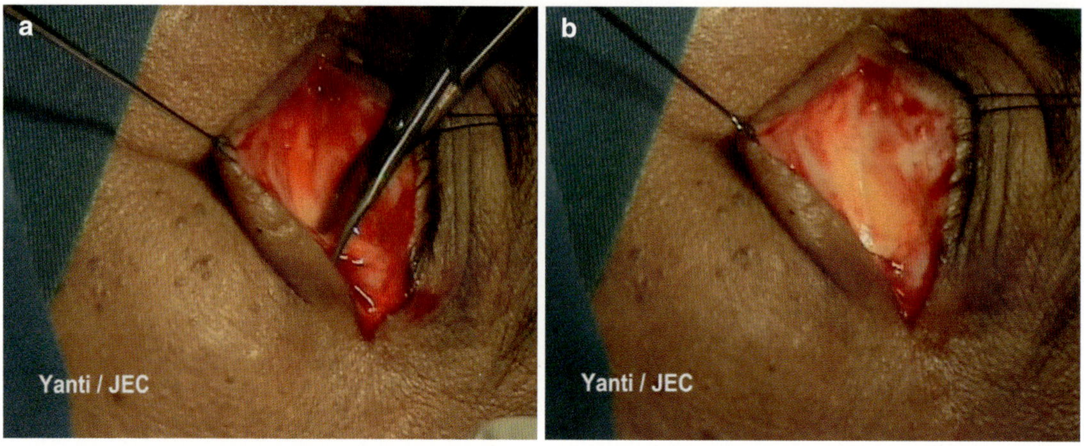


**Fig. 50.13** (**a**) Subciliaris muscle dissection. (**b**) Inferior orbital rim exposed

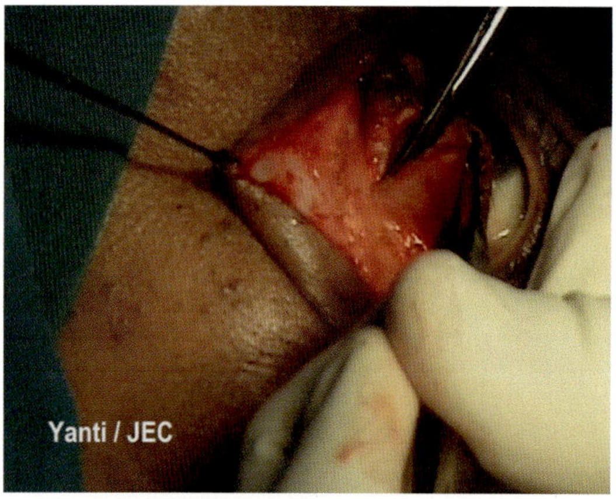


**Fig. 50.14** Nasal lower lid cut

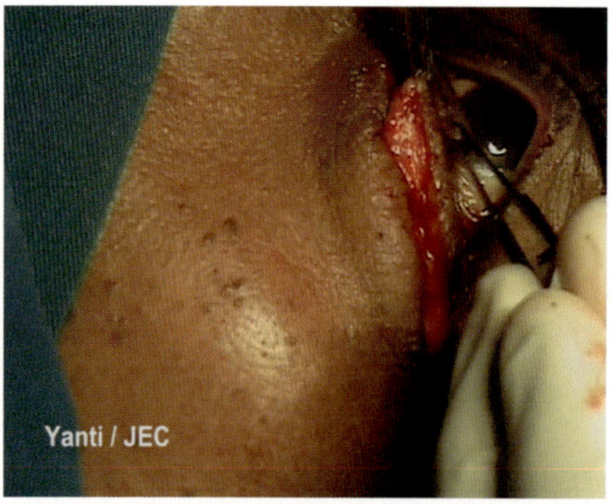


**Fig. 50.15** Tarsal plate foldedover

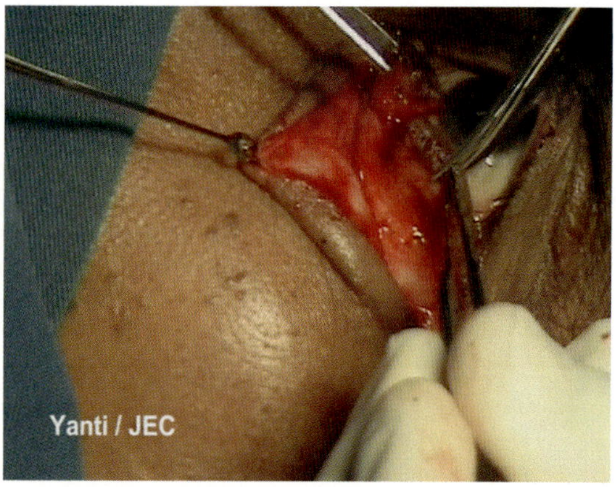


**Fig. 50.16** Lateral lower lid cut

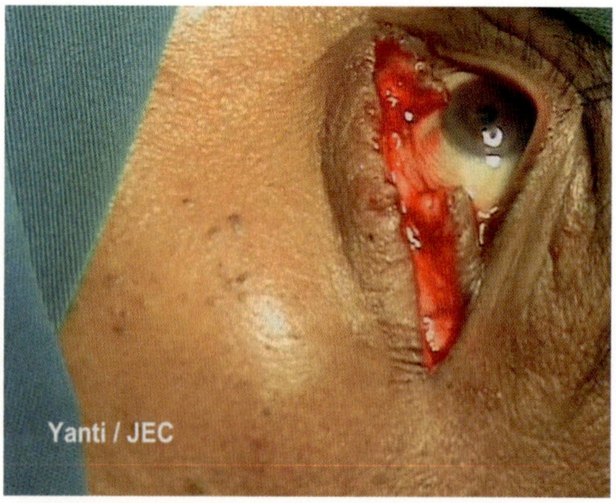


**Fig. 50.17** Pentagonal excision complete

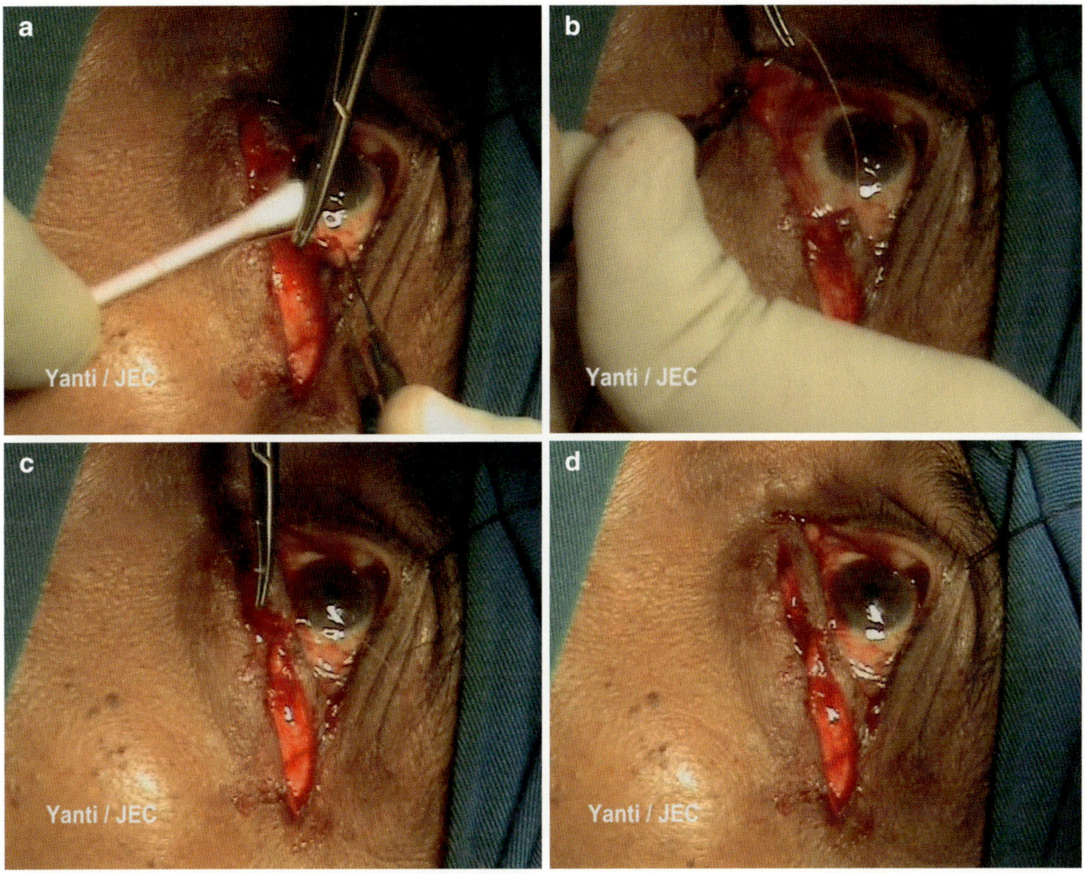


**Fig. 50.18** (**a**) First suture. (**b**) *Gray line*. (**c**) Suture tightened. (**d**) Suture cut

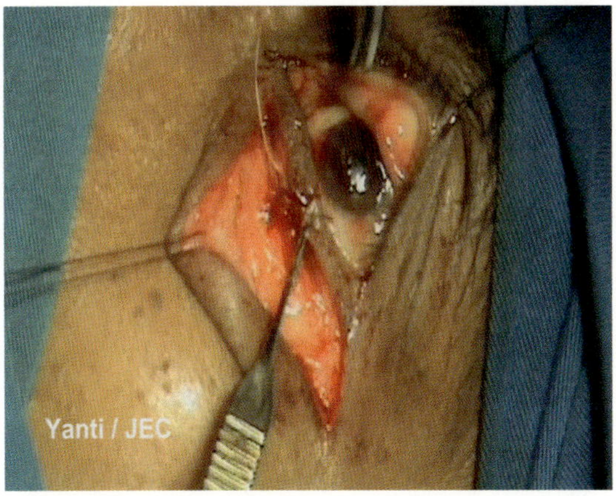


**Fig. 50.19** Skin border

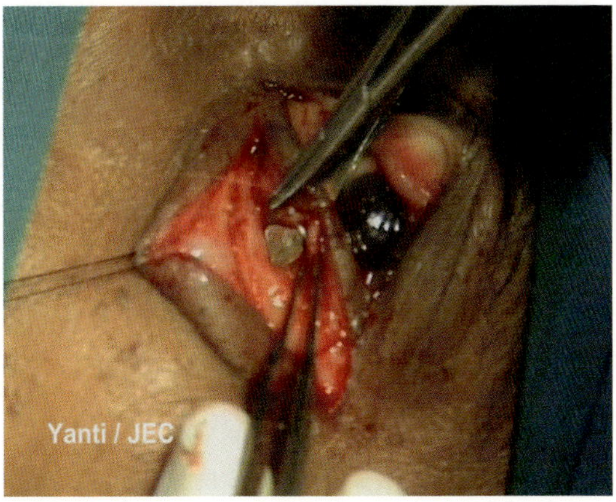


**Fig. 50.20** Instrument placed

9. Place the instrument to prevent damage to the eyeball when suturing the wound. Suture the tarsal plate. The tarsal plate should be sutured with two to three interrupted sutures with 6.0 absorbable sutures (Fig. 50.20).

10. Suture the conjunctiva, orbicularis muscle with absorbable suture 6.0, until the entire conjunctiva and orbicularis muscle is sutured (Fig. 50.21).
11. Harvest the graft from ear cartilage [5] (Fig. 50.22). Measure the length and height of the ear cartilage that will be harvested; mark it and then inject a small amount of xylocaine and epinephrine subdermally for hemostasis and separation of tissue planes to make the dissection easy. Cut the skin and then dissect under the skin to expose the cartilage.
12. Cut the cartilage carefully, not to cut the underlying skin at the lower incision (Fig. 50.23a) and at the upper incision (Fig. 50.23b). Gently dissect to separate the cartilage from the underlying skin (Fig. 50.23c) and then remove the graft (Fig. 50.23d).
13. Place the graft at the central lower lid (Fig. 50.24).
14. Suture the upper part of the graft to the lower edge of the tarsal plate with three sutures – central, medial, and lateral (Fig. 50.25a) – and then suture the lower part of the graft to the periosteum of the inferior orbital rim (Fig. 50.25b). After the graft has been placed, the position of the lower lid margin is seen exactly at the lower limbus (Fig. 50.25c).
15. Facial nerve paralysis causes laxity of all facial tissues, aggravating the laxity of the lower lid. Strengthening and upward fixation of the facial tissues will strengthen the lower lid structures. Midface lift: Dissect the submuscular aponeurotic system (SMAS) downward until the periosteum over maxillary bone is exposed (Fig. 50.26).
16. Take a bite of the periosteum at the upper part of the maxillary bone with 4-0 absorbable suture, then bite through the muscle tissues at the lower part to pull the facial tissues upward (Fig. 50.27a), and then tighten the sutures (Fig. 50.27b).
17. Take another bite through the periosteum at the upper part (Fig. 50.28a), bite the muscle tissue at the lower part (Fig. 50.28b), and then tighten the suture.
18. Excise the excess tissues (Fig. 50.29a). After excision of the excess tissues (Fig. 50.29b), suture the muscle and the periosteum at the level of incision with 5-0 absorbable suture; tighten the suture (Fig. 50.29c) and then suture the skin with continuous or interrupted sutures with 6-0 nonabsorbable suture (Fig. 50.29d).

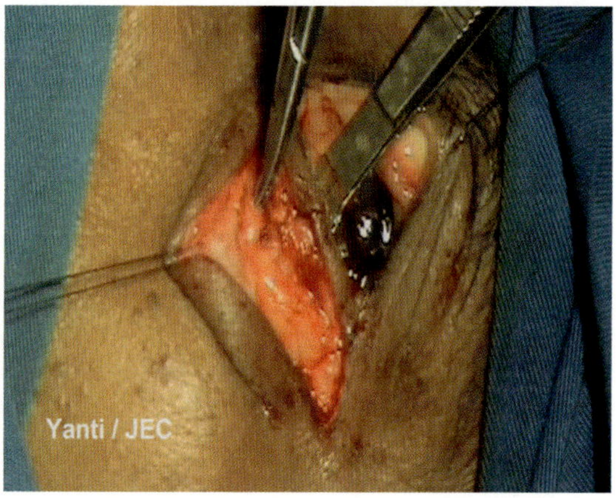


**Fig. 50.21** Sutured conjunctiva, orbicularis muscle

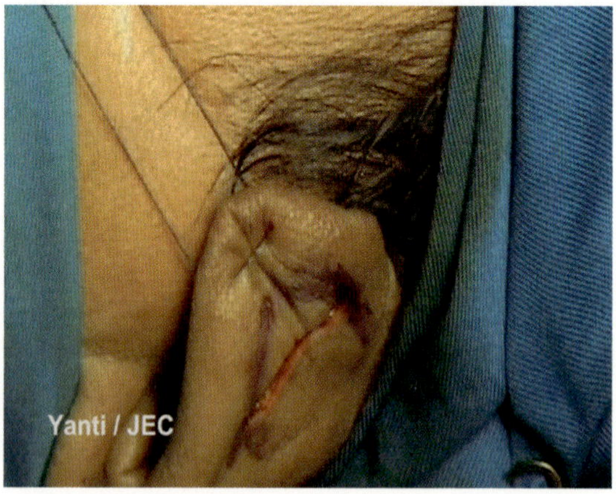


**Fig. 50.22** Graft harvested

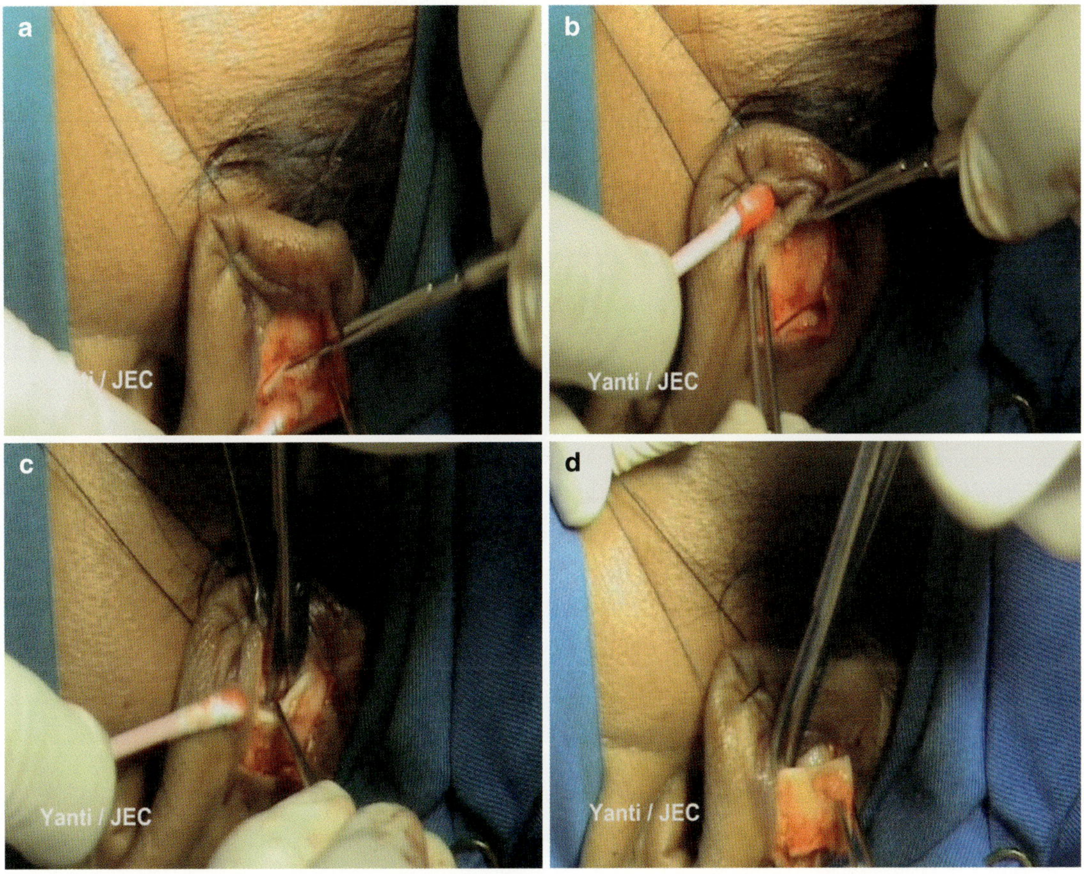


**Fig. 50.23** (**a**) Cartilage cut carefully, not to cut the underlying skin at the lower incision. (**b**) Cartilage cut carefully, not to cut the underlying skin at the upper incision. (**c**) Gentle dissection. (**d**) Graft removed

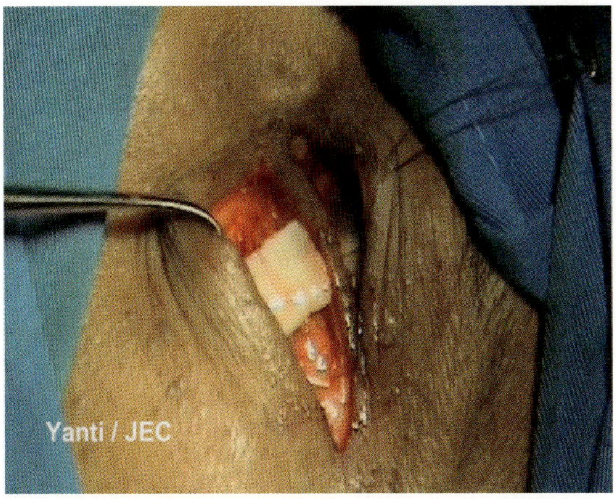


**Fig. 50.24** Graft placed at central lower lid

## Management of Corneal Perforation Caused by Lagophthalmos Due to Seventh Nerve Palsy

Patient with seventh nerve palsy caused by brain tumor excision 2 years prior (Figs. 50.30, 50.31, and 50.32a). She came with lagophthalmos (Fig. 50.32b) and severe keratopathy (Fig. 50.3) with corneal perforation on the right eye (Fig. 50.33c).

Corneal perforation (Fig. 50.33a). Viscoelastic material was injected into the anterior chamber just to form the anterior chamber

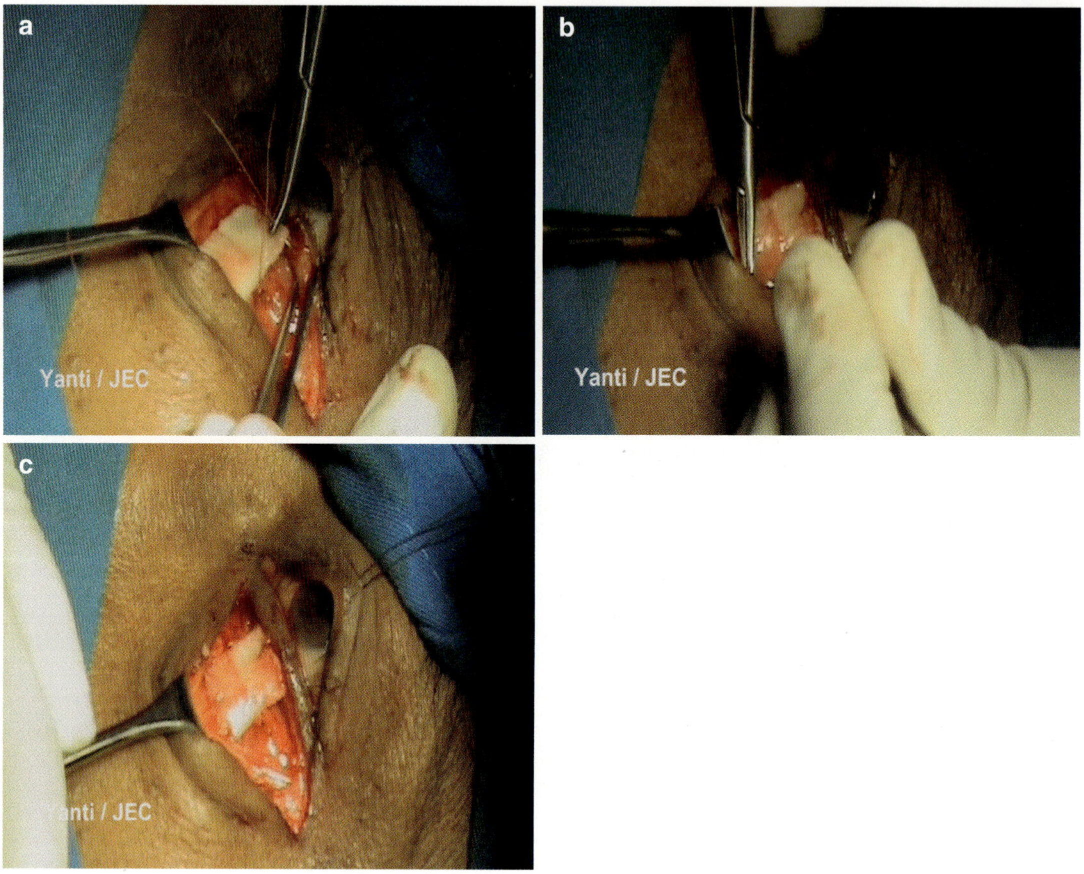


**Fig. 50.25** (**a**) Upper part of graft sutured to lower edge of the tarsal plate. (**b**) Lower part of graft sutured to periosteum of inferior orbital rim. (**c**) After graft is placed, the position of the lower lid margin is seen exactly at the lower limbus

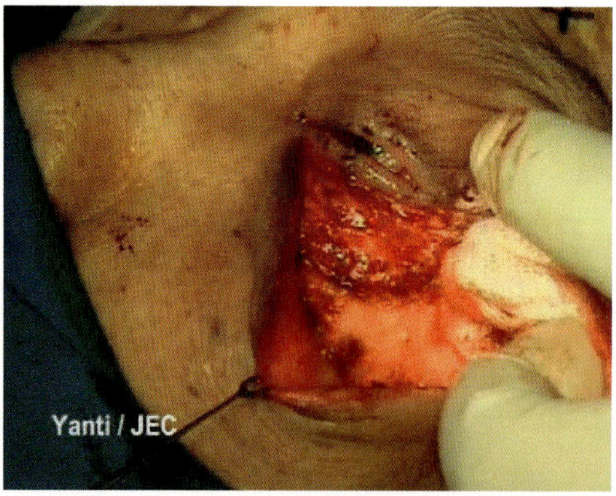


**Fig. 50.26** Submuscular aponeurotic system (SMAS) dissected downwards until periosteum over maxillary bone is exposed

(Fig. 50.33b). Once the anterior chamber formed (Fig. 50.33c), one piece of amniotic membrane was placed upon the perforate cornea (Fig. 50.33d). Then, piece by piece, amniotic membrane added until seven pieces of amniotic membrane were placed upon the perforate cornea. Then one large piece of amniotic membrane was placed over to cover those seven layers of amniotic membrane (Fig. 50.33e), sutured to the episclera at the limbal area just to fix the position of those amniotic membranes (Fig. 50.33f). Then conjunctival flap was performed (Fig. 50.33g) to tighten the position of the amniotic membrane and give nutrition. Lastly, a bandage contact lens was placed on for 2 weeks.

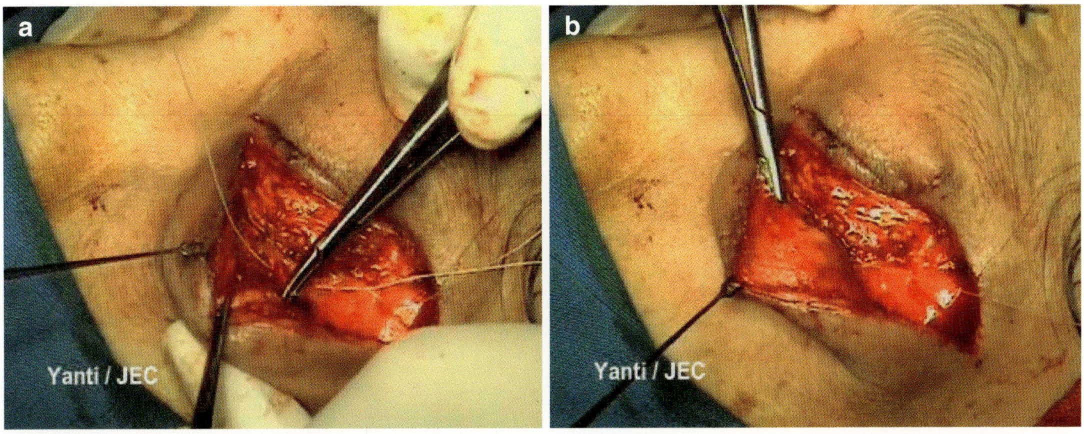


**Fig. 50.27** (**a**) Bite of the periosteum taken at the upper part of the maxillary bone with 4-0 absorbable suture, followed by bite taken through the muscle tissues at the lower part to pull the facial tissues upward. (**b**) Sutures tightened

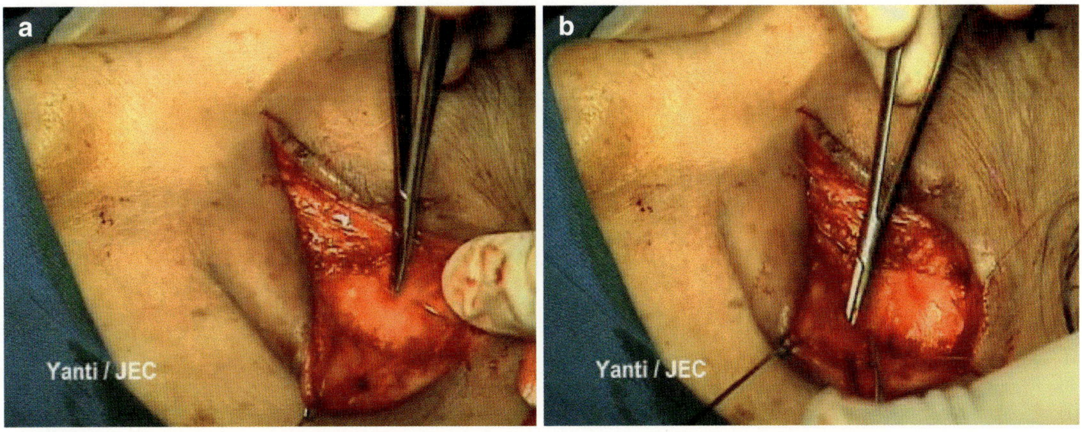


**Fig. 50.28** (**a**) Bite taken through the periosteum at the upper part. (**b**) Sutures tightened

The same patient 1 week after amnion graft and conjunctival flap on the cornea and shortening of the lower lid enhanced with ear cartilage graft (Fig. 50.34a, b).

The same patient 3 months after surgery, with no lagophthalmos (Fig. 50.35a, b). Conjunctival flap has separated itself, clear cornea at the upper area and corneal scar at the lower area with deep anterior chamber (Fig. 50.35c).

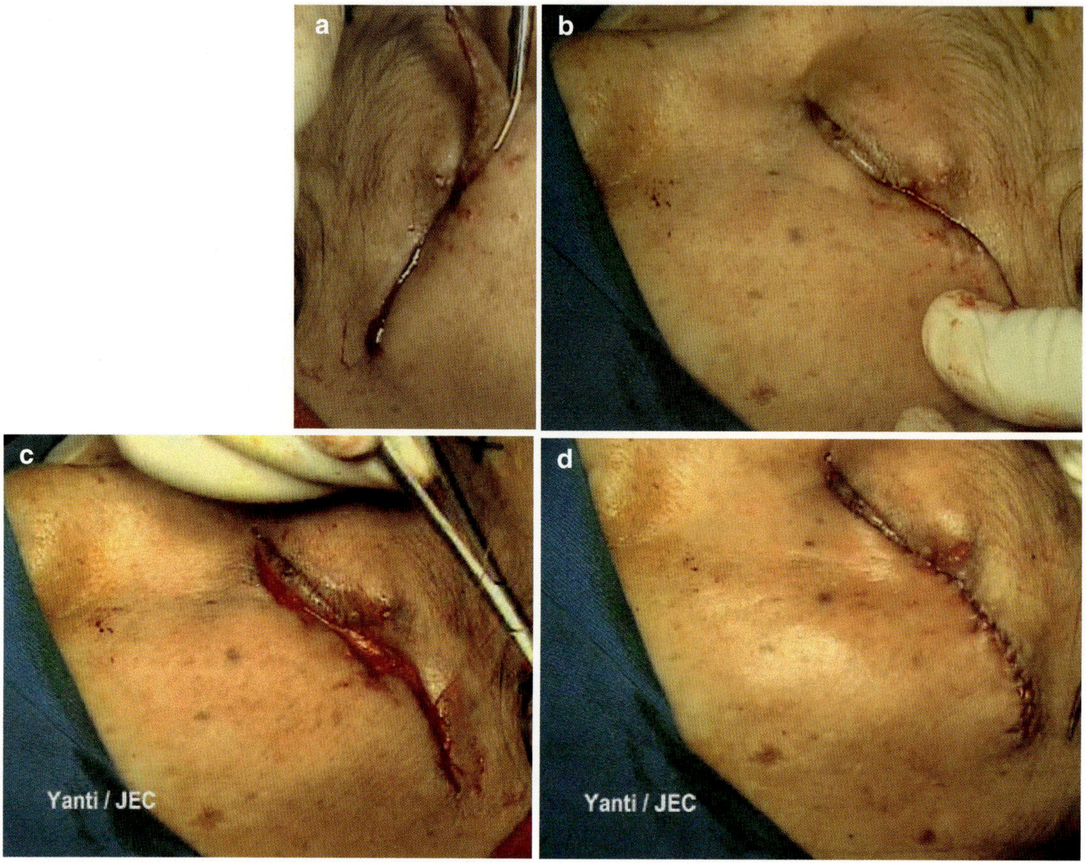


**Fig. 50.29** (**a**) Excess tissues excised. (**b**) After excision of the excess tissues. (**c**) Muscle and periosteum sutured at the level of incision with 5-0 absorbable suture and then tightened. (**d**) Skin sutured with continuous or interrupted sutures with 6-0 nonabsorbable

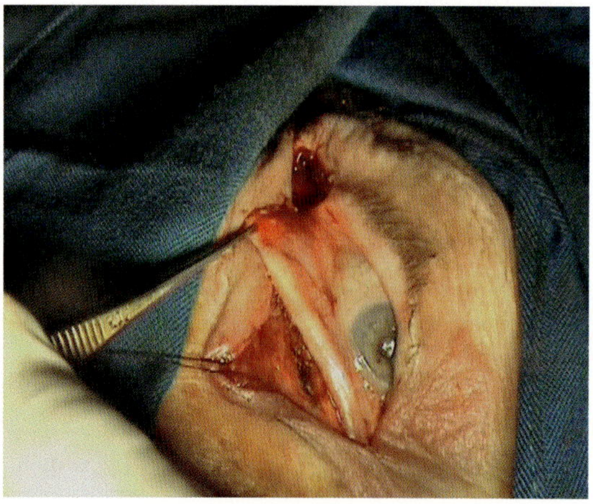

**Fig. 50.30** Residual mucosa on posterior surface of the tarsus deepithelized

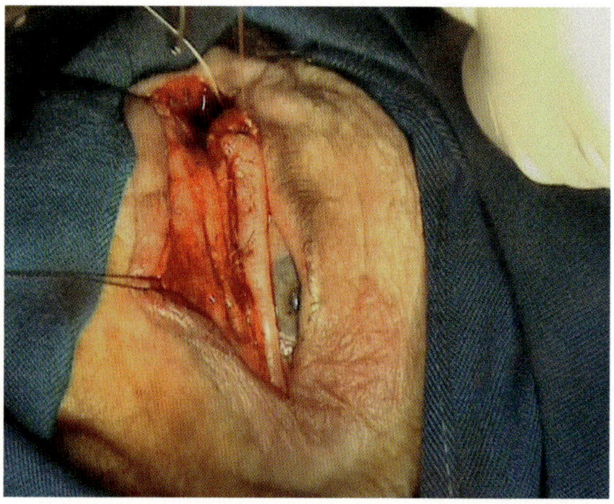

**Fig. 50.31** Lateral lower eyelid tarsal and orbicularis reinforced to the periorbita with two or three additional sutures to tighten all lower lid tissues

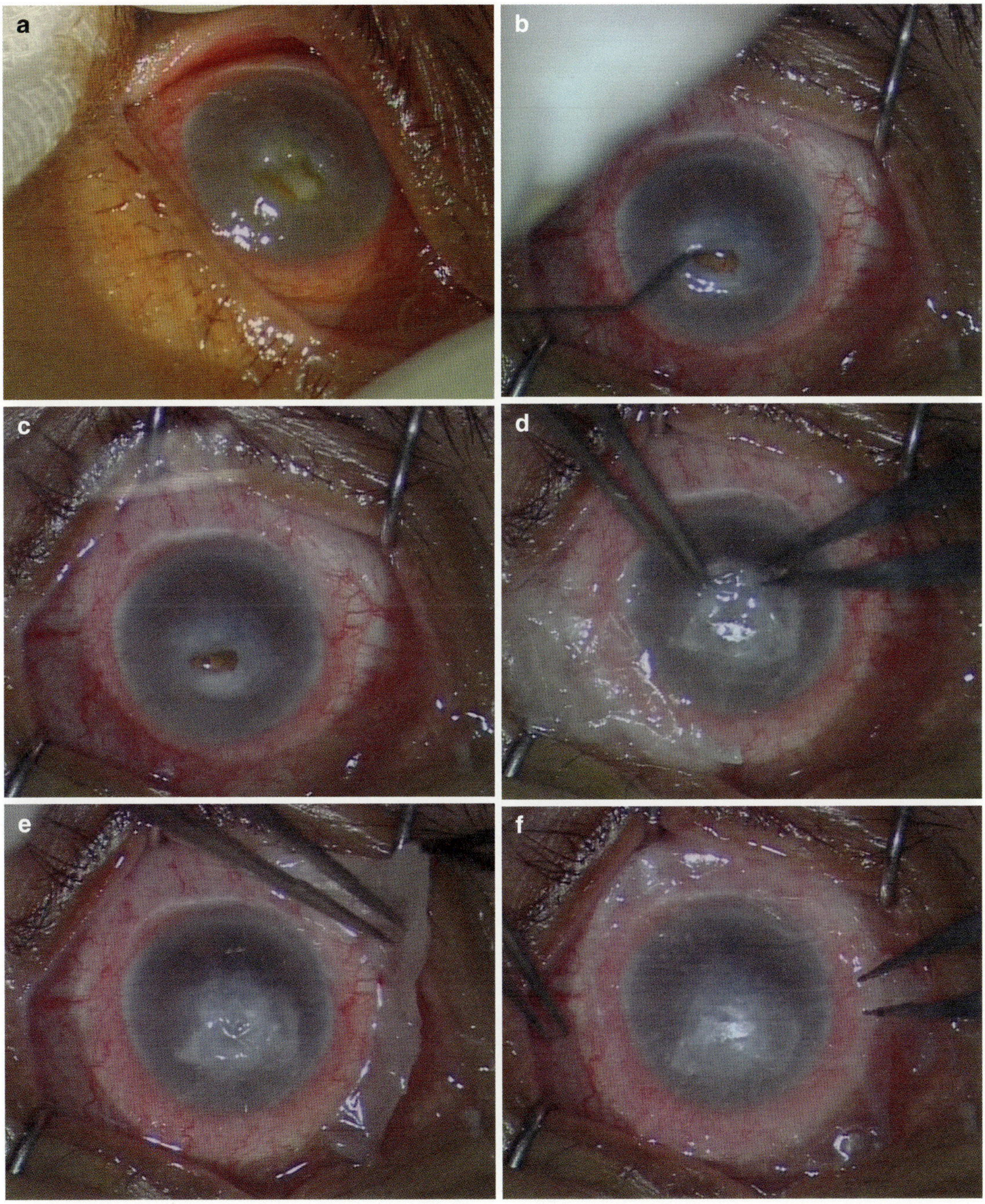


**Fig. 50.32** (**a**) Corneal perforation. (**b**) Viscoelastic material has been injected into the anterior chamber just to form the anterior chamber. (**c**) Anterior chamber has formed. (**d**) One piece of amniotic membrane has been placed upon the perforate cornea. (**e**) One large piece of amniotic membrane has been placed to cover seven layers of amniotic membrane. (**f**) Sutured to the episclera at the limbal area just to fix the position of the amniotic membranes. (**g**) Conjunctival flap performed

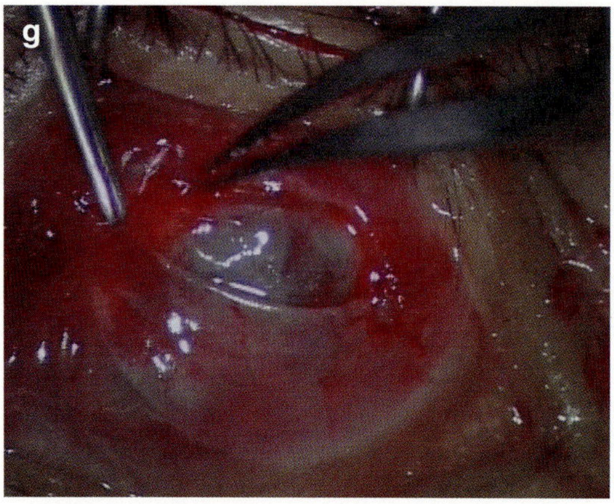


**Fig. 50.32** (continued)

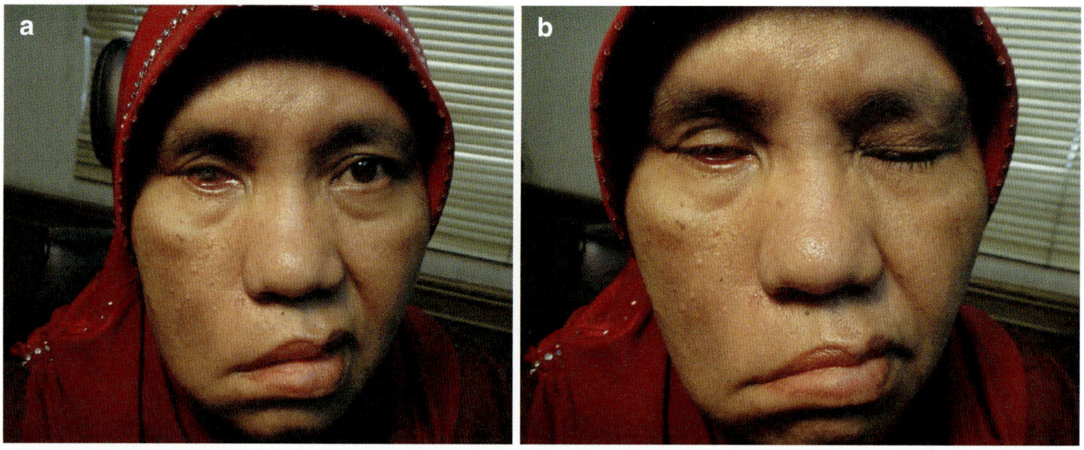


**Fig. 50.33** (**a**) Patient with seventh nerve palsy presenting lagophthalmos and severe keratopathy with corneal perforation on the right eye. (**b**) Right eye lagophthalmos

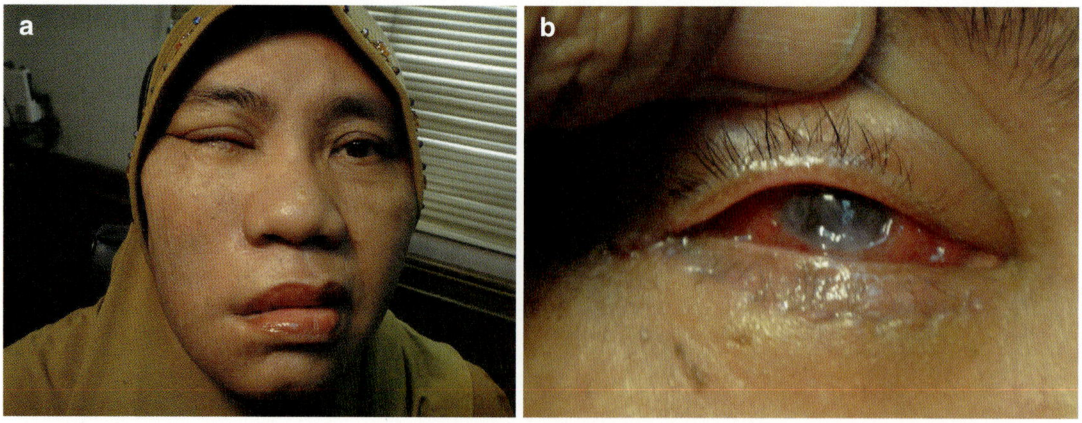


**Fig. 50.34** (**a**, **b**) Same seventh nerve palsy patient 1 week after amnion graft and conjunctival flap on the cornea and shortening of the lower lid enhanced with ear cartilage graft

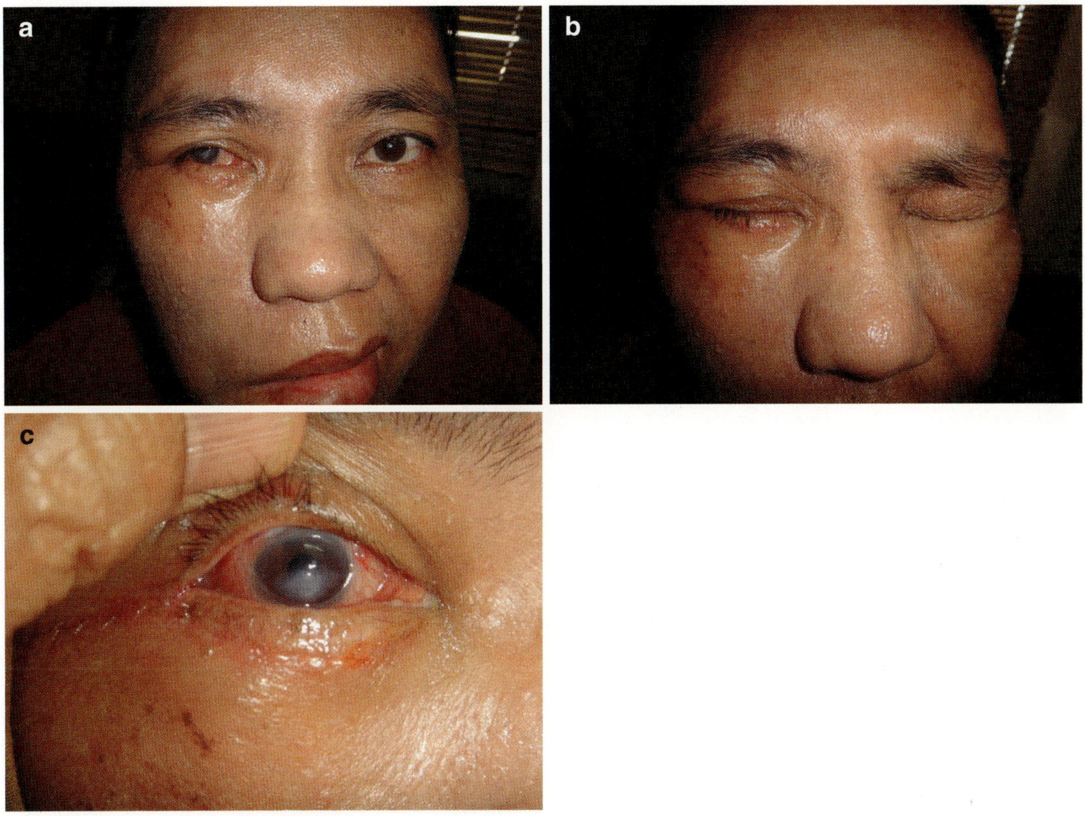

**Fig. 50.35** (**a**) Same patient 3 months after surgery with no lagophthalmos; conjunctival flap has separated itself; clear cornea at the upper area and corneal scar at the lower area with deep anterior chamber. (**b**) No lagophthalmos on the right eye. (**c**) Corneal scar with deep anterior chamber

## Lower Lid Reconstruction Is Mandatory in Facial Nerve Palsy but Not the Upper Lid. Some Patients Experience Much Better Results with Just Lower Lid Reconstruction and Upward Fixation of the Facial Tissues

### Management of Upper Lid in Facial Nerve Palsy

There are two alternatives for easy upper lid reconstruction: gold weight implant and horizontal lid shortening.

1. Gold weight implant [3, 7, 8]: place the implant with the hole at each side of the implant over the upper tarsal plate. Suture the gold implant with 6-0 nonabsorbable sutures to the tarsal plate at the medial (Fig. 50.36a) and lateral (Fig. 50.36b) sides. Once the gold implant has been sutured to the tarsal plate (Fig. 50.36c), suture the incision with continuous or interrupted sutures incorporating a bite through the upper tarsal border to create a lid fold (Fig. 50.36d).
2. The other alternative is horizontal lid shortening for patients with lax upper lids. Pull the upper lateral tarsal plate to estimate how much the whole thickness of the lateral upper lid should be removed and then mark the skin. Remove the whole thickness of the upper lateral lid and suture the upper lid margin just like suturing the lower lid margin. Suture layer by layer (Fig. 50.37).

Patient with left facial nerve palsy with severe lagophthalmos (Fig. 50.38a, b).

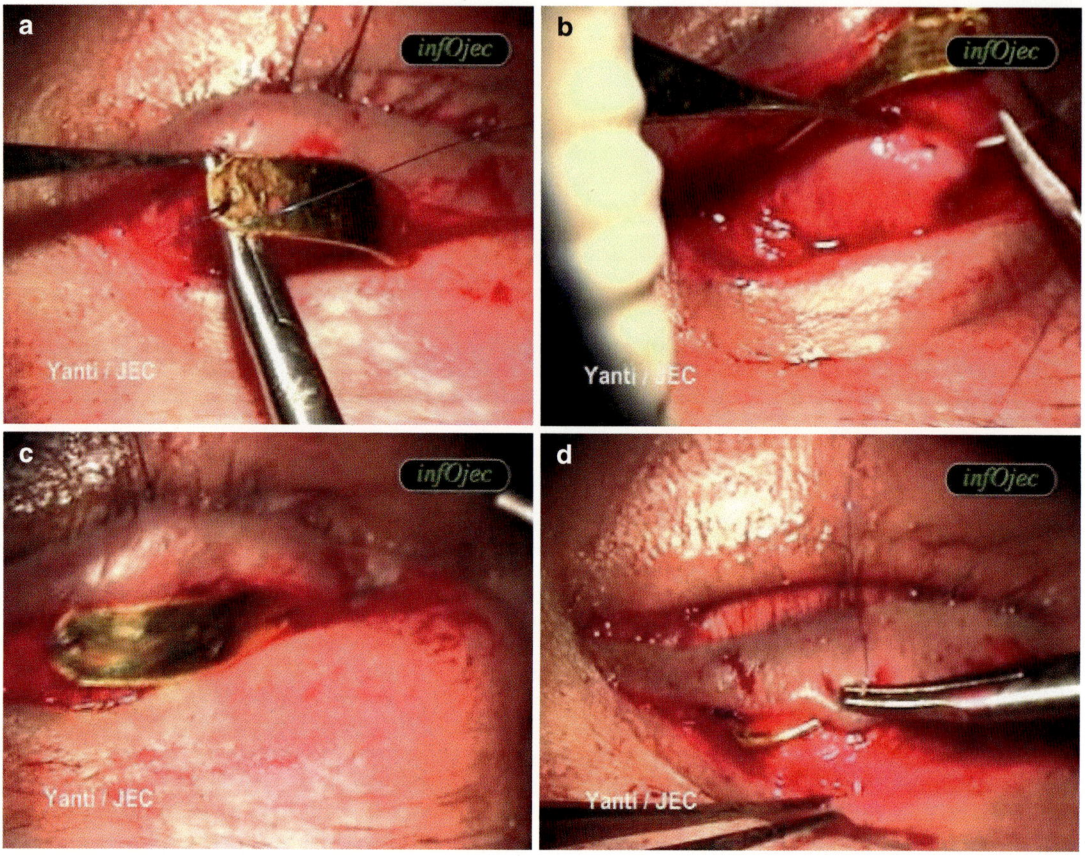


**Fig. 50.36** (**a**) Gold weight implant placed with a hole at each side of the implant to insert a needle and then sutured with 6-0 nonabsorbable suture to the tarsal plate. (**b**) Gold implant sutured to the lateral tarsal plate. (**c**) Gold implant has been sutured to the medial tarsal plate. (**d**) Lower skin incision sutured to the upper tarsal border and to the upper skin incision to create a lid fold

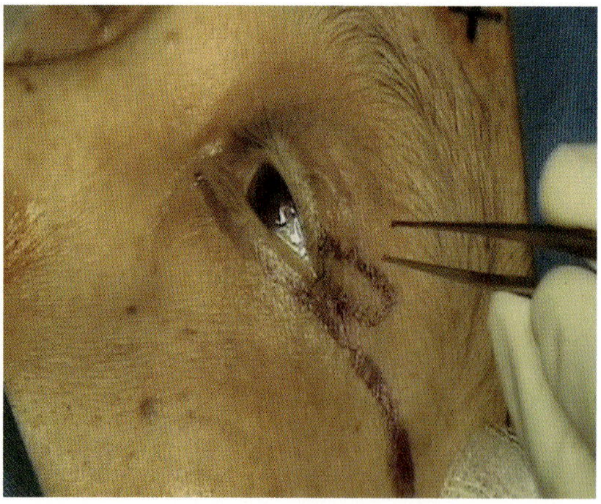

**Fig. 50.37** Upper lid excision

Lateral upper lid pentagonal excision and central lower lid pentagonal excision enhanced with ear cartilage graft was performed. The lower lid position is good; upper lid can close just a mild lagophthalmos (Fig. 50.38c, d).

Patient with left facial nerve palsy in 2004.

Gold weight implant at the upper lid and central lower lid pentagonal excision enhanced with ear cartilage graft was done in 2005, but the gold implant was extruded in 2006 (8 months after surgery). These pictures were taken 9 years after surgery; the position of the lower lid is still good with just a mild lagophthalmos (Fig. 50.39a, b).

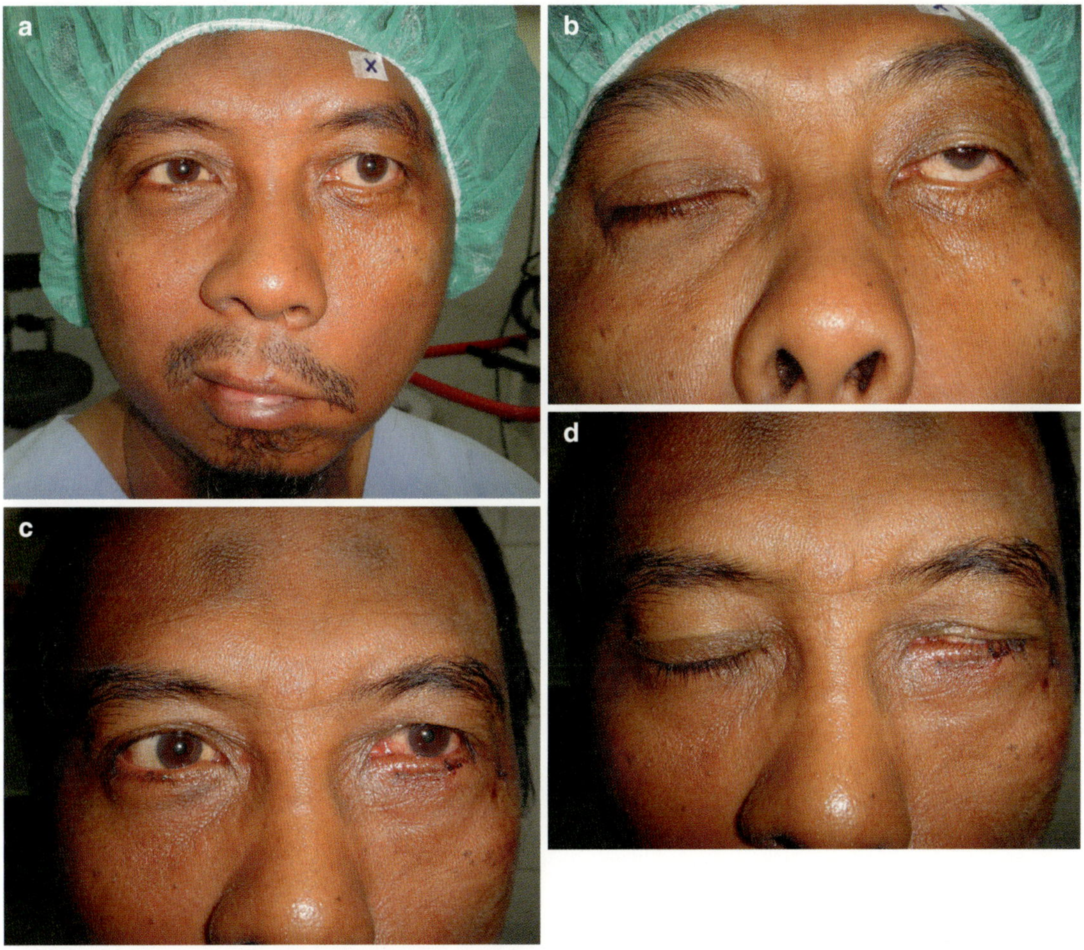

**Fig. 50.38** (**a**, **b**) Patient with left facial nerve palsy, with severe lagophthalmos. (**c**, **d**) Lateral upper lid pentagonal excision and central lower lid pentagonal excision enhanced with ear cartilage graft were performed; lower lid position is good; upper lid can close with just a mild lagophthalmos

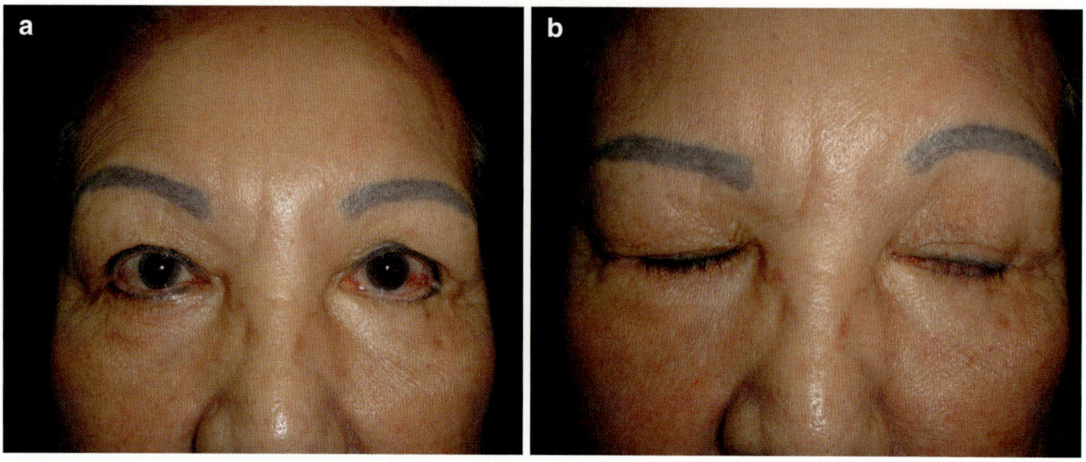

Fig. 50.39 (a, b) Patient with left facial nerve palsy in 2004; gold implant at the upper lid and central lower lid. Pentagonal excision enhanced with ear cartilage graft was done in 2005, but the gold implant was extruded in 2006 (8 months after surgery). These pictures were taken 9 years after surgery. The position of the lower lid is still good with just a mild lagophthalmos

## References


1. Bosnial SL. Cosmetic blepharoplasty. New York: Raven Press; 1990. p. 60–2.
2. Collin JRO. A manual of systematic eyelid surgery, facial palsy, thyroid eye disease and corneal protection. Edinburg: Churchill Livingstone; 1989. p. 139–42.
3. Cunningham SJ, Teller DC. Facial nerve paralysis: management of the eye, grand rounds presentation March 29, 2006.
4. Dutton JJ. Clinical and surgical orbital anatomy. The eyelids and anterior orbit, W.B. Saunders Co. p. 113–38.
5. Fox S. Ophthalmic plastic surgery, cartilage grafts. New York: Grune & Straton; 1970. p. 98–100.
6. Portelinha J, Passarincho M, Costa JM. Neuro- ophthalmological approach to facial nerve palsy. Saudi J Ophthalmol. 2015;28(1):39–47.
7. Lawrence FH, Steven LG, Alan EW, Jeffrey CP. Facial paralysis: diagnosis and management. In: Bosniak, editor. Principles and practice of ophthalmic plastic and reconstructive surgery, vol. 1. Philadelphia: W.B. Saunders Co; 1996. p. 465–83.
8. Lawrence SD, Orris CL. In: Scott IU, Fekrat S, Nelson CC, editors. Lagophthalmos evaluation and treatment, ophthalmic pearls: oculoplastic. Eye Net Magazine; April 2008.
9. Gilbord SM. Involutional and paralytic ectropion. In: Bosniak A, editor. Principle and practice of ophthalmic plastic and reconstructive surgery, vol. 1. Philadelphia: W.B Saunders co; 1996. p. 427–9.


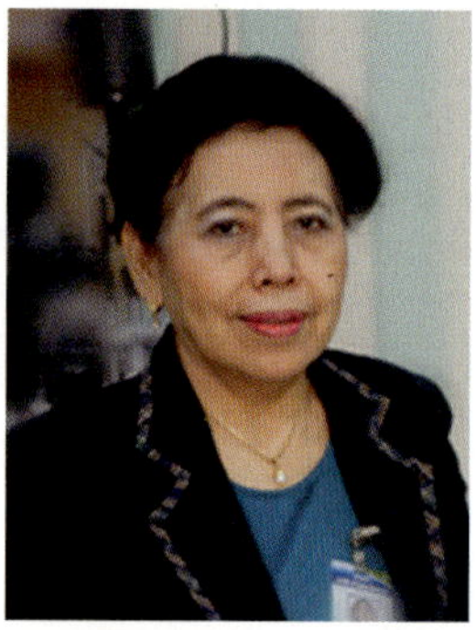


**Darmayanti Siswoyo** Dr. Darmayanti Siswoyo is currently consultant of Ophthalmic Plastic & Reconstructive Surgery, Jakarta Eye Center Hospital, Indonesia.

She was the past Head of Ophthalmic Plastic & Reconstructive Surgery Division, Department of Ophthalmology, Faculty of Medicine, University of Indonesia.

She was also the past Head of Indonesian Ophthalmic Plastic & Reconstructive Surgery & Eye Tumor Surgery Association.

She graduated from Department of Ophthalmology University of Indonesia in 1987.

She underwent orbital reconstruction training at Cranio Facial Center, Department of Plastic surgery, Royal Adelaide Hospital, South Australia in 1987.

She also underwent Oculoplastic & Reconstructive Surgery training at Department of Plastic Surgery, Kansai Medical Faculty and Department of Ophthalmology, Hamamatsu Hospital, Japan in 1992.

She was an Observer at Moorfield Eye Hospital London, England, 1993.

She is also National Speaker, Didactic Course Instructor, Wet Lab Instructor in Oculoplastic and Reconstructive Surgery in Indonesia since 1988 and International Speaker in Oculoplastic & Reconstructive Surgery since 1996.

# Complications of Botulinum Toxin and Facial Fillers

51

Leslie A. Wei, Ann Q. Tran, and Cat N. Burkat

## Introduction

In 2013, 13.4 million minimally invasive cosmetic procedures were performed in the USA, over 60 % of which were injectables such as botulinum toxin (BTX) and dermal fillers [1]. Botulinum toxin procedures alone accounted for almost 1.5 billion dollars spent on cosmetic procedures [2]. These types of aesthetic procedures are gaining popularity because of their relatively quick effects but shorter procedure and recovery time compared to incisional surgery. The overall complication rate of such procedures is low; however, knowledge of both complications and treatments are vital to a safe and successful cosmetic practice.

C.N. Burkat, MD, FACS (✉) • L.A. Wei, MD
Department of Ophthalmology and Visual Sciences, University of Wisconsin Hospitals and Clinics, 2870 University Ave, Suite 108, Madison, WI 53705, USA
e-mail: catburkat@yahoo.com; leslieweimd@gmail.com

A.Q. Tran, BSc, MD
Department of Ophthalmology and Visual Sciences, University of Wisconsin-Madison School of Medicine and Public Health, 2870 University Ave, Madison, WI 53705, USA
e-mail: vtran2@wisc.edu

## Complications of Botox (BTX)

The US Food and Drug Administration approved the cosmetic use of BTX for glabellar rhytids in 2002 and for crow's feet in 2013, although off-label uses of BTX for face and neck rejuvenation continue to be popular [3, 4]. Commercially available forms of BTX in the USA include onabotulinumtoxinA (Botox), abobotulinumtoxinA (Dysport), incobotulinumtoxinA (Xeomin), and rimabotulinumtoxinB (Myobloc) (Table 51.1) [5]. No long-term adverse complications have been reported from BTX for cosmetic indications, although transient side effects may occur (Table 51.2) [6]. While highly debated, Dysport encompasses a larger area of diffusion compared to Botox, which may lead to less localization of clinical effects and increase potential for adverse effects [7].

## Contraindications

Absolute contraindications include active infection at injection site and a history of allergic reaction to the constituents of BTX [8]. No deaths have occurred with cosmetic BTX; however, a case of lethal anaphylaxis to a Botox-lidocaine mixture has been reported [9].

Exclusion criteria include patients with neuromuscular conditions (such as myasthenia gravis, amyotrophic lateral sclerosis) who may be at increased risk of neuromuscular crises even with low doses of toxin [10].


B. Mukherjee, H. Yuen (eds.), *Emergencies of the Orbit and Adnexa*, DOI 10.1007/978-81-322-1807-4_51

**Table 51.1** Commercially available forms of botulinum toxin

| Trade name | Company | Toxin component | Other components | FDA approved uses |
|---|---|---|---|---|
| Botox | Allergan Inc. | OnabotulinumtoxinA | Human serum albumin, NaCl | Blepharospasm, cervical dystonia, glabellar lines, chronic migraine, etc. |
| Dysport | Medics Pharmaceutical Corp. | AbobotulinumtoxinA | Human serum albumin, lactose | Blepharospasms, cervical dystonia, glabellar lines |
| Xeomin | Merz Pharmaceuticals | IncobotulinumtoxinA | Human serum albumin, sucrose | Blepharospasms, cervical dystonia, glabellar lines |
| Myobloc | Solstice Neuroscience Inc. | RimabotulinumtoxinB | Human serum albumin, NaCl, disodium succinate water | Cervical dystonia |

**Table 51.2** Complications of Botox

| |
|---|
| Undertreatment |
| Injection site pain and bruising |
| Asymmetry |
| Headache |
| Allergic reaction |
| Dry eyes |
| Brow ptosis |
| Eyelid ptosis |
| Lip ptosis |
| Lower face complications: drooling, dysphagia, and neck weakness |

Women currently pregnant, lactating, or planning on becoming pregnant should avoid BTX, as it is a category C medication with little knowledge of breast milk absorption of excretion [10].

Relative contraindications include immunocompromised patients at increased risk of infection, over the age of 65, those with unrealistic expectations or with body dysmorphic disorder [10, 11]. BTX should be avoided in patients taking medications that interfere or interact with the metabolism of the drug such as aminoglycosides or cholinesterase inhibitors (Table 51.3).

**Table 51.3** Contraindications to botulinum toxin injection

| |
|---|
| *Absolute contraindications* |
| Active infection at injection site |
| Sensitivity or allergy to constituents of botulinum toxin product |
| *Relative contraindications* |
| Age >65 – safety and efficacy unknown |
| Actors or singers dependent on facial expression |
| Botulinophilia (body dysmorphic disorder) |
| Immunocompromised states (e.g., diabetes or alcoholism) |
| Inflammatory skin diseases (e.g., eczema, psoriasis, history of keloid scarring) |
| Medication use with aminoglycoside antibacterials (e.g., streptomycin or neomycin), cholinesterase inhibitors, calcium channel antagonist, local anesthetics, curane depolarizing agents, chloroquine, cyclosporine A, and penicillamine |
| Neuromuscular disorder (e.g., amyotrophic lateral sclerosis, Lambert-Eaton syndrome, myasthenia gravis, or other peripheral motor neuropathies) |
| Pregnancy or lactation |
| Pre-existing eyelid or brow ptosis |

## Relative Complications

### Undertreatment

Undertreatment may often result in consumer dissatisfaction, as residual lines or redundant skin in surrounding areas may become more noticeable. Clinicians should counsel patients for realistic expectations, need for additional treatment or adjunctive therapy with soft tissue augmentation or skin laser treatments, especially for maximal correction of rhytids. In addition, patient sensitivity and resistance vary; thus, more BTX may be needed for some compared to others.

Over time, repeated doses of BTX injections can elicit an immune response leading to the development of neutralizing antibodies against the neurotoxin in 0.49 % of patients [12]. These patients may become unresponsive despite increasing doses of BTX [13]. A trial of a different serotype can be beneficial in refractory cases as neutralizing antibodies against one serotype do not appear to block the activity of others [14, 15]. To prevent future loss of efficacy, current practices advocate for the lowest effective dose and the longest time interval between treatments.

## Bruising

In clinical trials, treating crow's feet, bruising, and pain were reported in 10–25 % of patients [16, 17]. The lateral canthal region is particularly susceptible as the orbicularis oculi is very thin with a rich network of superficial veins. To minimize bruising:

- Stop herbal products such as vitamin E, garlic, ginger, ginseng, *Ginkgo biloba*, and St. John's Wort and aspirin 1–2 weeks prior to treatment [18]. Take a thorough medication history as half of cosmetic patients may report using herbal supplements [19].
- Use small needles (30–32 gauge) on a tuberculin syringe.
- Inject in areas with minimal vascularity.
- Inject on top rather than into the muscle in periocular region.
- Apply ice to the areas of increased vascularity for vasoconstriction.

## Injection Site Pain

To reduce injection pain:

- Apply topical anesthetic cream 15–30 min prior to injection, if needed [20].
- Place cool compresses or ice before and after the procedure to minimize discomfort [20].
- Pinch the skin or tap a finger nearby injection site as a distraction technique.
- Preservative-containing saline as the diluent produces less pain with no difference in efficacy than non-preservative formulations [21].

## Asymmetry

Facial asymmetry can be reduced with dosing adjustments based on the preexisting muscle activity, proper technique, and knowledge of facial anatomy. Inappropriate injection to the glabella and frontalis may lead to an upside-down V-shaped or "cocked" eyebrow from incomplete weakening of the lateral frontalis that can be corrected with additional BTX to the lateral frontalis muscle [22]. Injection in close proximity to the orbicularis oris in the treatment of sad lines may produce flaccid cheek or asymmetric smile. To minimize, place injections 1 cm away from the lateral caudal lip at the jaw angle behind the nasolabial folds [22].

## Headache

BTX may cause headaches due to microtrauma from needle insertion or neurotoxin-induced muscle spasm [23]. Headache frequency varies from 11 % to 15 % [24, 25]. Most headaches are mild lasting for a few hours and relieved by over-the-counter analgesics [24]. Only 1 % of patients experience severe debilitating headaches lasting 2–4 weeks [23].

## Moderate Complications

### Allergic Reaction

Hypersensitivity and allergic reaction to BTX are extremely rare and typically manifest as pruritus or unspecified rash [26]. Skin rashes such as psoriasiform eruption, pseudo-segmental exanthema, and sarcoid nodules after intramuscular injection have been seen [27–29]. Systemic reactions such as botulinum toxicity have only been reported in four cases [30]. The use of epinephrine and methylprednisolone for management of severe allergic reactions is recommended over diphenhydramine (Benadryl) due to the anticholinergic effects [31].

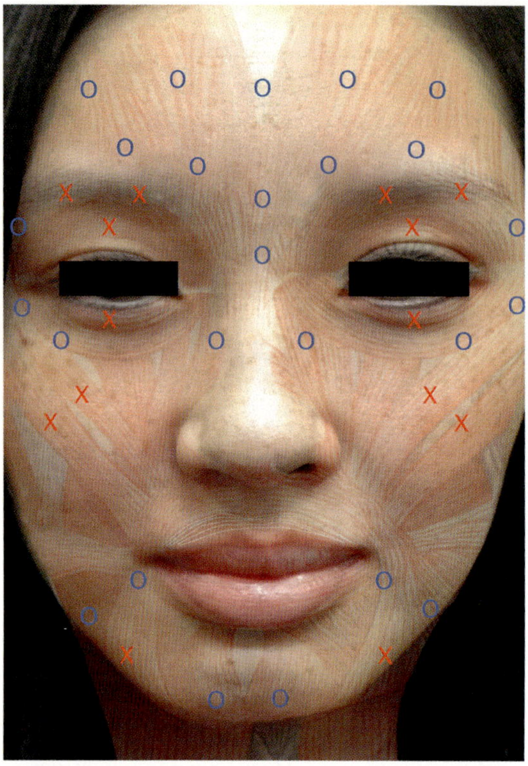

**Fig. 51.1** Muscles of facial expression. *X* = high-risk injection areas – injections here should be performed with caution and expertise. *O* = typical injection sites in cosmetic BTX treatment

## Upper Face Complications

Brow ptosis occurs in up to 5 % of patients treated for glabellar and forehead rhytids leading to partial obstruction in vision [32]. Older patients with increased hooding and brow laxity may develop pseudo-ptosis. To avoid this complication, injections should be placed approximately 1 cm above the supraorbital rim for glabellar rhytids, and no lower than the mid-forehead level for frontalis creases (Fig. 51.1).

Eyelid ptosis can occur after injection to any number of areas, including the lateral orbicularis oculi, glabella, and forehead. Blepharoptosis after crow's feet injection occurred in 5.4 % patients in early studies but has decreased to 0.3 % in later studies [33, 34]. Symptomatic patients can be treated with α-adrenergic agonist drops to contract Muller's muscle and produce 1–2 mm of eyelid elevation [10]. In refractory cases, apraclonidine drops can be used [35].

Injection too close to the lateral orbicularis oculi is associated with an increased risk of dry eyes, diplopia, ectropion, and lagophthalmos. The mechanism of dry eyes is thought to be secondary to decreased tear production and tear film stability [36]. Anti-inflammatory drops can be prescribed to alleviate this condition [37]. Diplopia from diffusion to the lateral rectus can develop into diplopia that can be symptomatically relieved with patching of the affected eye and follow-up with an ophthalmologist [38]. Ectropion can occur from lower orbicularis oculi paralysis, particularly if injected near or into the pretarsal orbicularis oculi portion. Performing the snapback test to assess lower eyelid laxity will allow for better patient selection.

## Midface and Lower Face Complications

Lip ptosis is a rare complication of BTX treatment of crow's feet and bunny lines and can last up to 6 weeks with no real treatment options. Injections too close to the zygomatic arch can weaken the zygomaticus major muscle and create an appearance similar to Bell's palsy [39]. Treatment of fine lateral nasal smile lines, known as bunny lines, can cause weakening of the levator labii superioris [40].

Treatment of vertical platysmal bands can lead to side effects such as neck stiffness, weakness, and dry mouth that may last up to 3 weeks [41]. Severe complications such as dysphagia and dysphonia arise if diffusion or direct injection occurs into the sternocleidomastoid. Superficial, small dose injections can avert accidental paralysis.

## Complications of Fillers

Dermal fillers, also called soft tissue fillers, are one of the most sought-after minimally invasive procedures, second only to Botulinum toxin [42]. 2.2 million soft tissue fillers were administered in the USA in 2013, an increase of 13 % compared to 2012 [1]. Commonly used fillers types

**Table 51.4** Dermal fillers

| | Nonabsorbable | Absorbable synthetic | | Absorbable natural | |
|---|---|---|---|---|---|
| Major component | PMMA | Hydroxylapatite | Poly-L-lactic acid | Hyaluronic acid | Collagen |
| Brand name | Artefill<br>Artecoll | Radiesse | Sculptra | Juvederm<br>Restylane<br>Perlane<br>Belotero<br>Hylaform<br>Elevess<br>Prevelle<br>Captique<br>Voluma | Zyderm<br>Cosmoderm<br>Evolence<br>Fibrel |

Adapted from Food and Drug Administration Office of Device Evaluation 2008 Executive Summary Dermal Filler Devices
Selected fillers are most commonly used in the USA; this table does not list all currently available fillers in all countries
*PMMA* polymethylmethacrylate

**Table 51.5** Complications of dermal fillers

| |
|---|
| Undertreatment |
| Overtreatment |
| Asymmetry |
| Bruising |
| Edema and erythema |
| Contour irregularities/ridging/beading |
| Tyndall effect |
| Granuloma formation |
| Allergic reaction |
| Skin necrosis |
| Blindness |

are listed in Table 51.4. Complications range from mild transient effects such as bruising and erythema to sequelae as severe as skin necrosis and blindness (Table 51.5). Judicious administration by an experienced injector is crucial to avoid complications. Should a complication occur, timely treatment and close follow-up are warranted to obtain an acceptable cosmetic outcome.

## Contraindications

Absolute contraindications to dermal fillers are an active infection at the injection site, history of allergy/hypersensitivity to filler or an allergy to lidocaine, and bleeding disorders [43, 44]. Relative contraindications include a history of herpetic eruption at injection sites and history of keloid formation, hyperpigmentation, or hypertrophic scarring (Table 51.6) [44]. Women who are pregnant or breastfeeding should delay elective cosmetic procedures, as there is a lack of controlled trials assessing the safety of fillers during pregnancy and postpartum periods [45].

**Table 51.6** Contraindications to dermal fillers [44]

| |
|---|
| *Absolute contraindications* |
| Active infection at injection site |
| Sensitivity or allergy to filler OR lidocaine |
| Bleeding disorders |
| *Relative contraindications* |
| History of herpetic eruptions at injection site |
| History of keloid formation, skin hyperpigmentation, or hypertrophic scarring |
| Pregnancy or lactation |

## Relative Complications

### Undertreatment

Undertreatment with facial fillers is a relative complication in the sense that it results in an unhappy patient. It is the easiest complication to fix by augmenting with additional filler. The most common areas for patients to complain of undertreatment are the nasolabial folds and marionette lines [46].

### Overtreatment

Overfilling an area of the face, particularly the lips or tear troughs, can give an unnatural appearance and also result in a dissatisfied patient. Hyaluronic acid fillers can be quickly reversed

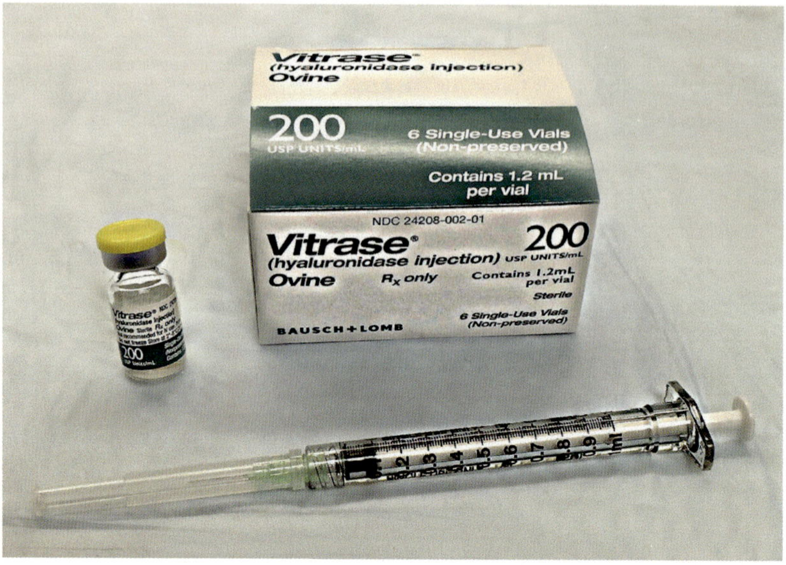


**Fig. 51.2** Unreconstituted hyaluronidase (Vitrase, Ista Pharmaceuticals, Inc). Inject 30–75 units directly into areas of unwanted filler using a 1-mL syringe and 30 or 32-gauge needle

using hyaluronidase, which will start reversing the filler immediately and achieve maximal results in 2–3 days (Fig. 51.2) [47, 48]. Several authors have recommended using 75 units, on average, for treatment of overfilled areas [46, 49]. However, the patient should be informed that hyaluronidase may lead to more dissolution of the filler than desired, resulting in recurrence of rhytids. Prevention via conservative injections to avoid overfilling is the best management. In extreme circumstances of overtreatment, areas that are overfilled can be surgically excised [46, 50].

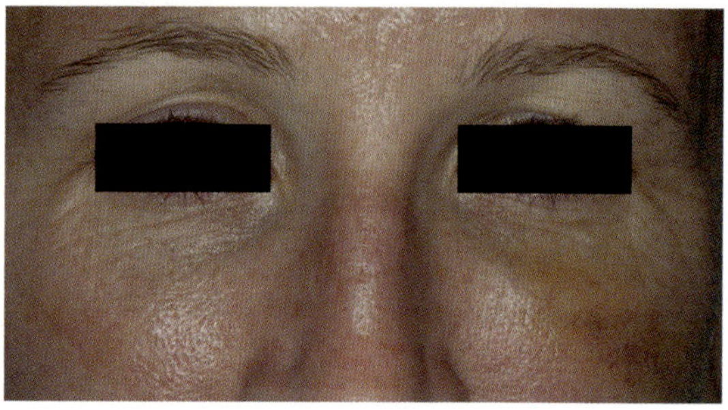

**Fig. 51.3** Bruising 1 week after injection of hyaluronic acid filler for malar augmentation

### Asymmetry

Asymmetry is a common, harmless complication after facial filler administration and is usually addressed by augmenting the side that appears underfilled [51]. Careful pre-injection counseling and follow-up visits for possible touch-ups will minimize patient dissatisfaction.

## Mild Complications

### Bruising

One of the most common complications associated with fillers (5–10 %), bruising, is bothersome but can be managed conservatively without affecting the final cosmetic outcome (Fig. 51.3) [42, 52, 53]. The lips and periocular area are highly vascular and prone to bruising even with appropriate injection techniques. Avoidance of visible cutaneous vessels, use of smaller gauge needles (27 gauge or smaller), and icing prior to and immediately after injection decrease the risk of bruising and hematoma formation [46, 50]. Patients should also be advised to stop any blood thinners (aspirin, nonsteroidal anti-inflammatory drugs, and vitamin supplements such as vitamin E, ginseng, ginkgo biloba, garlic, kava kava, and fish oils) 1 week prior to receiving filler [54]. Oral and topical *Arnica montana* may be given if bruising does occur to speed resolution of ecchymoses [55]. Intense pulsed light therapy can also be useful for prolonged bruising.

## Edema and Erythema

Some edema and erythema will occur naturally at injection sites, especially if the injection was too superficial. Postinjection icing will speed resolution. A short course of oral steroids, intralesional Kenalog, intense pulsed light therapy, or even dermabrasion can be given in severe circumstances [47, 50, 51].

## Contour Irregularities/Ridging/Beading

Unnatural contours and lumps are the result of poor filler placement. Injecting filler too superficially (calcium hydroxylapatite and poly-L-lactic acid) can result in palpable lumps. Light massaging during the injection session is very important to smooth out contour irregularities, particularly in the perioral region [46]. Most contour irregularities will resolve on their own over time; however, intralesional corticosteroids, surgical excision, and laser resurfacing or dermabrasion are reasonable management options, particularly for permanent filler lumps [43, 51].

## Tyndall Effect

The Tyndall effect (also known as the Rayleigh effect) describes the blue-gray appearance of filler under the skin (Fig. 51.4) resulting from a 10× higher scattering of blue light in comparison to red light [49]. Placing filler too superficially in areas with thinner skin (tear troughs) can result in a Tyndall effect that may last for several months or longer. To avoid this occurrence, dermal fillers in the periorbital area should be placed deeper, preferably in the pre-periosteal plane. Treatment includes observation, removal of filler (hyaluronidase or incision and expression), and Nd:YAG laser [56].

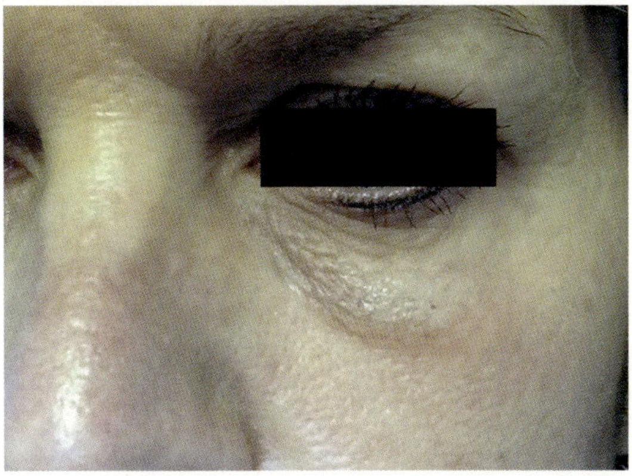

**Fig. 51.4** Tyndall effect still visible 1 year after tear trough injection of dermal filler

# Moderate Complications

## Granuloma Formation

All facial fillers activate a tissue foreign body response, ranging from mild inflammation to intense fibrosis and nodule formation [57]. Granuloma formation occurs mostly with silicon-based fillers, collagen, calcium hydroxylapatite, and poly-L-lactic acid 6–24 months after injection [50, 58]. True granulomas are rare, occurring in 0.01–1 % of patients [51]. Both host tissue inflammation and chronic low-grade infection are thought to be involved in the pathogenesis of filler-associated granulomas [57]. Increasing the time between injections as well as the dilution of the filler may decrease the risk of granulomas. Most granulomas will resolve with conservative management within 2 years [59]. Occasionally, granulomas will require intralesional steroid injection, topical tacrolimus, or surgical excision [54].

## Infection

Viral or bacterial infection may rarely complicate filler injections, particularly herpes simplex and skin flora such as *Staphylococcus aureus* [60]. Bacterial infections manifest as fluctuating painful erythematous nodules in the area of injection with or without fever and should be cultured if possible before placing the patient on empiric antibiotic therapy [61]. Prophylactic treatment for herpes is indicated for patients receiving lip filler who have a history of recurrent outbreaks [60].

## Severe Complications

### Systemic Allergic Reaction

True allergic reaction to dermal fillers is rare. Angioedema is reported to occur in one to five cases per 10,000, and anaphylaxis has been reported [62, 63]. Hyaluronic acid fillers have been shown to elicit a cellular or humoral immune response in only 2 % of individuals, with minimal IgE sensitization, IgG formation, and lymphocytic inflammatory reactions [64]. Acute type I hypersensitivity reactions should be treated with antihistamines, steroids, epinephrine, beta-agonists, and hemodynamic support [65].

### Skin Necrosis

Direct injection of a facial artery can result in skin necrosis, which is by far the most disfiguring complication of dermal fillers. It is fortunately very rare (<0.001–0.5 %) but has been reported for every type of filler [61, 66]. The risk is highest in the glabellar area due to limited collateral circulation, with the most vulnerable arteries being the supraorbital, supratrochlear, infraorbital, and angular [67, 68]. Prevention is the best treatment:

- Aspiration prior to injection
- The use of a blunt-tipped cannula rather than a needle
- Injection of small filler volumes
- Injection during withdrawal of cannula/needle

Early signs of arterial vascular compromise are pain and skin pallor, while signs of venous occlusion are often delayed and present as dull pain and discoloration [68]. When recognized, immediately:

- Stop injection.
- Massage area aggressively.
- Apply warm compresses.
- Apply topical 2 % nitroglycerin paste [67, 69].
- Inject hyaluronidase as expeditiously as possible (within 4 h) to dissolve the product [70].
- Administer daily aspirin and steroid taper [71].
- Consider the use of molecular weight heparin or other thrombolytics [67, 72].

If partial or full thickness skin necrosis occurs, attentive wound care with debridement as necessary will minimize the resultant scarring. After scar maturation (approximately 3 months), laser scar revision or surgical excision can be offered.

### Blindness

The most devastating functional adverse outcome of soft tissue fillers is blindness from occlusion of the ophthalmic artery and its branches. An intravascular bolus of filler can reach the ophthalmic artery via retrograde flow from any number of facial arteries, particularly the dorsal nasal, supratrochlear, or supraorbital vessels (Fig. 51.5). The dissemination of filler in a facial artery can eventually reach the brain, resulting in focal infarctions with corresponding neurologic symptoms such as hemiplegia and dysarthria [73]. Vision loss is often profound and permanent. In large series of iatrogenic ophthalmic artery occlusions from facial

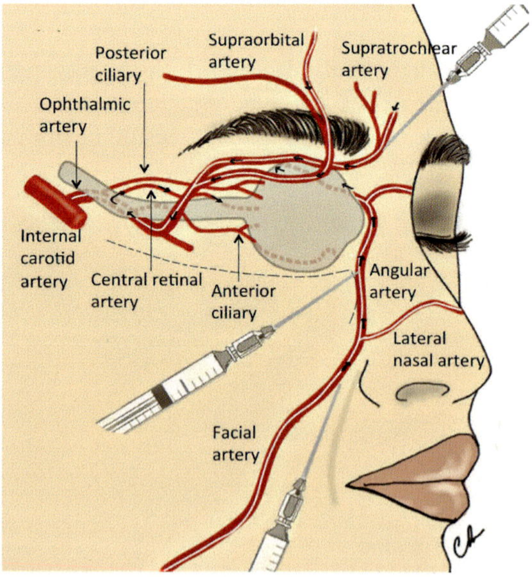


**Fig. 51.5** Arteries of the face at high risk for intravascular injection of filler

fillers, 60 % of patients had a final visual acuity of NLP (no light perception) [73, 74]. Vascular occlusions in the orbital and periorbital area can also result in other severe ophthalmic complications such as ophthalmoplegia and ptosis [75, 76]. The same preventative measures as outlined above to avoid skin necrosis should be undertaken. Should an ophthalmic artery occlusion occur, anterior chamber paracentesis, ocular massage, and hyperbaric oxygen may be attempted; however, the visual outcomes remain poor [77].

In summary, cosmetic chemodenervation with botulinum toxin and soft tissue filler augmentation can be done safely with appropriate knowledge of facial anatomy and specific filler characteristics. Understanding the breadth of complications and their treatment will improve injection safety and maximize patient satisfaction.

## References


1. American Society of Plastics Surgeons. ASPS National Clearinghouse of Plastic Surgery Procedural Statistics. Plast Surg Stat Rep. 2013;2014:1–23. http://www.plasticsurgery.org/Documents/news-resources/statistics/2013-statistics/plastic-surgery-statistics-full-report-2013.pdf
2. American Society of Aesthetic Plastic Surgeons. Cosmetic Surgery National Data Bank Statistics.; 2013:1–23.
3. U.S. Food and Drug Administration. FDA approves botox cosmetic to improve the appearance of Crow's feet lines. 2013.
4. Kaltreider SA, Kennedy RH, Woog JJ, Bradley EA, Custer PL, Meyer DR. Cosmetic oculofacial applications of botulinum toxin: a report by the American Academy of Ophthalmology. Ophthalmology. 2005;112(6):1159–67.
5. Walker TJ, Dayan SH. Comparison and overview of currently available neurotoxins. J Clin Aesth Dermatol. 2014;7(2):31–9.
6. Coté TR, Mohan AK, Polder JA, Walton MK, Braun MM. Botulinum toxin type A injections: adverse events reported to the US Food and Drug Administration in therapeutic and cosmetic cases. J Am Acad Dermatol. 2005;53(3):407–15.
7. de Trinda de Almeida AR, Marques E, de Almeida J, Cunha T, Boraso R. Pilot study comparing the diffusion of two formulations of botulinum toxin type A in patients with forehead hyperhidrosis. Dermatol Surg. 2007;33:S37–43.
8. Allergan. BOTOX® Cosmetic Prescribing Information. 1989:1–36. http://www.allergan.com/assets/pdf/botox_cosmetic_pi.pdf
9. Li M, Goldberger B, Hopkins C. Fatal case of BOTOX-related anaphylaxis? J Forensic Sci. 2005;50:169–72.
10. Klein AW. Contraindications and complications with the use of botulinum toxin. Clin Dermatol. 2003;22(1):66–75.
11. Harte W, Linse R. Botulinophilia: contraindication for therapy with botulinum toxin. Int J Clin Pharmacol Ther. 2001;39(10):460–3.
12. Naumann M, Carruthers A, Carruthers J, et al. Meta-analysis of neutralizing antibody conversion with onabotulinumtoxinA (BOTOX®) across multiple indications. Mov Disord. 2010;25(13):2211–8.
13. Dressler D, Munchau A, Bhatia K, Quinn N, Bigalke H. Antibody-induced botulinum toxin therapy failure: can it be overcome by increased botulinum toxin doses? Eur Neurol. 2002;47:118–21.
14. Alster TS, Lupton JR. Botulinum toxin type B for dynamic glabellar rhytides refractory to botulinum toxin type A. Dermatol Surg. 2003;29(5):516–8.
15. Dertzbaugh MT, West MW. Mapping of protective and cross-reactive domains of the type A neurotoxin of Clostridium botulinum. Vaccine. 1996;14(16):1538–44.
16. Lowe NJ, Lask G, Yamauchi P, Moore D. Bilateral, double-blind, randomized comparison of 3 doses of botulinum toxin type A and placebo in patients with crow's feet. J Am Acad Dermatol. 2002;47(6):834–40.
17. Ascher B, Rzany BJ, Grover R. Efficacy and safety of botulinum toxin type A in the treatment of lateral crow's feet: double-blind, placebo-controlled, dose-ranging study. Dermatol Surg. 2009;35(10):1478–86.
18. Dinehart SM, Henry L. Dietary supplements: altered coagulation and effects on bruising. Dermatol Surg. 2005;31(7 Pt 2):819–26.
19. Zwiebel SJ, Lee M, Alleyne B, Guyuron B. The incidence of vitamin, mineral, herbal, and other supplement use in facial cosmetic patients. Plast Reconstr Surg. 2013;132(1):78–82.
20. Elibol O, Ozkan B, Hekimhan PK, Cağlar Y. Efficacy of skin cooling and EMLA cream application for pain relief of periocular botulinum toxin injection. Ophthal Plast Reconstr Surg. 2007;23(2):130–3.
21. Alam M, Dover J, Arndt K. Pain associated with injection of botulinum a exotoxin reconstituted using isotonic sodium chloride with and without preservative: a double-blind, randomized controlled trial. Arch Dermatol. 2002;138(4):510–4.
22. Wollina U, Konrad H. Managing adverse events associated with botulinum toxin type A: a focus on cosmetic procedures. Am J Clin Dermatol. 2005;6(3):141–50.
23. Alam M, Arndt KA, Dover JS. Severe, intractable headache after injection with botulinum a exotoxin: report of 5 cases. J Am Acad Dermatol. 2002;46(1):62–5.
24. Carruthers JD, Lowe NJ, Menter MA, Gibson J, Eadie N. Double-blind, placebo-controlled study of the safety and efficacy of botulinum toxin type A for patients with glabellar lines. Plast Reconstr Surg. 2003;112(4):1089–98.

25. Carruthers JA, Lowe NJ, Menter MA, et al. A multicenter, double-blind, randomized, placebo-controlled study of the efficacy and safety of botulinum toxin type A in the treatment of glabellar lines. J Am Acad Dermatol. 2002;46(6):840–9.
26. Cohen D, Kaufman J. Hypersensitivity reactions to products and devices in plastics surgery. Facial Plast Surg Clin N Am. 2003;11(2):253–65.
27. Bowden JB, Rapini RP. Psoriasiform eruption from intramuscular botulinum A toxin. Cutis. 1992;50(6):415–6.
28. Brüggemann N, Dögnitz L, Harms L, Moser A, Hagenah J. Skin reactions after intramuscular injection of Botulinum toxin A: a rare side effect. J Neurol Neurosurg Psychiatry. 2008;79:231–2.
29. Ahbib S, Lachapelle J, Marot L. Sarcoidal granulomas following injections of botulic toxin A (Botox) for corrections of wrinkles. Ann Dermatol Venereol. 2006;133:43–5.
30. Chertow DS, Tan ET, Maslanka SE, et al. Botulism in 4 adults following cosmetic injections with an unlicensed, highly concentrated botulinum preparation. JAMA. 2006;296(20):2476–9.
31. Small R. Botulinum toxin injection for facial wrinkles. Am Fam Physician. 2014;90(3):168–75.
32. Mack WP. Complications in periocular rejuvenation. Facial Plast Surg Clin N Am. 2010;18(3):435–56.
33. Keen M, Blitzer A, Aviv J, et al. Botulinum toxin A for hyperkinetic facial lines: results of a double-blind, placebo-controlled study. Plast Reconstr Surg. 1994;94(1):94–9.
34. Hanke CW, Narins RS, Brandt F, et al. A randomized, placebo-controlled, double-blind phase III trial investigating the efficacy and safety of incobotulinumtoxinA in the treatment of glabellar frown lines using a stringent composite endpoint. Dermatol Surg. 2013;39(6):891–9.
35. Yazici B, Beden U. Use of 0.5% apraclonidine solution in evaluation of blepharoptosis. Ophthal Plast Reconstr Surg. 2008;24(4):299–301.
36. Ho M-C, Hsu W-C, Hsieh Y-T. Botulinum toxin type a injection for lateral canthal rhytids : effect on tear film stability and tear production. JAMA Ophthalmol. 2014;132(3):332–7.
37. Ferreira M, Salles A, Gimenez R, Soares M. Complications with the use of botulinum toxin type A in facial rejuvenation: report of 8 cases. Aesthet Plast Surg. 2004;28:441–4.
38. Emer J, Levy L. Complications of minimally invasive cosmetic procedures: prevention and management. J Cutan Aesthet Surg. 2012;5:121–32.
39. Matarasso S, Matarasso A. Treatment guidelines for botulinum toxin type A for the periocular region and a report on partial upper lip ptosis following injections to the lateral canthal rhytids. Plast Reconstr Surg. 2001;108(1):208–14.
40. Carruthers J, Carruthers A. Aesthetic botulinum A toxin in the mid and lower face and neck. Dermatol Clin. 2004;22(2):151–8.
41. Brandt FS, Boker A. Botulinum toxin for the treatment of neck lines and neck bands. Dermatol Clin. 2004;22(2):159–66.
42. McCracken MS, Khan JA, Wulc AE. Hyaluronic acid gel (Restylane) filler for facial rhytids: lessons learned from American Society of Ophthalmic Plastic and Reconstructive Surgery member treatment of 286 patients. Ophthal Plast Reconstr Surg. 2006;22(3):188–91.
43. La Faille P, Benedetto A. Fillers: contraindications, side effects and precautions. J Cutan Aesthet Surg. 2010;3:16–9.
44. Lim LM. Executive summary dermal filler devices. 2008. FDA general and plastic surgery devices panel. http://www.fda.gov/ohrms/dockets/ac/08/briefing/2008-4391b1-01%20-%20FDA%20Executive%20Summary%20Dermal%20Fillers.pdf
45. Lee KC, Korgavkar K, Dufresne RG, Higgins HW. Safety of cosmetic dermatologic procedures during pregnancy. Dermatol Surg. 2013;39(11):1573–86.
46. Niamtu J. Complications in fillers and Botox. Oral Maxillofac Surg Clin N Am. 2009;21:13–21.
47. Steinsapir KD, Steinsapir SMG. Deep-fill hyaluronic acid for the temporary treatment of the nasojugal groove: a report of 303 consecutive treatments. Ophthal Plast Reconstr Surg. 2006;22(5):344–8.
48. Ista Pharmaceuticals. Vitrase (HYALURONIDASE) injection, powder, lyophilized, for solution. 2006. https://dailymed.nlm.nih.gov/dailymed/archives/fdaDrugInfo.cfm?archiveid=1655
49. Hirsch RJ, Brody HJ, Carruthers JD. Hyaluronidase in the office: a necessity for every dermasurgeon that injects hyaluronic acid. J Cosmet Laser Ther. 2007;9(3):182–5.
50. Hassouneh B, Newman JP. Lasers, fillers, and neurotoxins: avoiding complications in the cosmetic facial practice. Facial Plast Surg Clin N Am. 2013;21(4):585–98.
51. Lemperle G, Rullan PP, Gauthier-Hazan N. Avoiding and treating dermal filler complications. Plast Reconstr Surg. 2006;118(3 Suppl):92S–107.
52. Cohen JL, Dayan SH, Brandt FS, et al. Systematic review of clinical trials of small- and large-gel-particle hyaluronic acid injectable fillers for aesthetic soft tissue augmentation. Dermatol Surg. 2013;39(2):205–31.
53. Goldberg RA, Fiaschetti D. Filling the periorbital hollows with hyaluronic acid gel: initial experience with 244 injections. Ophthal Plast Reconstr Surg. 2006;22(5):335–41.
54. Cohen JL. Understanding, avoiding, and managing dermal filler complications. Dermatol Surg. 2008;34 Suppl 1:S92–9.
55. Kouzi S, Nuzum D. Alternative therapies arnica for bruising and swelling. Am J Health Syst Pharm. 2007;64(23):2434–43.
56. Hirsch RJ, Narurkar V, Carruthers J. Management of injected hyaluronic acid induced Tyndall effects. Lasers Surg Med. 2006;38(3):202–4.

57. Christensen L. Normal and pathologic tissue reactions to soft tissue gel fillers. Dermatol Surg. 2007;33 Suppl 2:S168–75.
58. Holzapfel AM, Mangat DS, Barron DS. Soft-tissue augmentation with calcium hydroxylapatite: histologic analysis. Am J Ophthalmol. 2014;10(5):335–8.
59. Carruthers A, Carruthers JD. Polymethylmethacrylate microspheres/collagen as a tissue augmenting agent: personal experience over 5 years. Dermatol Surg. 2005;31(11 Pt 2):1561–4.
60. Alijotas-Reig J, Fernández-Figueras MT, Puig L. Inflammatory, immune-mediated adverse reactions related to soft tissue dermal fillers. Semin Arthritis Rheum. 2013;43(2):241–58.
61. Narins RS, Jewell M, Rubin M, Cohen J, Strobos J. Clinical conference: management of rare events following dermal fillers--focal necrosis and angry red bumps. Dermatol Surg. 2006;32(3):426–34.
62. Sclafani AP, Fagien S. Treatment of injectable soft tissue filler complications. Dermatol Surg. 2009;35 Suppl 2:1672–80.
63. Leonhardt J, Lawrence N, Narins R. Angioedema acute hypersensitivity reaction to injectable hyaluronic acid. Dermatol Surg. 2005;31(5):577–9.
64. Hamilton RG, Strobos J, Adkinson NF. Immunogenicity studies of cosmetically administered nonanimal-stabilized hyaluronic acid particles. Dermatol Surg. 2007;33 Suppl 2:S176–85.
65. Sampson HA, Muñoz-Furlong A, Campbell RL, et al. Second symposium on the definition and management of anaphylaxis: summary report – second national institute of allergy and infectious disease/food allergy and anaphylaxis network symposium. J Allergy Clin Immunol. 2006;117(2):391–7.
66. Daines SM, Williams EF. Complications associated with injectable soft-tissue fillers: a 5-year retrospective review. JAMA Facial Plast Surg. 2013;15(3):226–31.
67. Glaich A, Cohen J, Goldberg L. Injection necrosis of the glabella: protocol for prevention and treatment after use of dermal fillers. Dermatol Surg. 2006;32:276–81.
68. Park T-H, Seo S-W, Kim J-K, Chang C-H. Clinical experience with hyaluronic acid-filler complications. J Plast Reconstr Aesthet Surg. 2011;64(7):892–6.
69. Kleydman K, Cohen JL, Marmur E. Nitroglycerin: a review of its use in the treatment of vascular occlusion after soft tissue augmentation. Dermatol Surg. 2012;38(12):1889–97.
70. Kim D-W, Yoon E-S, Ji Y-H, Park S-H, Lee B-I, Dhong E-S. Vascular complications of hyaluronic acid fillers and the role of hyaluronidase in management. J Plast Reconstr Aesthet Surg. 2011;64(12):1590–5.
71. Tracy L, Ridgway J, Nelson JS, Lowe N, Wong B. Calcium hydroxylapatite associated soft tissue necrosis: a case report and treatment guideline. J Plast Reconstr Aesthet Surg. 2014;67(4):564–8.
72. Schanz S, Schippert W, Ulmer A, Rassner G, Fierlbeck G. Arterial embolization caused by injection of hyaluronic acid. Br J Dermatol. 2002;146(5):928–9.
73. Park KH, Kim Y-K, Woo SJ, Kang SW, Lee WK. Iatrogenic occlusion of the ophthalmic artery after cosmetic facial filler injections: a national survey by the Korean Retina Society. JAMA Ophthalmol. 2014;132(6):714–23.
74. Park SW, Woo SJ, Park KH, Huh JW, Jung C, Kwon O-K. Iatrogenic retinal artery occlusion caused by

cosmetic facial filler injections. Am J Ophthalmol. 2012;154(4):653–662.e1.
75. Kim S, Byun D, Park J, Han S, Baik J, Kim J. Panophthalmoplegia and vision loss after cosmetic nasal dorsum injection. J Clin Neurosci. 2014;21:678–80.
76. Kwon SG, Hong JW, Roh TS, Kim YS, Rah DK, Kim SS. Ischemic oculomotor nerve palsy and skin necrosis caused by vascular embolization after hyaluronic acid filler injection: a case report. Ann Plast Surg. 2013;71(4):333–4.
77. Lazzeri D, Agostini T, Figus M, Nardi M, Pantaloni M, Lazzeri S. Blindness following cosmetic injections of the face. Plast Reconstr Surg. 2012;129(4): 995–1012.

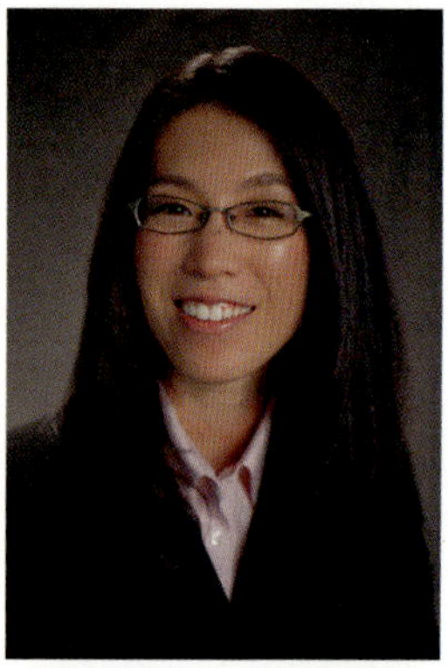

**Dr. Leslie Wei** is a board-certified ophthalmologist specializing in ophthalmic plastic and reconstructive surgery. She completed both her undergraduate and medical degrees at Brown University, followed by residency at University of Colorado and fellowship at University of Wisconsin. She is currently in private practice in upstate New York.

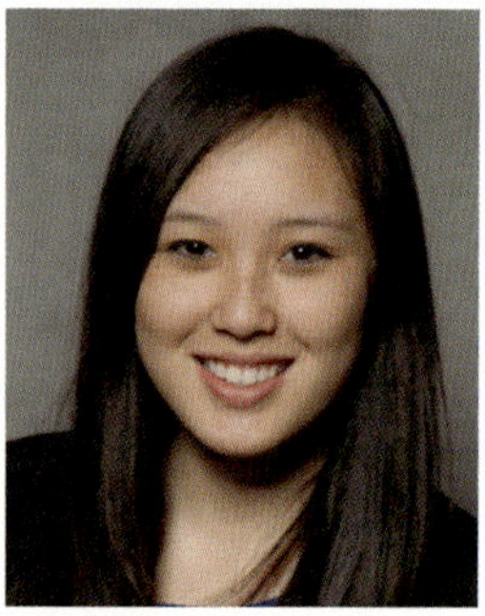

**Dr. Ann Tran** is currently a first year ophthalmology resident at the University of Miami Bascom Palmar Eye Institute. She completed her undergraduate degrees in biochemistry at the University of Wisconsin-Madison and pursued her medical degree at the University of Wisconsin School of Medicine and Public Health.

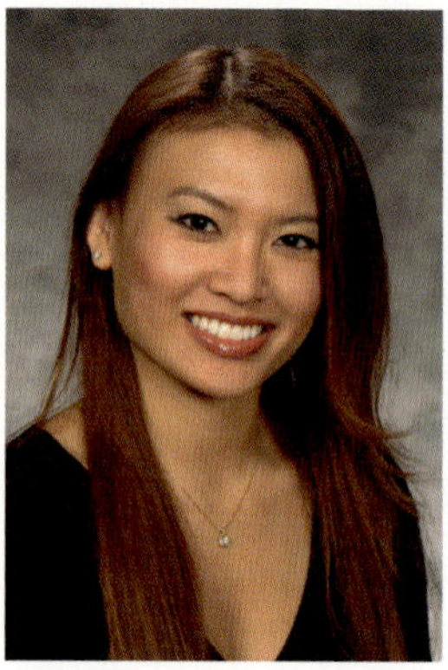

**Cat N. Burkat** Dr. Cat Burkat is a board-certified ophthalmologist with expertise in plastic and reconstructive surgery and aesthetic surgery around the eyes. Dr. Burkat has been uniquely dual-fellowship trained in both ophthalmic plastic and reconstructive surgery, as well as cosmetic facial surgery, which allows her to offer an approach that combines the microsurgical precision of ophthalmology with the concepts of aesthetic facial surgery. She graduated from Harvard University and University of Rochester, followed by a dual-fellowship at the University of Wisconsin.

Dr. Burkat specializes in a broad range of conditions, with particular interest in surgical repair of droopy eyelids, congenital eyelid abnormalities, tear duct abnormalities, and cancer reconstruction. She also offers a wide array of non-surgical and surgical cosmetic procedures for enhancing the natural beauty of the face, including cosmetic eyelid and forehead surgery, Asian blepharoplasty, cosmetic botulinum and soft tissue filler injections, facial laser resurfacing and other related procedures.

In addition to her clinical practice, Dr. Burkat has published numerous peer-reviewed articles and over 35 book chapters, and is on the editorial board and review board of many prestigious journals. She is active in several committees in the American Society of Ophthalmic Plastic and Reconstructive Surgery Society, and leads several courses and breakfast expert roundtables at the annual AAO scientific meeting. She has been invited to speak and teach at numerous national and international courses, and actively participates in volunteer medical trips in Southeast Asia, India, Africa, Central America, and the South Pacific. She has also received multiple awards including the American Academy of Ophthalmology Achievement Award, the American Journal of Cosmetic Surgery Richard B. Aronsohn Founder's Award for the year's Best Scholarly Manuscript published, and several Outstanding Surgical Teaching Awards from Ophthalmology Residents. She is also an Associate Preceptor for the University of Wisconsin Fellowship in Ophthalmic Facial Plastic and Reconstructive Surgery, the American Academy of Cosmetic Surgery Fellowship, and is the Administrative Director of the International Fellowship in Ophthalmic Facial Plastic and Reconstructive Surgery at the University of Wisconsin.

# Iatrogenic Orbital Injury Associated with Adnexal Intervention

# 52

Kelvin Kam-lung Chong and Bipasha Mukherjee

## Introduction

Orbital injuries are important surgical complications to be considered in any eyelid, lacrimal, orbital, socket, sinus, and even neurosurgical procedures. The increasingly popular periocular injections of fillers or autologous tissues may also cause problems due to periorbital tissue reaction and/or needle-related injuries.

## Retrobulbar Hemorrhage

Retrobulbar hemorrhages can occur while injecting (sub-Tenon, peribulbar, or retrobulbar) or operating around the periocular region, e.g., blepharoplasties [1] and ptosis correction, or when the orbit is inadvertently entered during lacrimal (medial orbit), sinus (medial or inferior) [2], dental (inferior), or neurosurgical (superior or lateral orbit) operations. Details of managing retrobulbar hemorrhage have been covered elsewhere and will not be repeated here.

K.K.-l. Chong, MB, ChB (Hon), FHKAM, FCOphth (✉)
Ophthalmology and Visual Science,
The Chinese University of Hong Kong,
Prince of Wales Hospital, Alice Ho Miu Ling
Nethersole Hospital, 4/F Hong Kong Eye Hospital,
Hong Kong, SAR, China
e-mail: chongkamlung@cuhk.edu.hk

B. Mukherjee, MS, DNB(Ophthalmology), FICO
Department of Orbit, Oculoplasty,
Reconstructive & Aesthetic Services,
Sankara Nethralaya, 18, College Road,
Chennai, Tamil Nadu 600006, India
e-mail: drbpm@snmail.org

## Extraocular Muscles and Levator Injuries

### During Eyelid Operations

The superior rectus muscle may rarely be injured or even transected during levator resection, while injuries to the superior oblique, inferior rectus, or more commonly inferior oblique muscle were reported during fat removal in upper or lower lid blepharoplasties [3]. Injury or disinsertion of the underlying levator aponeurosis causing postoperative ptosis may occur if orbital fat is aggressively removed during upper lid blepharoplasties [4].

### During Sinus or Orbital Operations

Most often, medial rectus (MR) [5] and rarely inferior rectus and superior and inferior oblique [6] injuries have been reported during functional endoscopic sinus surgery (FESS). Extraocular muscles may be injured during fracture repair, orbitotomies, or orbital decompression.


B. Mukherjee, H. Yuen (eds.), *Emergencies of the Orbit and Adnexa*,
DOI 10.1007/978-81-322-1807-4_52

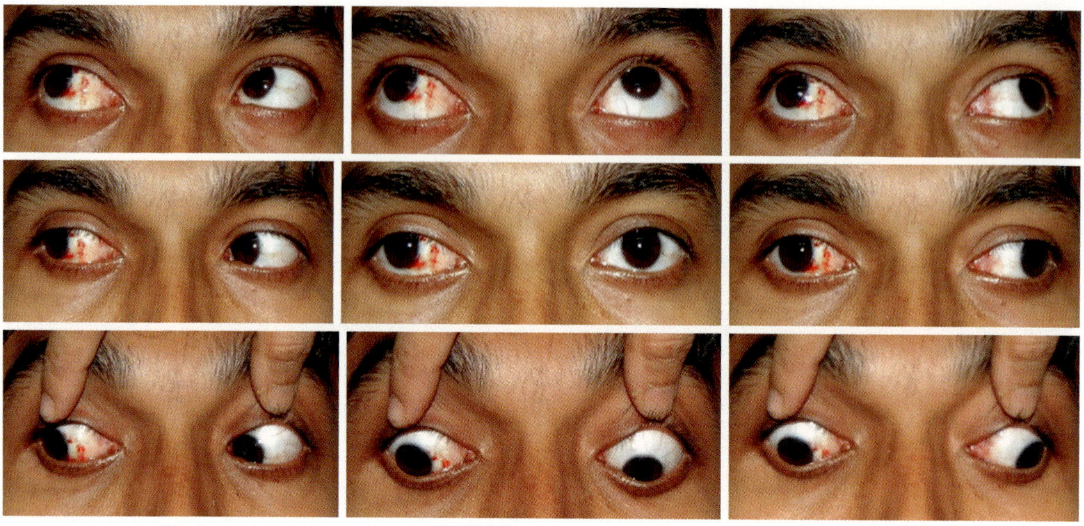

**Fig. 52.1** Nine positions of gaze showing restricted adduction in type I injury to MR during FESS

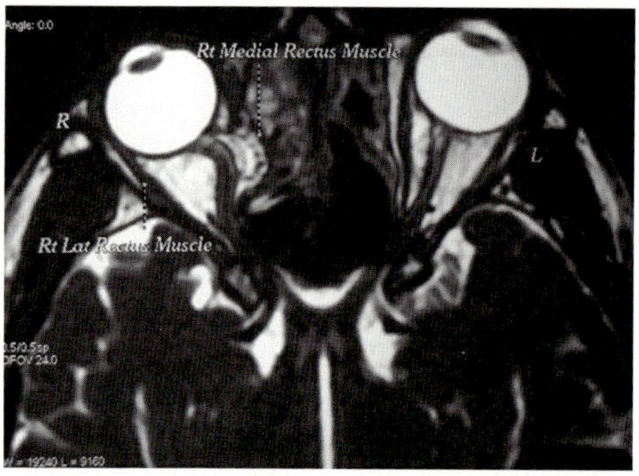


**Fig. 52.2** T2-weighted axial MRI image of transected right medial rectus (RMR) in the same patient (Figure reprinted with permission from © Association of Otolaryngologists of India 2015)

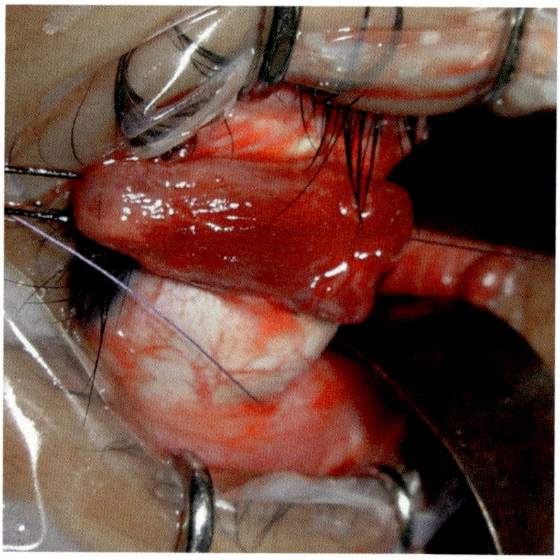

**Fig. 52.3** Operative view of the transected RMR during exploration

Four types of MR injury have been proposed from one study [5]. Type I involves a large-angle exotropia (25 prism diopters) and marked adduction deficit with relatively intact abduction and little or no entrapment (Figs. 52.1 and 52.2). These cases were typically associated with complete transection of the midportion of the MR muscle (Fig. 52.3). Early exploration with suturing of the muscle remnants [7], along with botulinum toxin injection to the ipsilateral (antagonist) lateral rectus (LR), may improve primary ocular alignment. Severe restriction in the range of horizontal ductions usually persisted. Type II cases revealed a moderate- to large-angle exotropia with combined adduction and abduction deficits suggesting partial MR transection or severe contusion with moderate MR and orbital soft-tissue entrapment. Treatment entailed early repair of the medial wall defect and release of the entrapped MR. Type III cases generally demonstrated no or only mild ocular deviation (typically small esotropia) in primary gaze but a marked

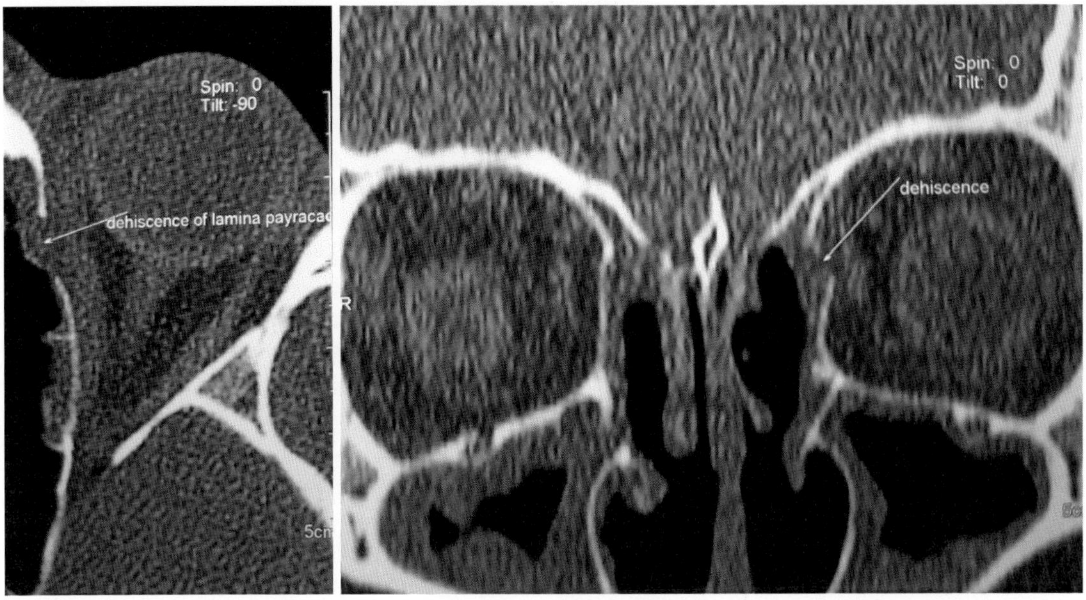


**Fig. 52.4** Small left medial wall fracture with no entrapment after FESS

abduction deficit, suggestive of a grossly intact or modestly contused muscle with marked bony entrapment. Management is by orbital exploration, release of entrapped orbital tissue, and/or repair of the orbital wall defect. Type IV cases were characterized by only mild degrees of ocular misalignment caused by muscle contusion without entrapment. Conservative management is recommended (Fig. 52.4).

In cases where there is concomitant medial and inferior rectus injury, transposition procedures may not be possible. Inactivation of the antagonist and use of an apically based orbital periosteal flap as a globe tether to center it may be an alternative [8]. Tse et al. reported the use of a suture/titanium T-plate anchoring platform system for one case of medial rectus injury with good improvement [9].

## Lacrimal Gland and Nasolacrimal Injuries

The lacrimal gland may be mistaken as orbital fat during upper lid blepharoplasties which, if inadvertently removed or resected, may lead to significant bleeding due to its vascularity. Dry eye, lateral eyelid drooping due to levator disinsertion, and numbness around the lateral upper lid are other possibilities [10]. Lacrimal sac or nasolacrimal duct injury may occur during medial/inferomedial orbital procedure (fracture repair, orbitotomy, decompression) when the incision on the periorbita (posterior lacrimal crest) is placed too anteriorly.

## Optic or Periorbital Nerve Injuries

Visual loss due to direct optic nerve injury is rare, but indirect causes, e.g., compressive or ischemic optic neuropathy, often associated with retrobulbar hemorrhage, are the most dreaded complication of all adnexal procedures, particularly that at the orbital apex or alongside the optic nerve [11, 12]. Details of iatrogenic visual loss can be found elsewhere in the book (Chap. 21). Oculomotor, trochlear, and abducens nerves and ciliary ganglions can be injured at orbital or maxillofacial procedures [13]. The infraorbital nerve may be injured during floor fracture repair while supraorbital nerve in different brow-elevating procedures.

## Iatrogenic Orbital Bony Injuries

Sino-orbital fistula may occur if medial or inferior wall is violated during orbital exenteration [14] (Fig. 52.5). On the other hand, iatrogenic orbital fracture may happen during orbitotomy, decompression, or fracture repair or when the orbit is inadvertently entered during lacrimal (medial orbit), sinus (medial or inferior, see above Sect. 10.2.2), dental (inferior), or neurosurgical (superior or lateral orbit) operations.

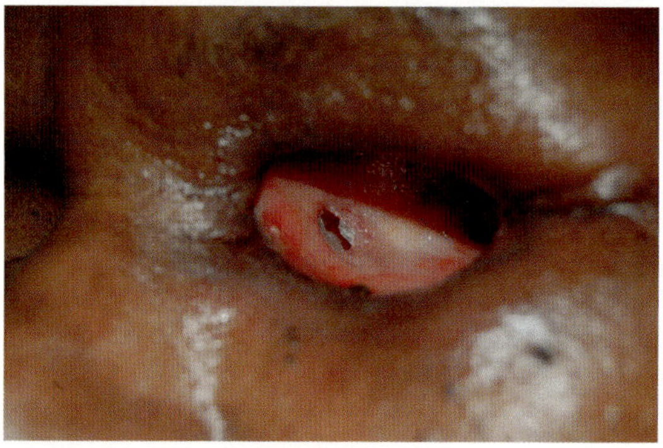

**Fig. 52.5** Left sino-orbital fistula after exenteration (Figure reprinted with permission from © Association of Otolaryngologists of India 2015)

## Implant-Related Orbital Injuries

Apart from infection and peri-implant hemorrhages [15], fracture or socket implant may migrate and cause sinusitis [16], injury to the optic nerve, extraocular muscle, or globe itself causing motility and visual disturbances.

## Injection-Related Orbital Injuries

Periocular injections may cause needle-related injuries to the globe, extraocular muscles, and lacrimal gland. Hyaluronidase used as part of the anesthetic compound may cause an allergic reaction in the periocular region [17] (Figs. 52.6 and 52.7).

Infectious [18] or sterile granuloma [19] or even visual loss due to retinal artery occlusion [20, 21] can occur during cosmetic fillers or autologous fat injections.

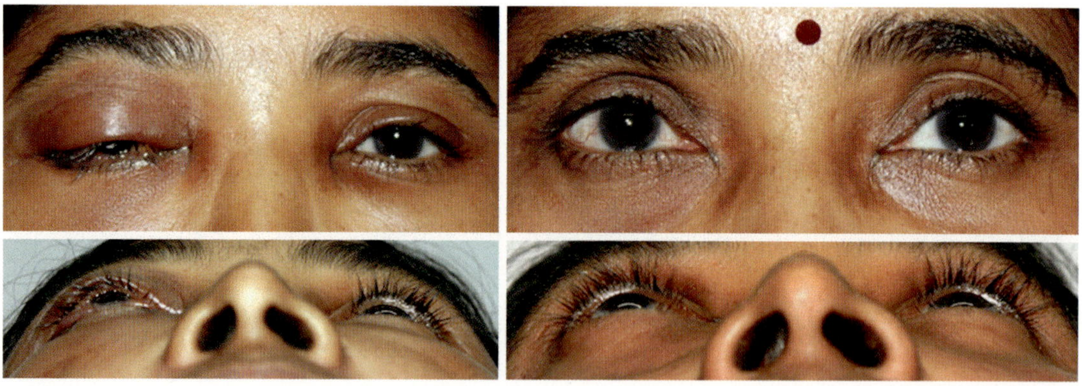

**Fig. 52.6** (**a**) *Left*: suspected hyaluronidase allergy 1 day post cataract extraction under local anesthesia with right eye periocular swelling and 2 mm proptosis. (**b**) *Right*: resolution of periorbital swelling after 5 days with systemic steroids

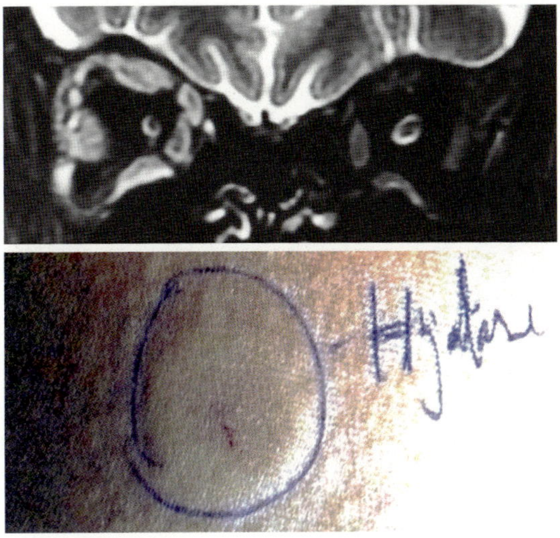

**Fig. 52.7** (**a**) T1 fat-suppressed contrast MRI orbit showing diffuse swelling of right extraocular muscles and fat enhancement of subject from Fig. 52.6. (**b**) Positive intradermal test after hyaluronidase injection in the same patient

## References


1. Wolfort FG, Vaughan TE, Wolfort SF, Nevarre DR. Retrobulbar hematoma and blepharoplasty. Plast Reconstr Surg. 1999;104(7):2154–62.
2. Sood V, Rejali D, Stocker J, Pagliarini S, Ahluwalia H, Mehta P. A case report of orbital haemorrhage associated with endoscopic sinus surgery and reversible sight loss: a multidisciplinary approach to management. Orbit. 2013;32(1):73–5.
3. Syniuta LA, Goldberg RA, Thacker NM, Rosenbaum AL. Acquired strabismus following cosmetic blepharoplasty. Plast Reconstr Surg. 2003;111(6):2053–9.
4. Baylis HI, Sutcliffe T, Fett DR. Levator injury during blepharoplasty. Arch Ophthalmol. 1984;102(4): 570–1.
5. Huang CM, Meyer DR, Patrinely JR, Soparkar CN, Dailey RA, Maus M, Rubin PA, Yeatts RP, Bersani TA, Karesh JW, Harrison AR, Shovlin JP. Medial rectus muscle injuries associated with functional endoscopic sinus surgery: characterization and management. Ophthal Plast Reconstr Surg. 2003;19(1): 25–37.
6. Rosenbaum AL, Astle WF. Superior oblique and inferior rectus muscle injury following frontal and intranasal sinus surgery. J Pediatr Ophthalmol Strabismus. 1985;22(5):194–202.
7. Pineles SL, Laursen J, Goldberg RA, Demer JL, Velez FG. Function of transected or avulsed rectus muscles following recovery using an anterior orbitotomy approach. J AAPOS. 2012;16(4):336–41.
8. Goldberg RA, Rosenbaum AL, Tong JT. Use of apically based periosteal flaps as globe tethers in severe paretic strabismus. Arch Ophthalmol. 2000;118(3):431–7.
9. Tse DT, Shriver EM, Krantz KB, Tse JD, Capo H, McKeown CA. The use of titanium T-plate as platform for globe alignment in severe paralytic and restrictive strabismus. Am J Ophthalmol. 2010;150(3): 404–11.
10. Lelli Jr GJ, Lisman RD. Blepharoplasty complications. Plast Reconstr Surg. 2010;125(3):1007–17.
11. Rose GE. The "devil's touch"; visual loss and orbital surgery. A synopsis of the Mustardé Lecture, 2006. Orbit. 2007;26(3):147–58.
12. Hass AN, Penne RB, Stefanyszyn MA, Flanagan JC. Incidence of postblepharoplasty orbital hemorrhage and associated visual loss. Ophthal Plast Reconstr Surg. 2004;20(6):426–32.
13. Chrcanovic BR, Custódio AL. Optic, oculomotor, abducens, and facial nerve palsies after combined maxillary and mandibular osteotomy: case report. J Oral Maxillofac Surg. 2011;69(6):e234–41.
14. Limawararut V, Leibovitch I, Davis G, Rees G, Goldberg RA, Selva D. Sino-orbital fistula: a complication of exenteration. Ophthalmology. 2007;114(2):355–61.
15. Gilhotra JS, McNab AA, McKelvie P, O'Donnell BA. Late orbital haemorrhage around alloplastic orbital floor implants: a case series and review. Clin Exp Ophthalmol. 2002;30(5):352–5.
16. Lee DH, Joo YE, Lim SC. Migrated orbital silastic sheet implant mimicking bilateral sinusitis. J Craniofac Surg. 2011;22(6):2158–9.
17. Delaere L, Zeyen T, Foets B, Van Calster J, Stalmans I. Allergic reaction to hyaluronidase after retrobulbar anaesthesia: a case series and review. Int Ophthalmol. 2009;29(6):521–8.
18. Ross AH, Malhotra R. Long-term orbitofacial complications of polyalkylimide 4% (bio-alcamid). Ophthal Plast Reconstr Surg. 2009;25(5):394–7.
19. Sa HS, Woo KI, Suh YL, Kim YD. Periorbital lipogranuloma: a previously unknown complication of autologous fat injections for facial augmentation. Br J Ophthalmol. 2011;95(9):1259–63.
20. Park SW, Woo SJ, Park KH, Huh JW, Jung C, Kwon OK. Iatrogenic retinal artery occlusion caused by cosmetic facial filler injections. Am J Ophthalmol. 2012;154(4):653–62.
21. Carle MV, Roe R, Novack R, Boyer DS. Cosmetic facial fillers and severe vision loss. JAMA Ophthalmol. 2014;132(5):637–9.

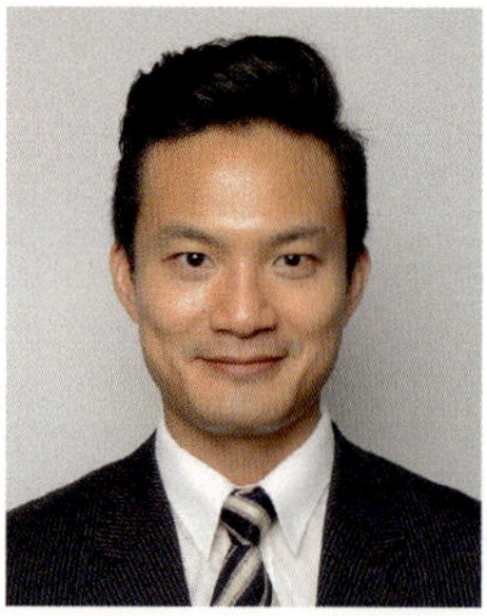

**Kelvin Kam-lung Chong** Dr Kelvin Chong is a surgeon-scientist in orbital and oculoplastic surgery and related cell biology. He graduated at the top of his class in the Bachelor of Medicine and Surgery (CUHK) program. He was awarded the Li Po Chun Charitable Trust Fund Overseas Postgraduate Scholarship where he continued later as an international clinical and research fellow at the University of California at Los Angeles (UCLA) (preceptor: Prof. Robert Goldberg) and LA Biomedical Institute (Preceptor: Prof. Terry Smith and Dr Raymond Douglas). His awards included the City Lion Club Gold Medal, Action for Vision Eye Foundation Young Researcher of the Year, Exemplary Eye Resident Award, Achievement Awards from American Academy of Ophthalmology and Asia Pacific Academy of Ophthalmology. Dr. Chong serves as the Coordinator of Orbital and Oculoplastic Surgery at the teaching hospital of the CUHK, the Prince of Wales Hospital and the CUHK Eye Center. He is the current vice President of Hong Kong Society of Ophthalmic Plastic and Reconstructive Surgery (HKSOPRS), Secretary of the Asia-Pacific Society of Ophthalmic Plastic and Reconstructive Surgery (APSOPRS).

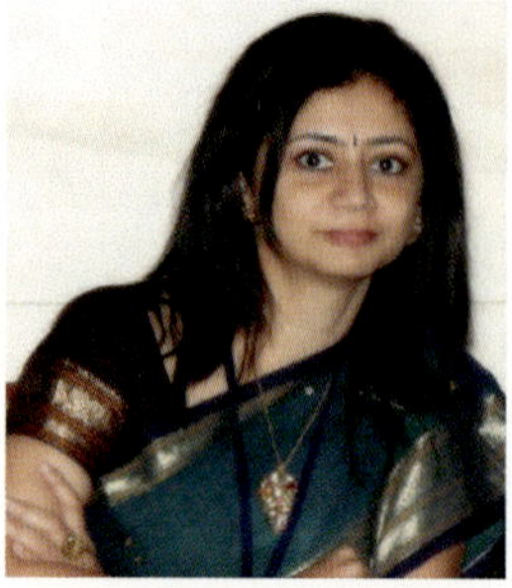

**Bipasha Mukherjee** Dr. Bipasha Mukherjee is a fellow in Orbit & Oculoplasty from Aravind Eye Hospitals, India, and ICO fellow from University Hospital of Limoges, France, under Prof. Jean-Paul Adenis. She has undergone clinical observerships with stalwarts like Jack Rootman, Richard Collins, Geoff Rose, Mark Duffy, and Robert Goldberg.

She currently heads the department of Orbit, Oculoplasty, Aesthetic & Reconstructive services in Medical Research Foundation, Chennai. She has numerous presentations in national and international conferences and publications in peer-reviewed journals and text books. Her areas of interest include diseases of the orbit and adnexa including tumors, lacrimal surgery, socket reconstruction, traumatic lid and adnexal injuries, training residents and fellows, and photography.

Printed by Printforce, the Netherlands